Advance Praise for *Advancing the Science of Implementation Across the Cancer Continuum*

"A book that harnesses the promise of D&I science on our country's second leading cause of death could not be better timed. The guidance in these pages will significantly boost our ability to translate rapidly accruing evidence on how to prevent, detect, control, and treat cancer. It's all here: the why and the how of extending cancer research breakthroughs to the benefit of health systems, communities of care, and population health. The case studies convey the imperative for D&I cancer research, and the authors provide the agenda and tools for advancing implementation science in this field as well as others."

— **Enola K. Proctor, PhD**, Shanti K. Khinduka Distinguished Professor and Director of Implementation Science, Washington University Institute for Clinical and Translational Science, St. Louis, MO

"Advancing the Science of Implementation across the Cancer Continuum provides a terrific overview of the state of the science in cancer control including what we know and what we don't yet know. Particularly valuable are the case studies to illustrate the concepts, which offer rich contextual detail about implementation including what works and what may not. The integration of theory, evidence and case studies from across the cancer control continuum makes for a terrific resource for those interested in implementation science."

—**Sharon Straus, MD, FRCPC, MSc, HBSc**, Professor of Medicine, University of Toronto, Director of the Knowledge Translation Program, St. Michael's Hospital, Toronto, Canada

"The authors of this engaging and timely book balance a focus on research methods with real world examples across the cancer care continuum to further advance our goals for health equity and reduction in the burden of cancer. The emerging issues summarized in this volume set an agenda for prevention research for the coming years. An extremely important guide to maximizing our return on investment in past cancer prevention and control discoveries through timely integration into practice."

—**Graham A. Colditz, MD, DrPH**, Associate Director of Prevention and Control, Siteman Cancer Center, Niess-Gain Professor, Washington University School of Medicine, St. Louis, MO

"The evolution of implementation science can, in principle, be traced to roots as far back in medical history as Semmelweis. But the explosion of interest in the application of scientific knowledge for the benefit of patients and populations has been playing out only in recent decades. Chambers, Vinson, and Norton, who themselves have been key actors in this recent evolution, have made an enormous contribution to the field by pulling together historical context, theory, practical case studies, and forward-looking challenges from almost a hundred members of the large supporting cast active in this field. This volume is a must for anyone interested in the application of scientific evidence for the benefit of better patient outcomes and population health."

—**Robert A. Hiatt, MD, PhD**, Professor and Chair of the Department of Epidemiology and Biostatistics, Associate Director of Population Sciences, Leader of the Cancer Control Program, University of California, San Francisco, Helen Diller Family Comprehensive Cancer Center, San Francisco, CA

ADVANCING THE SCIENCE OF IMPLEMENTATION ACROSS THE CANCER CONTINUUM

Edited by
David A. Chambers, DPhil
DEPUTY DIRECTOR FOR IMPLEMENTATION SCIENCE
DIVISION OF CANCER CONTROL AND POPULATION SCIENCES
NATIONAL CANCER INSTITUTE
ROCKVILLE, MD

Cynthia A. Vinson, PhD, MPA
SENIOR ADVISOR FOR IMPLEMENTATION SCIENCE
DIVISION OF CANCER CONTROL AND POPULATION SCIENCES
NATIONAL CANCER INSTITUTE
ROCKVILLE, MD

Wynne E. Norton, PhD
PROGRAM DIRECTOR, IMPLEMENTATION SCIENCE
DIVISION OF CANCER CONTROL AND POPULATION SCIENCES
NATIONAL CANCER INSTITUTE
ROCKVILLE, MD

OXFORD
UNIVERSITY PRESS

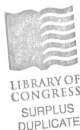

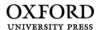
OXFORD
UNIVERSITY PRESS

Oxford University Press is a department of the University of Oxford. It furthers
the University's objective of excellence in research, scholarship, and education
by publishing worldwide. Oxford is a registered trade mark of Oxford University
Press in the UK and certain other countries.

Published in the United States of America by Oxford University Press
198 Madison Avenue, New York, NY 10016, United States of America.

Library of Congress Cataloging-in-Publication Data
Names: Chambers, David A., DPhil, editor. | Vinson, Cynthia A., editor. |
Norton, Wynne E., editor.
Title: Advancing the science of implementation across the cancer continuum /
edited by David A. Chambers, Cynthia A. Vinson, Wynne E. Norton.
Description: New York, NY : Oxford University Press, [2019] |
Includes bibliographical references and index.
Identifiers: LCCN 2018007924 | ISBN 9780190647421 (hardback) /
Subjects: | MESH: Neoplasms | Translational Medical Research | Diffusion of Innovation |
Evidence-Based Medicine
Classification: LCC RC267 | NLM QZ 206 | DDC 362.196/9940072—dc23
LC record available at https://lccn.loc.gov/2018007924

9 8 7 6 5 4 3 2 1

Printed by Sheridan Books, Inc., United States of America

For Jessica, Jordan, and Eva Chambers
—D.A.C.

For my husband and son—Dave and Jaden Mower
—C.A.V.

For Paul, Elyse, Andy, and Erik Norton
—W.E.N.

CONTENTS

FOREWORD: THE IMPLEMENTATION OF CANCER CONTROL IN THE 21ST CENTURY (PART 1)

Otis W. Brawley

CANCER IS the second leading cause of death for Americans and will surpass heart disease to become the most common cause of death within the next decade. Cancer has been a major health concern for a very long time. From 1900 to 1991, the annual cancer death rate rose by a factor of 3.6 from 60 per 100,000 to 215 per 100,000 (age-adjusted to the 2000 standard).[1]

Cancer control efforts began in the early 20th century. An early proponent was the American Society for the Control of Cancer (ASCC). It was formed in 1913 to provide public education regarding the early signs and symptoms of cancer. The ASCC would change its name to the American Cancer Society in the 1940s and go on to champion a number of cancer control efforts.[2]

Today, cancer control is a medical science critical to public health. The "cancer control continuum" is a phrase that has been used since at least the mid-1970s to describe a spectrum of activities from the study of cancer etiology, cancer prevention, early detection, diagnosis, treatment, survivorship, and end of life. It is often a struggle to remove the emotion and politics caused by cancer's devastation and to use the scientific method to define the pertinent issues and the solutions to reduce death and suffering from cancer.

Despite the dramatic rise in mortality in the past century, cancer control efforts have borne some success. There has been a 26% decline in the age-adjusted cancer death rate since 1991 from 215 per 100,000 to 159.1 per 100,000 in 2014.[1] The 26% decline means that 2.38 million cancer deaths were prevented over 23 years.

The largest driver of the decline is through preventive intervention, smoking cessation, and tobacco control. Smoking prevalence declined from 55% among American adult males in 1955 to 16.7%

in 2015 and from 35% of American adult females in 1965 to 13.6% in 2015.[1] This led to dramatic declines in the lung cancer death rate, but it also caused reductions in the incidence and death rates of at least 16 other cancers. Improvements in treatment and screening also contributed to the decline in colorectal and breast cancer death rates. The decline in the death rate of prostate cancer is due to improvements in treatment, and some of it is likely due to screening.

There is evidence that we can do better. College-educated Americans have a lower risk of cancer death compared to the non-college educated.[3] Indeed, if one applies the cancer mortality rate of the college educated to all Americans, one-fourth of all cancer deaths would not occur.[4] This means that more than 150,000 cancer deaths would not have occurred in 2018 if we had applied all that we know. This is not the effect of new prevention technologies, new screening or diagnostic tests, or new treatments. This is the effect of more fully implementing what we already know.

There is both overuse and underuse of health care technologies. Medical history tells us we have often wasted resources by implementing interventions that were later proven ineffective and, in some cases, even net harmful. The philosopher George Santayana famously stated, "Those who do not remember the past are condemned to repeat it." For example, for years many advocated widespread use of the dietary supplement beta-carotene for cancer prevention. Eventually, several clinical trials suggested that beta-carotene users who were smokers were at an even greater risk of lung cancer compared to those who just smoked.[5] The 40 years of routine use of postmenopausal hormone replacement therapy until the results of the Women's Health Initiative were published is a similar example of exuberant overuse of a purported preventative therapy before critical assessment.[6]

Cancer control has repeatedly introduced promising but not fully evaluated interventions, with the result that people were hurt. For example, Pap testing was promoted before the difference between cervical dysplasia and cervical cancer was understood. From the 1920s through the 1950s, many women with dysplasia, what is now termed CIN 1, were aggressively treated with radical hysterectomy or radiation therapy.[7] Today, CIN 1 is rarely observed because most spontaneously regress. Similar examples of premature use leading to people being harmed include lung cancer screening using chest X-ray, neuroblastoma screening using serum vanillylmandelic acid, and thyroid cancer screening using ultrasound.[8]

Appropriate cancer screening and treatment should be supported and widely disseminated. Fortunately, there are data to show that cancer screening tests are being used more responsibly today, but there is still room for improvement. Newer screening technologies, including genetic screening, present today's challenges for assessment and validation. Unfortunately, the population data show that a substantial proportion of Americans who would benefit from breast and colorectal screening are not receiving it.[9,10] Even among those who get it, there is evidence of variable quality of screening and treatment. This trend has not been documented in cancer screening for other diseases (especially lung screening) but likely exists. This is where the science of implementation can help.

A concerted effort to get high-quality screening and treatment to more Americans could spare many more people a cancer death. Cancer Intervention and Surveillance Modeling Network (CISNET) investigators estimate that increasing screening prevalence from its current 60% to 90% would eventually reduce the number of deaths due to breast cancer by approximately 5,100–6,100 deaths per year.[9] Getting adequate appropriate therapy to all women diagnosed (with no change in screening pattern) would prevent 11,400–14,500 deaths per year. Providing all women high-quality screening, in addition to indicated therapy, would eventually prevent 18,100–20,400 deaths per year.[9]

Cancer prevention is a long-term high-value investment. In a recent review, Islami and colleagues estimated that more than 45% of cancer deaths are attributed to modifiable risk factors.[11] Among them, smoking cessation and tobacco control could have prevented approximately 28% of cancer deaths (approximately 170,000 in 2018). Tobacco control remains the area in which the most cancer deaths can be prevented. It is estimated that 16% of all cancers (approximately 98,000 in 2018) are attributed to energy balance, poor food choices, and alcohol consumption. If smoking rates continue to decline, it is likely that the combination of diet (too many calories), not enough exercise, and obesity will become the leading cause of cancer death in the next decade or two.

Cancer control science can benefit from the implementation of a range of effective interventions to decrease significant cancer risk factors and improve prevention, screening, treatment, and survivorship. Clearly, interventions at multiple levels of society need to be assessed, with implementation of those that show promise.[12] These might include changes in zoning at a governmental or community level to decrease opportunities to consume tobacco, increase opportunities for physical activity (the built environment), and increase availability of healthy foods. It involves interventions to influence health care providers, families, and individuals at other levels of society.

Science is a search for truth; it is about inquiry and learning. Its ultimate goal is to better the human condition. Cancer control science is defining the problems and the solutions in cancer health care. Epidemiologic study has shown us what can be achieved with implementation of those solutions. Implementation of cancer control interventions is central to most efficiently reducing human suffering from cancer. It is only right that we study the implementation of cancer prevention and control interventions, improving the uptake of those that benefit patient health and reducing the use of those that do not, and that the study of implementation has become an academic interest. Indeed, the most pressing question in cancer medicine is

How do we get the fruits of already conducted research in cancer prevention and treatment to the people who need it?

REFERENCES

1. Siegel RL, Miller KD, Jemal A. Cancer statistics, 2017. *CA Cancer J Clin.* 2017;67(1):7–30.
2. Eyre HJ. National Cancer Act 1971–1996. National Cancer Institute/American Cancer Society relationship—June 1996. *Cancer.* 1996;78(12):2609–2610.
3. Ma J, Siegel RL, Ward EM, Jemal A. State-level educational disparities in mortality in the United States, 2010–2014. *Prev Med.* 2018;106:53–59.
4. Siegel R, Ward E, Brawley O, Jemal A. Cancer statistics, 2011: The impact of eliminating socioeconomic and racial disparities on premature cancer deaths. *CA Cancer J Clin.* 2011;61(4):212–236.
5. The Alpha-Tocopherol Beta Carotene Cancer Prevention Study Group. The effect of vitamin E and beta carotene on the incidence of lung cancer and other cancers in male smokers. *N Engl J Med.* 1994;330(15):1029–1035.
6. Krieger N, Lowy I, Aronowitz R, et al. Hormone replacement therapy, cancer, controversies, and women's health: Historical, epidemiological, biological, clinical, and advocacy perspectives. *J Epidemiol Community Health.* 2005;59(9):740–748.
7. Lowy I. Cancer, women, and public health: The history of screening for cervical cancer. *Hist Cienc Saude Manguinhas.* 2010;17(Suppl 1).
8. Croswell JM, Ransohoff DF, Kramer BS. Principles of cancer screening: Lessons from history and study design issues. *Semin Oncol.* 2010;37(3):202–215.
9. Mandelblatt J, van Ravesteyn N, Schechter C, et al. Which strategies reduce breast cancer mortality most? Collaborative modeling of optimal screening, treatment, and obesity prevention. *Cancer.* 2013;119(14):2541–2548.
10. Meester RG, Doubeni CA, Lansdorp-Vogelaar I, et al. Colorectal cancer deaths attributable to nonuse of screening in the United States. *Ann Epidemiol.* 2015;25(3):208–213.
11. Islami F, Goding Sauer A, Miller KD, et al. Proportion and number of cancer cases and deaths attributable to potentially modifiable risk factors in the United States. *CA Cancer J Clin.* 2018;68(1):31–54.
12. Taplin SH, Anhang Price R, Edwards HM, et al. Introduction: Understanding and influencing multilevel factors across the cancer care continuum. *J Natl Cancer Inst Monogr.* 2012;2012(44):2–10.

FOREWORD: THE IMPLEMENTATION OF CANCER CONTROL IN THE 21ST CENTURY (PART 2)

Electra D. Paskett

DURING MY doctoral training, I became enamored with the notion that as an epidemiologist I did not merely want to discover what caused cancer but also how to prevent it and reduce the burden it caused in terms of effects and death. Thus, I became a behavioral epidemiologist, developing and testing interventions to prevent, detect, and manage side effects of cancer. Early in my career, during my tenure at Wake Forest University School of Medicine, I realized that most of the efficacious interventions scientists, like myself, were developing went no further than being reported in scientific meetings and journals. Soon afterward, the National Cancer Institute initiated Cancer Control *Plan, Link, Act, Network* with *Evidence-based Tools* (P.L.A.N.E.T.),[1] developed as a portal to provide access to cancer-related data and resources, including a clearinghouse of evidence-based interventions (Research-Tested Intervention Programs, or RTIPs). Thus, implementation science (IS) was awakened in the cancer field. However, a question still remains: How can we advance implementation research and practice?

WHY IS IMPLEMENTATION SCIENCE IMPORTANT IN THE CANCER WORLD?

There are a number of areas in which implementation science can be most influential in the cancer world, and many topics along the cancer control continuum[2] that are ripe for research. We know much about how to prevent cancer; however, the problem has been and still is that these proven interventions are not being delivered to populations at risk. Prime examples are chemoprevention strategies for women at risk of developing breast cancer and the human papillomavirus (HPV) vaccine.[3-6] Tamoxifen can reduce the risk of developing breast cancer by 50% if taken appropriately;[7] however, uptake is approximately 35% in eligible, high-risk women.[8,9] Likewise, the HPV vaccine can reduce the risk of developing up to six types of cancers,[4] yet less than 50% of eligible female teens and less than 40% of male teens aged 13 years are up-to-date with the series.[10] Colon cancer screening not only reduces late-stage cancer but also can prevent cancers if adenomatous polyps are found and removed; less than 60% of adults aged 50 years or older are adherent to screening guidelines.[11] For treatment, aromatase inhibitors reduce the likelihood of recurrence after a primary breast cancer,[12,13] yet adherence to recommended therapy is as low as 50%.[14] Smoking cessation in healthy people, as well as cancer patients, will prevent disease and death: The Cancer Moonshot Blue Ribbon Panel reported that 30% of cancer deaths are due to tobacco use.[15] Implementation science might be especially relevant to address the growing disparities in cancer incidence, morbidity, and mortality rates. In many cases, the uptake of innovations is not equal among all sectors of society or the medical communities. As demonstrated in the amenability index[16] with regard to cancers for which there are known early detection modalities and/or efficacious treatments, people in underserved communities are less likely to be exposed to those innovations and thus have worse outcomes. For example, there are no efficacious early detection tests or treatments for pancreatic cancer; thus, mortality rates are similar for Black and White populations. For other cancers, such as breast cancer, for which early detection and treatments impact outcomes, there are disparities in mortality. Interventions across the cancer control continuum have been developed for many underserved populations; however, there are also barriers that inhibit both testing intervention efficacy in these populations and testing the implementation of efficacious interventions. Thus, these populations should be a priority for this research because implementing successful interventions might have the greatest impact in these underserved and more vulnerable communities.

Expanding upon this area of disparities is the need to disseminate efficacious interventions for cancer prevention and control to address the global burden of cancer. This brings IS to a new level, adapting efficacious interventions for multiple countries—understanding cultures and languages to adapt interventions where they were not originally developed. Moreover, in many less developed countries, the cancer burden includes cancers not as common in more developed countries—bringing new meaning to implementation science. Different health care systems, cultures, customs, and political systems also bring unique challenges.

HOW CAN THIS BOOK HELP BRING IMPLEMENTATION SCIENCE TO BEAR ON OPPORTUNITIES ACROSS THE CANCER CONTROL CONTINUUM?

For many of the areas discussed previously, efficacious interventions tested in controlled situations exist. The challenge is to move these interventions into the real world and sustain them to impact disease rates. This is where this book can help. In the subsequent chapters, one can better understand the history of IS at the National Cancer Institute; understand how to identify, adapt, and implement evidence-based interventions across the cancer continuum; review theories, frameworks, models, measures, outcomes, study designs, data collection methods, and analytic approaches commonly used in implementation studies; and examine case studies of IS in primary prevention, uptake of screening tests and treatment, care delivery, survivorship, and global health. Thus, the why and the how of designing implementation studies are followed by real examples of how to conduct this type of research. This information is helpful because it does not exist in one easy-to-access place, tailored to the cancer world.

WHAT ABOUT THE FUTURE?

The one constant factor we can rely on is change. The future will bring us new challenges in this field as well as others. This book also provides helpful hints for addressing unanswered questions. Although there are many examples of precision medicine in treatment and detection, ensuring that all populations have equal access to these revolutionary strategies requires IS solutions. How to make big data relevant in all clinical settings is also a challenge for IS. Questions remain within this science, specifically with regard to effectively scaling-up and sustaining interventions, as well as determining the overuse of and knowing when to de-implement an intervention. Last, partnerships and assessment of cost-effectiveness are needed for true implementation and sustainability. The hope is that this book will direct more researchers to embark on and conduct implementation studies to address the burden of cancer in all populations, leading to sustaining cost-effective strategies that are employed in full partnership with communities and clinical partners. This is the only way to win the war on cancer.

REFERENCES

1. Agency for Healthcare Research and Quality, Centers for Disease Control and Prevention, International Cancer Control Partnership, National Cancer Institute, and Substance Abuse and Mental Health Services Administration. Cancer Control P.L.A.N.E.T. https://cancercontrolplanet.cancer.gov/index.html. Accessed October 12, 2017.
2. Best A, Hiatt RA, Cameron R, Rimer BK, Abrams DB. The evolution of cancer control research: An international perspective from Canada and the United States. *Cancer Epidemiol Biomarkers Prev.* 2003;12(8):705–712.
3. Cuzick J. Preventive therapy for cancer. *Lancet Oncol.* 2017;18(8):e472–e482.
4. Joura EA, Giuliano AR, Iversen OE, et al. A 9-valent HPV vaccine against infection and intraepithelial neoplasia in women. *N Engl J Med.* 2015;372(8):711–723.
5. Ropka ME, Keim J, Philbrick JT. Patient decisions about breast cancer chemoprevention: A systematic review and meta-analysis. *J Clin Oncol.* 2010;28(18):3090–3095.
6. Finkelstein J, Wood J, Crew KD, Kukafka R. Introducing a comprehensive informatics framework to promote breast cancer risk assessment and chemoprevention in the primary care setting. *AMIA Jt Summits Transl Sci Proc.* 2017;2017:58–67.
7. Fisher B, Costantino JP, Wickerham DL, et al. Tamoxifen for prevention of breast cancer: Report of the National Surgical Adjuvant Breast and Bowel Project P-1 Study. *J Natl Cancer Inst.* 1998;90(18):1371–1388.
8. Narod SA, Sopik V, Sun P. Which women decide to take tamoxifen? *Breast Cancer Res Treat.* 2017;164(1):149–155.
9. Skandarajah AR, Thomas S, Shackleton K, Chin-Lenn L, Lindeman GJ, Mann GB. Patient and medical barriers preclude uptake of tamoxifen preventative therapy in women with a strong family history. *Breast.* 2017;32:93–97.
10. Walker TY, Elam-Evans LD, Singleton JA, et al. National, regional, state, and selected local area vaccination coverage among adolescents aged 13–17 years—United States, 2016. *MMWR Morb Mortal Wkly Rep.* 2017;66(33):874–882.
11. Sabatino SA, White MC, Thompson TD, Klabunde CN; Centers for Disease Control and Prevention. Cancer screening test use—United States, 2013. *MMWR Morb Mortal Wkly Rep.* 2015;64(17):464–468.
12. Boccardo F, Rubagotti A, Puntoni M, et al. Switching to anastrozole versus continued tamoxifen treatment of early breast cancer: Preliminary results of the Italian Tamoxifen Anastrozole Trial. *J Clin Oncol.* 2005;23(22):5138–5147.
13. Breast International Group 1-98 Collaborative Group, Thurlimann B, Keshaviah A, et al. A comparison of letrozole and tamoxifen in postmenopausal women with early breast cancer. *N Engl J Med.* 2005;353(26):2747–2757.
14. Murphy CC, Bartholomew LK, Carpentier MY, Bluethmann SM, Vernon SW. Adherence to adjuvant hormonal therapy among breast cancer survivors in clinical practice: A systematic review. *Breast Cancer Res Treat.* 2012;134(2):459–478.
15. National Cancer Institute. Cancer Moonshot Blue Ribbon Panel Report 2016. 2016. https://deainfo.nci.nih.gov/advisory/ncab/0916/singer.pdf
16. Tehranifar P, Neugut AI, Phelan JC, et al. Medical advances and racial/ethnic disparities in cancer survival. *Cancer Epidemiol Biomarkers Prev.* 2009;18(10):2701–2708.

PREFACE

As I approached the field, carefully laid out according to the specifications of the International Sporting Society, I noted the pristine markings, the carefully attended hills, the manicured zones of grandeur. It was assumed that the mass populace would flock to such a scene, but nary a soul had visited this majestic wonderland before me. It was clearly not just the construction, but the demand for its utilization that would ultimately determine its societal impact. I sighed, drawing slowly in the oxygen that would fuel my future path toward diffusional understanding. And in the background, a flicker of movement caught my eye. A solitary crustacean casually traversed the bases.
—Lord Harry Henry (1897)

WE ARE in a time of rich discovery for the etiology, prevention, detection, diagnosis, treatment, and survivorship from cancer. Incredible advances in technology, data collection, analysis, and biological insights have positioned our field to have powerful tools to reduce the burden of cancer on the global population. However, true population-level impact can only come with increased understanding of how best to utilize and integrate the results of our biomedical research studies into everyday health care and public health settings.

It is with this significant challenge in mind that we see the need for this edited volume on implementation science across the cancer control continuum. Implementation science, broadly defined as the scientific study of how best to integrate evidence-based interventions, practices, programs, treatments, and other innovations into routine health care and public health settings[1], has gained considerably traction over the past decade, and particularly in cancer. For example, the recent Cancer Moonshot initiative identified implementation science as one of a handful of top priorities for cancer research. To best make use of the opportunities that lie ahead, we believed that a comprehensive publication that not only reviewed products from the implementation science field but also oriented readers to the next generation of themes needed to better integrate evidence into clinical and community settings would be of significant value moving forward.

We are in a new era of communication, access to information, and access to tools that can more precisely meet the needs of people across the cancer continuum. Without sufficient attention to the fit of these advances with the populations, settings, and individual needs, however, our progress will be limited. This book offers several paths forward, along with a wealth of examples from cancer prevention, detection, diagnosis, treatment, care delivery, and survivorship that we hope will illustrate the importance of attending to the science of implementation. It is in this spirit that we offer this book, a snapshot of what has been accomplished and what more there is to do.

D.A.C.
C.A.V.
W.E.N.

---

1. Although there are many terms associated with this definition, we use the term *implementation science* throughout this book for consistency and clarity. Related terms include *implementation research, dissemination and implementation research,* or *dissemination and implementation science.* Simiarly, we use the term *evidence-based interventions* to generally refer to evidence-based practices, evidence-based programs, evidence-based treatments, and other evidence-based health-focused innovations. See glossary for additional terms and definitions.

ACKNOWLEDGMENTS

WE ARE grateful to many individuals who were instrumental in the creation and publication of this text.

We thank the amazing collection of authors who contributed to the content of this edited text. We are fortunate to have so many leaders and experts in the field of implementation science in cancer be part of this collection, and we are grateful for their time, contribution, and deep thinking on these issues for this text.

We are indebted to Drs. Barbara Rimer and Robert Croyle for their leadership in the Division of Cancer Control and Population Sciences at the National Cancer Institute and for their foresight in recognizing and prioritizing implementation science within cancer control and population sciences. We are greatly appreciative of former leaders of the Implementation Science team at the National Cancer Institute—Drs. Jon Kerner and Russell Glasgow—for establishing a foundation in this area and paving the way for cancer researchers to help advance the science of implementation.

We thank the staff at Oxford University Press (OUP) for their efforts throughout the development process. In particular, we thank Tiffany Lu, Assistant Editor of Clinical Medicine, for her superb organizational skills, timely responses, detail-oriented correspondence, and excellent management from the inception through the production of this text. We also thank Marta Moldvai, Editor of Emergency Medicine and Palliative Care, for her continued support and expert advice on maximizing the utility of the text. In addition, we acknowledge two OUP editors, Andrea Knobloch and Rebecca Suzan, who provided wonderful guidance and encouragement during the initial stages.

Finally, we are grateful to the community of implementation scientists, both in cancer and in other health areas, who have dedicated their careers to helping bridge the gap between evidence and practice to make a measurable impact on patient outcomes and population health. In particular, we thank Drs. Ross Brownson, Graham Colditz, and Enola Proctor for the formative textbook, *Dissemination and Implementation Research in Health*, which has remained invaluable in our efforts to build capacity in the field.

CONTRIBUTORS

Gregory A. Aarons, PhD
Professor, Department of Psychiatry
University of California, San Diego
La Jolla, CA
Director, Child and Adolescent Services Research
   Center
San Diego, CA

Prajakta Adsul, MBBS, MPH, PhD
Cancer Prevention Fellow, Implementation Science
Division of Cancer Control and Population Sciences
National Cancer Institute
Rockville, MD
Research Fellow, Public Health Research Institute
   of India
Mysore, India

Linda J. Ahrendt, MEd
Director, Child and Family Services
Division of Family and Community Health
South Dakota Department of Health
Pierre, SD

Catherine M. Alfano, PhD
Vice President, Cancer Survivorship
American Cancer Society
Atlanta, GA

Karla Alfaro, MD, MPH
Medical Director
Basic Health International
San Salvador, El Salvador

Peg M. Allen, PhD, MPH
Research Assistant Professor
Prevention Research Center in St. Louis
Brown School
Washington University in St. Louis
St. Louis, MO

Rinad Beidas, PhD
Assistant Professor, Department of Psychiatry
Director, Implementation Research
Center for Mental Health Policy and Services
   Research
Perelman School of Medicine
University of Pennsylvania
Philadelphia, PA

Michelle Betts, MSW
Social Worker
St. Luke's Mountain States Tumor Institute
Boise, ID

Sarah A. Birken, PhD
Assistant Professor, Department of Health Policy
   and Management
UNC Gillings School of Global Public Health
Associate Member, UNC Lineberger
   Comprehensive Cancer Center
Faculty Research Fellow, Cecil G. Sheps Center for
   Health Services Research
University of North Carolina
Chapel Hill, NC

Heather M. Brandt, PhD, CHES
Associate Professor, Department of Health
   Promotion, Education, and Behavior
Arnold School of Public Health
University of South Carolina
Columbia, SC

Otis W. Brawley, MD, MACP
Chief Medical Officer
American Cancer Society
Professor of Hematology, Medical Oncology,
   Medicine and Epidemiology
Emory University
Atlanta, GA

Laura Brossart, BA
Assistant Director of Communications and
    Dissemination
Center for Public Health Systems Science
Brown School
Washington University in St. Louis
St. Louis, MO

Ross C. Brownson, PhD
Bernard Becker Professor of Public Health
Director, Prevention Research Center in St. Louis
Brown School and Department of Surgery
    (Division of Public Health Sciences)
School of Medicine
Alvin J. Siteman Cancer Center
Washington University in St. Louis
St. Louis, MO

Mindy Clyne, MHS
Research Assistant, Implementation Science
Division of Cancer Control and Population
    Sciences
National Cancer Institute
Rockville, MD

Todd B. Combs, PhD
Assistant Director of Research
Center for Public Health Systems Science
Brown School
Washington University in St. Louis
St. Louis, MO

Alex Conway, BS
Research Assistant
George Washington University
Washington, DC

Gloria D. Coronado, PhD
Senior Investigator, Mitch Greenlick Endowed
    Scientist for Health Disparities
Kaiser Permanente Center for Health Research
Portland, OR

Miriam Cremer, MD, MPH
President and Founder
Basic Health International
San Salvador, El Salvador
Associate Professor
Department of Obstetrics and Gynecology
Cleveland Clinic Lerner College of Medicine
Cleveland, OH

Janet S. de Moor, PhD, MPH
Behavioral Scientist and Program Director,
    Healthcare Assessment Research Branch
Healthcare Delivery Research Program
Division of Cancer Control and Population
    Sciences
National Cancer Institute
Rockville, MD

James W. Dearing, PhD
Professor and Chairperson
Department of Communication
Michigan State University
East Lansing, MI

Maryam Doroudi, MPH, PhD
Cancer Prevention Fellow
Division of Cancer Prevention
National Cancer Institute
Bethesda, MD

Caitlin N. Dorsey, BA
Research Specialist
MacColl Center for Health Care Innovation
Kaiser Permanente Washington Health Research
    Institute
Seattle, WA

Nancy C. Edwards, RN, PhD
Professor and Distinguished Professor
School of Nursing
University of Ottawa
Ottawa, Canada

Cam Escoffery, PhD, MPH, CHES
Associate Professor, Department of Behavioral
    Sciences and Health Education
Rollins School of Public Health
Emory University
Atlanta, GA

Maria E. Fernandez, PhD
Professor, Department of Health Promotion and
    Behavioral Sciences
Lorne Bain Distinguished Professor in Public
    Health and Medicine
Director, Center for Health Promotion and
    Prevention Research
School of Public Health
University of Texas Health Science Center
Houston, TX

Harold P. Freeman, MD
Founder and President/CEO
Harold P. Freeman Patient Navigation Institute
New York, NY

Julia C. Gage, PhD, MPH
Staff Scientist, Clinical Genetics Branch
Division of Cancer Epidemiology and Genetics
National Cancer Institute
Bethesda, MD

Krystal G. Garcia, BS
Graduate Student
Department of Health Policy and Management
UNC Gillings School of Global Public Health
University of North Carolina
Chapel Hill, NC

Russell E. Glasgow, PhD
Research Professor, Family Medicine
Director, Dissemination and Implementation
    Science Program of ACCORDS (Adult and
    Child Consortium for Health Outcomes
    Research and Delivery Science)
University of Colorado School of Medicine
Aurora, CO

Heather Taffet Gold, PhD
Associate Professor, Department of Population
    Health, Department of Orthopedic Surgery
Director, Population Health Research
New York University School of Medicine
NYU Langone Health
New York, NY

Vicky Gomez, MPH
Research Associate
Division of Research
Kaiser Permanente Northern California
    Health Care
Oakland, CA

Lawrence W. Green, DrPH
Professor Emeritus, Epidemiology and
    Biostatistics
Helen Diller Family Comprehensive
    Cancer Center
School of Medicine
University of California, San Francisco
San Francisco, CA

Melvin Grimes, BS
Graduate Student
School of Science and Mathematics
Mississippi College
Clinton, MS

Erin E. Hahn, PhD, MPH
Research Scientist, Division of Health Services
    Research and Implementation Science
Department of Research and Evaluation
Kaiser Permanente Southern California
Pasadena, CA

Emily Haines, BA
Public Health Analyst
RTI International
Research Triangle Park, NC

Alison B. Hamilton, PhD, MPH
Associate Director for Implementation Science
Veterans Affairs Health Services Research and
    Development Service
Center for the Study of Healthcare Innovation,
    Implementation, and Policy
Veterans Affairs, Greater Los Angeles
    Healthcare System
Associate Anthropologist, Department of
    Psychiatry and Biobehavioral Sciences
David Geffen School of Medicine
University of California, Los Angeles
Los Angeles, CA

Kathy J. Helzlsouer, MD, MHS
Associate Director
Epidemiology and Genomics Research Program
Division of Cancer Control and Population
    Sciences
National Cancer Institute
Rockville, MD

Kiley A. Hump, MS
Administrator, Office of Chronic Disease
    Prevention and Health Promotion
Division of Family and Community Health
South Dakota Department of Health
Pierre, SD

Vivian Jiang, MD
Fellow, Family Medicine for America's Health
Virginia Commonwealth University
Richmond, VA

Amy Kennedy, PhD, MPH
Health Scientist Administrator
Center for Research Strategy
National Cancer Institute
Rockville, MD

Erin E. Kent, PhD
Scientific Advisor, Outcomes Research Branch
Healthcare Delivery Research Program
Division of Cancer Control and Population
    Sciences
National Cancer Institute
Rockville, MD

Jon Kerner, PhD
Expert Advisor, Knowledge Mobilization and
    Evaluation
Strategy Division, Canadian Partnership
    Against Cancer
Toronto, Ontario, Canada

Muin J. Khoury, MD, PhD
Director, Office of Public Health Genomics
Centers for Disease Control and Prevention
Atlanta, GA

Debbie Kirkland, BA
Director, Prevention and Early Detection
Co-Chair, National Council on Skin Cancer
    Prevention
American Cancer Society
Atlanta, GA

Lisa M. Klesges, PhD, MS
Professor, Division of Epidemiology, Biostatistics and
    Environmental Health School of Public Health
University of Memphis
Memphis, TN

Sarah C. Kobrin, PhD, MPH
Branch Chief, Health Systems and Interventions
    Research Branch
Healthcare Delivery Research Program
Division of Cancer Control and Population
    Sciences
National Cancer Institute
Rockville, MD

Racquel E. Kohler, PhD, MSPH
Research Fellow, Department of Social and
    Behavioral Sciences
Harvard T. H. Chan School of Public Health
Harvard University
Center for Community-Based Research
Dana–Farber Cancer Institute
Boston, MA

Barnett S. Kramer, MPH, MD
Director
Division of Cancer Prevention
National Cancer Institute
Rockville, MD

Alex H. Krist, MD, MPH
Professor, Department of Family Medicine and
    Population Health
Fairfax Family Medicine Residency
Director, Ambulatory Care Outcomes Research
    Network
Virginia Commonwealth University
Fairfax, VA

Jennifer Leeman, PhD
Associate Professor, Systems/Policy/Informatics
School of Nursing
University of North Carolina
Chapel Hill, NC

Cara C. Lewis, PhD
Associate Investigator
Kaiser Permanente Washington Health Research
    Institute
Seattle, WA

Edwin A. Lomotan, MD
Medical Officer and Chief of Clinical Informatics
Division of Health Information Technology
Center for Evidence and Practice Improvement
Agency for Healthcare Research and Quality
Rockville, MD

Douglas A. Luke, PhD
Professor and Director
Center for Public Health Systems Science
Brown School
Washington University in St. Louis
St. Louis, MO

Purnima Madhivanan, MBBS, MPH, PhD
Associate Professor, Department of Epidemiology
Robert Stemple College of Public Health and
    Social Work
Florida International University
Miami, FL
Public Health Research Institute of India
Mysore, India

Deborah K. Mayer, PhD, RN, AOCN, FAAN
Professor, Adult and Geriatric Health Division
School of Nursing
Director, Cancer Survivorship
UNC Lineberger Comprehensive Cancer Center
University of North Carolina
Chapel Hill, NC

Mauricio Maza, MD, MPH
Executive Director
Basic Health International
San Salvador, El Salvador

Kayne D. Mettert, BA
Research Specialist
Kaiser Permanente Health Research Institute
Seattle, WA

Brian Mittman, PhD
Research Scientist, Division of Health Services
    Research and Implementation Science
Department of Research and Evaluation
Kaiser Permanente Southern California
Pasadena, CA

Paul Montgomery, MD, FACP
Clinical Assistant Professor of Medicine
University of Washington
Seattle, WA
Hematologist/Oncologist
Boise Veterans Affairs Medical Center
Boise, ID

Kathi Mooney, PhD, RN, FAAN
Louis S. Peery and Janet B. Peery Presidential
    Endowed Chair in Nursing
College of Nursing
Distinguished Professor, College of Nursing
University of Utah
Co-Leader, Cancer Control and Population
    Sciences
Huntsman Cancer Institute
Salt Lake City, UT

Joanna C. Moullin, PhD
Lecturer, Faculty of Health Sciences
Curtin University
Perth, Western Australia
Investigator, Child and Adolescent Services
    Research Center
San Diego, CA

Patricia Dolan Mullen, DrPH, MLS
Distinguished Teaching Professor of the University
    of Texas System
UTHealth President's Scholar
Professor, Department of Health Promotion and
    Behavioral Sciences
University of Texas School of Public Health
Houston, TX

Jamie S. Ostroff, PhD
Chief, Behavioral Sciences Service and Vice Chair
    for Research
Department of Psychiatry and Behavioral Sciences
Memorial Sloan Kettering Cancer Center
Professor of Psychology, Department of Healthcare
    Policy and Research
Weill Cornell Medical College
New York, NY

Lynne Padgett, PhD
Health Psychologist
Veterans Affairs Medical Center
Washington, DC

Mark Parascandola, PhD, MPH
Epidemiologist and Program Director, Tobacco
    Control Research Branch
Behavioral Research Program
Division of Cancer Control and Population
    Science
National Cancer Institute
Rockville, MD

Electra D. Paskett, PhD
Marion N. Rowley Professor of Cancer Research
Division of Cancer Prevention and Control
Department of Internal Medicine
College of Medicine Epidemiology
The Ohio State University College of Public
    Health
Columbus, OH

Jane Peredo, ScM
Research Associate and Genetic Counselor
Veterans Affairs Greater Los Angeles
    Healthcare System
Los Angeles, CA

Meagan R. Pilar, MPH
Graduate Research Assistant
Prevention Research Center in St. Louis
Washington University in St. Louis
St. Louis, MO

Paul F. Pinsky, PhD
Branch Chief, Early Detection Research Branch
Division of Cancer Prevention
National Cancer Institute
Rockville, MD

Michael B. Potter, MD
Professor, Department of Family and Community
    Medicine
School of Medicine
University of California, San Francisco
San Francisco, CA

Byron J. Powell, PhD, LCSW
Assistant Professor, Department of Health Policy
    and Management
UNC Gillings School of Global Public Health
Fellow, Cecil G. Sheps Center for Health Services
    Research
Fellow, Frank Porter Graham Child Development
    Institute
University of North Carolina
Chapel Hill, NC

Shoba Ramanadhan, ScD, MPH
Research Scientist, Department of Social and
    Behavioral Sciences
Harvard T. H. Chan School of Public Health
Senior Scientist, Center for Community-Based
    Research
Dana–Farber Cancer Institute
Boston, MA

Gurvaneet S. Randhawa, MD, MPH
Medical Officer, Health Systems and Interventions
    Research Branch
Healthcare Delivery Research Program
Division of Cancer Control and Population Sciences
National Cancer Institute
National Institutes of Health
Rockville, MD

Kurt M. Ribisl, PhD
Professor and Department Chair, Department of
    Health Behavior
UNC Gillings School of Global Public Health
Program Leader, Cancer Prevention and Control
UNC Lineberger Comprehensive Cancer Center
University of North Carolina
Chapel Hill, NC

Barbara L. Riley, PhD
Executive Director
Propel Centre for Population Health Impact
Faculty of Applied Health Sciences
University of Waterloo
Waterloo, Ontario, Canada

Julia H. Rowland, PhD
Senior Strategic Advisor
Smith Center for Healing and the Arts
Washington, DC

Marcia Russell, MD
Veterans Affairs Health Services Research and
    Development
Veterans Affairs Greater Los Angeles
    Healthcare System
Department of Surgery
David Geffen School of Medicine
University of California, Los Angeles
Los Angeles, CA

Anne E. Sales, RN, PhD
Professor, Department of Learning Health
    Sciences
Associate Chair for Educational Programs and
    Health System Innovations
Director, Health Infrastructures and Learning
    Systems MS and PhD Programs
University of Michigan Medical School
Research Scientist, Center for Clinical
    Management Research
Veterans Affairs Ann Arbor Healthcare System
Ann Arbor, MI

Maren T. Scheuner, MD, MPH
Chief, Medical Genetics
Center for the Study of Healthcare Innovation,
    Implementation and Policy
Veterans Affaris Health Services Research and
    Development
Veterans Affairs Greater Los Angeles Healthcare
    System
Professor, Department of Medicine
David Geffen School of Medicine
University of California, Los Angeles
Los Angeles, CA

**Kathryn H. Schmitz, PhD, MPH,
FACSM, FTOS**
Professor, Public Health Sciences
Penn State College of Medicine
Associate Director of Population Sciences
Penn State Cancer Institute
Hershey, PA

Donna Shelley, MD, MPH
Associate Professor of Medicine and
    Population Health
Co-Director, Section on Tobacco, Alcohol and
    Drug Use
Department of Population Health
New York University School of Medicine
New York, NY

Melissa A. Simon, MD, MPH
Vice Chair for Clinical Research, Department of
    Obstetrics and Gynecology
George H. Gardner, MD, Professor of Clinical
    Gynecology
Professor of Obstetrics and Gynecology (General
    Obstetrics and Gynecology)/Preventive
    Medicine and Medical Social Sciences
Northwestern Medicine, Feinberg School of
    Medicine
Chicago, IL

Sudha Sivaram, MPH, DrPH
Branch Chief, Public Health, Networks and
    Research Branch
Center for Global Health
National Cancer Institute
Rockville, MD

Marisa Sklar, PhD
Project Scientist, Department of Psychiatry
University of California, San Diego
La Jolla, CA
Child and Adolescent Services Research Center
San Diego, CA

Ted A. Skolarus, MD, MPH, FACS
Associate Professor, Department of Urology
University of Michigan
Core Investigator, Center for Clinical Management
    Research
Veterans Affairs Health Services Research and
    Development
Veterans Affairs Ann Arbor Healthcare System
Ann Arbor, MI

C. Scott Smith, MD, MACP
Professor of Medicine
Adjunct Professor, Biomedical Informatics and
    Medical Education
University of Washington
Seattle, WA
Section Head
Boise Veterans Affairs Medical Center
Boise, ID

Carol P. Somkin, PhD
Associate Professor
University of California, San Francisco School of
    Nursing
San Francisco, CA
Division of Research
Kaiser Permanente Northern California
Oakland, CA

Shannon Wiltsey Stirman, PhD
Assistant Professor, Department of Psychiatry and
    Behavioral Sciences
Stanford University School of Medicine
Acting Deputy Director, Dissemination and
    National Center for PTSD Dissemination and
    Training Division
VA Palo Alto Health Care System
Palo Alto, CA

Angela M. Stover, PhD
Assistant Professor, Department of Health Policy
and Management
UNC Gillings School of Global Public Health
Associate Member, UNC Lineberger
Comprehensive Cancer Center
University of North Carolina
Chapel Hill, NC

Rachel G. Tabak, PhD
Research Assistant Professor
Prevention Research Center in St. Louis
Brown School
Washington University in St. Louis
St. Louis, MO

Nicole Thurston, MD
Psychiatrist
St. Luke's Mountain States Tumor Institute
Boise, ID

Robin C. Vanderpool, DrPH, CHES
Associate Professor, Department of Health,
Behavior, and Society
University of Kentucky College of Public Health
Lexington, KY

Arti Patel Varanasi, PhD, MPH
President and CEO
Advancing Synergy, LLC
Baltimore, MD

K. Viswanath, PhD
Lee Kum Kee Professor of Health Communication
Harvard T. H. Chan School of Public Health
(HSPH)
Dana–Farber Cancer Institute (DFCI)
Director, Center for Translational Health
Communication Science, DFCI/HSPH
Director, Harvard Chan India Research Center
Co-Director, Lee Kum Sheung Center for Health
and Happiness
Boston, MA

Timothy J. Walker, PhD
Postdoctoral Research Fellow, Department of
Health Promotion and Behavioral Sciences
School of Public Health
University of Texas Health Science Center
Houston, TX

Judith M. E. Walsh, MD
Primary Care Internist
Department of Medicine
University of California, San Francisco School of
Medicine
San Francisco, CA

Bryan J. Weiner, PhD
Professor of Global Health and Health Services
University of Washington
Seattle, WA

Stephanie B. Wheeler, PhD, MPH
Associate Professor, Department of Health Policy
and Management
UNC Gillings School of Global Public Health
University of North Carolina
Chapel Hill, NC

Meagan Whisenant, PhD, APRN
Postdoctoral Fellow, Department of Symptom
Research
University of Texas MD Anderson Cancer Center
Department of Symptom Research, Division of
Internal Medicine
Houston, TX

Cameron D. Willis, PhD
Cause Communications Researcher
The Movember Foundation
Melbourne, VIC, Australia
Scientist and Research Assistant Professor
Propel Centre for Population Health Impact
University of Waterloo
Waterloo, Ontario, Canada

Elizabeth M. Yano, PhD, MSPH
Director, Center for the Study of Healthcare
Innovation, Implementation and Policy
Veterans Affairs Health Services Research and
Development
Veterans Affairs Greater Los Angeles
Healthcare System
Adjunct Professor, Department of Health Policy
and Management
UCLA Fielding School of Public Health
University of California, Los Angeles
Los Angeles, CA

Yan Yu, MD
Resident Family Physician
Alberta Health Services
Calgary, Alberta, Canada

SECTION I

AN INTRODUCTION TO IMPLEMENTATION SCIENCE ACROSS THE CANCER CONTROL CONTINUUM

1A

AN ORIENTATION TO IMPLEMENTATION SCIENCE IN CANCER

David A. Chambers, Wynne E. Norton, and Cynthia A. Vinson

THE ROOTS of implementation science (IS) in cancer in some sense date back to the earliest days of uncovering cancer's etiology, diagnosis, prevention, and treatment, although it was not called that. Indeed, unlocking the mysteries of cancer and determining effective ways to intervene began not in the lab but, rather, the clinic. As Mukherjee recounted in the seminal work, *The Emperor of All Maladies*,[1] cancer had been the subject of clinical examination for centuries, and the drive to optimize care began in those early days. As opposed to the largely separate worlds of research discovery and care delivery that exist today, scientific research and cancer treatment coexisted. In addition, epidemiologic observations of risk factors affecting oncogenesis developed targets for what types of prevention programs needed to be implemented. Naturally, the challenges of what exactly to implement and how best to implement have been with us throughout time.

CONTEXT FOR THIS BOOK

This book has been compiled at an exciting time. Just 2 years ago, Vice President Joseph R. Biden launched the Cancer Moonshot initiative (https://www.cancer.gov/research/key-initiatives/www.cancer.gov/research/key-initiatives/

moonshot-cancer-initiative), a broad-based effort to drive accelerated progress toward the reduction of burden of cancer in the population. A key component of the Cancer Moonshot initiative was the formation of a Blue Ribbon Panel, advisory to the National Cancer Institute (NCI), that would identify the key next steps for cancer research that could be targeted for rapid growth. Of the many possible areas of focus across the cancer research enterprise, the panel chose seven to form work groups around. Implementation science took its place alongside tumor evolution and progression, clinical trials, precision prevention and early detection, pediatric cancer, enhanced data sharing, and cancer immunology as one of a select set of themes. The Implementation Science working group's discussions yielded two key recommendations that were described in the final report: (1) Expand use of proven cancer prevention and early detection strategies and (2) minimize cancer treatment's debilitating side effects (which focused on the implementation of evidence-based symptom management strategies) (https://www.cancer.gov/research/key-initiatives/moonshot-cancer-initiative/blue-ribbon-panel).

The first wave of concepts released by NCI to solicit research studies based on the Blue Ribbon Panel's recommendations included three that emerged from the recommendations of the Implementation Science group. The first sought to test "Approaches to Identify and Care for Individuals with Inherited Cancer Syndromes" (RFA-CA-17-041; https://grants.nih.gov/grants/guide/rfa-files/RFA-CA-17-041.html). The second focused on improving the uptake and sustainment of evidence-based colorectal cancer screening, follow-up, and referral to care (RFA-CA-17-039/040; https://grants.nih.gov/grants/guide/rfa-files/RFA-CA-17-038.html). The third focused on implementing effective strategies for symptom management across stages of cancer care (RFA-CA-17-042/043; https://grants.nih.gov/grants/guide/rfa-files/RFA-CA-17-042.html). All are expected to have contributions to our understanding of implementation science in cancer during the next 5 years.

Contemporaneous with the Cancer Moonshot activity, multiple professional organizations and advocacy groups seized upon implementation science as a major focus. The annual meetings of the American Society of Preventive Oncology, the American Society of Clinical Oncology's Quality of Care Symposium, and the American Association for Cancer Research all brought implementation science to the forefront in plenary sessions within a single calendar year. The American Cancer Society, in partnership with NCI and the Centers for Disease Control and Prevention and the Comprehensive Cancer Control National Partnership (https://www.cccnationalpartners.org), conducted a series of technical assistance forums to help state teams improve implementation of evidence-based programs to promote colorectal cancer screening and human papillomavirus vaccination uptake. Finally, the National Academy of Medicine's Roundtable on Genomics and Precision Health has formed an action collaborative seeking to improve the integration of genomic medicine within health care and public health settings. One of the work groups, now in its third year, specifically focuses on advances in the implementation of genetic and genomic testing and follow-up care (http://www.nationalacademies.org/hmd/Activities/Research/GenomicBasedResearch/Innovation-Collaboratives/Genomics-and-Population-Health.aspx). These implementation science-related activities collectively represent work across the cancer continuum, from advances in prevention and diagnostics to early detection and treatment, as well as survivorship care.

At NCI, implementation science is largely concentrated within the Division of Cancer Control and Population Sciences (https://cancercontrol.cancer.gov). Through ongoing funding opportunity announcements, training programs, workshops and conferences, and theoretical and empirical advances, implementation science in cancer continues to spread. Much of this work is done in concert with other institutes and centers within the National Institutes of Health (NIH; the trans-NIH funding opportunity announcements, for example, involve 18 institutes, centers, and offices; https://grants.nih.gov/grants/guide/pa-files/PAR-18-007.html), enabling the steady progress of implementation science in overall health as well as specifically in cancer. Recent history of implementation science in cancer, through the eyes of leadership at NCI, is chronicled in Chapter 1b of this volume.

BRIEF HISTORY OF IMPLEMENTATION SCIENCE IN HEALTH

Although Chapter 2 focuses on the history governing NCI's investment in implementation science, we thought it would be helpful to briefly touch upon the long history of implementation science in health overall. Similar to our view of implementation science in cancer, it would be disingenuous to declare that implementation science in health dates back only a few decades, as the overall intention of making optimal care into standard care for patients has been present as far back as we can document. It is arguable that the foundation of clinical research had, at its core, the purpose of providing new opportunities for treatment, prevention, and palliation.

The roots of evidence-based medicine, it is said, can be viewed in Semelweis' work to reduce maternal mortality during childbirth and in Dr. Lind's work to identify the cause of scurvy among sailors in the British Navy.[2] In these examples from past centuries, the systematic effort to understand how clinical practice could be improved and how disease could be averted suggested that research can be harnessed to reduce illness and prolong life. It caught steam many decades later in the work of Archibald Cochrane, whose seminal book, *Effectiveness and Efficiency*,[3] brought epidemiology into the clinical setting and established key targets for clinical research to concentrate on in efforts to improve medical practice.

This was furthered by David Sackett and colleagues[4] in the mid-1990s in the enumeration of "scientific evidence, clinical expertise, and patient preferences" as the three legs of the evidence-based medicine stool, which bred an entire range of efforts to translate research into practice.

Sackett et al.'s[4] identification of "evidence-based medicine" was recognized as having the potential to achieve what would later be considered the triple aim[5]—improved clinical practice, reduced costs, and improved patient outcomes—and stimulated worldwide efforts to implement evidence-based medicine. In the United States, the Agency for Healthcare Policy Research (later renamed the Agency for Healthcare Research and Quality [AHRQ]) funded a set of evidence-based practice centers that would review clinical evidence, make recommendations for implementation, and carry out local projects to change clinical practice (https://www.ahrq.gov/research/findings/evidence-based-reports/overview/index.html). In the United Kingdom, the National Health Service funded a series of demonstration projects with the goal of improving the management of clinical practice change across a range of health topics.[6] And in the final years of the last millennium, a new emphasis at the National Institute of Mental Health, AHRQ, and the Veterans Administration (VA) on translating research into practice led to multiple calls for research applications to advance the science of dissemination and implementation in health.

The most recent era has seen tremendous expansion in efforts to standardize the knowledge base for implementation science, with a number of flagship activities leading the way. Since 2005, NIH (with the majority of NIH institutes and centers participating) has steadily solicited applications to develop the implementation science knowledge base, as well as build capacity for studies to increase in quality and quantity. The 10th in a series of annual conferences on the science of dissemination and implementation was held in 2017; this is a partnered effort among NIH, Academy Health, the Patient-Centered Outcomes Research Institute, AHRQ, the VA, and others. We also have seen increased efforts in the training of interested investigators, with the NIH/VA Training Institute for Dissemination and Implementation Research in Health[7] providing training for more than 7 years, along with a range of other programs both within the United States and internationally.[8] The field has also benefitted greatly from the founding of the journal *Implementation*

Science[9] as well as the increased opportunities to publish in high-impact clinical research journals and the use of a variety of approaches to share updates with the field (social media, listservs, etc.).

THE RAPID EVOLUTION OF IMPLEMENTATION SCIENCE IN HEALTH

The collective activities mentioned previously are only made possible by the steady march of implementation scientists to devise and execute studies of increased complexity, rigor, and relevance to health and health care practice. Early implementation studies seemed primarily to wrestle with identification of barriers and facilitators, prominently centered on "Why doesn't it work?" With the long-standing assumption that the high-impact publication concludes the research process,[10] investigators were looking to identify what went wrong and what could be done about it.

A few years later, the balance of studies, at least those coming into a number of funding agencies, shifted to focus more on the development and testing of implementation strategies, typically with multiple components, to overcome the barriers to practice change so that implementation of evidence-based practices would be more successful than the oft-tried initial training and limited support. We had moved as a field from "Why doesn't implementation work?" to "Can we make implementation efforts work?" kitchen sink and all. Quickly, investigators began to devise alternate strategies for implementation, and in line with expanded focus on comparative effectiveness research (framed at the center of the development of the Patient-Centered Outcomes Research Institute), we have seen a shift to "How can we make our implementation strategies work better?"

Along a different axis, we have also seen implementation scientists expand the range of "implementation stages" under focus. Early emphasis on the adoption of evidence-based health interventions moved to enumerate the influences and strategies governing implementation, followed swiftly by a drive to understand determinants of sustainability. The field has more recently sought to build additional expertise in scale-up and spread, as well as to give more thoughtful attention to the adaptability and evolution of our interventions over time and across space. These indicators of progress form much of the enthusiasm that surrounds the development of this book, which we offer as a signpost of where we have been and, more important, where the cancer research field can go in the future.

ORGANIZATION OF THIS BOOK

This book is divided into three major sections. The first set of chapters in Section I (including this chapter) focus on an introduction to implementation science in cancer across the cancer control continuum (i.e., covering a range of topics related to cancer prevention, early detection, screening, diagnosis, treatment, survivorship, and palliative care). The intention is to summarize the core components of implementation science with a specific lens on their use within the cancer domain. Following the historical perspective on implementation science in cancer (Chapter 1b), the next chapters review the evidence base for interventions, practices, and programs in cancer control (Chapter 2) and summarize the range of existing theories, frameworks, and models used in implementation science in cancer (Chapter 3). Subsequent chapters introduce progress in measures and outcomes (Chapter 4), study designs and methods (Chapter 5), and the definition and examples of implementation strategies (Chapter 6). From this series of chapters, we intend for the reader to get a foundation in the development of the field and the major components of the growing portfolio of studies building empirical support for implementation science in cancer.

Section II uses a case study format to relate lessons learned from implementation science on specific topics in cancer prevention and control that are designed to illuminate multiple implementation opportunities and challenges. Each chapter includes an overview that provides an introduction to the set of cases as well as the content area within which the cases reside. The implementation science case studies center around examples in cancer prevention and public health promotion (Chapter 7), cancer detection and screening (Chapter 8), provider-level factors influencing implementation (Chapter 9), organization- and system-level factors influencing implementation (Chapter 10), cancer survivorship (Chapter 11), and cancer in a global health context (Chapter 12). Each chapter presents several cases that illustrate progress in implementation science and challenges with moving the evidence base for cancer prevention and control into practice. It is our hope that these cases are instructive not only to researchers seeking to apply them to their next studies but also to a range of participants in cancer control planning and care delivery.

Section III focuses on a set of emerging issues in implementation science across the cancer control continuum that will likely form the next generation of activity in this field. Each chapter takes on a specific priority area, summarizing the challenges and opportunities, current progress, and next steps. Topics include precision medicine (Chapter 13), big data and technological advances (Chapter 14), scaling-up cancer programs (Chapter 15), sustainability of cancer programs (Chapter 16), overuse and de-implementation (Chapter 17), and partnerships and networks for implementation science (Chapter 18). The volume concludes with a chapter on cost-effectiveness analysis for implementation science (Chapter 19) and a chapter on future directions in the field from the perspectives of the three editors (Chapter 20).

Although we know that even a full-length volume cannot possibly capture the sum and substance of the field of implementation science as it seeks to advance all aspects of the cancer control continuum, we hope that it well characterizes the vibrancy of past and current activities and the promise of those to come. We are gratified by the many researchers, practitioners, policymakers, advocates, patients, and families who commit themselves daily to making optimal cancer care the reality for everyone, and we hope this serves as a signpost that we are making progress toward that important goal.

REFERENCES

1. Mukherjee S. *The Emperor of All Maladies: A Biography of Cancer*. New York: Simon & Schuster; 2010.
2. Greenstone G. The roots of evidence-based medicine. *Br Columbia Med J*. 2009;51:342–344.
3. Cochrane AL. *Effectiveness and Efficiency: Random Reflections on Health Services*. London: Nuffield Provincial Hospitals Trust London; 1972.
4. Sackett DL, Rosenberg WM, Gray JM, Haynes RB, Richardson WS. Evidence based medicine: What it is and what it isn't. *Br Med J*. 1996;312(7023):71–72.
5. Berwick DM, Nolan TW, Whittington J. The triple aim: Care, health, and cost. *Health Aff (Millwood)*. 2008;27:759–769.

6. Dopson S, Locock L, Chambers D, Gabbay J. Implementation of evidence-based medicine: Evaluation of the Promoting Action on Clinical Effectiveness programme. *J Health Serv Res Policy.* 2001;6:23–31.

7. Meissner HI, Glasgow RE, Vinson CA, Chambers D, Brownson RC, Green LW, Ammerman AS, Weiner BJ, Mittman B. The U.S. training institute for dissemination and implementation research in health. *Implement Sci.* 2013;8:12.

8. Proctor EK, Chambers DA. Training in dissemination and implementation research: A field-wide perspective. *Transl Behav Med.* 2017;7:624–635.

9. Eccles MP, Mittman BS. Welcome to implementation science. *Implement Sci.* 2006;1:1.

10. Balas EA, Boren SA. Managing clinical knowledge for health care improvement. *Yearb Med Inform.* 2000; 312(1):65–70.

1B

A HISTORY OF THE NATIONAL CANCER INSTITUTE'S SUPPORT FOR IMPLEMENTATION SCIENCE ACROSS THE CANCER CONTROL CONTINUUM

CONTEXT COUNTS

Jon Kerner, Russell E. Glasgow, and Cynthia A. Vinson

INTRODUCTION

This chapter reviews the historical development of the National Cancer Institute's (NCI) Implementation Science Program. It discusses the history of implementation science at the NCI and the co-author's personal and professional contributions to the development of NCI's Division of Cancer Control and Population Science (DCCPS). All three authors played key roles (and CV continues to play a key role) in the evolution of the NCI's DCCPS Implementation Science Program, and each brought a different background and perspective to the factors that contributed to the development of implementation science at NCI.

THE ROOTS OF IMPLEMENTATION SCIENCE IN CANCER CONTROL RESEARCH: FROM DISCOVERY TO DELIVERY

The history of cancer control in the United States is documented in multiple places on the NCI's website.[1] This history has directly impacted the growth of the field of implementation science in cancer. Figure 1B.1 provides an overview of the key events in the development of cancer control and implementation science at NCI.

In 1971, President Richard M. Nixon signed the National Cancer Act, which for the first time specified a role for the NCI that included a focus on cancer control. At the time of the passage of the Act, "the scientific community and the Congress thought . . . that many research advances existed which could affect cancer, but these advances were not being disseminated and used. The cancer control program was intended to bridge this gap."[2] From 1972 to 1982, the cancer control program budget was largely allocated to contract programs in professional education whereby NCI-designated cancer centers were provided cancer control program funds to conduct professional education with hospitals and clinical centers in each center's self-designated catchment area. The transition of the cancer control program from a "diffusion of innovations"[3]

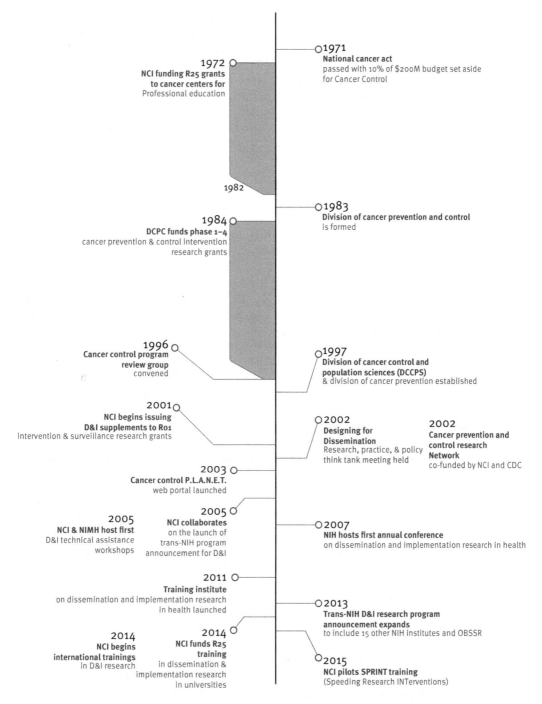

FIGURE 1B.1 Overview of the key events in the development of cancer control and implementation science at NCI.

professional education model to a cancer prevention and control intervention research model took place in 1983 when the Division of Cancer Prevention and Control was established and a new definition and framework for cancer control research were developed that included a linear series of phases from hypothesis generation to demonstration and implementation projects.[4]

This research framework represented the first reference to eventual, long-term implementation science within the context of the NCI's cancer research programs. During the 15-year lifespan of the Division of Cancer Prevention and Control, there was considerable growth in the number and diversity of NCI-funded intervention testing research grants (Phase 3) and defined population intervention studies (Phase 4) across the cancer control continuum. Based in part on this growth, in 1986, Dr. Vincent Devita, then director of the NCI, stated that a reduction in the cancer mortality rate by as much as 50% was possible "if current recommendations regarding smoking reduction, diet changes, screening, and state-of-the-art treatment are effectively applied."[5]

Partially in response to this optimistic objective of reducing overall cancer mortality by 50% in 14 years, some in the research, practice, and policy communities remained concerned that the war on cancer was not making sufficient progress.[6] In addition, the gap between what was known from these research investments and what was being done in practice and policy to reduce the burden of cancer for all Americans was continuing to grow.[7] In response to these concerns and to important trends (e.g., an aging population, exponential expansion of electronic communications, health care management, and molecular biology), the Cancer Control Program Review Group was convened by NCI in 1996.[8] The review group recommended that NCI make a long-term commitment to develop a more balanced partnership between the biomedical and behavioral/public health paradigms to reverse the upward trend in cancer mortality. It was also recommended that research should aim to reduce the burden and improve the quality of life of those who will get cancer despite our best efforts at prevention and the early detection and removal of precursor lesions. The review group recommended several organizational changes in NCI's areas of research opportunity that required focused attention, including the creation or enhancement of four major research initiatives in basic behavioral science, primary prevention, screening, and rehabilitation and survivorship.

NCI'S DIVISION OF CANCER CONTROL AND POPULATION SCIENCE

In 1997, DCCPS was established to enhance NCI's ability to alleviate the burden of cancer through research in epidemiology, behavioral sciences, health services, surveillance, and cancer survivorship. First under the leadership of Dr. Barbara Rimer and then Dr. Robert Croyle, the division grew and evolved. The division aimed to generate basic knowledge about how to monitor and change individual and collective behavior and also to ensure that knowledge is translated into practice and policy rapidly, effectively, and efficiently. It was this latter mission that led to the recruitment of the first author (JK) in the 2000 to serve as deputy director for research dissemination and diffusion and implementation science and the second author (RG) in 2010 to serve as the deputy director for implementation science, respectively. The third author (CV) has played key leadership roles with the program throughout its duration.

Two factors influenced the growth of research dissemination and diffusion and implementation science within NCI. First was the growing accumulation of intervention studies that were being published in the peer-reviewed literature with little or no evidence that the lessons learned from this science were being translated into evidence-based practice or policy. The unequal burden of cancer incidence and mortality among many low-income and racially diverse populations strongly suggested that the gap between what was known and what was done to prevent and control cancer among medically underserved populations was not being closed by the passive diffusion of new research knowledge.[9] Second, the methods used to integrate the lessons learned from cancer prevention and control intervention science with the lessons learned from practice and policy were not based on rigorous scientific methods nor in many cases even on careful evaluations.

Reflecting on these two different but related factors, the NCI, in partnership with the Center for the Advancement of Health and the Robert Wood Johnson Foundation, held a 2-day think tank meeting of researchers, practitioners, and intermediary research, practice, and policy funding agencies in September 2002 titled "Designing for Dissemination."[10] A key framework for understanding the challenges of integrating the lessons learned from science with the lessons learned from practice and policy was presented by Dr. Tracy Orleans from the Robert Wood Johnson Foundation (Figure 1B.2). As noted by Dr. Orleans, the continued emphasis on "pushing" scientific findings

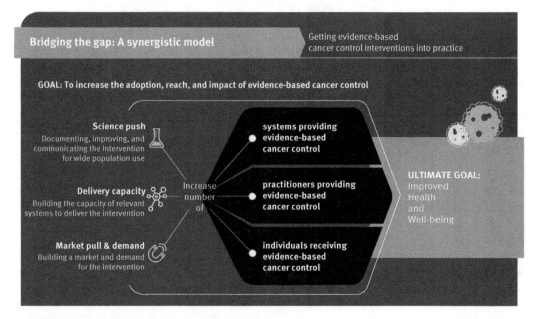

FIGURE 1B.2   Bridging the gap: A synergistic model.

Source: Adapted from presentation given by Tracey Orleans, PhD (Robert Wood Johnson Foundation), at NCI-sponsored Designing for Dissemination meeting, 2002.

out through publication and presentation, although necessary, was not sufficient to increase uptake of evidence-based interventions (EBIs). Research would need to address both what practitioners and policymakers want (pull) and the infrastructure resources and contexts that exist to deliver these EBIs (delivery capacity).[10] This was, at the time, referred to as dissemination research.

The meeting was also informed by an evidence review.[11] At the meeting, a brief presentation was made of the systematic review of the literature specific to the dissemination of EBIs in five areas of cancer control:

• Tobacco control
• Dietary change
• Mammography screening for breast cancer
• Pap smear testing for cervical cancer
• Cancer pain management

The evidence review identified the following recommendations for future dissemination research:

1. Increase the amount of research.
2. Focus the research on the dissemination of effective cancer control interventions.

3. Examine the best research designs and the best measures of outcome effectiveness.
4. Define what constitutes a reasonable decline of effectiveness after an intervention is extended to more diverse populations and settings beyond a controlled clinical trial.
5. Explore how qualitative research methods may help capture contextual factors that can serve as barriers to or facilitators for the adoption of EBIs.
6. Explore establishing criteria for reporting dissemination research.

In addition, think tank participants were invited to participate in an online concept mapping exercise.[12] The concept mapping data showed that each group of think tank participants (i.e., researchers, practitioners, and funding/policy agency intermediaries) held very different ideas about its own role and the roles of the other groups in disseminating and implementing EBIs. Researchers were the least likely to believe that translation and dissemination of research findings were their responsibility; because they were not trained in the science of dissemination and communication, their research grants generally did not pay for this type of work, and their interests and strengths lay elsewhere. Practitioners, whether clinicians or public health professionals, generally assigned responsibility for the synthesis and dissemination of research elsewhere. They viewed their job as acting on findings that are readily available and formatted for easy use. Intermediaries, whether public or private funders or of non-profit policy organizations, were most likely to describe translation and dissemination as activities for which they could provide leadership, but they were adamant that researchers and practitioners must play important partnership roles.

With respect to action steps that NCI should specifically take, the theme most commonly suggested for NCI was to join with other research and service funding agency intermediaries and take responsibility for supporting a nationwide permanent, community-based infrastructure for supporting the implementation of research findings (see, as an example, the US Department of Agriculture's cooperative extension service).[13] Other recommendations included the following:

- Increase funding for dissemination components in grants.
- Build dissemination requirements into requests for research grant applications.
- Require and fund the dissemination of effective interventions in existing intervention studies.
- Require research dissemination and diffusion in all applicable requests for proposals, and allocate resources for this component.
- Issue requests for applications on dissemination research, but also provide funds for the actual dissemination of research findings.
- NCI-funded comprehensive cancer centers should build in dissemination cores as a shared resource in future cancer center support grant applications.*
- Ensure that study review groups will better understand and appreciate this much-needed field of study.
- Train/educate NCI/National Institutes of Health (NIH) study sections regarding how to evaluate dissemination research using criteria other than those used for randomized controlled trials.
- Training and support should be provided to researchers and practitioners regarding how to disseminate and evaluate the impact of their research.

- NCI should provide more opportunities to develop a broader group of practitioners, researchers, and intermediaries exposed to this dissemination research and practice information.
- Involve practitioners and community partners in the research design stage, and promote research/practice partnerships.
- Develop systems for the dissemination of effective ideas, programs, and interventions by acting as a clearinghouse for state-of-the art dissemination methods and best practices.
- Promote online dissemination of knowledge and process assistance by developing a dissemination. gov website.

NCI was also urged to provide a clear vision and a specific action plan for necessary stakeholder collaboration.

Many of the aforementioned recommendations became the foundation for NCI's commitment to the emerging concepts of dissemination and implementation (D&I) research and research dissemination and diffusion. To engage the large cancer prevention and control intervention research community in D&I research, NCI initially supported D&I research through the Dissemination and Diffusion Supplements program. This administrative supplement program provided small, short-term awards to existing NCI intervention research grantees (and, later, surveillance research grantees) engaged in cancer control research. A total of 20 supplements were issued between 2001 and 2008 (12 focused on cancer risk or prevention and 8 focused on surveillance).[14] NCI's sponsorship of these supplements paved the way for its participation in future more robust research initiatives.[15]

In parallel with the effort to seed the field of D&I research, and in response to the 2002 think tank meeting recommendation that NCI act as a clearinghouse for state-of-the-art dissemination methods and best practices and develop a dissemination.gov website, in 2003 NCI launched Cancer Control P.L.A.N.E.T. (Plan, Link, Act, Network with Evidence-Based Tools). The P.L.A.N.E.T. web portal was designed to provide access to data and resources to help planners, program staff, and researchers design, implement, and evaluate evidence-based cancer control programs.[16]

---

*. It is noteworthy that the growth of population science within NCI-funded comprehensive cancer centers increased dramatically when guidelines for comprehensive cancer center status were changed to require evidence of substantial peer-reviewed NCI grant funding for population science.

It was developed in partnership with the Centers for Disease Control and Prevention (CDC), the American Cancer Society (ACS), the Substance Abuse and Mental Health Services Administration (SAMHSA), the American College of Surgeons Commission on Cancer, and the Agency for Healthcare Research Quality (AHRQ). Later, under Dr. Glasgow's leadership, the Research-Tested Intervention Programs (RTIPs) section of the Cancer Control P.L.A.N.E.T. was expanded in 2012 to include reviews of the reach, adoption, implementation, and maintenance findings of the relevant research on RTIPs programs into data summaries and implementation guides.[16]

A key recommendation from the 2002 think tank meeting included that NCI should provide a clear vision and a specific action plan for necessary stakeholder collaboration, providing more opportunities to develop a broader group of practitioners, researchers, and intermediaries; involve practitioners and community partners in the research design stage; and promote researcher–practitioner partnerships. In response, the Cancer Prevention and Control Research Network (CPCRN) was initiated in October 2002, with funding from the CDC and NCI as part of their joint effort to more effectively translate research into practice. As a federally funded, national network of academic, public health, and community partnerships, CPCRN provided resources for these partners to work together to reduce the burden of cancer, especially among those disproportionately affected. The initial five CPCRN sites were selected through a competition among the CDC-funded Prevention Research Centers.

Since 2002, the network has focused on conducting community-based research to accelerate the adoption and implementation of evidence-based cancer prevention and control and advance the implementation science and practice.[17] Members of the network have successfully collaborated on multiple implementation science grants. They have developed community-based grants designed to increase the adoption of EBIs and have tested and delivered training on how to identify, adapt, and implement evidence in public health practice (see http://cpcrn.org/pub/evidence-in-action). In 2007, the network piloted a research partnership with the Missouri 2-1-1 service that provides information and linkages to social services via a telephone exchange similar to 9-1-1. The network built on initial pilot work to study adaptation of evidence-based health programs

and scale-up of the program with other state 2-1-1 systems.[18,19] The CPCRN is currently focusing efforts on two signature projects: (1) strengthening colorectal cancer screening rates in populations served by Federally Qualified Health Centers and (2) contributing to the science and evidence base supporting community–clinical linkages to increase human papillomavirus vaccination initiation and completion.

As noted previously, NCI issued supplements to existing NCI funded R01, P01, P50, U01, and U19 grants to study the implementation of efficacious interventions and surveillance research. Based on success with the supplement program, NCI collaborated with other institutes and centers (ICs) in the development and launch of the first trans-NIH Program Announcements on Dissemination and Implementation Research in Health (PAR-06-039, PAR-06-071, and PAR-06-072) in 2005. These program announcements were designed to encourage transdisciplinary research on models for implementation science that would be applicable across diverse practice settings and studies that would assess the outcomes of implementation science efforts.

The PARs have been reissued four times since the original announcements were released in 2005. Participation from ICs at NIH has increased from 8 ICs in 2005 to 17 ICs, and the Office of Behavioral and Social Sciences and the Office of Disease Prevention also participate. This funding mechanism has been the single largest funder of major implementation science projects since its inception in 2005. Key themes emphasized in the 2013 revision of the PARs included calls for the study of adaptations during the implementation of evidence-based programs; health equity, health policy, and global health research; investigation of sustainability; and "de-implementation" (reduction in wasteful, harmful, and ineffective practices). To date, NCI has awarded 51 R01's, 13 R03's, and 48 R21's under these program announcements. Because implementation science was a relatively new area of research, grants under the initial PARs were reviewed by Special Emphasis Panels (SEPs). Leaders from NCI and the National Institute of Mental Health (NIMH) had the opportunity to orient SEP peer reviewers on the focus of the program announcements. In 2010, the Dissemination and Implementation Research in Health standing study section was established at NIH, and all grants submitted under the PARs along with other implementation science-associated grants are now reviewed by this group.

NCI has spearheaded work to expand technical assistance by developing and co-sponsoring the annual D&I Science Conference and also by leading various D&I training courses for investigators. In 2005 and 2006, NCI and NIMH hosted joint technical assistance workshops for investigators interested in D&I research. The goal of these workshops was to provide an opportunity for researchers to learn more about the field of implementation science and also share the work that they were doing in this area. These workshops evolved from having invited speakers presenting on key topics in the field combined with technical assistance feedback sessions provided to investigators in 2005 to a moderately sized conference held on the NIH campus in 2007 attended by approximately 100 people. The annual NIH and Veterans Administration (VA) D&I science meeting grew to more than 1,200 by 2011. Themes at this meeting addressed key evolving issues within the implementation science field, including multilevel interventions, innovative implementation science designs, de-implementation, and global health. In 2013 (for that year only), the annual meeting changed format to a small invited working group meeting of implementation science experts that focused on consolidating research findings to date and identifying key areas for future research. Figure 1B.3 presents the conclusions of

this meeting as summarized in Neta et al.[20] In brief, key issues included measures and understanding of multilevel interventions, partnership research, fidelity to key intervention components, and external validity. Participants also identified priorities for future research, including the need for better understanding of contextual factors; economic issues; evolution, sustainability, and adaptation of programs; and pragmatic research designs.[20]

This annual conference has grown in size and scope throughout the years. A record 702 abstracts were submitted for consideration for the 2017 annual conference. More than 1,000 people continue to participate each year, and the conference is now co-sponsored by NIH, Academy Health, AHRQ, the Patient Centered Outcomes Research Institute (PCORI), the Robert Wood Johnson Foundation, and the US Department of Veterans Affairs.

Dr. Glasgow's appointment as Deputy Director for Implementation Science at DCCPS in 2010 coincided with an increased focus on implementation science. During Dr. Glasgow's tenure at NCI (2010–2013), there were several implementation science activities within DCCPS as well as many new "external" collaborations and advances in the field to which the NCI group made substantial contributions; these are summarized in a 2012 trans-NIH publication.[21] Examples of interagency activities

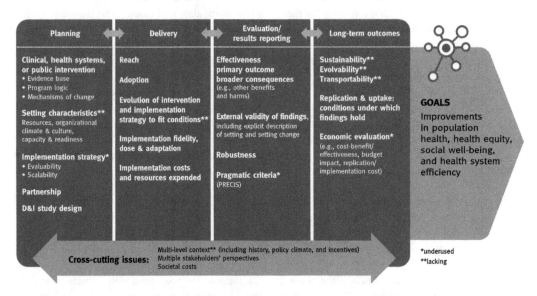

FIGURE 1B.3   Framework for enhancing the value of research for dissemination and implementation.

Source: Adapted from Neta G, Glasgow RE, Carpenter CR, et al. A framework for enhancing the value of research for dissemination and implementation. *Am J Public Health.* 2015; 105(1): 49–57.

during 2010–2013 include a key interagency conference co-sponsored by the NCI Implementation Science (IS) team with then new PCORI on key contextual factors and challenges faced by patients with multiple chronic conditions.[22]

Several activities revolved around expanding the implementation science focus of existing DCCPS programs and activities. Several papers were published that reviewed, presented models for, and discussed cancer-related future directions for implementation science within the context of areas such as genomics and public health,[23] comparative effectiveness research,[24,25] cancer survivorship,[26] cancer surveillance,[27,28] advances in and the need for practical patient-report measures,[29] and global health,[30] as well as the general field of implementation science.[31] Implementation science approaches across these areas emphasized cancer research that was pragmatic, rapid, and contextual and that produced results that were generalizable, equitable, and sustainable.

The NCI IS team played an important and often seminal role in terms of both scientific and programmatic leadership and also in funding of several trans-NIH and cross-agency initiatives. An important goal during this time was to extend the cancer-specific focus of DCCPS to a broader view of cancer as a chronic illness that related to and shared many of the same behavioral and biological determinants as other chronic illnesses. These included common psychosocial issues (e.g., disease distress and depression); the importance of physical activity and disease self-management;[32] interactions with the health care system; health inequities;[33] and the impact of health policy issues, especially family stress and financial hardships, on chronic illness development and management.

Possibly the most important cross-agency project during this period was the My Own Health Report (MOHR) project.[34,35] This project culminated in an NCI DCCPS- and AHRQ-funded cluster randomized pragmatic trial in 18 diverse, primary care clinics throughout the country that collaborated to assess the feasibility, cost, and impact of efforts to systematically collect and act upon brief patient report questions assessing health behaviors (eating patterns, smoking, physical activity, and drug use), mental health issues (distress, depression, anxiety, and alcohol use), quality of life, and patient preferences. Although led by NCI, MOHR included active involvement from AHRQ, NIMH, the Office of Behavioral and Social Sciences Research (OBSSR), CDC, and the Society

of Behavioral Medicine, among other partners. Approximately half of the clinic sites were associated with the CPCRN.

The goal of MOHR was to evaluate the consistency with which such patient-report measures could be collected, used to set patient-driven goals, and provide feedback to patients, primary care providers, and staff among a wide variety of patient populations and clinical settings. These settings included community health centers, rural offices, and inner-city clinics as well as academic-affiliated clinics serving underserved populations. MOHR utilized rapid research practices[36] to accomplish its goals within a very short period of time and with very limited funding.[37]

Key findings from MOHR included that it was feasible to collect and provide feedback on these patient-centered issues in diverse settings.[38] This was only possible by allowing local clinics to tailor the timing (a few days before a visit, at the beginning of a visit, or in the exam room), modality (e.g., web based, computer tablet, phone call, or read to low-literacy patients), and language (English and Spanish). Initial reports on the patterns and interrelationship of different health behaviors,[37] time and costs required, and initial results have been published,[39] and papers on other implementation issues are forthcoming.

TRAINING IN D&I RESEARCH

In 2011, NCI, NIMH, OBSSR, and VA led efforts to develop the week-long Training Institute on Dissemination and Implementation Research in Health (TIDIRH).[40] The goal of the training was to provide participants with a thorough grounding in implementation science across all areas of health and health care. Faculty and guest lecturers consisted of leading experts (researchers, practitioners, and educators) in implementation and evaluation approaches to implementation science; creation of partnerships and multilevel transdisciplinary research teams; research design, methods, and analyses appropriate for implementation science investigations; and conducting research at multiple levels of intervention (e.g., clinical, community, and policy). Participants were expected to return to their home institutions and share what they had learned to grow the field of implementation science (e.g., giving scientific presentations, forming new collaborations, mentoring, and submitting grant proposals).

Since 2011, more than 1,250 investigators have applied to TIDIRH, and approximately 200 investigators have participated in training. Since 2014, based on the success of the TIDIRH program, less centralized and more focused training programs, such as the Mentored Training in Dissemination and Implementation Research in Cancer at Washington University in St. Louis[41,42] and the Implementation Research Training Program in Cancer Prevention and Control at the University of Massachusetts Medical School, have been funded by NCI to further expand the pool of implementation scientists.

In 2014, NCI began developing a number of important international collaborations to help foster the growth and understanding of implementation science methodological challenges and research methods. International collaboration has primarily focused on training investigators. NCI collaborated with Argentina's Ministry of Health on a implementation science workshop. The aim was to build a critical mass of cancer control researchers, program managers, and decision-makers with a knowledge of implementation science to promote the systematic uptake of EBIs to reduce the cancer. Sixty-three trainees participated in the 3-day training in Buenos Aires in November 2014. At least one of the trainees was awarded a competitive grant from the Argentina Ministry of Health for the proposal developed at this training.

Also in 2014, NCI began collaborating with the Union for International Cancer Control (UICC) to deliver master's courses on implementation science. The first master's course was designed to deliver a condensed version of the annual TIDIRH training to researchers who attended the 2014 UICC World Cancer Congress in Melbourne, Australia. A second master's course was delivered in 2016 as part of the UICC World Cancer Congress in Paris. These master's courses consisted of six webinars delivered between 3 and 6 months with an online interactive course component managed on a wiki site where participants could engage with faculty and other trainees on the development of research proposals. The course concluded with a 1-day in-person training session the day before the World Cancer Congress convened.

Based on evaluation and feedback from the initial UICC master's course, NCI modified the online/in-person training and developed a different master's course in implementation science for a new partnership with the US Agency for International Development (USAID) Partnerships for Enhanced Engagement in Research (PEER) program. A modified version of the course was open to eligible investigators from low- and middle-income countries in Southeast Asia (2015) and the Middle East (2016). The course was redesigned so that six webinars were delivered over 3 months. The webinars were prerecorded, and participants were able to complete assigned coursework over the 3-month period. All coursework had to be submitted via an online wiki platform in order for in-person training to be supported. The in-person training was extended to a 3-day in-person training with ample time spent in small groups working on individual implementation science grant proposals. Fifty investigators have participated in these trainings. To date, one of the investigators has received funding for her research project by the Ministry of Health in her country, and a second has received funding from the Conquer Cancer Foundation for her research.

In 2016, based on the experience from the international trainings with UICC and USAID, a new TIDIRH training model was piloted that delivered key trainings via webinars over a 3-month period and required trainees to engage in online coursework prior to participating in a 2-day in-person training. The goal of this pilot was to increase reach, reduce costs, and enhance sustainability to meet the growing demand for this training. Results from this pilot will be reported once the program has been completed.

SUMMARY AND FUTURE DIRECTIONS

The NCI has played a leadership role in the development of cancer prevention and control intervention and surveillance research, and implementation science more generally. Within NCI, the growth of its cancer prevention and control intervention research portfolio from 1982 through 1996 led to the recognition that absent a new focus on implementation science and a new infrastructure to integrate the lessons learned from research with the lessons learned from practice and policy, the limited diffusion of research evidence through publications and scientific presentations alone would not be sufficient to reduce the burden of cancer for all Americans.

With respect to more action-oriented research dissemination, NCI has also played a leadership role in developing and nurturing research, practice, and policy partnerships both within government (e.g., AHRQ, CDC, Health Resources and Services Administration, SAMHSA, and the VA) and with outside organizations and agencies (e.g., ACS, Robert Wood Johnson Foundation, PCORI, and the National Commission on Aging) sharing a concern for how the lessons learned from science can better influence cancer and chronic disease prevention and control practices and policies. Examples of these collaborations include the Cancer Control P.L.A.N.E.T. web portal, including the RTIPs component;[16] the CPCRN;[17] and a series of scientific and think tank meetings to engage the research, practice, and policy communities in helping identify new and innovative approaches to integrating the lessons learned from science with those from practice and policy.

Although this chapter has focused on the development of research dissemination and diffusion tools and resources, and the growth and development of implementation science coordinated and led by NCI domestically and internationally (see Figure 1B.1), the research funding framework for implementation science and its translation into practice and policy also bear some commentary.

Soon after his arrival in 2001 as the director of NCI, Dr. Andrew von Eschenbach articulated a new vision of how NCI-funded science could lead to the *elimination of death and suffering* from cancer by 2015.[43] Although 2015 has passed without having achieved this laudable goal, Dr. von Eschenbach's editorial laid out an ambitious plan to seamlessly link discovery, development, and delivery of cancer research findings to reduce the time between "bench and bedside." Discovery was described as the process that generates new knowledge about fundamental cancer-related processes at the genetic, molecular, cellular, organ, person, and population levels. Development was the process of creating and evaluating tools and interventions to reduce cancer burden, including the prevention, detection, diagnosis, and treatment of cancer and its sequelae. Delivery was the process of disseminating, facilitating, and promoting evidence-based prevention, early detection, diagnosis, and treatment practices and policies to reduce the burden of cancer in all segments of the population. To reach all segments of the population, NCI must especially focus its efforts on those populations who bear the greatest burden of disease.

In the first author's work in Canada for the Canadian Partnership Against Cancer, Dr. Kerner employed this three D model and led a transdisciplinary Canadian research working group to adapt it into a framework for collaborative action in cancer prevention research funding for the Canadian Cancer Research Alliance.[44]

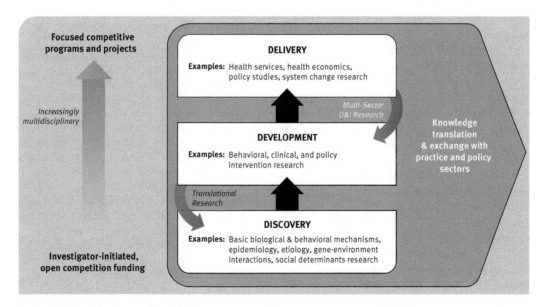

FIGURE 1B.4   Conceptual model: Dissemination and implementation research funding context.

Source: Adapted from Canadian Cancer Research Alliance. *Canadian Cancer Research Alliance (2012). Cancer Prevention Research in Canada: A Strategic Framework for Collaborative Action.* Toronto: CCRA.

Figure 1B.4 provides a further adaptation of this three D framework to fit what we view as the challenge for NCI of finding the right balance between investments in fundamental discovery, translational, and intervention development research in relation to delivery and implementation science. As reflected in Figure 1B.4, much of discovery, translational, and intervention research is investigator initiated and obtains its funding through open competition pools of available research dollars. Conversely, much of delivery and implementation science is driven by focused requests for application funding announcements and by necessity requires greater cooperation and collaboration between researchers, practitioners, and policymakers to ensure that the science being proposed is well aligned with the contextual factors and local community conditions so as to translate delivery and implementation science findings into practical programs and policies.

Currently, the balance of research investment is heavily weighted in the area of discovery, translational, and intervention development research. As the research investment in applied (e.g., delivery and implementation) science has grown, some concerns have been voiced among basic scientists and clinical investigators that resources for their important foundational and translational research priorities are being reduced because of this growth.[45] Although it is difficult to discern the trends in the exact funding proportions for basic, translational, intervention development, delivery, and implementation science at NCI, two overall trends are clear. First, whereas overall NIH funding for basic discovery research has declined from approximately $18 billion in 2003 to approximately $15 billion in 2016, applied research funding has plateaued to approximately $13 billion in 2016.[46] Second, within NCI, although there has been considerable growth in implementation science funding from 2001 to 2016, largely from the grants funded through the NIH D&I PAR, it remains an extremely small proportion of the overall research funding envelope of NCI (2016 congressionally enacted budget of $5,213,509M) and will probably remain so for the foreseeable future.

Thus, NCI must work together even more assiduously with other research, practice, and policy intermediary organizations to ensure that the emerging implementation science findings do not simply "gather dust" in libraries or in online publication repositories. In particular, health policy issues have received very modest funding. NCI-funded implementation science must be translated into evidence-based implementation practices and policies that accelerate the adoption, adaptation, and implementation of evidence-based interventions to more rapidly and more equitably reduce the burden of cancer for all Americans. Future implementation science efforts in cancer research should build on and enhance the activities summarized in this chapter, including a focus on multisector partnerships; pragmatic research models, methods, and measures; and integration of research, practice, and policy activities that are culturally and contextually appropriate, sustainable, and reduce health inequities.

REFERENCES

1. National Cancer Institute. National Cancer Act of 1971. https://www.cancer.gov/about-nci/legislative/history/national-cancer-act-1971. Accessed June 28, 2017.
2. Ahart, GJ. *The Objectives of the Cancer Control Program and the National Cancer Institute's Administration of Program Contracts*. Washington, DC: US Government Accountability Office; June 13, 1980.
3. Rogers EM. *Diffusion of Innovations*. 5th ed. New York: Free Press; 2003.
4. Greenwald P, Cullen JW. The scientific approach to cancer control. *CA Cancer J Clin*. 1984;34(6):328–332.
5. Devita V, ed. Cancer control objectives for the nation: 1985–2000. *NCI Monogr*. 1986; (2) vii.
6. Bailer JC, Smith EM. Progress against cancer? *N Engl J Med*. 1986;314(19):1226–1232.
7. Kerner J, Dusenbury L, Madelblatt J. Poverty and cultural diversity: Challenges for health promotion among the medically underserved. *Annu Rev Public Health*. 1993;14:355–377.
8. Division of Extramural Affairs. *A New Agenda for Cancer Control Research: Report of the Cancer Control Advisory Group*. Bethesda, MD: National Cancer Institute; 1997.
9. Kerner JF, Hall KL. Research dissemination and diffusion: Translation within science and society. *Res Soc Work Pract*. 2009;19(5):519–530.
10. National Cancer Institute. Designing for Dissemination conference summary report. https://cancercontrol.cancer.gov/IS/pdfs/d4d_conf_sum_report.pdf. Accessed July 28, 2017.
11. Ellis P, Robinson P, Ciliska D, et al. Diffusion and dissemination of evidence-based cancer control interventions. *Evid Rep Technol Assess (Summ)*. 2003 May; (79): 1–5.

12. Trochim WM, McLinden D. An introduction to a special issue on concept mapping. *Eval Program Plann.* 2017;60:166–175.

13. USDA. Co-op research and extension services. https://www.usda.gov/topics/rural/cooperative-research-and-extension-services. Accessed July 12, 2017.

14. National Cancer Institute. Dissemination and diffusion supplements (2002–2008). https://maps.cancer.gov/overview/DCCPSGrants/grantlist.jsp?method=portfolio&program=is&owner=cvinson&portfolio=DandD%20Supplements&status=archive. Accessed July 14, 2017.

15. Eckstein E. NCI's Dissemination and Diffusion Administrative Supplement Program: Lessons learned and recommendations. 2012. https://cancercontrol.cancer.gov/is/pdfs/Dissemination-and-Diffusion-Supplements-Analysis-Final.pdf. Accessed July 28, 2014.

16. Sanchez MA, Vinson CA, LaPorta M, Viswanath K, Kerner JF, Glasgow RE. Evolution of Cancer Control P.L.A.N.E.T.: Moving research into practice. *Cancer Causes Control.* 2012;23(7):1205–1212.

17. Harris JR, Brown PK, Coughlin S, et al. The cancer prevention and control research network. *Prev Chronic Dis.* [serial online] 2005.

18. Purnell JQ, Kreuter MW, Eddens KA, et al. Cancer control needs of 2-1-1 callers in Missouri, North Carolina, Texas and Washington. *J Health Care Poor Underserved.* 2012;23:752–67.

19. Savas LS, Fernandez ME, Jobe D, Carmack CC. Human papillomavirus vaccine: 2-1-1 helplines and minority-parent decision-making. *Am J Prev Med.* 2012;43(6S5):S490–S496.

20. Neta G, Glasgow RE, Carpenter CR, et al. A framework for enhancing the value of research for dissemination and implementation. *Am J Public Health.* 2015;105(1):49–57.

21. Glasgow RE, Vinson C, Chambers D, Khoury MJ, Kaplan RM, Hunter C. National Institutes of Health approaches to dissemination and implementation science: Current and future directions. *Am J Public Health.* 2012;102(7):1274–1281. doi:10.2105/AJPH.2012.300755

22. Bayliss EA, Bonds DE, Boyd CM, et al. Understanding the context of health for persons with multiple chronic conditions: Moving from what is the matter to what matters. *Ann Fam Med.* 2014;12(3):260–269.

23. Khoury M, Clauser SB, Freedman AN, et al. An enhanced population science agenda in translational genomics to reduce the burden of cancer in the 21st century. *Cancer Epidemiol Biomarkers Prev.* 2011;20(10):2105–2114.

24. Glasgow RE, Doria-Rose VP, Khoury MJ, Elzarrad M, Brown ML, Stange KC. Comparative effectiveness research in cancer: What has been funded and what knowledge gaps remain. *J Natl Cancer Inst.* 2013;105(11):766–773.

25. Glasgow RE, Rabin BA. Implementation science and comparative effectiveness research: A partnership capable of improving population health. *J Comp Effectiveness Res.* 2014;3(3):237–240.

26. Alfano CM, Smith T, de Moor JS, et al. An action plan for translating cancer survivorship research into care. *J Natl Cancer Inst.* 2014;106(11):1–9.

27. Rabin BA, Purcell P, Naveed S, et al. Advancing the application, quality, and harmonization of implementation science measures. *Implement Sci.* 2012;7:119.

28. Rabin B, Purcell P, Glasgow RE. Harmonizing measures for implementation science using crowd-sourcing. *Clin Med Res.* 2013;11(3):158.

29. Glasgow RE, Kaplan RM, Ockene J, Fisher EB, Emmons KM. Patient-reported measures of psychosocial issues and health behavior should be added to electronic health records. *Health Aff.* 2013;31:3497–3504.

30. Sivaram S, Sanchez MA, Rimer BK, Samet JM, Glasgow RE. Implementation science in cancer prevention and control: A framework for research and programs in low- and middle-income countries. *Cancer Epidemiol Biomarkers Prev.* 2014;23(11):2273–2284.

31. Glasgow RES, Sanchez MA. News from NIH: Global Health. *Transl Behav Med.* 2011;1(2):201–202.

32. Phillips SM, Alfano CM, Perna FM, Glasgow RE. Accelerating translation of physical activity and cancer survivorship research into practice: Recommendations for a more integrated and collaborative approach. *Cancer Epidemiol Biomarkers Prev.* 2014;23(5):687–699.

33. Breen N, Scott S, Percy-Laurry A, Lewis D, Glasgow RE. Health disparities calculator: A methodologically rigorous tool for analyzing inequalities in population health. *Am J Public Health.* 2014;104(9):1589–1591.

34. Krist AH, Glenn BA, Glasgow RE, et al. Designing a valid, pragmatic primary care implementation trial: The My Own Health Report (MOHR) project. *Implement Sci.* 2014;25(8):73.

35. Glasgow RE, Kessler RS, Ory M, Roby D, Sheinfeld-Gorin S, Krist A. Conducting rapid,

relevant, research: Lessons learned from the My Own Health Report (MOHR) project. *Am J Prev Med.* 2014;47(2):212–219.

36. Kessler R, Glasgow RE. A proposal to speed translation of healthcare intervention research into practice: Dramatic change is needed. *Am J Prev Med.* 2011;40(6):637–644.

37. Phillips SM, Glasgow RE, Bello G, et al. Frequency and prioritization of patient health risks from a structured health risk assessment. *Ann Fam Med.* 2014;12(6):505–513.

38. Krist AH, Glasgow RE, Heurtin-Roberts S, et al.; MOHR Study Group. The impact of behavioral and mental health risk assessments on goal setting in primary care. *Transl Behav Med.* 2016 June;6(2):212–219.

39. Krist AH, Phillips SM, Sabo RT, et al. Adoption, reach, implementation, and maintenance of a behavioral and mental health assessment in primary care. *Ann Fam Med.* 2014 November;12(6):525–533.

40. Meissner HI, Glasgow RE, Vinson CA, et al. The U.S. Training Institute for Dissemination and Implementation Research in Health. *Implement Sci.* 2013;8:12.

41. Tabak RG, Padek MM, Kerner JF, et al. Dissemination and Implementation Science Training Needs: Insights From Practitioners and Researchers. *Am J of Prev Med.* 2017 March;52(3):S322–S329.

42. Padek M, Mir N, Jacob RR, et al. Training scholars in dissemination and implementation research for cancer prevention and control: a mentored approach. *Implement Sci.* 2018;13:18.

43. Von Eschenbach AC. NCI sets goal of eliminating suffering and death from cancer by 2015. *J Natl Med Assoc.* 2003;95(7):637–639.

44. Canadian Cancer Research Alliance. *Cancer Prevention Research in Canada: A Strategic Framework for Collaborative Action.* Toronto, Ontario, Canada: Author; 2012. http://www.ccra-acrc.ca/index.php/publications-en/strategy-related-publications. Accessed July 28, 2017.

45. Arnold E, Giarracca F. Getting the balance right: Basic research, missions and governance for horizon 2020. 2012. http://www.earto.eu/fileadmin/content/03_Publications/FINAL_TECH_REPORT2012.pdf

46. American Association for the Advancement of Science. Historical trends in federal R & D. https://www.aaas.org/page/historical-trends-federal-rd. Accessed July 14, 2017.

2

EVIDENCE-BASED CANCER PRACTICES, PROGRAMS, AND INTERVENTIONS

Maria E. Fernandez, Patricia Dolan Mullen, Jennifer Leeman, Timothy J. Walker, and Cam Escoffery

INTRODUCTION

Research on cancer prevention and control has led to the development of numerous evidence-based cancer control practices, programs, clinical care guidelines, and interventions. Although additional research is needed to fill gaps in cancer control best practices, the field has both produced many evidence-based interventions (EBIs) with demonstrated efficacy or effectiveness and made them more widely available.[1] The ultimate impact of these research innovations on reducing the cancer burden and cancer-related health disparities, however, is limited by failures in implementation and scale-up. Implementation challenges are related to the development of EBIs that are not easily implemented in real-world settings, difficulties in understanding and identifying EBIs, limited planning of strategies to enhance their delivery, and problems adapting existing EBIs for new settings and populations. Determining which EBIs are best to use and how they might be adapted to fit a new context can be a substantial challenge for practitioners charged with addressing a cancer control issue in their community or practice setting.[2] Implementation science seeks to better understand why some EBIs are successfully adopted, implemented, and maintained, whereas others are not; and how to intervene to enhance adoption, adaptation, and use of EBIs to improve cancer control.[3,4]

The implementation of EBIs is critical for public health efforts focused on cancer prevention. Unfortunately, many EBIs never make it beyond the research setting and into practice.[5] Even when an EBI is adopted, implementers often face challenges, which can impact delivery and the desired effects.[6] These challenges are in part due to the gap between prevention science and implementation practice.[7]

This chapter describes the types of evidence-based cancer control interventions available; highlights issues related to the adoption and implementation of EBIs such as fidelity and adaptation; and describes processes that can be used to enhance the development, adaptation, and implementation of evidence-based cancer control interventions.

WHAT TYPES OF EVIDENCE-BASED CANCER CONTROL INNOVATIONS ARE AVAILABLE FOR IMPLEMENTATION?

In the implementation science literature, the term *evidence-based intervention* (EBI) has been broadly defined to include programs, practices, policies, packaged programs, and clinical practice guidelines with demonstrated efficacy and/or effectiveness to achieve an intended outcome.[1] Differentiating these terms is important because they have distinct characteristics; are derived from different types of evidence bases; and present unique considerations for adoption, adaptation, and implementation. Here, and consistent with the literature,[8,10] we define three types of research innovations that result from the translation of research findings for use in practice: clinical practice guidelines, general interventions, and specific interventions or programs. We refer to the latter two collectively as evidence-based interventions.

Clinical Practice Guidelines

The Institute of Medicine defines *clinical practice guidelines* (CPGs) as "statements that include recommendations intended to optimize patient care."[8] In other words, CPGs provide recommendations for what care should be delivered to provide optimal benefits for health and well-being. The evidence base for CPGs is typically generated through systematic reviews and meta-analyses of reports of research studies that meet prespecified quality criteria, although some are still based on expert opinion that may or may not reflect systematic reviews. The US Preventive Services Task Force, for example, reviewed research and recommended "screening for colorectal cancer starting at age 50 years and continuing until age 75 years."[9] CPGs play a central role in defining *what* should be done in practice; however, CPGs do not provide guidance on *how* to intervene with individuals, providers, or systems to ensure that optimal care is delivered and received. Indeed, this is an important focus of implementation science—the development of implementation strategies to increase the adoption, implementation, and sustainment of CPGs.

Evidence-Based Interventions

Evidence-based interventions (EBIs) include any action or set of actions that has been shown to be effective at improving individual- or population-level health behaviors or outcomes. EBIs may target individual behaviors and/or changes at the level of the environment, including the interpersonal (providers, teachers, and parents), organizational (schools, worksites, and clinics), and/or policy (public or organization) environments, with the goal of changing environmental conditions that impact health directly (exposure to second-hand smoke) or creating external conditions that support and promote recommended behaviors (provider recommendation of screening). An EBI may target organization-level changes that create contextual and environmental conditions that make behavioral changes more likely, such as creating more flexible clinic hours to increase patients' access to health services or implementing provider reminders to prompt recommendation for colorectal cancer screening. An EBI might also target changes to public policy governing public funding for screening, diagnosis, and treatment. EBIs may be grouped into one of two broad categories: general interventions and specific intervention programs.

GENERAL INTERVENTIONS

Like CPGs, general interventions, called "strategies" in The Guide to Community Preventive Services (Community Guide) also are generated through systematic reviews of the literature. The Community Guide and the Cochrane Collaboration are two organizations that conduct systematic reviews to identify all studies that test the effectiveness of a category of intervention (e.g., provider-oriented interventions to increase cancer screening) and meet prespecified quality criteria.[10,11] The identified studies are reviewed and findings synthesized and translated into recommendations for which general interventions have sufficient evidence in support of their effectiveness and which do not. For example, the Community Guide recommends the general intervention approach of "one-on-one education" to increase colorectal cancer (CRC) screening with fecal occult blood testing based on sufficient evidence of effectiveness.[12] General interventions are essentially broad approaches to change that fall within a particular category (i.e., one on one education, mass media, face to face, and provider reminders) and may be at various levels (patient, provider, and system) but are not specifically designed to "implement" an innovation. Instead, they are designed to create change in behaviors or environmental conditions influencing the health problem. Thus, "general interventions" here represent the innovation to be implemented, and those interested in using them would need to design implementation strategies to ensure their appropriate delivery.

SPECIFIC INTERVENTION PROGRAMS

The second type of EBI are specific intervention program such as those available on Research Tested Intervention Programs (RTIPs). These can include specific policies or programs that have peer-reviewed, documented evidence of efficacy and/or effectiveness. The review criteria applied are similar to systematic reviews but rather than looking *across* specific interventions to produce a general conclusion related to a "type" of intervention as in general intervention described above, here the criteria are applied to individual intervention programs. The criteria are based on the design and execution of the study, the methods used to analyze efficacy and/or effectiveness, and the size of the effect. For example, Reuland and associates[13] developed and tested an intervention that included a video of a CRC screening decision aid shown immediately before a clinic visit that promoted screening and provided information on colonoscopy and fecal occult blood testing. Following the visit, a patient navigator contacted participants to support screening completion. Those who received the intervention were more likely to complete CRC screening within 6 months compared to those who received usual care (68% vs. 27%, respectively).

Specific intervention programs have identifiable and clearly defined components and may include one or more materials, activities, and delivery approaches. Some specific intervention programs have been "packaged" for dissemination and made available for others. Packaged programs may include a description of the intervention components, protocols and materials, a summary of the evidence of its effectiveness, and guidance and resources to support the intervention's implementation into practice. The National Cancer Institute provides access to packaged programs through its Research-Tested Intervention Programs (RTIPs) website. This compendium of peer-reviewed intervention programs, which have a demonstrated positive outcome within the past 10 years, provides a description of the program, implementation guidance, information on the time and resources required, guidelines for adaptation, and links to intervention materials that users can download and use (print and video

educational materials, evaluation tools, intervention manuals and protocols, etc.). Both the RTIPs and the Community Guide websites[14,15] provide cross-referencing that allows potential adopters to match packaged programs to recommended general intervention approaches. By doing so, potential adopters can build on both the strong evidence base in support of a general intervention and the materials and protocols provided by a packaged program.

Table 2.1 provides examples of the types of evidence-based innovations described above (CPBs and EBIs) for breast cancer control that are available for implementation across the cancer continuum from prevention to survivorship. The clinical practice guidelines derive from recommendations by the US Preventive Services Task Force, American Cancer Society, and American Society of Clinical Oncology, whereas the general intervention approaches derive from systematic reviews published by the Cochrane Collaboration and the Community Guide. The programs listed in the table are National Cancer Institute RTIPs.

IMPORTANT CONSIDERATIONS WHEN IMPLEMENTING DIFFERENT TYPES OF RESEARCH INNOVATIONS

Because CPGs play a central role by establishing targets for optimal clinical care, the development of implementation strategies to increase use of CPGs is an important area of research and clinical quality improvement. In fact, there is a large body of scientific literature related to implementation science and knowledge translation (KT) that focuses on the implementation of clinical guidelines (CPGs) in practice settings.[31] Influenced historically by conceptualizations of evidence-based medicine, the process of implementation of CPGs was primarily focused at the individual (provider) level and described as changes that the provider has to make to "implement" CPGs. More recently, researchers and practitioners recognize that for guideline implementation, changes need to occur at the team, organization, and policy levels.[31] Therefore, implementation strategies aimed at creating change at multiple levels to increase implementation of CPGs can have the greatest impact. An important consideration when thinking about the implementation of CPGs is that once strategies are developed (e.g., audit and feedback, practice facilitation, and provider reminders),

Table 2.1. Examples of Evidence-Based Products Across the Breast Cancer Control Continuum

	PREVENTION	EARLY DETECTION	TREATMENT	SURVIVORSHIP
Guidelines	*Topic:* Breast cancer: medications for risk reduction (US Preventive Services Task Force) *Recommendation:* Clinicians should engage in shared, informed decision-making and offer to prescribe medications (e.g., tamoxifen or raloxifene) to women who are at increased risk for breast cancer and low risk for adverse medication effects in order to reduce their risk of breast cancer.[16]	*Topic:* Breast cancer: screening (US Preventive Services Task Force) *Recommendation:* Women aged 50–74 years should undergo screening mammography every 2 years.[17]	*Topic:* Sentinel lymph node biopsy for patients with early stage breast cancer (American Society of Clinical Oncology Clinical Practice Guideline Update) *Recommendation:* For women with early stage breast cancer, sentinel lymph node dissection—rather than auxiliary lymph node dissection—is recommended as the first step in lymph node biopsy.[18]	*Topic:* Breast cancer survivorship care guideline (American Cancer Society/American Society of Clinical Oncology) *Recommendation:* Primary care clinicians should educate and counsel female adult breast cancer survivors regarding signs and symptoms of local or regional recurrence of breast cancer.[19]
Intervention strategies	*Topic:* Physical activity interventions in community settings to promote and maintain weight loss (*Community Guide*) *Brief summary:* Breast cancer has been linked to increased weight.[20] Using a combination of counseling or coaching with technologies such as video conferencing, computer applications, or wearable technologies has been effective in promoting and maintaining weight loss.[21]	*Topic:* Reducing out-of-pocket costs for breast cancer screening (*Community Guide*) *Brief summary:* Reducing the cost of breast cancer screening through vouchers, reimbursements, reduced co-pays, or other means increases breast cancer screening practices in target populations.[22]	*Topic:* Psychological interventions for women with nonmetastatic breast cancer (*Cochrane Review*) *Brief summary:* A psychological intervention, namely cognitive-behavioral therapy, produced favorable effects on some psychological outcomes, particularly anxiety, depression, and mood disturbance.[23]	*Topic:* Home-based, multidimensional breast cancer survivorship programs (*Cochrane Review*) *Brief summary:* Survivorship programs that include multiple components—physical, educational, and psychological—and are conducted in breast cancer survivors' homes may increase quality of life, measured through physical, cognitive, emotional, and social well-being.[24]

Programs	Topic: Program to maintain weight loss (RTIPs)	Topic: Community-based program to increase mammogram use by African American women (RTIPs)	Topic: Psychosocial treatment for women with metastatic or recurrent breast cancer (RTIPs)	Topic: Education for breast cancer survivors (RTIPs)
	Brief summary: Increased weight is associated with breast cancer risk.[20] This 2-hour telephone-based weight loss maintenance coaching program targets adults who have recently lost weight and aims to help them maintain weight loss through awareness building, behavior modification, and self-efficacy. In the initial intervention, the intervention group gained significantly less weight than the control group at 12 and 24 months after baseline.[25-27]	*Brief summary:* The Witness Program is targeted to African American women aged ≥40 years and uses a church setting, role modeling, and active learning to increase knowledge and awareness of breast cancer screening and motivation to be screened. Intervention participants increased their use of mammography at 6-month follow-up.[28]	*Brief summary:* The program uses weekly, 90-minute therapist-led supportive-expressive group psychotherapy sessions to help women cope with concerns and emotions related to the disease and improve relationships, social support, and symptom management. The treatment group showed reductions in trauma symptoms and pain and improvements in mood disturbances.[29]	*Brief summary:* The Breast Cancer Education Intervention provides one-on-one teaching and support (three 1-hour sessions plus two 30-minute telephone and face-to-face follow-ups) to women with ≤1 year of treatment. The experimental group showed significant improvements in quality of life—defined as physical, social, psychological, and spiritual well-being—at 3- and 6-months follow-up.[30]

RTIPs, Research-Tested Intervention Programs.

these in turn need to be adopted and implemented to bring about the desired changes.

Where one stands on the research to practice continuum and also one's interpretation of the innovation to be implemented (e.g., a guideline or an intervention program to ensure guideline use) influences the name one uses to describe the intervention or strategy. For example, some may call approaches to implement CPGs "implementation strategies." Others would consider these general interventions or specific intervention programs at the environmental level (e.g., materials and methods to increase provider recommendation for mammography screening) designed to change provider or system behavior. Indeed, multilevel interventions for cancer control that include components targeting the health care organization, providers, and patients are often developed and considered to be among the most powerful for effecting change.[32] Health promotion professionals accustomed to developing interventions at various levels would likely consider a program designed to change provider behavior (e.g., recommend colorectal cancer screening for all patients aged 50 years or older) a provider-level intervention. By contrast, KT and D&I scientists may call that same program an "implementation strategy" because it is influencing the implementation of a particular guideline. It is difficult to reach consensus on various terms, particularly across disciplines. Therefore, it is important to be aware of these different uses of terms when working in multidisciplinary teams and to define them explicitly to ensure common understanding. Within this book, authors have largely used the term "implementation strategy" to cover all of these approaches that are intended to result in the improved uptake of the various types of health innovations (CPGs, general interventions, and specific intervention programs).

Previously, we mentioned some of the characteristics of general interventions versus specific intervention programs. Each of these has strengths and weaknesses.[33] General interventions may be based on multiple studies that often have been conducted across diverse settings and populations; therefore, they typically have a stronger evidence base both for their effectiveness and for their generalizability compared to specific intervention programs. To the extent that they focus on general approaches (e.g., reminder systems and small media), they also have greater flexibility compared to programs with specific materials and protocols. Practitioners might assess barriers and facilitators to breast screening

across multiple levels of their practice context and then select and combine general interventions to target factors at different levels. For example, they might combine a general intervention that targets patients' knowledge and attitudes (one-on-one education) with one that targets environmental barriers to participation (mobile mammography) and another that targets providers' awareness of the patient's need for screening (reminders).

General interventions strategies, however, may be challenging to use in practice because they provide recommendation for broad approaches rather than specific materials and messages. In addition, to reach consensus about the evidence base supporting a particular strategy, studies are often grouped into broad categories—for example, by delivery format (e.g., one-on-one education)—and may include heterogeneous elements across studies, such as population group, type of person delivering the intervention (e.g., a doctor or lay health worker), and specific methods and content used (e.g., didactic or motivational interviewing style). As a result, practitioners are left only with general guidance of what should be implemented and little detail on specific components (materials, protocols, etc.) of the intervention approach or how to implement it in practice.[33,34]

Practitioners wanting to use implement a specific EBI (intervention program) may get more information by searching the list of publications included in the systematic review that generated the recommendation. The evidence tables included in most reviews provide a brief description of the intervention program, including the population and setting, and, often, data on effectiveness. If the practitioner can find a publication(s) that describes a program conducted in a similar setting and with a similar population as his or her own, that publication will provide some additional guidance on how to implement the program into practice but often will fall short of providing a full description of the program and its implementation.

In contrast, specific EBIs have the advantage of arming the practitioner with a tested intervention that often includes materials, protocols, and guidance on implementation. Specific EBIs provide more detailed information on the intervention and how it was implemented. This information is available, to a limited extent, in publications reporting on the intervention, but more details may be found in compilations of programs such as RTIPs (described previously). A potential disadvantage of implementing specific intervention programs is that they often have been designed and tested with a population and setting that differ from those for which the practitioner seeks to implement an EBI. As a result, they may target some factors that were not identified as barriers and facilitators to screening in the new context and population and may fail to target others, thus requiring adaptation.

The program's materials may need to be adapted for a new population and its protocols for implementation may need to be adapted to fit the resources available in a new setting.[35] Because an individual program comprises a specific set of activities, cancer control planners may be limited in their ability to revise those activities or incorporate new activities that they have identified as effective ways to engage their populations.[36] In addition, specific EBIs tested in highly controlled trials with external funding may require more extensive resources than the new context can support. For these reasons, the provision of programs with detailed guidance and materials to support implementation has not led cancer control planners to favor them over general EBIs. When surveyed, cancer control planners report greater use of Community Guide recommended interventions than RTIPs packaged programs.[3,14,37] To address these challenges, several websites disseminate implementation guidance along with their general EBIs.[33,38] Robert Wood Johnson's Using What Works for Health website, for example, disseminates general interventions together with a summary of the systematic reviews that recommended them and also provides links to implementation examples and implementation resources.[38] Also, the cross-referencing between the Community Guide and RTIPs allows potential adopters the same benefits.

EVALUATING THE SOURCES OF EVIDENCE-BASED INTERVENTIONS

Numerous organizations are disseminating EBIs on the internet.[33] To date, there is no consistent set of criteria for determining when an intervention is evidence based and ready for dissemination and implementation. Although there are several potential sources of EBIs including books and published reviews, websites are perhaps the most accessible and important resource for locating cancer control EBIs. Practitioners need to critically assess each website to evaluate the evidence in support of the interventions being disseminated. Websites differ across several dimensions that are important to consider when evaluating them as a potential source of EBIs. The following questions should be considered:[33]

1. Who created the website?
2. What types of EBIs are they disseminating?
3. What methods did they use to review the evidence?
4. What criteria did they apply to determine when an intervention was evidence-based and ready to be disseminated?
5. How current is the evidence base?
6. What information is available to support EBI implementation?

1. Who created the website? Identifying the website creator is a first step toward identifying potential sources of bias. If information about the website's creator is not evident on the home page, it is generally available through a link from the home page. The potential for bias is increased if the website's creators have a profit motive or an ideological position that might influence their selection of interventions.

2. What types of EBIs are they disseminating? The home pages of most websites identify the site's priority health conditions or factors that contribute to those health conditions. More searching may be required to identify whether they disseminate general or specific EBIs or both and what additional resources they provide to support implementation.

3. What methods did they use to review the evidence? Ideally, the website's home page will have a link to the methods used to review the evidence. Systematic reviews of peer-reviewed intervention studies are generally considered the strongest source of evidence for effectiveness; however, producing them is resource intensive. (The continuum of efficacy and effectiveness and their importance is discussed later.) To speed the translation of evidence to practice, some websites use less rigorous review methods. Although these websites are a valuable source of current information, users should use caution and consider how review methods may influence their confidence in recommendations.

After systematic reviews, summaries of research findings for interventions are the next strongest source of information on effective interventions. RTIPs summaries, for example, are provided by external reviewers who independently apply predefined criteria to determine whether an intervention is ready for dissemination. Some websites also review and disseminate interventions that have been evaluated in practice but have not been re-search tested.[33,39] Although these "practice-based" interventions do not provide evidence of "effectiveness," when disseminated as packaged interventions, they may offer guidance and resources for how to implement evidence-based strategies in real-world practice settings.

4. What criteria did they apply to determine when an intervention was evidence-based and ready to be disseminated? Websites use a range of criteria to designate different levels of "evidence-based." An intervention is considered "evidence-based" contingent on the strength and consistency of research findings supporting its efficacy or effectiveness at achieving intended outcomes.[19] Assessments of effectiveness may include the number of studies reviewed, study design and execution, magnitude of effects, and consistency of findings across studies. Criteria may also address cost, priority of the population for whom the intervention is intended, and potential for broad-scale adoption and implementation. Consensus is lacking, however, on criteria that qualify an intervention for "evidence-based" designation. In 2000, the working group Grading of Recommendations Assessment, Development and Evaluation (GRADE) began as an informal collaboration of people with an interest in addressing the shortcomings of grading systems in health care, and it is increasingly influencing criteria for guiding decisions about which interventions are "evidence-based" (http://www.gradeworkinggroup. org). Building on GRADE recommendations, the Community Guide has recognized that criteria may need to vary for interventions targeting different levels. This is because intervention studies that target the individual level are more numerous and more likely to use randomized controlled designs than are studies that target organizational, community, or policy levels.[40]

For an intervention to improve health, it must not only be effective but also be adopted by those with the potential to put it into practice. To achieve maximal impact, an intervention also needs to be implemented with fidelity and maintained over time.[41,42] For this reason, some websites apply criteria from RE-AIM (Reach, Effectiveness, Adoption, Implementation, Maintenance; described later) or similar frameworks to assess the evidence in support of an intervention's potential to reach intended beneficiaries and to be adopted, implemented, and maintained by those providers and settings that serve the intended beneficiaries.[34,41]

5. How current is the evidence base? Most websites provide information on when the evidence in support of an EBI was last reviewed. It is not unusual for websites to disseminate EBIs based on evidence that was reviewed more than a decade ago. These EBIs may still be of value to cancer control planners. However, planners will benefit from searching for more recent systematic reviews or conducting a review themselves of reports of more recent studies testing the EBI. They will also want to consider changes to CPGs or the policy context (e.g., changes in policy governing coverage of screening tests) that may require that the EBI be adapted or replaced.

6. What information is available to support EBI implementation? Websites vary in how much detail they provide about an EBI and whether they include materials to support implementation (i.e., implementation manual, facilitator's guide, patient materials, etc.). In some cases, materials are readily accessible for free through website links. In other cases, websites may include information about how to purchase the EBI from the developer or other sources. Therefore, it is important to assess the information that the website provides about its EBIs, what materials are available, whether those materials are readily accessible, and whether implementation resources will be available.

SELECTING AN EVIDENCE-BASED INTERVENTION

In making decisions to select EBIs, cancer control planners must weigh various features of the intervention, such as the strength of the evidence in support of the EBI's effectiveness and its fit with local needs and resources, including its potential to reach the intended recipients and the likelihood that it could be adopted and implemented with integrity.

Strength of the Evidence and Potential for Impact

As discussed previously, not all evidence is created equal, and it is important to understand the strength of the evidence and how a website defines its terms. By applying the criteria outlined previously, planners can compare the evidence in support of the effectiveness of their menu EBI options. If a website applies the RE-AIM framework to evaluate its interventions, then planners can use that information to assess an EBI's potential for reach, adoption or adaptation, and implementation. Even when websites do not provide this information, planners can consider RE-AIM criteria (Reach, Effectiveness, Adoption, Implementation, and Maintenance) to identify EBIs more likely to make an enduring impact.[43] Reach is defined as the number, proportion, and representativeness of individuals who participate in a given intervention. It is influenced by an intervention's acceptability, penetration, and ability to impact the intended beneficiaries. Thus, considerations of reach may favor less efficacious interventions that are more feasible and acceptable for a much broader group than highly efficacious EBIs that may be more intensive and/or work very well for a highly select group of individuals who may be unusually motivated and able to accept and stick with the intervention. Adoption is the number, proportion, and representativeness of the settings and/providers that have agreed to use the intervention. Implementation is the actual use of the intervention and may include consistency and skill with which various intervention components are implemented. Maintenance is the sustainment of the intervention over time.[44] Thus, an EBI tested in a real-world setting with good reach to a representative group and delivered by individuals already part of the setting or readily integrated and without special incentives or monitoring (evidence of effectiveness) may have more potential for impact than one tested in a highly controlled efficacy trial.[45]

Another way that planners can judge the relevance of a particular study's findings to one's own practice setting is to apply the pragmatic–explanatory continuum indicator summary (PRECIS) criteria. PRECIS offers an assessment of the balance between multiple qualities valuable in experimental studies and those valuable in practical, real-world settings. The PRECIS model can be visually displayed, with intervening characteristics such as follow-up intensity and practitioner adherence depicted as the spokes of a wheel and levels of explanatory power and pragmatism charted on each spoke.[46,47] Thus, it can provide a graphic depiction of an intervention's potential for implementation in settings to which the results are intended to apply.

Determining an Evidence-Based Intervention's Fit with Local Needs and Resources

In addition to appraising the evidence in support of an EBI's potential impact, cancer control planners also need to determine how well the EBI fits local needs and resources that, ideally, have been identified in a thorough needs and resource assessment. Determining fit involves consideration of the EBI's match with the local health problem, factors contributing to that problem, setting and organizational capacity, and characteristics of the population.[48,49]

Health Problem and Influencing Factors

Is there a match between the focus of the EBI and the locally identified health problem and behavioral and environmental factors influencing that problem? Considering match with the health problem is usually the first criterion because it is at the most basic level a way to assess whether a particular EBI fits the local need and is usually fairly straightforward. For example, if the community assessment identified low CRC screening rates as a problem, planners will identify EBIs that effectively increase screening rates. Identifying an EBI that fits local behavioral and environmental factors and the determinants of these, however, is more challenging. The available EBIs may target some but not all of the locally identified behavioral or environmental determinants. For example, an EBI may have included intervention components to increase knowledge of guidelines and attitudes about screening but may not have included a component that is designed to influence provider recommendation or communication skills. Often, the goal is to find the best rather than the perfect match and then to adapt the EBI to improve its fit.

Organizational Capacity

Does the organization or coalition have the capacity required to carry out the intervention? Are the content, delivery method, and resources required in keeping with the organizational mission, strategic goals, and resources? It must be feasible to implement the intervention in the new setting with the current resources or with new resources available through partnerships or coalitions. If organizational capacity is limited but all other aspects of the EBI are a match, planners might want to consider modifications in intervention delivery or intensity as long as the key components of the program that contributed to its effectiveness remain intact.

Population

Is the at-risk population with whom the EBI was originally tested the same or similar to the one in the new site? This criterion is last because a priority population with a different population and/or culture may have similar influencing factors ("determinants") as the population with whom a specific EBI was originally tested. For example, Vietnamese nail salon workers and low-income Latinas may have more in common with respect to Pap/human papillomavirus testing and screening mammography than might be immediately obvious.[50,51] Cultural adaptation of images, language, and relevant statistics and resources might be the only adaptation required, or surface structure modifications. Therefore, EBIs tested in a "general" or a different population might still be useful and examined more closely for the fit of determinants. On the other hand, there may be important behaviors or environmental conditions that make it more difficult for one group to access screening than another, or the behaviors may be influenced by different beliefs, attitudes and other determinants, some of which may be culturally influenced (deeper structure modifications). Therefore, a careful examination of factors influencing the behavior in the new population and setting will provide guidance for what may need to be adapted.

INTERVENTION FIDELITY AND ADAPTATION

Both fidelity and adaptation play important roles in EBI implementation. Finding the right balance between the two has led to healthy debate in the field.[52–55] Some researchers believe fidelity is the central concern for implementation because of the risk associated with changing intervention elements that can negatively impact outcomes.[56–59] In a review assessing implementation impact on intervention outcomes, researchers noted that higher levels of fidelity were associated with better outcomes.[6] Unintentional changes may lead to program drift, resulting in the loss of core components required to achieve outcomes.[60] However, implementing interventions with high fidelity may not always be realistic or desirable. There can be negative consequences if researchers do not make intentional adaptations to improve fit. For example, adaptation may occur from challenges faced during implementation. As a result, some researchers suggest adaptation is an unavoidable process necessary to meet the needs of a specific context.[61] Furthermore, some studies that have monitored adaptation have found positive effects on intervention outcomes.[6]

The Definition/Conceptualization of Fidelity

Fidelity has been defined as the degree to which an intervention is implemented as it is prescribed in the original protocol.[1] Given the focus on a specific intervention protocol, fidelity is readily applied to the implementation of specific than general EBIs. Multiple studies have identified or acknowledged five key elements of fidelity, which help inform the conceptualization of the term and its measurement: adherence, exposure or dose, quality of delivery, participant responsiveness, and program differentiation.[62–64] Adherence refers to whether an intervention is delivered as designed or written. Exposure is the amount of the program received by participants, which can be the frequency, number, or length of sessions. Quality of delivery is the manner in which an interventionist delivers the program, such as the skill, techniques, and methods of delivery used. Participant responsiveness refers to how engaged and involved participants are with the program content. Last, program differentiation is defined by unique features of components that are distinguished from one another.

Monitoring the different elements of intervention fidelity is important for multiple reasons. As a moderator between interventions and their outcomes, fidelity can alter the strength of the relation between an intervention and its potential success.[62] Well-implemented (with high fidelity) EBIs can be highly effective. However, if they are poorly implemented, they can lose their effectiveness.

Fidelity also plays an important role in understanding intervention results. If fidelity is not monitored and an intervention is determined to have a significant effect, then it is impossible to know whether the results were due to an effective intervention or to unknown elements that were added or removed.[56] Likewise, if a nonsignificant effect is observed, then it is unclear if the findings resulted from an ineffective intervention or poor fidelity.

Balancing Fidelity and Adaptation

Although fidelity plays an important role in implementation, adaptations are often required to better suit the setting or target population. Finding a balance between fidelity and adaptation is critical to the success of an EBI. Researchers have proposed that the fidelity–adaption debate does not have to be an either–or proposition.[6] Instead, adopters and implementers need to think about fidelity in terms of what must remain the same to ensure effectiveness (e.g., behavior change techniques used and mode of delivery) and what needs to change to better fit the needs and resources of the new population and setting. Therefore, it is possible to strike a balance between adaptation and fidelity to maximize the reach, effectiveness, and sustainability of cancer control interventions.

CORE COMPONENTS

One way to help achieve a proper balance between fidelity and adaptation is to identify core components of a specific EBI. Core components include "the functions or principles and related activities necessary to achieve outcomes."[65] They are directly related to the theoretical basis behind an intervention and provide the mechanisms driving intervention effectiveness. Ideally, but not frequently, the core components have been tested through research and have evidence supporting their impact on short- and potentially long-term outcomes.[65]

Identifying core components is critical for researchers and practitioners. Poor specification of core components makes it difficult to evaluate an intervention and disseminate it to other populations and settings. Adopters often cannot identify elements that must be maintained for an intervention to be effective. While it is not always clear what the core components are, they likely include the change mechanisms or methods used to influence key determinants of behavior. In a recent report, four criteria were identified as elements that comprise a well-operationalized intervention that includes the core components or elements.[65] First, there must be a clear description of the intervention's context. This includes the principles and values that provide a basis for the intervention as well as a clear definition of the target population. Second, there needs to be a clear description of core components, including the essential functions that are necessary for success. Third, there should be a description of active ingredients that further define the core components. Last, there needs to be a practical assessment for assessing the implementation as it relates to core components.

Balancing adaptation and fidelity has also been likened to baking a cake with variations, where core components are categorized as ingredients, methods, and equipment.[60] Core ingredients include the main program elements, such as behavior change techniques and processes for change (e.g., supporting participant well-being). Core methods include how the program was delivered (e.g., home visits and group activities). Core equipment includes the necessary resources, such as effective management, trained staff, and data tools/systems for quality monitoring. Variations are additions to enhance the core program related to goals and context of the intervention. Overall, there is a need to understand what the core components of interventions are as well as what elements need to be adapted.

Conceptualization of Adaptation

Adaptation has been defined as the degree to which an EBI is changed or modified by a user during adoption and implementation to suit the needs of the setting or to improve the fit to local conditions.[1] Adaptations are a specific type of modification that are planned and purposeful to help improve intervention fit while intending to maintain fidelity.[66] Wiltsey-Stirman and associates[66] developed a system for classifying adaptations by grouping them into five different categories: (1) by whom modifications are made, (2) what is modified, (3) at what level of delivery, (4) context modifications, and (5) the nature of the content modification. These categories were based on reviewing numerous studies and were proposed to help characterize different types of adaptations that may occur. Given the importance of balancing fidelity and adaptation, an organized, systematic approach to adaptation is critical.

IMPORTANCE OF A SYSTEMATIC APPROACH TO ADAPTATION

The need for a systematic approach to adaptation was recognized as a way to promote dissemination and better fit with the new setting while remaining conscious of core components. After a review of the literature on sustainable programs in substance abuse, in 2002 one of the most influential thinkers in the field, T. E. Backer, wrote, "The fundamental conclusion is that attention to BOTH program fidelity and adaptation during the complex process of program implementation is critical to successful, sustained implementation of science-based substance abuse prevention programs."[67,68] This conclusion was reached simultaneously by several US governmental agencies that were actively interested in scaling-up interventions whose development and testing they had sponsored, and frameworks for the adaptation of EBIs ensued. A systematic approach to adaptation thus helps resolve the tension between those who consider adaptation an essential and natural step to implementation and those who argue for strict fidelity. Systematic approaches or frameworks increase the likelihood that reports will include the rationale for adaptation, a clear description of the process, and an accurate inventory of the changes. They also call attention to evaluation of the adapted EBI.

ADAPTATION FRAMEWORKS

Four US agencies provided the primary support and leadership in the past 15 years for systematic approaches to adaptation: the National Institute for Child Health and Human Development, the National Institute of Allergy and Infectious Diseases, the Center for Substance Abuse Prevention in the Substance Abuse and Mental Health Services Administration, and the Centers for Disease Control and Prevention (CDC).[68] The first three sponsored seminal conferences/ workshops in 2002, with CDC's participation. A recent scoping study of adaptation frameworks led by Escoffery identified 13 frameworks introduced into the literature or on websites beginning in 2002 and traced the history of mutual citation and acknowledgment.[68] Half of these frameworks attributed their sponsorship to one or more of the four agencies, with several positioning their guidance as more suitable for use by practitioners than

academics.[67,69–73] Others indicated awareness of the agency-sponsored work but either were not focused on a particular health topic, as with the framework based on the intervention mapping approach, or were drilling down into specific steps in the process. The remainder did not cite the other frameworks but cited key sources on cultural adaptation.[7,74–77]

Common Steps

Eleven steps could be identified across the frameworks in the review by Escoffery and associates, although not all included every step.[68] They are generally described as follows:

1. *Assess the community.* Collect data to learn about the target population, including risk behaviors and their environmental and behavioral determinants. This can include the community context and organizational capacity to implement a program.

2. *Understand the EBI program.* Review the program and then gather all available materials (protocols, training manuals, print materials, participant notebooks, etc.) to help identify the core components. Clarify the program objectives, theory, and/or strategies.

3. *Select the intervention.* Choose the EBI that best matches the target population and context.

4. *Consult the experts.* Work with experts or advisors to learn more about the selected EBI and receive guidance on core components and culture/ context. Contact with the intervention developer(s) enables discussion of the "core components" and ensures that the adapted products maintain fidelity to the original program.

5. *Consult with stakeholders.* Seek input from a variety of stakeholders, particularly professionals who know about the population of interest or members of the community in which EBI implementation occurs. These stakeholders can also identify partners who can champion program adoption.

6. *Decide what needs to be adapted.* Identify whether the EBI needs to be adapted by comparing the assessment of the new community to the one in which the EBI was tested. If adaptation is necessary, identify areas in which EBI needs to be adapted and include possible changes in program structure, content, provider, or delivery methods. Also, systematically reduce mismatches between the program

and the new context while retaining fidelity to core elements.

7. *Adapt the original program.* Make an adaptation plan that includes collaboration and continuous pilot testing, avoiding modification of core components. Make cultural adaptations continuously through pilot testing.

8. *Train staff.* Select and train staff about the overall intervention, its delivery, and the evaluation of key outcomes. This helps ensure quality implementation.

9. *Test the adapted materials.* Conduct pretests and readability tests of the adapted materials with stakeholders as well as a full pilot test of the entire intervention and its evaluation with the new target population.

10. *Implement.* Develop an implementation plan based on results generated in previous steps. Implementation includes both adoption and implementation of the adapted program with the population(s) of interest. The implementation plan includes the scope, sequence, and instructions, as well as identification of the implementers and the intended behaviors and outcomes.

11. *Evaluate.* Document the adaptation process, and evaluate the process and outcomes of the adapted intervention as implemented. Write evaluation questions; choose indicators, measures, and the evaluation design; and plan data collection, analysis, and reporting. Employ the empowerment evaluation approach framework to improve program implementation.

This overview of the common steps identified in Escoffery et al.'s scoping review suggests there is consensus on the basic process of adaptation.[68] It does not, however, provide the details and "how to" guidance offered by the various frameworks on specific steps. Most of the frameworks provide an overview, with more or less depth.[49,70–73,77] Other frameworks have a particular focus; for example, four frameworks take up cultural adaptation exclusively, examining both the surface and the deep structure of culture.[7,69,76,78] The framework by Chen and associates represents a new generation in frameworks given they observe that it is "now both possible and necessary to focus on articulating separate steps of the process rather than offering broad models that cover many steps."[74] These authors suggest that participant feedback has received too little attention and advocate using this method to identify population differences. They also provide a process

for deciding what to change, noting the wide variability of actors across previous frameworks, and they illustrate their framework with arthritis self-help programs. The adaptation framework based on Intervention Mapping first debuted in 2005 with an example from a sexual health intervention and was refined in later editions of the textbook, with the most recent iteration known as IM Adapt.[77,79,80] IM Adapt attends to each step in depth, with a strong emphasis on understanding "how to," using a intervention mapping approach.

COMMUNITY ENGAGEMENT DURING ADAPTATION PLANNING

As described previously, virtually all the adaptation framework authors have pointed to the importance of consulting the at-risk or priority group to identify community needs and gain perspectives on needed adaptation.[68] This may be particularly relevant in cases in which the original EBI was developed for and tested with a population or context that differs from the new target. Yet, to increase the potential for adoption, implementation, and maintenance in the new settings, the concept of community engagement should also include engagement of stakeholders who are responsible for program use. Only 3 of the 12 frameworks described previously explicitly mentioned potential implementers as stakeholders, and 5 described implementation as a step.[68] In addition, only 3 frameworks identified assessment of organizational capacity as important, and only 3 mentioned staff preparation and training as steps in adapting an EBI.[68] An enlarged group of stakeholders that includes potential adopters and implementers would also be in a stronger position to point out needed adaption that will maximize implementation and maintenance. For example, a cervical cancer control intervention developed by Colombia's National Cancer Institute was adapted to a local community during a needs assessment process. The intervention succeeded in increasing colorectal cancer screening among uninsured women because local knowledge provided key information, such as the need for a lab to process cervical cancer screening tests and the idea to frame cancer control as a human right.[81] Community-based participatory research (CBPR), when used to its fullest capacity, is a strong framework to engage communities in evidence-based programs, adapted to be useful in specific contexts.[81]

Testing changes to the adapted EBI with intended users is another aspect of community engagement that also has long been a feature of program development in health promotion and cancer prevention and control, whether formalized as part of community participatory research or basic health promotion practice.[82-88]

DESIGNING FOR DISSEMINATION

Issues related to the identification, assessment of fit, adaptation, and implementation of EBIs for cancer control are essential for increasing the relevance and impact of research and research products. These issues, however, are all focused on what happens after interventions are developed and available. One of the major challenges to overcome to increase the impact of cancer control EBIs is that even when interventions are effective, they are often unready for widespread use, and it typically takes a long time for these interventions to be used consistently in practice or to influence policy.[4,89,90] Part of the problem is that they were not initially developed with implementation and dissemination in mind. To make the largest strides in increasing both the effectiveness and the dissemination of cancer control EBIs, researchers and program planners must consider issues of feasibility, practicality, context, and implementation during the development of interventions. Thus, the concept of "designing for dissemination,"[91] which encourages consideration of and planning for implementation during the initial development of an intervention, is a key strategy for improving the use of cancer control interventions in practice. Kegles and colleagues offer questions to consider in the development of an intervention to help with its future scalability.[92]

Unfortunately, for some EBI development efforts, planning for program use and scale-up are often an afterthought, primarily addressed after the intervention has already been developed. This approach can lead to implementation challenges or failure. Instead, program planners should pay careful attention during the design and development phase of an intervention to ensure that it includes characteristics that make it more likely to be adopted, implemented, and maintained. Development efforts should also include implementation planning that includes the development of materials and strategies to facilitate program use.

Importance of Participatory Planning

Using CBPR approaches during the development of an intervention can greatly enhance its potential for successful implementation and maintenance. CBPR is a framework for research in which an equal partnership is formed between a research team and a community, and all members of this partnership have equal ownership in the direction, collection, analysis, and products of the research. In a CBPR approach, the first step for a research project is to form a community advisory board that includes local stakeholders and directs all aspects of the research project.[93,94] This grounds the project's methods—including the intervention's contents, theoretical methods, and practical applications—within the community's context, effectively "designing for dissemination" as the intervention is conceived.[49,91-94] In addition, creating a program in partnership with a community can help leverage community networks for implementation.[95]

Translation of an intervention to a new setting requires thought about that setting. Common challenges include issues relating to external validity, origins of knowledge, language, power-sharing, trust, and sustainability. When individuals who may adopt, implement, or use the program are included in the community advisory board, CBPR is uniquely positioned to address these issues through integration of the local community's priorities, perspectives, and practices.[96] This also helps ensure that program materials, methods, and strategies fit the local context to which an intervention is disseminated.[49,92,94]

Engaging potential EBI *implementers* as key stakeholders in planning has received less attention, despite its importance in successful adoption, implementation, and program maintenance in new settings. In their chapter in an intervention mapping textbook on program implementation, Fernandez and co-authors highlight a participatory approach to implementation planning that includes potential adopters, implementers, and maintainers from the beginning of the planning process.[75] They also point to the notion of a linkage system and provide numerous examples in which new members with relevant and fresh views on program implementation are added to the planning group.[49,97,98] Ideally, these include not only change agents or program champions but also representatives of those with actual responsibility for implementation. Doing so can help planners gain a realistic understanding of what is needed for implementation of an EBI, including organizational resources, staffing needs, financial constraints, and other factors. Bringing them into the planning group to exchange ideas and information with other planners contributes to user-friendly programs and improves the likelihood of successful implementation.

Guidance from Theoretical Models and Frameworks

Theoretical models and frameworks from behavioral and social sciences and from implementation science can all help inform both intervention development (to enhance its potential future use) and EBI implementation. There are numerous theoretical models and frameworks that can be used for designing for dissemination.[100] Research suggests Diffusion of Innovations is commonly used for this purpose, although RE-AIM, social cognitive theory, social marketing, network theory, and others have also been used.[101] Interventions that use theoretical models and frameworks are more likely to be successful because they help focus developers and evaluators on key aspects to consider during the intervention development process. For example, Diffusion of Innovations and the Consolidated Framework for Implementation Research (CFIR) articulate characteristics of Interventions (innovations) that make them more likely to be adopted and implemented.[102,103] The Diffusion of Innovations model describes intervention characteristics that make an innovation more likely to be adopted and implemented. These include intervention source, evidence strength and quality, relative advantage, compatibility, adaptability, trialability, complexity, design quality and packaging, and cost. If planners keep these characteristics in mind and apply these concepts during intervention development, they will increase the likelihood of successful adoption and implementation. Overall, using theories and frameworks can provide critical information to focus on during intervention development, implementation, and dissemination.

SYSTEMATIC INTERVENTION PLANNING

A good way to integrate information from theories, empirical evidence, and new data is to use a systematic planning approach. Systematic planning approaches can greatly increase the potential that

interventions will be implemented and maintained. PRECEDE–PROCEDE is one such planning approach that was designed to provide a systematic method for applying theories during the development of interventions.[104] PRECEDE–PROCEDE consists of planning phases, an implementation phase, and evaluation phases. Using the PRECEDE–PROCEDE approach helps ensure an organized process that incorporates theories during all stages of intervention development to better achieve desired outcomes, including an intervention that can be more easily implemented.

Intervention Mapping is another approach that, when used appropriately, can enhance implementation in a number of ways, including development, implementation planning, and adaptation planning.[46] First, it helps planners develop programs using a process that will enhance the program 'sir potential for use. Intervention mapping is based on principles of participatory planning (described previously) and provides a step-by-step approach to understanding the problem at multiple levels. It then proceeds to the development of a multilevel logic model of change, the selection of appropriate methods, and practical applications that will create change in the determinants of behaviors and environmental conditions influencing the cancer control problem. Second, intervention mapping guides planners through steps that provide explicit guidance on planning for program implementation. This can be used to plan strategies to enhance the initial implementation of an intervention, or after the intervention has been evaluated, it can be used to plan strategies for scale-up and spread. Finally, intervention mapping can guide users through a systematic process of comparing information about a new population, setting, or context with elements of the existing intervention to inform adaptation decisions.[104]

Critical questions for planning implementation approaches (whether during development or for scale-up and spread of existing interventions) include the following: Who is responsible for the adoption of this intervention? Who will deliver it? (The answer to this question may differ by intervention components, particularly if they are targeting different levels.) What do they have to do to deliver the intervention? What factors (both personal and contextual) influence program adoption, implementation, and maintenance? What methods and practical strategies can be used to influence these?

SUMMARY

Improving the implementation of EBIs is critical to move the field of cancer control forward. Understanding the different types of cancer control products and their advantages and disadvantages for adoption and implementation can help improve the selection of EBIs as well as the development of strategies to increase their use and sustainability. There are many existing websites and resources, so being able to effectively evaluate these sources is also critical for program selection. However, selecting an intervention is only one step in the process. Several challenges with implementation must be addressed. For example, balancing fidelity and adaptation is necessary for delivering EBIs that are appropriate for priority populations and settings while maintaining the core components that make them efficacious. Adaptations of EBIs should use frameworks to guide the process. Doing so will help ensure EBIs are implemented effectively in addition to providing documentation to the process. Overall, considering dissemination during the intervention development process is necessary for improving the dissemination of EBIs. Use of CBPR and systematic intervention planning approaches that are theory informed will help when taking an EBI to scale. Furthermore, there needs to be a greater emphasis on interventions that are effective and scalable. Thus, in order to bridge the research-to-practice gap and ultimately improve cancer control, we must continue to build the evidence base of both general and specific EBIs; improve access to them; provide guidance on how they can be adopted, adapted, and implemented; and develop implementation approaches to accelerate their use.

REFERENCES

1. Rabin BA, Brownson RC, Haire-Joshu D, Kreuter MW, Weaver NL. A glossary for dissemination and implementation research in health. *J Public Health Manag Pract.* 2008;14(2):117–123.
2. Biglan A, Ogden T. The evolution of evidence-based practices. *Eur J Behav Anal.* 2008;9(1):81–95.
3. Hannon PA, Fernandez ME, Williams RS, et al. Cancer control planners' perceptions and use of evidence-based programs. *J Public Health Manag Pract.* 2010;16(3):E1–8.
4. Neta G, Glasgow RE, Carpenter CR, et al. A framework for enhancing the value of research for dissemination and implementation. *Am J Public Health.* 2015;105(1):49–57.
5. Brownson RC, Fielding JE, Maylahn CM. Evidence-based public health: A fundamental concept for public health practice. *Annu Rev Public Health.* 2009;30:175–201.
6. Durlak JA, DuPre EP. Implementation matters: A review of research on the influence of implementation on program outcomes and the factors affecting implementation. *Am J Community Psychol.* 2008;41(3–4):327–350.
7. Lee SJ, Altschul I, Mowbray CT. Using planned adaptation to implement evidence-based programs with new populations. *Am J Comm Psych.* 2008;41(3):290–303.
8. Graham R, Mancher M, Wolman DM, Greenfield S, Steinberg E. Committee on Standards for Developing Trustworthy Clinical Practice Guidelines; Board on Health Care Services. Clinical Practice Guidelines We Can Trust. Washington, DC: National Academies Press; 2011.
9. US Preventive Task Force. Colorectal cancer: Screening. 2016. https://www.uspreventiveservicestaskforce.org/Page/Document/UpdateSummaryFinal/colorectal-cancer-screening2?ds=1&s=colorectal%20cancer
10. Community Preventive Services Task Force. *The Community Guide.* September 2017 version that can be retrieved from https://www.thecommunityguide.org/
11. The Cochrane Collaboration. Cochrane. 2017. http://www.cochrane.org.
12. Community Preventive Services Task Force. Increasing cancer screening: One-on-one education for clients. 2013. https://www.thecommunityguide.org/sites/default/files/assets/Cancer-Screening-One-on-One-Education.pdf
13. Reuland DS, Brenner AT, Hoffman R, et al. Effect of combined patient decision aid and patient navigation vs usual care for colorectal cancer screening in a vulnerable patient population: A randomized clinical trial. *JAMA Intern Med.* 2017;177(7):967–974.
14. National Cancer Institute. Research-Tested Intervention Programs (RTIPs): Moving science into programs for people. n.d.; https://rtips.cancer.gov
15. National Cancer Institute. Cancer Control PLANET: Plan, Link, Act, Network with Evidence-based Tools. n.d.; https://cancercontrolplanet.cancer.gov

16. US Preventive Task Force. Breast cancer: Medications for risk reduction. 2013. https://www.uspreventiveservicestaskforce.org/Page/Document/UpdateSummaryFinal/breast-cancer-medications-for-risk-reduction?ds=1&s=breast%20cancer. Accessed September 5, 2017.

17. US Preventive Services Task Force. Breast cancer: Screening. 2016. https://www.uspreventiveservicestaskforce.org/Page/Document/UpdateSummaryFinal/breast-cancer-screening1

18. Lyman GH, Somerfield MR, Bosserman LD, Perkins CL, Weaver DL, Giuliano AE. Sentinel lymph node biopsy for patients with early-stage breast cancer: American Society of Clinical Oncology clinical practice guideline update. *J Clin Oncol.* 2017;35(5):561–564.

19. Runowicz CD, Leach CR, Henry NL, et al. American Cancer Society/American Society of Clinical Oncology breast cancer survivorship care guideline. *J Clin Oncol.* 2016;34(6):611–635.

20. American Cancer Society. How your weight affects your risk of breast cancer. 2014. https://www.cancer.org/latest-news/how-your-weight-affects-your-risk-of-breast-cancer.html. Accessed September 5, 2017.

21. The Community Guide. Obesity: Technology-supported multicomponent coaching or counseling interventions—to reduce weight. 2009. https://www.thecommunityguide.org/findings/obesity-technology-supported-multicomponent-coaching-or-counseling-interventions-reduce. Accessed September 5, 2017.

22. The Community Guide. Cancer screening: Reducing client out-of-pocket costs—breast cancer. 2009. https://www.thecommunityguide.org/findings/cancer-screening-reducing-client-out-pocket-costs-breast-cancer. Accessed September 5, 2017.

23. Jassim GA, Whitford DL, Hickey A, Carter B. Psychological interventions for women with non-metastatic breast cancer. *Cochrane Database Syst Rev.* 2015;2015(5):CD008729.

24. Cheng KKF, Lim YTE, Koh ZM, Tam WWS. Home-based multidimensional survivorship programmes for breast cancer survivors. *Cochrane Database Syst Rev.* 2017;2017(8):561–564CD011152.

25. Shaw PA, Yancy WS, Jr., Wesby L, et al. The design and conduct of Keep It Off: An online randomized trial of financial incentives for weight-loss maintenance. *Clin Trials.* 2017;14(1):29–36.

26. Sherwood NE, Crain AL, Martinson BC, et al. Enhancing long-term weight loss maintenance: 2 year results from the Keep It Off randomized controlled trial. *Prev Med.* 2013;56(3–4):171–177.

27. Research-Tested Intervention Programs (RTIPS). Keep It Off. 2015. https://rtips.cancer.gov/rtips/programDetails.do?programId=16899086. Accessed September 5, 2017.

28. Research-Tested Intervention Programs (RTIPS). The Witness Project. 2015. https://rtips.cancer.gov/rtips/programDetails.do?programId=270521. Accessed September 6, 2017.

29. Research-Tested Intervention Programs (RTIPS). Effects of psychosocial treatment on cancer survivorship. 2014. https://rtips.cancer.gov/rtips/programDetails.do?programId=297250. Accessed September 5, 2017.

30. Research-Tested Intervention Programs (RTIPS). Breast Cancer Education Intervention (BCEI). 2013. https://rtips.cancer.gov/rtips/programDetails.do?programId=1416306. Accessed September 5, 2017.

31. Grimshaw J, Eccles M, Tetroe J. Implementing clinical guidelines: Current evidence and future implications. *J Contin Educ Health Prof.* 2004;24(S1):S31–S37.

32. National Cancer Institute. Understanding and influencing multilevel factors across the cancer care continuum. *J Natl Cancer Inst Monogr.* 2012;44:1–144.

33. Mullen PD, Leeman J, Escoffery CT, Wood R, Dube S, Fernandez ME. Tools for improving searches for evidence-based interventions (EBIs) and assessing their basic fit. Paper presented at the annual meeting of the American Public Health Association, Atlanta, GA; 2017.

34. Leeman J, Sommers J, Leung MM, Ammerman A. Disseminating evidence from research and practice: A model for selecting evidence to guide obesity prevention. *J Public Health Manag Pract.* 2011;17(2):133–140.

35. Lipsey MW. The challenges of interpreting research for use by practitioners: Comments on the latest products from the Task Force on Community Preventive Services. *Am J Prev Med.* 2005;28(2 Suppl 1):1–3.

36. Leeman J, Moore A, Teal R, Barrett N, Leighton A, Steckler A. Promoting community practitioners' use of evidence-based approaches to increase breast cancer screening. *Public Health Nurs.* 2013;30(4):323–331.

37. Escoffery C, Hannon P, Maxwell AE, Vu T, Leeman J, et al. Assessment of training and technical assistance needs of Colorectal Cancer Control Program Grantees in the U.S. *BMC Public Health.* 2015;15(1):49. doi:10.1186/s12889-01501386-01501381

38. County Health Rankings and Roadmaps. Using what works for health. http://www.countyhealthrankings.org/roadmaps/what-works-for-health/using-what-works-health

39. Leeman J, Aycock N, Paxton-Aiken A, et al. Policy, systems, and environmental approaches to obesity prevention: Translating and disseminating evidence from practice. *Public Health Rep.* 2016 130(6):616–622.

40. Briss PA, Mullen PD, Hopkins DP. Methods used for reviewing evidence and linking evidence to recommendations in the Community Guide. In: Zaza S, Briss P, Harris K, eds. *Guide to Community Preventive Services: What Works to Promote Health?.* New York: Oxford University Press; 2005:431–448.

41. Glasgow RE, Lichtenstein E, Marcus AC. Why don't we see more translation of health promotion research to practice? Rethinking the efficacy-to-effectiveness transition. *Am J Public Health.* 2003;93(8):1261–1267.

42. Rychetnik L, Frommer M, Hawe P, Shiell A. Criteria for evaluating evidence on public health interventions. *J Epidemiol Community Health.* 2002;56(2):119–127.

43. Glasgow RE, Vogt TM, Boles SM. Evaluating the public health impact of health promotion interventions: The RE-AIM framework. *Am J Public Health.* 1999;89(9):1322–1327.

44. Glasgow RE, Klesges LM, Dzewaltowski DA, Estabrooks PA, Vogt TM. Evaluating the impact of health promotion programs: Using the RE-AIM framework to form summary measures for decision making involving complex issues. *Health Educ Res.* 2006;21(5):688–694.

45. Glasgow RE. What does it mean to be pragmatic? Pragmatic methods, measures, and models to facilitate research translation. *Health Educ Behav.* 2013;40(3):257–265.

46. Bartholomew Eldredge LK, Markham CM, Kok G, Ruiter RA, Parcel GS. *Planning Health Promotion Programs: An Intervention Mapping Approach.* San Francisco, CA: Jossey-Bass; 2016.

47. Thorpe KE, Zwarenstein M, Oxman AD, et al. A pragmatic–explanatory continuum indicator summary (PRECIS): A tool to help trial designers. *J Clin Epidemiol.* 2009;62(5):464–475.

48. Cancer Prevention and Control Network. Putting Public Health Evidence in Action training workshop. 2015; http://cpcrn.org/pub/evidence-in-action

49. Bartholomew Eldredge LK, Markham CM, Kok G, et al. *Using Intervention Mapping to Adapt Evidence-Based Interventions.* San Francisco, CA: Jossey-Bass; 2016.

50. Fernandez-Esquer M, Le Y-C, Huynh, TN, Tran V, et al. Sức Khỏe là Hạnh Phúc—Health is happiness: A breast and cervical cancer prevention program for Vietnamese nail salon workers. Paper presented at the meeting of the American Public Health Association, Denver, CO; 2016.

51. Schick V, Tran V, Huynh, TN, et al. Exploring opportunities for cancer screening promotion at nail salons: Increasing healthcare access and utilization among Vietnamese women outside of recommended cancer screening guidelines. Paper presented at the meeting of the American Public Health Association, Denver, CO; 2016.

52. Carvalho ML, Honeycutt S, Escoffery C, Glanz K, Sabbs D, Kegler MC. Balancing fidelity and adaptation: Implementing evidence-based chronic disease prevention programs. *J Public Health Manag Pract.* 2013;19(4):348–356.

53. Bopp M, Saunders RP, Lattimore D. The tug-of-war: Fidelity versus adaptation throughout the health promotion program life cycle. *J Prim Prev.* 2013;34(3):193-207.

54. Castro FG, Barrera M, Jr., Martinez CR, Jr. The cultural adaptation of prevention interventions: Resolving tensions between fidelity and fit. *Prev Sci.* 2004;5(1):41–45.

55. Morrison DM, Hoppe MJ, Gillmore MR, Kluver C, Higa D, Wells EA. Replicating an intervention: The tension between fidelity and adaptation. *AIDS Educ Prev.* 2009;21(2):128.

56. Bellg AJ, Borrelli B, Resnick B, et al. Enhancing treatment fidelity in health behavior change studies: Best practices and recommendations from the NIH Behavior Change Consortium. *Health Psychol.* 2004;23(5):443–451.

57. Breitenstein SM, Gross D, Garvey CA, Hill C, Fogg L, Resnick B. Implementation fidelity in community-based interventions. *Res Nurs Health.* 2010;33(2):164–173.

58. Cohen DJ, Crabtree BF, Etz RS, et al. Fidelity versus flexibility: Translating evidence-based research into practice. *Am J Prev Med.* 2008;35(5 Suppl):S381–389.

59. Dumas JE, Lynch AM, Laughlin JE, Phillips Smith E, Prinz RJ. Promoting intervention fidelity: Conceptual issues, methods, and

preliminary results from the EARLY ALLIANCE prevention trial. *Am J Prev Med.* 2001;20(1 Suppl):38–47.

60. Kemp L. Adaptation and fidelity: A recipe analogy for achieving both in population scale implementation. *Prev Sci.* 2016;17(4):429–438.

61. Ringwalt CL, Ennett S, Johnson R, et al. Factors associated with fidelity to substance use prevention curriculum guides in the nation's middle schools. *Health Educ Behav.* 2003;30(3):375–391.

62. Carroll C, Patterson M, Wood S, Booth A, Rick J, Balain S. A conceptual framework for implementation fidelity. *Implement Sci.* 2007;2:40.

63. Dane AV, Schneider BH. Program integrity in primary and early secondary prevention: Are implementation effects out of control? *Clin Psychol Rev.* 1998;18(1):23–45.

64. Mihalic S. The importance of implementation fidelity. *Emotion Behav Disord Youth.* 2004;4(4):83–105.

65. Blase K, Fixsen D. Core intervention components: Identifying and operationalizing what makes programs work. ASPE Research Brief. Washington, DC: US Department of Health and Human Services; 2013.

66. Stirman SW, Miller CJ, Toder K, Calloway A. Development of a framework and coding system for modifications and adaptations of evidence-based interventions. *Implement Sci.* 2013;8(1):65.

67. Backer TE. *Finding the Balance: Program Fidelity and Adaptation in Substance Abuse Prevention: A State-of-the-Art Review.* Rockville, MD: US Department of Health and Human Services, Substance Abuse and Mental Health Services Administration, Center for Substance Abuse Prevention; 2001;1.

68. Escoffery C, Lebow-Skelley, E, Udelson, H, Boing, E, Fernandez, M, Wood, R, Mullen PD. A scoping study of frameworks for adapting evidence-based interventions. *Translational Behavioral Medicine.* 2018 Jan 16. doi:10.1093/tbm/ibx067. E Pub ahead of print.

69. Card JJ, Solomon J, Cunningham SD. How to adapt effective programs for use in new contexts. *Health Promot Pract.* 2011;12(1):25–35.

70. McKleroy VS, Galbraith JS, Cummings B, et al. Adapting evidence-based behavioral interventions for new settings and target populations. *AIDS Educ Prev.* 2006;18(4 Suppl A):59–73.

71. Rolleri LA, Fuller TR, Firpo-Triplett R, Lesesne CA, Moore C, Leeks KD. Adaptation guidance for evidence-based teen pregnancy and STI/HIV prevention curricula: From development to practice. *Am J Sex Educ.* 2014;9(2):135–154.

72. Solomon J, Card JJ, Malow RM. Adapting efficacious interventions: Advancing translational research in HIV prevention. *Eval Health Prof.* 2006;29(2):162–194.

73. Wingood GM, DiClemente RJ. The ADAPT-ITT model: A novel method of adapting evidence-based HIV Interventions. *J AIDS.* 2008;47(Suppl 1):S40–S46.

74. Chen EK, Reid MC, Parker SJ, Pillemer K. Tailoring evidence-based interventions for new populations: A method for program adaptation through community engagement. *Eval Health Prof.* 2013;36(1):73–92.

75. Bartholomew Eldredge LK, Markham CM, Kok G, Ruiter RA, Parcel GS. *Intervention Mapping Step 5: Program Implementation Plan.* San Francisco, CA: Jossey-Bass; 2016.

76. Kumpfer KL, Pinyuchon M, Teixeira de MA, Whiteside HO. Cultural adaptation process for international dissemination of the strengthening families program. *Eval Health Prof.* 2008;31(2):226–239.

77. Williams AB, Wang H, Burgess J, Li X, Danvers K. Cultural adaptation of an evidence-based nursing intervention to improve medication adherence among people living with HIV/AIDS (PLWHA) in China. *Int J Nurs Stud.* 2013;50(4):487–494.

78. Smith E, Caldwell L. Adapting evidence-based programs to new contexts: What needs to be changed? *J Rural Health.* 2007;23(s1):37–41.

79. Bartholomew LK, Fernandez M, James S, Leerlooijer J, Markham C, Reinders J, Mullen PD. Using Intervention Mapping to adapt evidence-based programs to new settings and populations. In: Bartholomew LK, Parcel GS, Kok G, Gottlieb NH, Fernandez ME. *Planning Health Promotion Programs: An Intervention Mapping Approach.* San Francisco: Jossey-Bass; 2011.

80. Bartholomew Eldredge LK, Highfield L, Hartman M, Mullen PD, Leerlooijer J, Fernandez M. Chp 10, Int Map Adapt: Using Intervention Mapping to adapt evidence-based interventions. In: Bartholomew Eldredge LK, Markham C, Ruiter RAC, Fernandez ME, Kok G, Parcel GS. *Planning Health Promotion Programs: An Intervention Mapping Approach.* San Francisco: Jossey-Bass. 2016.

81. Wiesner-Ceballos C, Cendales-Duarte R, Tovar-Murillo SL. Applying a cervical cancer

control model in Soacha, Colombia. *Rev Salud Publica*. 2008;10(5):691–705.

82. Israel B, Schulz A, Parker E, Becker A, Allen A, Guzman J. *Critical Issues in Developing and Following Community-Based Participatory Research Principles*. San Francisco, CA: Jossey-Bass; 2008.

83. Minkler M. *Community Organizing with the Elderly Poor in San Francisco's Tenderloin District*. Piscataway, NJ: Rutgers University Press; 2004.

84. Minkler M. Community-based research partnerships: Challenges and opportunities. *J Urban Health*. 2005;82(2 Suppl 2):ii3–12.

85. Wallerstein NB, Duran B. Using community-based participatory research to address health disparities. *Health Promot Pract*. 2006;7(3):312–323.

86. Green LW, Kreuter MW. *Health Program Planning: An Educational and Ecological Approach*. 3rd ed. Mountain View, CA: Mayfield; 1999.

87. Green LW, Kreuter MW. *Health Program Planning: An Educational and Ecological Approach*. 4th ed. New York: McGraw-Hill; 2005.

88. Green LW, Mercer SL. Can public health researchers and agencies reconcile the push from funding bodies and the pull from communities? *Am J Public Health*. 2001;91(12):1926–1929.

89. Balas EA, Boren SA. Managing clinical knowledge for health care improvement. *Yearb Med Inform*. 2000(1):65–70.

90. Glasgow RE, Emmons KM. How can we increase translation of research into practice? Types of evidence needed. *Annu Rev Public Health*. 2007;28:413–433.

91. Kerner J, Rimer B, Emmons K. Introduction to the special section on dissemination: Dissemination research and research dissemination: How can we close the gap? *Health Psychol*. 2005;24(5):443.

92. Klesges LM, Estabrooks PA, Dzewaltowski DA, Bull SS, Glasgow RE. Beginning with the application in mind: designing and planning health behavior change interventions to enhance dissemination. *Annals of Behavioral Medicine*. 2005 Apr 1;29(2):66–75.

93. Coughlin SS, Smith SA, Fernández ME. *Handbook of Community-Based Participatory Research*. New York: Oxford University Press; 2017.

94. Fernandez ME, Bartholomew LK, Vidrine JI, Reininger B, Kransy S, Wetter DW. *The Role of Translational Research in Behavioral Science and Public Health*. Hackensack, NJ: World Scientific; 2014.

95. Glasgow RE, Marcus AC, Bull SS, Wilson KM. Disseminating effective cancer screening interventions. *Cancer*. 2004;101(5 Suppl):1239–1250.

96. Wallerstein N, Duran B. Community-based participatory research contributions to intervention research: The intersection of science and practice to improve health equity. *Am J Public Health*. 2010;100(Suppl 1):S40–S46.

97. Havelock RG. The utilisation of educational research and development. *Br J Educ Technol*. 1971;2(2):84–98.

98. Orlandi MA. The diffusion and adoption of worksite health promotion innovations: An analysis of barriers. *Prev Med*. 1986;15(5):522–536.

99. Tabak RG, Khoong EC, Chambers DA, Brownson RC. Bridging research and practice: Models for dissemination and implementation research. *Am J Prev Med*. 2012;43(3):337–350.

100. Brownson RC, Jacobs JA, Tabak RG, Hoehner CM, Stamatakis KA. Designing for dissemination among public health researchers: Findings from a national survey in the United States. *Am J Public Health*. 2013;103(9):1693–1699.

101. Damschroder LJ, Aron DC, Keith RE, Kirsh SR, Alexander JA, Lowery JC. Fostering implementation of health services research findings into practice: A consolidated framework for advancing implementation science. *Implement Sci*. 2009;4(1):50.

102. Rogers EM. *Diffusion of Innovations*. 5th ed. New York: Free Press; 2003.

103. Glanz K, Rimer BK, Viswanath K. *Health Behavior and Health Education: Theory, Research, and Practice*. 4th ed. San Francisco, CA: Wiley; 2008.

104. Bartholomew Eldredge LK, Markham CM, Kok G, Ruiter RA, Parcel GS. *Intervention Mapping Step 2: Program Outcomes and Objectives—Logic Model of Change*. San Francisco, CA: Jossey-Bass; 2016.

3

THEORIES, FRAMEWORKS, AND MODELS IN IMPLEMENTATION SCIENCE IN CANCER

Ted A. Skolarus, Rachel G. Tabak, and Anne E. Sales

INTRODUCTION

There is growing recognition of the importance of implementation science across the continuum of cancer care.[1-4] Our evolving understanding of the richness of all phases of cancer care from prevention and diagnosis to treatment, survivorship, and palliation further supports the necessity of effective implementation if we are to translate research to practice for the benefit of cancer patients.[4] Indeed, as our paradigm shifts from basic and discovery-based research to include more clinical and translational research,[5] researchers, public health experts, and clinicians will need a variety of tools to implement effective innovations into a variety of complex contexts across the oncology continuum and delivery system. These tools include tailored interventions, multifaceted implementation strategies, process re-engineering, and even structural changes to the delivery system.[1,6] However, unless the building blocks for these implementation efforts are rooted in behavioral theories, conceptual models, and operational frameworks, the successes and failures of interventions in cancer prevention and care delivery will lack generalizability, limiting the capacity to advance implementation science and, more

important, steward resources to effectively improve cancer patient care across the continuum. The goals of this chapter are to introduce models, theories, and frameworks to the cancer community interested in implementation; discuss examples of their use; provide resources to help guide selection for cancer-related interventions; and highlight future directions to increase the impact of evidence-based practices across the cancer continuum, and ultimately decrease the burden of cancer.

IMPLEMENTATION THEORIES, MODELS, AND FRAMEWORKS ACROSS THE CANCER CARE CONTINUUM

Theories, models, and frameworks are increasingly recognized as critical instruments to the mission of implementation science.[1,7] We use the term "model" to encompass all three entities—theories, models, and frameworks—which play roles in supporting implementation science. Each of these distinct instruments serves as a resource for researchers to advance our understanding of complex interventions and how and why they succeed or fail. Moreover, as the constructs (building blocks) of these models become ingrained in everyday implementation practice, the benefits to implementation practitioners, as well as public health experts, oncology providers, and patients, include systematic approaches to planning, designing, implementing, and sustaining interventions in routine public health and oncology practice. These will be increasingly recognized, including the ability to predict implementation outcomes.

To begin, we describe each of these model categories (theory, model, and framework), followed by some approaches to conceptualize their use in implementation science and practice across the cancer control continuum. In many cases, these resources, especially frameworks, represent an amalgamation of theoretical constructs from social sciences, business, engineering, network theory, organizational theory, education theory, behavioral psychology, and marketing and economics, among others. Taking advantage of constructs across disciplines creates opportunities to hasten implementation efforts in complex cancer control and oncology care delivery contexts, as well as to learn about how best to describe, explain, and predict implementation outcomes.[6]

Although commonly referred to as interchangeable given their often overlapping domains, constructs, and considerations, it is important to note that theories, models, and frameworks are not synonymous. Moreover, a given model might be related more to dissemination, implementation, or treat both relatively equally. The constructs and factors making up a model might be flexible and broad versus operational and defined for a given oncology context and activity. The socioecologic level at which the model is targeted can vary from the individual, organization, and health care system levels to the community and policy levels, with many operating at more than one level. The current cadre of theories, models, and frameworks are increasingly dissected down to their core and adaptive components to identify causal relationships between their use and implementation outcomes.[7]

Figure 3.1 illustrates the cancer control continuum as endorsed by the National Cancer Institute (NCI), highlighting key focus areas of prevention, detection, diagnosis, treatment, and survivorship.[8] As shown in the figure and encountered in clinical practice, cross-cutting issues include communications, surveillance, decision-making, quality of care, and epidemiology. To conceptualize integration of implementation science models across this matrix, it is important to consider the socioecologic level and dissemination to implementation spectrum for cancer control implementation activities.[7] For example, implementation strategy targets can range from the individual level to the policy level and focus across the spectrum from dissemination to implementation. Therefore,

THE CANCER CONTROL CONTINUUM				
Focus				
PREVENTION	DETECTION	DIAGNOSIS	TREATMENT	SURVIVORSHIP
Tobacco control	Pap/HPV testing	Shared and informed decision making	Health care delivery and outcomes research	Coping
Diet	Mammography			Health promotion for survivors
Physical activity	Fecal occult blood test			
Sun protection	Colonoscopy			
HPV vaccine	Lung cancer screening			
Limited alcohol use				
Chemoprevention				
Crosscutting issues				
Communications				
Surveillance				
Social determinants of health disparities				
Genetic testing				
Decision-making				
Dissemination of evidence-based interventions				
Quality of cancer care				
Epidemiology				
Measurement				

FIGURE 3.1   The NCI cancer control continuum.[2]

Source: Adapted from David B. Abrams, Brown University School of Medicine.

implementation considerations are vast depending on the focus area of cancer control, cross-cutting issues, socioecologic level(s), and the implementation spectrum, necessitating significant early investment in a relevant implementation model (theory, model, and framework) and how it applies to a particular effort. For instance, if implementation is focused at the individual provider level to improve appropriate neoadjuvant chemotherapy administration, one might consider use of cognitive, educational, or stage of change theories depending on known or anticipated contextual barriers.[6] On the other hand, if the effort is targeting low rates of colon cancer screening at the organizational or population level, one might choose to base implementation in social network, organizational learning, process re-engineering, or economic theory depending on the resources and scope of one's efforts.[6] In some cases, multiple models are needed to capture the relevant predisposing, enabling, and reinforcing factors to implement and sustain innovation in cancer control and practice. Without systematic use and study of models to guide implementation activities, the likelihood that the oncology community can efficiently learn how best to address cancer control and cancer patient needs across the focus areas and cross-cutting issues is arguably low.

To help with understanding differences among theories, models, and frameworks as implementation instruments, we briefly define and discuss each here. *Theory* is defined as "a plausible or scientifically acceptable general principle or body of principles offered to explain phenomena."[9] Theory generally provides a structured means of understanding and explaining the world around us. Using theory in implementation science allows for description and explanation of relationships and events such as implementation or clinical outcomes, thereby facilitating prediction and causal inference. A *model* is defined as "a description or analogy used to help visualize something that cannot be directly observed."[9] In general, model use in implementation guides efforts to translate research into practice, often in practical steps, rather than emphasizing causal determinants as in theory. A *framework* is defined as "a basic conceptual structure (as of ideas)"[9] and perhaps the most descriptive of the model types. Many implementation science frameworks exist to describe and categorize factors believed to influence implementation outcomes.

Categorization of Implementation Theories, Models, and Frameworks

To help implementation researchers in selection and use of implementation models during their research, Tabak et al.[7] categorized 61 common theories, models, and frameworks according to their socioecologic level, construct flexibility, and dissemination to implementation focus. As shown in Table 3.1, the models' constructs range from broad to operational, and implementation activities range from dissemination to implementation. This review is an increasingly cited resource for the implementation science community given its comprehensive, pragmatic approach to categorization.

Another comprehensive effort sought to develop a taxonomy and guidance for implementation researchers and practitioners.[10] Nilsen identified three primary goals of using theories, models, and frameworks to guide implementation activities (Figure 3.2). First, they can be used to describe and guide the process of translating research into practice as *process models*. These theoretical approaches tend to specify steps in implementation activities. *Action models* are process models with more discrete guidance for planning an intervention or implementation strategy. Second, they can be used to understand and explain influences on implementation outcomes, retrospectively or prospectively, through understanding relationships among variables. The three categories included in this aim are *"classic"* *theories* from fields outside implementation science, such as the social sciences and psychology; *implementation theories* through adaptation of existing theoretical approaches or theories to understand implementation; and *determinant frameworks* of various domains and factors acting as barriers and facilitators influencing implementation outcomes. Third, they can be used as *evaluation frameworks* to determine aspects associated with implementation success or failure. Examples of implementation evaluation frameworks include RE-AIM (Reach, Effectiveness, Adoption, Implementation, Maintenance);[11] PRECEDE–PROCEED;[12] and a model by Proctor et al.[13] that draws distinctions between implementation, clinical, and Institute of Medicine service-related outcomes Table 3.2. Figure 3.2 illustrates these five categories of theoretical approaches used in implementation science. Using both of these resources can help with model selection as one decides a study question and goals for the implementation effort.

Table 3.1. Implementation Science Models According to Construct Flexibility and Dissemination & Implementation Focus

CONSTRUCT FLEXIBILITY	DISSEMINATION ONLY	DISSEMINATION AND IMPLEMENTATION			IMPLEMENTATION ONLY
		I > D	D > I	D = I	
Broad 1	1. Diffusion of Innovation 2. RAND Model of Persuasive Communication and Diffusion of Medical Innovation	—	1. Health Promotion Technology Transfer Process 2. Real-World Dissemination	—	—
2	1. Effective Dissemination Strategies 2. Model for Locally Based Research Transfer Development 3. Streams of Policy Process	1. A Framework for Spread 2. Collaborative Model for Knowledge Translation Between Research and Practice Settings 3. Coordinated Implementation Model 4. Framework for Analyzing Adoption of Complex Health Innovations 5–Model for Improving the Dissemination of Nursing Research	1. A Framework for the Transfer of Patient Safety Research into Practice 2. Interactive Systems Framework 3. Interacting Elements of Integrating Science, Policy, and Practice 4. Push–Pull Capacity Model 5. Research Development Dissemination & Utilization Framework 6. Utilization-Focused Surveillance Framework	1. FAB Model	—

3	1. A Conceptual Model of Knowledge Utilization 2. Conceptual Framework for Research Knowledge Transfer and Utilization 3. Conceptualizing Dissemination Research and Activity: Canadian Heart Health Initiative 4. Policy Framework for Increasing Diffusion of Evidence-Based Physical Activity Interventions	1. Framework for the Dissemination and Utilization of Research for Health-Care Policy and Practice 2. Framework of Dissemination in Health Services Intervention Research 3. Linking Systems Framework 4. Marketing and Distribution System for Public Health 5. OPTIONS Model	1. "4E" Framework for Knowledge Dissemination and Utilization 2. CRARUM 3. Davis' Pathman-PRECEED Model 4. Dissemination of Evidence-Based Interventions to Prevent Obesity 5. Knowledge Translation Model of TUMS 6. Multi-level Conceptual Framework of Organizational Innovation Adoption	1. Pathways to Evidence Informed Policy 2. Six-Step Framework for International Physical Activity Dissemination	1. Active Implementation Framework 2. An Organizational Theory of Innovation Implementation 3. Conceptual Model of Implementation Research 4. Implementation Effectiveness Model 5. Normalization Process Theory 6. PARIHS 7. Pronovost's 4E's Process Theory 8. Sticky Knowledge
4	1. Blueprint for Dissemination	1. Conceptual Model for the Diffusion of Innovations in Service Organizations 2. HPRC Framework 3. Knowledge Exchange Framework 4. Research Knowledge Infrastructure	1. OMRU 2. RE-AIM	1. CDC DHAP's Research-to-Practice Framework 2. PRISM	1. CFIR 2. REP Plus

(continued)

Table 3.1 Continued

CONSTRUCT FLEXIBILITY	DISSEMINATION ONLY	DISSEMINATION AND IMPLEMENTATION			IMPLEMENTATION ONLY
		I > D	D > I	D = I	
Operational 5	1. Framework for Knowledge Translation	1. A Convergent Diffusion and Social Marketing Approach for Dissemination 2. Framework for Dissemination of Evidence-Based Policy	1. PRECEDE–PROCEED	—	1. ARC Model 2. Conceptual Model of Evidence-Based Practice Implementation in Public Service Sectors

ARC, Availability, Responsiveness, and Continuity; CFIR, Consolidated Framework for Implementation Research; CRARUM, Critical Realism and the Arts Research Utilization Model; D, dissemination; DHAP, Divisions of HIV/AIDS Use and HIV Testing in Reducing HIV Risk Behavior and Prevention; D&I, dissemination and implementation; FAB, Facilitating Adoption of Best Practices; HPRC, Health Promotion Research Center; I, implementation; OMRU, Ottawa Model of Research Use; OPTIONS, OutPatient Treatment in Ontario Services; PARIHS, Promoting Action on Research Implementation in Health Services; PRISM, Practical, Robust Implementation and Sustainability Model; Pronovost's 4E's, engage, educate, execute, evaluate; RE-AIM, Reach, Effectiveness, Adoption, Implementation, Maintenance; REP Plus, Replicating Effective Programs Plus Framework; TUMS, Tehran University of Medical Sciences.

Source: Adapted from Tabak et al.[7]

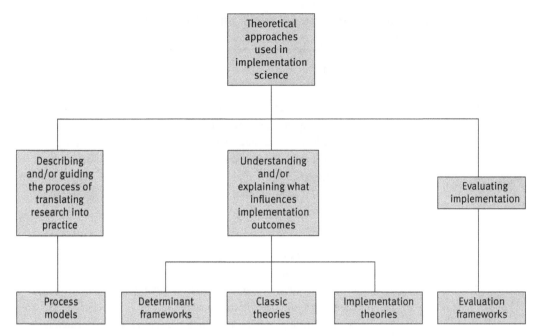

FIGURE 3.2 Aims and categories of theoretical approaches used in implementation science according to Nilsen.[10]

A Checklist for Determinants Frameworks

Although there are many uses for the other types of implementation frameworks described previously, *determinants frameworks* are particularly useful in supporting design of implementation strategies—interventions explicitly designed to overcome or resolve barriers to implementation of specific evidence-based practices or innovations or to maximize use of facilitators to implementation. For this purpose, determinants frameworks serve as checklists, sometimes organized or classified into specific groupings of determinants. The most notable and likely most useful determinants frameworks are those that consolidate findings from empirical research or related theories, often from what Nilsen[10] refers to as "classic theories"—those derived from disciplines that underlie implementation science, such as sociology, psychology, economics, and others (see Figure 3.2).

Three major consolidations of determinant frameworks are widely cited in the implementation science literature in health. One, originally published in 2005, consolidated more than 30 psychological theories related to health behavior change at the individual (patient) level.[14–16] This consolidation, the Theoretical Domains Framework (TDF), was subsequently revised through a process of engaging experts, and it now contains more than 90 constructs organized into 14 domains (knowledge, skills, social/professional role and identity, beliefs about capabilities, optimism, beliefs about consequences, reinforcement, intentions, goals, memory/attention/decision processes, environmental context and resources, social influences, emotions, and behavioral regulation).

The second,[17] published in 2009, consolidated a number of existing reviews and frameworks, notably Rogers' Diffusion of Innovation theory[18] and work led by Greenhalgh in the United Kingdom,[19] which covered factors affecting implementation in social service organizations. This framework, the Consolidated Framework for Implementation Research (CFIR), contains 39 constructs organized into five domains: (1) intervention characteristics (e.g., evidence, complexity, and relative advantage), (2) outer setting (e.g., peer pressure and external policies), (3) inner setting (e.g., structural characteristics, readiness for implementation, and culture), (4) individual characteristics (e.g., knowledge about intervention and self-efficacy), and (5) process (e.g.,

Table 3.2. Five Categories of Theories, Models, and Frameworks Used in Implementation Science

CATEGORY	DESCRIPTION
Process models	Specify steps (stages and phases) in the process of translating research into practice, including the implementation and use of research. The aim of process models is to describe and/or guide the process of translating research into practice. An action model is a type of process model that provides practical guidance in the planning and execution of implementation endeavors and/or implementation strategies to facilitate implementation. Note that the terms "model" and "framework" are both used, but the former appears to be the most common.
Determinant frameworks	Specify types (also known as classes or domains) of determinants and individual determinants, which act as barriers and enablers (independent variables) that influence implementation outcomes (dependent variables). Some frameworks also specify relationships between some types of determinants. The overarching aim is to understand and/or explain influences on implementation outcomes (e.g., predicting outcomes or interpreting outcomes, retrospectively).
Classic theories	Theories that originate from fields external to implementation science (e.g., psychology, sociology, and organizational theory), which can be applied to provide understanding and/or explanation of aspects of implementation.
Implementation theories	Theories that have been developed by implementation researchers (from scratch or by adapting existing theories and concepts) to provide understanding and/or explanation of aspects of implementation.
Evaluation frameworks	Specify aspects of implementation that could be evaluated to determine implementation success.

Source: Adapted from Nilsen.[10]

planning, engaging stakeholders, champions, and execution).[17]

The most recent consolidation of existing frameworks was published in 2013[20,21] and covers both the TDF and the CFIR, as well as 10 other existing determinants frameworks and reviews. This consolidation, the Tailoring Interventions for Chronic Disease (TICD) checklist, contains more than 50 factors or determinants organized into 12 domains. The fact that this is the most recent consolidation and also the fact that it includes both the TDF and the CFIR are important strengths of this determinants framework and make it an important option for using a single determinants framework rather than requiring use of multiple frameworks.

IMPLICATIONS OF IMPLEMENTATION MODEL USE IN CANCER CONTROL INTERVENTIONS AND PRECISION ONCOLOGY

The reasons to use theory-based implementation models in cancer control activities mirror those for other interventions in health; however, there are at least three unique aspects of cancer that need to be considered. First, the diagnosis of cancer is perhaps one of the most critical life events an individual may face.[22,23] The implications not only impact the individual but also impact family, friends, and providers, and the course of the individual's life is altered as he or she transitions through the continuum from patient to survivor. Mortality is immediately contemplated. Cancer is different from most other chronic conditions that patients must face and for which implementation activities are employed. Second, although cancer is in many cases a chronic disease—making the TICD checklist,[20] for example, seemingly appropriate for intervention planning—it is a unique chronic disease with novel, expensive, constantly emerging treatments with little regulation regarding cost and ultimately value to patients, health systems, and populations, thus making implementation of high-value, evidence-based practices critical.[4] Last, cancer is treated by specialists in collaboration with primary care clinicians, making it inherently multidisciplinary. Transitions in cancer care are arguably the most complex and burdensome to the delivery system, and implications for implementation need to be considered with even the most straightforward care coordination interventions.[3] Taken together, these unique aspects of cancer care make use of implementation theories, models, and frameworks critical to improving cancer-related patient and population health, especially if the investments in understanding implementation are to be generalizable across cancer types and chronic diseases more broadly.

Implementation models can be used to plan for dissemination and guide each step of the scientific and even operational processes across the continuum shown in Figure 3.1. They can guide the study questions (e.g., Should survivorship care plans be incorporated into electronic medical records and how?); study design (e.g., interrupted time series, stepped wedge, and cluster randomization); the implementation measures and outcomes at the patient, provider, system, organizational, and population levels; and ultimately inform implementation strategy selection. Moreover, theoretical frameworks are useful for designing implementation strategies. Mapping barriers and facilitators to theoretical constructs, and theoretical constructs to evidence-based interventions (e.g., lack of evidence knowledge to knowledge gap to education) to facilitate individual behavior change, can support effective implementation strategy development.[24,25] Using a combination of individual, organizational, and population-based frameworks may also guide implementation efforts at multiple socioecologic levels, allow for mapping of findings to key constructs, and advance cancer care and implementation science. For example, a recent systematic review identified 12 protocols and completed studies that used a combination of TDF and CFIR to examine a variety of implementation strategies across different socioecologic levels.[26]

Precision Oncology Requires Precision Implementation

The Precision Medicine Initiative (PMI) is a program funded by a $215 million investment in President Obama's fiscal year 2016 budget. Its goals are to accelerate biomedical research and provide clinicians with new tools to select the therapies that will work best in individual patients.[27] The PMI's $70 million in funding for NCI is being used to advance the field of precision oncology with a particular focus on genetically targeted therapies. The key areas of the PMI are (1) developing a national cancer knowledge system, (2) expanding precision medicine clinical trials, (3) overcoming drug resistance, and (4) developing new laboratory models for research. The focus of these four broad areas is the discovery of unique therapies to treat patients' cancer based on the genetics of their tumors. This precision oncology initiative is intended to "accelerate the pace of discovery, and bring additional benefits to cancer patients."[27]

However, bringing these benefits to patients ultimately requires precision implementation across a variety of contexts, patients, and cancer types. Using implementation science models is critical to precision implementation to help guide the design and scope of the study, focus the study questions and hypotheses, understand how to select and measure clinical and implementation outcomes, and tailor implementation strategies to individual settings to benefit cancer patients. Using implementation science models to frame these implementation activities can help explain why the genetically targeted therapies borne out of this program do or do not work in real-world practice settings or at a population level. Moreover, advancing implementation science requires understanding how and why implementation strategies succeed and fail and also how to overcome voltage drop in effectiveness across clinical settings.[28] Precision implementation requires that these implementation strategies be grounded in theoretical approaches with selected constructs and measures that are able to account for a combination of factors impacting local implementation and that help determine how to select strategies focused on those factors acting as barriers and facilitators to evidence-based oncology practice.

Melding the Study Question and Implementation Model Selection

The active interplay between the study question and implementation model selection is necessary early in the study process to guide implementation efforts.[6] What is the socio-ecologic level target for the implementation strategy? Is this a dissemination- or implementation- focused cancer-related activity? Is the purpose of the study to translate research into practice after a Phase III clinical trial of a novel immunotherapy for pancreatic cancer in need of a process model, to evaluate implementation of survivorship care plans in hospitals participating in the American College of Surgeons Commission on Cancer Program, or to promote population-based sun protection best practices? The answers to these core questions can be complicated, creating challenges for model selection and use before, during, and after the implementation strategy. Fortunately, the results of efforts to clarify characteristics of theories, models, and frameworks in terms of their aims, taxonomy, socioecologic level, focus along the dissemination to implementation spectrum, flexibility of constructs, and determinants of clinical practice are now available to help practitioners and investigators with regard to their study questions (see Figure 3.2).

Guiding Study Design

After defining the study question and identifying candidate models for a study, learning more about the possible models and their use can help clarify possible study designs. For example, if the study question pertains to dissemination of an evidence-based colon cancer screening program among primary care practices in an integrated delivery system, learning more about dissemination models with operational-focused constructs and prior studies using these models can inform study design (e.g., the Blueprint for Dissemination[29] and the Conceptual Model for the Diffusion of Innovations in Service Organizations[19]). Indeed, a review of four national quality campaigns to improve evidence-based practices in cardiology, home health, and patient safety informed the Blueprint for Dissemination framework and its eight strategies.[29] In addition to helping tailor implementation strategies based on lessons learned from the studies informing this framework, study design and who to include in the study sample can also be informed. For example, there was continuous enrollment in the aforementioned national campaigns.

Choosing Outcomes

Implementation outcomes as distinctly defined by Proctor et al.[13] (acceptability, adoption, appropriateness, feasibility, fidelity, implementation cost, penetration, and sustainability) are commonly used in implementation science and practice. However, primary and secondary outcomes should also be based on what the model states is important to consider—for example, using the TDF[16] to measure determinants of adjuvant hormonal therapy in a study of breast cancer survivors or using the Health Belief Model[30] domains to understand cervical cancer screening patterns in anticipation of interventions. Study outcomes can also be related to processes, from the number of enrolled organizations to adoption of recommended practices. Moreover, implementation outcomes can be more or less the focus in combination with other service-related and clinical outcomes using hybrid study designs, as discussed elsewhere in this book.[31]

Selection and Tailoring of Implementation Strategies

As alluded to previously, one of the major implementation challenges is selection and tailoring of implementation strategies to context. Characterizing this context and the potential problematic areas facing implementation using theories, models, and frameworks to guide strategy selection and tailoring offers a structured means to address this complicated process. Moreover, as highlighted by Grol et al.[6] and in the Medical Research Council guidance statements,[32] robust pilot work and planning are necessary for the formative evaluation[33] and implementation strategy development very early on in implementation efforts. Basing this activity in theoretical approaches, as suggested by Nilsen[10] and others, can facilitate planning for dissemination and sustainability. In addition, using these models can help identify pitfalls and effective evidence-based strategies to address the most important barriers. In essence, an implementation model can identify areas that might be problematic and help select strategies to address those challenges. As discussed next, a growing experience with cancer-related interventions in implementation science provides unique resources and perspectives for implementation across the cancer control continuum.

CANCER-FOCUSED IMPLEMENTATION STUDIES ACROSS THE CONTINUUM

This section discusses examples of how various theories, frameworks, and models have been used within cancer-focused implementation studies.

Skin Cancer Prevention

The use of multiple theories, models, and frameworks to design, disseminate and implement a cancer prevention trial is demonstrated by the Pool Cool Diffusion Trial.[35,36] Glanz et al. developed this three-level cluster-randomized study grounded in individual and organizational theoretical constructs to understand implementation, maintenance, and sustainability of the program, changes to organizational context, and child sun protection patterns and sunburn in outdoor swimming pools. In the experimental condition, implementation strategies to increase use of Pool Cool included incentives, reinforcement, feedback, and skill building. The study was positive for the enhanced condition, which demonstrated greater program maintenance during three summer participation periods and indicated that higher intensity, theory-based implementation strategies can improve implementation and maintenance of cancer prevention activities. A process evaluation evaluated the implementation strategies and outcomes, including those related to staff training, a toolkit regarding program implementation, use of laminated lesson cards and cartoons to support sun protection activities, as well as environmental changes such as the use of a large sunscreen dispenser and tips signs. The toolkit, ease of implementation, and enjoyment of the program by children and staff supported program diffusion.[37]

Colon Cancer and Lynch Syndrome Screening

Lynch syndrome is the most common cause of hereditary colorectal cancer, and universal tumor screening for this syndrome is increasingly endorsed. However, variation exists in subsequent genetic counseling and germ line testing after a positive screening result. Using two complementary frameworks, RE-AIM and CFIR, to guide the survey and interview guide content, Cragun et al.[38] conducted a multiple case study with qualitative comparative analysis examining adoption, implementation, and effectiveness of universal tumor screening programs across several institutions. The results were mapped to RE-AIM dimensions and indicated that involvement of genetic counselors in the testing process and reducing barriers to patient contact can increase patient follow-through with this recommended practice.

Addressing Disparities in Mammography Screening

Given Korean American women have low rates of breast cancer screening with mammography, Maxwell et al.[39] developed a theory-based Korean-language print intervention to increase mammography screening with a plan for scale-up through the National Breast and Cervical Cancer Early Detection Program (NBCCEDP). After formative evaluation and development based on constructs from the Health Behavior Framework, the Health Belief Model, and the theory of planned behavior, the intervention was pilot tested in a community clinic in Koreatown, Los Angeles County, where mammograms were provided free of charge through support from the NBCCEDP. Using the RE-AIM framework to examine implementation outcomes, the investigators identified a slight increase in annual screening of 6%, and a post-intervention survey indicated one-third of patients remembered getting the brochure and slightly more than half had appropriate addresses documented. The pilot study indicated that using NBCCEDP to disseminate print materials was feasible; however, the incorrect address information limited the intervention's reach and effectiveness. This study underscores the importance of intervention planning, pilot testing, and using an evaluation framework to help the oncology and implementation communities better understand barriers with respect to decreasing disparities in breast cancer screening, as well as promote generalizable implementation knowledge.

Using the Theoretical Domains Framework to Understand Cancer Staging and Survivorship Care Plans

Overuse in cancer care is increasingly relevant given costs and the expanding resources to stage and treat cancer as well as to conduct cancer surveillance. Implications of overuse include incidental findings leading to further testing in asymptomatic patients. To better understand overuse in prostate cancer staging, Makarov et al.[40] used TDF to explore linkages between themes from interviews with prostate cancer patients and their providers and TDF domains with respect to imaging (e.g., computerized tomography scan and bone scan) to search for metastatic disease spread at diagnosis. The investigators found that patient goals focused on disease treatment rather than staging and that many lacked *knowledge* about whether staging was performed. Patients' *beliefs about capabilities* tended to rely on the providers to make decisions about staging, and their *emotions* and anxiety about prostate cancer outweighed fears of radiation exposure from excessive staging. On the other hand, physician interviews were distilled into five TDF domains, including *knowledge* about the guideline recommendations for staging and their clinical experiences supporting their *beliefs about capabilities* with regard to recommended testing. Physicians also noted *beliefs about consequences* of not staging with respect to medicolegal implications, *social influences* of colleagues who tended to overuse staging imaging, and the *environmental context* of their facility. Based on this work, the investigators concluded that physicians are the primary decision-makers with regard to prostate cancer staging, indicating physician-targeted implementation strategies targeting the identified domains may improve concordance with prostate cancer staging and imaging guidelines to minimize overuse.

Survivorship care plans (SCPs) are increasingly recommended as part of quality oncologic care and required to meet the American College of Surgeons Commission on Cancer accreditation standards. These clinical documents include cancer treatment summaries, plans for cancer surveillance, and information on long-term and late effects of cancer and its treatments for patients and their providers.[3] However, SCP uptake in clinical practice has been poor, with a variety of barriers and determinants examined.[41-43] Using TDF to better characterize these barriers and inform implementation strategy development through mapping to evidence-based behavior change techniques, Birken et al.[42] discovered a variety of domains and constructs that could be targeted to promote SCP use moving forward. Relevant domains included health care professionals' beliefs about the consequences of SCP use, the motivation and goals of SCP implementation, how environmental context and resources enable use, and the social influences prompting SCP use. Using qualitative analyses, the

investigators mapped beliefs onto TDF constructs, including outcome expectations, intrinsic motivation, goal priority, resources, leadership, and teamwork. Taken together, these comprehensive approaches serve as prototypes for theory-based barrier assessment using a determinants framework to explain current challenges and to inform future implementation efforts.

Improving Implementation of Palliative Care

Using an integrative literature review approach, van Riet Paap et al.[44] examined implementation strategies to improve palliative care across 68 experimental and quasi-experimental studies. Although most studies demonstrated positive effects ($n = 53$), a variety of implementation strategies were found to be effective, including education, process mapping, feedback, multidisciplinary meetings, and multifaceted implementation strategies. The results of this review were used to inform the European Union's Seventh Framework IMPACT (IMplementation of quality indicators for PAlliative Care sTudy) study across 40 palliative care services in Europe according to the implementation of change model characterized by preparation, planning, and executing an implementation process.[6]

RESOURCES AND FUTURE EFFORTS

Building Implementation Science Capacity in Cancer Care and Use of Theories, Models, and Frameworks

Although there are examples of using theories, models, and frameworks to guide implementation activities in cancer control and care, much more needs to be done to build our evidence base and advance the field. One barrier is expertise in implementation science given it is an emerging field with the majority of experience outside of cancer-related interventions, with exceptions in tobacco control and other public health prevention strategies loosely tied to the cancer delivery system. Fortunately, leaders in implementation science have developed a program to build capacity in cancer prevention and control with the support of NCI and the Veterans Health Administration. The Mentored Training for Dissemination and Implementation Research in

Cancer (MT-DIRC) program aims to develop and refine a set of competencies and model curriculum in implementation science through enrolling post-doctoral applicants across various cancer-related disciplines in a 2-year fellowship program (http://mtdirc.org). Its goals include building capacity to conduct high-quality implementation science through state-of-the-art methods, including use of implementation theories, models, and frameworks, to ultimately speed translation of research to practice in cancer prevention and control. As part of this program, the next generation of cancer-focused implementation researchers are being produced, with more than 40 fellows in the first three fellow classes. Although this unique program is dependent on cyclical grant funding, the significant investment in implementation science by the funding agencies, faculty, and fellows is already contributing to advancing our understanding of theory-based approaches to improving cancer care.[38,40,45-47]

More broadly, NCI and its Implementation Science team in the Division of Cancer Control and Population Sciences provide a variety of tools and resources to advance implementation science and practice (https://cancercontrol.cancer.gov/IS/tools/research.html).[2] The tools included on the website are intended to assist implementation researchers to plan and conduct rigorous implementation studies in cancer care, including through the use of theories, models, and frameworks as discussed in this chapter. As part of their efforts, the NCI team also facilitated the development of an interactive website titled "Dissemination and Implementation Models in Health Research and Practice" (http://dissemination-implementation.org) based on the 61 theories, models, and frameworks from the 2012 review by Tabak et al.[7] and work by Mitchell et al.[48] This rich resource serves to assist implementation researchers and practitioners with model selection, adaptation, integration, and measurement of model constructs. Several other resources are available to help guide implementation instrument selection, including the Veteran Affairs' Quality Enhancement Research Initiative (http://www.queri.research.va.gov/implementation/default.cfm), the Training Institute for Dissemination and Implementation Research in Health (https://obssr.od.nih.gov/training/training-institutes/training-institute-on-dissemination-and-implementation-research-tidirh), and the Canadian Knowledge Translation Clearinghouse (http://ktclearinghouse.ca/ktcanada).

Collaboration to Support the Use of Theories, Models, and Frameworks in Cancer Care

As the capacity to conduct high-quality implementation studies across the cancer control continuum builds, collaboration across researchers, institutions, and funding agencies can help synergize these activities to hasten our understanding of how to translate research to practice across the cancer continuum. This collaboration can lead to work across various cancer types, from breast, lung, colon, and prostate cancer to more rare cancer types such as pancreatic and brain cancer, to build understanding of barriers and enablers to quality cancer care and population-based prevention and early detection in a generalizable manner. This also pertains to selection and use of implementation models because perhaps some are particularly well-suited to cancer-related implementation studies. Other opportunities for collaboration include working with colleagues involved in clinical trials to study implementation alongside randomized clinical trials to support planning for scale-up.[49] Finally, empirical testing of theories, models, and frameworks and their constructs can be facilitated through collaboration to ultimately help with prediction of how best to disseminate and implement innovations across the cancer care continuum.

Implementation of Patient-Reported Outcomes into Clinical Practice

Patient-reported outcomes (PROs) for cancer care are increasingly called for by patients, providers, and advocacy groups, with anticipation that payers and policymakers will soon be on board, thus raising the stakes for this complex aspect of cancer care delivery and its effective implementation into routine clinical practice. There is extensive operational and administrative effort to better understand and implement PROs across a variety of clinical contexts, institutions, and national oncology organizations. Both the National Institutes of Health, through its significant investment in the Patient-Reported Outcomes Measurement Information System (PROMIS) to support PRO measurement,[50] and the American Society of Clinical Oncology, through its dedicated PRO work group for oncology-based care,[51] are building the knowledge base around process and outcome measures for PROs. However, currently, there are no broad standards for development or implementation of PRO measures into clinical care. Planning for dissemination and implementation will be critical to the successful downstream efforts to implement these measures and conduct comparative effectiveness studies not only of their impact on clinical delivery system and patient outcomes but also of different theory-based interventions and implementation strategies on implementation outcomes. In particular, opportunities include add-on studies to PRO-based clinical trials to examine and potentially compare different implementation strategies, as well as formative and process evaluations based on the current cadre of theories, models, and frameworks to build our understanding of the best approaches to effective PRO implementation.

De-implementation to Decrease Low-Value Cancer Care

Unlearning routinized clinical practices is challenging even if they are no longer or never were considered effective.[52] This is particularly true with regard to treating patients with cancer, where provider reluctance to hold off on treatments is often a significant barrier to stopping or not initiating treatments, even when there are no symptoms. De-implementation, or stopping practices that are not evidence-based, has tremendous potential to improve patient outcomes and mitigate rising health care costs.[53,54] This is important given recent campaign attempts, including Choosing Wisely, to curb overuse of services. However, the best theories, models, and frameworks for de-implementation strategies in cancer care remain a work-in-progress with tremendous potential to improve quality and cost of care.

Measurement Across Models in Cancer Care Implementation

As discussed in Chapter 4, solidifying our understanding and systematic use of implementation measures and constructs is vital to advancing implementation science and practice. As the cancer community increases use and documentation of theories, models, and frameworks, we will be able to increase our understanding of the relationship to clinical and implementation outcomes across the cancer continuum and guide next-generation implementation efforts.

SUMMARY

In this chapter, we described implementation theories, models, and frameworks and justified their systematic use to build our understanding of implementation across the cancer care continuum and ultimately facilitate our stewardship of effective cancer care and spending across complex clinical and public health contexts. We offered several previously developed taxonomy and categorization schemes as well as resources to aid implementation researchers and practitioners in their implementation efforts. We discussed the importance of precision implementation using systematic theoretical approaches to coincide with precision oncology efforts and funding. After providing concrete examples of theory, model, and framework use across the continuum from prevention to palliative care, we highlighted relevant implementation science opportunities for collaboration, patient-reported outcomes research, de-implementation, and measurement with respect to these models as future directions. As our implementation science capacity builds in the oncology community, we construct a case for systematic use of theories, models, and frameworks in implementation science and practice.

REFERENCES

1. Brownson R, Colditz G, Proctor E, eds. *Dissemination and Implementation Research in Health: Translating Science to Practice.* New York: Oxford University Press; 2012.
2. National Cancer Institute. Implementation science. https://cancercontrol.cancer.gov/IS. Accessed January 5, 2017.
3. Committee on Cancer Survivorship: Improving Care and Quality of Life, National Cancer Policy Board; Hewitt M, Greenfield S, and Stovall E, eds. *From Cancer Patient to Cancer Survivor: Lost in Transition.* Washington, DC: National Academies Press; 2005.
4. Institute of Medicine. *Delivering High-Quality Cancer Care: Charting a New Course for a System in Crisis.* Washington, DC: National Academies Press; 2013.
5. Westfall JM, Mold J, Fagnan L. Practice-based research—"Blue highways" on the NIH roadmap. *JAMA.* 2007;297(4):403–406.
6. Grol R, Wensing M, Eccles M. *Improving Patient Care: The Implementation of Change in Clinical Practice.* New York: Elsevier; 2005.
7. Tabak RG, Khoong EC, Chambers DA, Brownson RC. Bridging research and

practice: Models for dissemination and implementation research. *Am J Prev Med.* 2012;43(3):337–350.

8. National Cancer Institute. Cancer control continuum. https://cancercontrol.cancer.gov/od/continuum.html. Accessed January 5, 2017.

9. Merriam–Webster. *The Merriam–Webster Dictionary.* https://www.merriam-webster.com. Accessed January 5, 2017.

10. Nilsen, P. Making sense of implementation theories, models and frameworks. *Implement Sci.* 2015;10:53.

11. Glasgow RE, Vogt TM, Boles SM. Evaluating the public health impact of health promotion interventions: The RE-AIM framework. *Am J Public health.* 1999;89(9):1322–1327.

12. Green LW, Kreuter MW, Green LW. *Health Program Planning: An Educational and Ecological Approach.* 4th ed. New York: McGraw-Hill; 2005.

13. Proctor E, Silmere H, Raghavan R, et al. Outcomes for implementation research: Conceptual distinctions, measurement challenges, and research agenda. *Adm Policy Ment Health.* 2011;38(2):65–76.

14. French SD, Green SE, O'Connor DA, et al. Developing theory-informed behaviour change interventions to implement evidence into practice: A systematic approach using the theoretical domains framework. *Implement Sci.* 2012;7:38.

15. Michie S, Johnston M, Abraham C, et al. Making psychological theory useful for implementing evidence based practice: A consensus approach. *Qual Saf Health Care.* 2005;14(1):26–33.

16. Cane J, O'Connor D, Michie S. Validation of the theoretical domains framework for use in behaviour change and implementation research. *Implement Sci.* 2012;7:37.

17. Damschroder LJ, Aron DC, Keith RE, Kirsh SR, Alexander JA, Lowery JC. Fostering implementation of health services research findings into practice: A consolidated framework for advancing implementation science. *Implement Sci.* 2009;7(4):50.

18. Rogers EM. *Diffusion of Innovations.* New York: Free Press of Glencoe; 1962.

19. Greenhalgh T, Robert G, Macfarlane F, Bate P, Kyriakidou O. Diffusion of innovations in service organizations: Systematic review and recommendations. *Milbank Q.* 2004;82(4):581–629.

20. Flottorp SA, Oxman AD, Krause J, et al. A checklist for identifying determinants of practice: A systematic review and synthesis of frameworks and taxonomies of factors that prevent or enable improvements in healthcare professional practice. *Implement Sci.* 2013;8:35.

21. Wensing M, Oxman A, Baker R, et al. Tailored Implementation for Chronic Diseases (TICD): A project protocol. *Implement Sci.* 2011;6:103.

22. The C word. http://thecwordmovie.com. Accessed January 5, 2017.

23. Institute of Medicine. *Cancer Care for the Whole Patient: Meeting Psychosocial Health Needs.* Washington, DC: National Academies Press; 2008.

24. Michie S, Atkins L, West R. *The Behaviour Change Wheel: A Guide to Designing Interventions.* London: Silverback; 2014.

25. French SD, Green SE, O'Connor DA, et al. Developing theory-informed behaviour change interventions to implement evidence into practice: A systematic approach using the theoretical domains framework. *Implement Sci.* 2012;7(1):38.

26. Birken SA, Powell BJ, Presseau J, et al. Combined use of the Consolidated Framework for Implementation Research (CFIR) and the Theoretical Domains Framework (TDF): A systematic review. *Implement Sci.* 2017;12(1):2.

27. National Cancer Institute. NCI and the Precision Medicine Initiative. https://www.cancer.gov/research/key-initiatives/precision-medicine. Accessed January 5, 2017.

28. Chambers DA, Glasgow RE, Stange KC. The dynamic sustainability framework: Addressing the paradox of sustainment amid ongoing change. *Implement Sci.* 2013;8:117.

29. Yuan CT, Nembhard IM, Stern AF, Brush JE, Jr, Krumholz HM, Bradley EH. Blueprint for the dissemination of evidence-based practices in health care. *Issue Brief (Commonw Fund).* 2010;86:1–16.

30. Janz NK, Becker MH. The Health Belief Model: A decade later. *Health Educ Q.* 1984;11(1):1–47.

31. Curran GM, Bauer M, Mittman B, Pyne JM, Stetler C. Effectiveness–implementation hybrid designs: Combining elements of clinical effectiveness and implementation research to enhance public health impact. *Med Care.* 2012;50(3):217–226.

32. Craig P, Dieppe P, Macintyre S, et al. Developing and evaluating complex interventions: The new Medical Research Council guidance. *BMJ.* 2008;337:a1655.

33. Stetler CB, Legro MW, Wallace CM, et al. The role of formative evaluation in implementation

research and the QUERI experience. *J Gen Intern Med.* 2006;21(Suppl 2):S1–S8.

34. Kegler MC, Bundy L, Haardorfer R, et al. A minimal intervention to promote smoke-free homes among 2-1-1 callers: A randomized controlled trial. *Am J Public Health.* 2015;105(3):530–537.

35. Glanz K, Geller AC, Shigaki D, Maddock JE, Isnec MR. A randomized trial of skin cancer prevention in aquatics settings: The Pool Cool program. *Health Psychol.* 2002;21(6):579–587.

36. Glanz K, Escoffery C, Elliott T, Nehl EJ. Randomized trial of two dissemination strategies for a skin cancer prevention program in aquatic settings. *Am J Public Health.* 2015;105(7):1415–1423.

37. Escoffery C, Glanz K, Elliott T. Process evaluation of the Pool Cool Diffusion Trial for skin cancer prevention across 2 years. *Health Educ Res.* 2008;23(4):732–743.

38. Cragun D, DeBate RD, Vadaparampil ST, Baldwin J, Hampel H, Pal T. Comparing universal Lynch syndrome tumor-screening programs to evaluate associations between implementation strategies and patient follow-through. *Genet Med.* 2014;16(10):773–782.

39. Maxwell AE, Jo AM, Chin SY, Lee KS, Bastani R. Impact of a print intervention to increase annual mammography screening among Korean American women enrolled in the National Breast and Cervical Cancer Early Detection Program. *Cancer Detect Prev.* 2008;32(3):229–235. doi:10.1016/j.cdp.2008.04.003. Epub 2008 Sep 16.

40. Makarov DV, Sedlander E, Braithwaite RS, et al. A qualitative study to understand guideline-discordant use of imaging to stage incident prostate cancer. *Implement Sci.* 2016;11(1):118.

41. Birken SA, Deal AM, Mayer DK, Weiner BJ. Determinants of survivorship care plan use in US cancer programs. *J Cancer Educ.* 2014;29(4):720–727.

42. Birken SA, Presseau J, Ellis SD, Gerstel AA, Mayer DK. Potential determinants of health-care professionals' use of survivorship care plans: A qualitative study using the theoretical domains framework. *Implement Sci.* 2014;9:167.

43. Birken SA, Mayer DK, Weiner BJ. Survivorship care plans: Prevalence and barriers to use. *J Cancer Educ.* 2013;28(2):290–296.

44. van Riet Paap J, Vernooij-Dassen M, Sommerbakk R, et al. Implementation of

improvement strategies in palliative care: An integrative review. *Implement Sci.* 2015;10:103.

45. Koczwara B, Birken SA, Perry CK, et al. How context matters: A dissemination and implementation primer for global oncologists. *J Global Oncol.* 2016;2(2):51–55.

46. Cragun D, Pal T, Vadaparampil ST, Baldwin J, Hampel H, DeBate RD. Qualitative comparative analysis: A hybrid method for identifying factors associated with program effectiveness. *J Mix Methods Res.* 2016;10(3):251–272.

47. Selove R, Birken SA, Skolarus TA, Hahn EE, Sales A, Proctor EK. Using implementation science to examine the impact of cancer survivorship care plans. *J Clin Oncol.* 2016;34(32):3834–3837.

48. Mitchell SA, Fisher CA, Hastings CE, Silverman LB, Wallen GR. A thematic analysis of theoretical models for translational science in nursing: Mapping the field. *Nurs Outlook.* 2010;58(6):287–300.

49. Brownson RC, Jacobs JA, Tabak RG, Hoehner CM, Stamatakis KA. Designing for dissemination among public health researchers: Findings from a national survey in the United States. *Am J Public Health.* 2013;103(9):1693–1699.

50. HealthMeasures. PROMIS (Patient-Reported Outcomes Measurement Information System). http://www.nihpromis.com. Accessed January 5, 2017.

51. Basch E, Snyder C, McNiff K, et al. Patient-reported outcome performance measures in oncology. *J Oncol Pract.* 2014;10(3):209–211.

52. Rushmer R, Davies HT. Unlearning in health care. *Qual Saf Health Care.* 2004;13(Suppl 2):ii10–ii15.

53. Montini T, Graham ID. "Entrenched practices and other biases": Unpacking the historical, economic, professional, and social resistance to de-implementation. *Implement Sci.* 2015;10:24.

54. Prasad V, Ioannidis JP. Evidence-based de-implementation for contradicted, unproven, and aspiring healthcare practices. *Implement Sci.* 2014;9:1.

55. National Cancer Institute. Grid Enabled Measures (GEM) database. https://www.gem-beta.org/Public/Home.aspx. Accessed January 5, 2017.

4

MEASURES AND OUTCOMES IN IMPLEMENTATION SCIENCE

Cara C. Lewis, Kayne D. Mettert, Caitlin N. Dorsey, and Bryan J. Weiner

EVALUATING IMPLEMENTATION OUTCOMES

The past several decades of intervention science resulted in hundreds of evidence-based behavioral interventions and clinical services, which we refer to collectively as evidence-based interventions (EBIs), for the prevention, diagnosis, treatment, survivorship, and palliative care needs of cancer patients. EBIs such as the Motivation and Problem Solving (MAPS) intervention (prevention),[1] functional imaging (diagnosis),[2] radiation therapy[3]/chemotherapy (treatment),[4] routine magnetic resonance imaging surveillance (survivorship),[5] and bereavement interventions (palliative care)[6,7,8] demonstrate marked improvements in clinical outcomes such as cancer incidence, early detection, morbidity, mortality, and quality of life, as well as service outcomes such as efficiency, safety, effectiveness, equity, patient-centeredness,

and timeliness (Figure 4.1).[9] Only recently has the focus shifted to the development and evaluation of strategies for implementing these EBIs in "real-world" settings to benefit the people for which they were created. As a new field, implementation science has identified its own set of outcomes for determining "success,"[10,11] beyond the clinical and service outcomes listed previously. This isolation and concrete operationalization of implementation outcomes importantly focuses on multiple, nested levels of analysis (e.g., individual, group, organization, and environment) that, in turn, affect outcomes at the lowest levels (e.g., consumer; see Table 4.1).[12] Accordingly, it is believed that an EBI will have the intended effect on clinical and service outcomes if implemented with "success." That is, the implementation strategies utilized and the clinical intervention should be viewed as separate, each with a distinct set of outcomes.

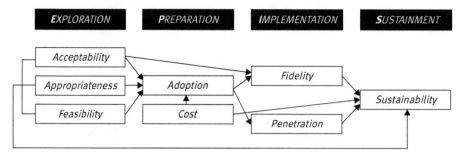

| EXPLORATION | PREPARATION | IMPLEMENTATION | SUSTAINMENT |

FIGURE 4.1   Temporal depiction of implementation outcomes as they intersect with EPIS. The relations among the implementation outcomes as depicted by the arrows are supported by extant research.[13–19]

Proctor and colleagues[10] put forth the Implementation Outcomes Framework (IOF) that conceptualizes the variables of interest in an implementation evaluation. This framework culminated from stage-pipeline models of change, multilevel models of change, and models of health service use. An extensive literature review was conducted to identify and synthesize prominent terms and themes surrounding key implementation concepts, with careful attention paid to definitional issues to avoid conflation or redundancy. The IOF was first introduced in 2009 with seven core outcomes (i.e., *acceptability, feasibility, uptake, penetration, cost, fidelity,* and *sustainment*), with a revision in 2011 that added *appropriateness* and renamed *uptake* as *adoption*. Importantly, the IOF provides a necessary common vernacular that, if used in implementation evaluations, has the potential to support the generation of cumulative knowledge allowing for fluent communication of findings across studies, contexts, and time. These eight outcomes are now viewed as the foundation of implementation science because they are what we seek to impact.

To evaluate the impact of a set of implementation strategies, separate from the effect of the EBI (the clinical intervention), quality measures of implementation outcomes across multiple levels of analysis are needed. At least 12 systematic reviews of measures of implementation-relevant constructs have been published.[20] Although each study has differed in its scope (e.g., mental health,[21] business,[22] and education/health[12]) and focus (e.g., predictors of adoption[23] and levels of

analysis[24]), a common finding has emerged: There is a dearth of high-quality measures for the study of implementation. There are (at least) three reasons for this state of the literature: (1) The field is so new that there simply has not been enough time for sufficient measure development; (2) researchers do not conduct psychometric testing, leaving a pool of unvalidated measures; and (3) existing measures perform poorly on tests of psychometrics.

Only one study has examined the state of measurement for implementation outcomes, albeit those emerging from the field of mental health. C. C. Lewis, Fischer, and colleagues[21] identified 104 measures of the eight variables in the IOF and subjected each to an evidence-based assessment rating process, which revealed profiles reflecting psychometric strength along the following dimensions: internal consistency, structural validity, predictive validity, norms, responsiveness, and usability. Similar to measures of other implementation-relevant constructs, information regarding psychometric properties of the IOF measures was limited and variable. Only a single measure had literature reporting information for all six of the evidence-based assessment rating criteria (Table 4.2). Of the remaining 103 measures, 4% were missing information for one criterion, 20% were missing information for two criteria, 29% were missing information for three criteria, and 46% were missing information for four or more criteria. In other words, nearly half of these instruments reported nothing pertaining to four of the six rating criteria. In terms of each specific criterion, 51% of

Table 4.1. Implementation Outcomes, Levels of Analysis, and Assessment

IMPLEMENTATION OUTCOME	LEVEL OF ANALYSIS				ASSESSMENT	
	PATIENT	FAMILY	PROVIDER	ORGANIZATION	EXAMPLE METHODS OF MEASUREMENT	EXAMPLE MEASURE
Acceptability	X	X	X		Surveys Key informant interviews Administrative data	Abernethy et al.[25]
Adoption			X	X	Surveys Observation Key informant interviews Focus groups Administrative data	Allen et al.[26]
Appropriateness	X		X	X	Surveys Key informant interviews Focus groups	Bloch[27]
Feasibility			X	X	Surveys Administrative data	Adelson et al.[28]
Fidelity			X		Observation Checklists Content analyses Self-report	Bast et al.[29]
Cost			X	X	Administrative data	Lairson, Huo, Ricks, Savas, and Fernandez[30]
Penetration				X	Surveys Case studies Key informant interviews	Steckler et al.[31]
Sustainability				X	Surveys Case studies Record and policy reviews Key informant interviews	Honeycutt, Carvalho, Glanz, Daniel, and Kegler[32]

Source: Adapted from Lewis et al.[33]

Table 4.2. Evidence-Based Assessment Rating Criteria Table

RELIABILITY INFORMATION

0   None (N): α values are not yet available OR are only available for subscales.

1   Minimal/Emerging (M): α values of <.60.

2   Adequate (A): α values of .60–.69.

3   Good (G): α values of .70–.79.

4   Excellent (E): α values of ≥.80.

N/A   Internal consistency measures are not applicable for this measure OR classical test theory anchors are not appropriate; results reported using item response theory.

STRUCTURAL VALIDITY

0   None (N): No exploratory or confirmatory analysis has yet been performed, nor have any item response theory tests of (uni-)dimensionality been conducted; OR, percept variance explained is not reported.

1   Minimal/Emerging (M): The sample consisted of less than five times the number of items AND an exploratory factor analysis explained less than 25% of the variance.

2   Adequate (A): The sample consisted of less than five times the number of items but is less than 100 in total AND
an exploratory factor analysis explained less than 50% of the variance
OR
a confirmatory factor analysis revealed an RMSEA = .08 to .05
OR
CFI or GFI = .90–.95.

3   Good (G): The sample consisted of five times the number of items and is greater than or equal to 100 in total OR the sample consisted of five to seven times the number of items but is less than 100 in total AND in either case
an exploratory factor analysis explained less than 50% of the variance
OR
a confirmatory factor analysis revealed an RMSEA or SRMR of = .05 to .03 OR
CFI or GFI = .95–.97.

4   Excellent (E): The sample consisted of seven times the number of items and is greater than 100 in total AND
an exploratory analysis explained greater than 50% of the variance
OR
a confirmatory factor analysis revealed an RMSEA or SRMR of <.03
OR
GFI or CFI >.97.

Table 4.2   Continued

CRITERION (PREDICTIVE) VALIDITY INFORMATION

| 0 | None (N): Predictive validity not yet tested or failed to be detected in evaluation. |

0   None (N): Predictive validity not yet tested or failed to be detected in evaluation.

1   Minimal/Emerging (M): Evidence of small correlation (range, 0.1–0.29) between measure and scores on another test (measuring a distinct construct of interest or outcome) administered at some point in the future.

2   Adequate (A): Evidence of medium correlation (range, 0.3–0.49) between measure and scores on another test (measuring a distinct construct of interest or outcome) administered at some point in the future.

3   Good (G): Evidence of strong correlation (range, 0.5–1.00) between measure and scores on another test (measuring a distinct construct of interest or outcome) administered at some point in the future.

4   Excellent (E): Evidence of medium–strong correlation (0.3 or higher) between measure and scores on at least two other tests (measuring a distinct construct of interest or outcome) administered at some point in the future.

NORMS

0   None (N): Norms are not yet available.

1   Minimal/Emerging (M): Measures of central tendency and distribution for the total score (and subscales if relevant) based only on a small ($n < 30$) sample are available.

2   Adequate (A): Measures of central tendency and distribution for the total score (and subscales if relevant) based on a moderate ($n = 30$–49) sample are available.

3   Good (G): Measures of central tendency and distribution for the total score (and subscales if relevant) based on a medium ($n = 50$–99) sample are available.

4   Excellent (E): Measures of central tendency and distribution for the total score (and subscales if relevant) based on a large ($n > 100$) sample are available.

RESPONSIVENESS (SENSITIVITY TO CHANGE)

0   None (N): The measure has either not been administered both pre- and post-implementation to evaluate sensitivity to change OR it has been administered and did not demonstrate responsiveness (change) across an implementation process.

1   Minimal/Emerging (M): The measure demonstrated change over time based on a small ($n < 50$) sample.

2   Adequate (A): The measure demonstrated EITHER clinically OR statistically significant change over time based on a medium sample ($n > 50$ but < 100).

3   Good (G): The measure demonstrated change over time reflective of BOTH clinically and statistically significant change based on a large sample ($n > 100$).

4   Excellent (E): The measure demonstrated BOTH clinically and statistically significant change over time based on at least two large ($n > 100$) samples.

(continued)

Table 4.2 Continued

USABILITY (MEASURE LENGTH)

0	None (N): The measure is not in the public domain.
1	Minimal (M): The measure has greater than 100 items.
2	Adequate (A): The measure has greater than 50 items but fewer than 100.
3	Good (G): The measure has greater than 10 items but fewer than 50.
4	Excellent (E): The measure has fewer than 10 items.

CFI, comparative fit index; GFI, goodness-of-fit index; N/A, not applicable; RMSEA, root mean square error of approximation; SRMR, standardized root mean square residual.

instruments had not provided information about reliability, 74% had not provided information about structural validity, 82% had not provided information about predictive validity, 28% had not provided information about norms, and 96% had not provided information about responsiveness. Total scores ranged from 2 to 19.5 (with the highest possible score being 24). Moreover, there was great variability across the IOF for the number of instruments each search returned. Fifty measures were used to assess *acceptability*, and 19 measures were used to assess *adoption*. The remaining six outcomes had fewer than 10 measures available. The growth of IOF measures appears to be evolving at a rapid rate since the initial Proctor et al.[10] publication.[21]

Although the aforementioned review set search parameters to reveal measures of implementation outcomes in mental and behavioral health, the majority of these measures demonstrate relevance to fields outside of mental health (i.e., the name of the intervention could be replaced for that of a cancer-related intervention) and therefore the results are summarized in greater detail here. No parallel systematic review of IOF measures exists in the field of cancer, or any field for that matter. However, we conducted an environmental scan to identify cancer-relevant measures and preliminarily report on their quality for the purposes of this chapter.[20] Specifically, PubMed, Google Scholar, NIH Reporter, *Implementation Science*,

and the National Cancer Institute Research Tested Intervention Programs[34] were accessed using search strings as broad as "implementation AND cancer AND outcome," with "outcome" replaced with each of the eight IOF terms.[1] We also searched the 1,800 articles published by researchers affiliated with the Cancer Prevention and Control Research Network. Across these diverse databases and outlets, only 40 measures of implementation outcomes used in the field of cancer research were identified. Table 4.3 contains all eight implementation outcomes, all measures that emerged from our environmental scan, as well as information regarding their use (number of citations) and quality (evidence-based assessment rating); see Box 4.1 for details about the quality rating process. What follows is an overview of each implementation outcome, synonyms, and the current state of measurement (at least with respect to mental health and cancer).

Acceptability refers to the extent to which an innovation or EBI is attractive, agreeable, or palatable.[11] Synonyms include *satisfaction* and *agreeability*. The systematic review by C. C. Lewis, Fischer, et al.[21] revealed 50 measures of *acceptability* both of the implementation strategies and of the clinical interventions, whereas 10 measures were identified in the field of cancer. Of those used in cancer research, measures appeared in an average of 1.2

---

1. The identical search terms as those used in the C. C. Lewis, Fischer, et al.[21] review were submitted to PubMed—for instance, replacing "mental health" with "cancer"—and fewer than 10 measures were identified across the eight implementation outcomes. Accordingly, broadening of the search terms was necessary to reveal additional measures. Note that although traditional search methods were used (i.e., using advanced search builders), crafting nuanced search strings with the help of health science librarians and PubMed experts may have yielded more results.

Table 4.3. Implementation Outcome Measures Used in Cancer Research[a]

MEASURE	NO. OF CITATIONS	NO. OF USES	INTERNAL CONSISTENCY	STRUCTURAL VALIDITY	PREDICTIVE VALIDITY	NORMS	RESPONSIVENESS	USABILITY	TOTAL SCORE	OUTCOME
Abernethy et al.[25]	68	1	0	0	0	3	0	4	7	Acceptability Feasibility
Adelson et al.[28]	12	N/A	N/A	N/A	N/A	N/A	N/A	N/A	N/A	Fidelity
Allen et al.[26]	3	1	3	0	0	4	0	3	10	Adoption
Bast et al.[29]	0	N/A	N/A	N/A	N/A	N/A	N/A	N/A	N/A	Fidelity
Beale et al.[35]	12	1	4	0	0	4	0	4	12	Acceptability
Berg and Schauer[36]	11	1	0	0	0	2	0	3	5	Acceptability
Bloch[27]	33	N/A	N/A	N/A	N/A	N/A	N/A	N/A	N/A	Appropriateness
Brouwers et al.[37]	26	3	4	3	0	4	0	4	15	Acceptability
Brouwers et al.[37]	26	3	3	3	0	4	0	4	14	Appropriateness
Doak, Doak, and Root[38]	1,431	N/A	N/A	N/A	N/A	N/A	N/A	N/A	N/A	Appropriateness

(continued)

Table 4.3   Continued

MEASURE	NO. OF CITATIONS	NO. OF USES	INTERNAL CONSISTENCY	STRUCTURAL VALIDITY	PREDICTIVE VALIDITY	NORMS	RESPONSIVENESS	USABILITY	TOTAL SCORE	OUTCOME
Duffy et al.[39]	0	N/A	N/A	N/A	N/A	N/A	N/A	N/A	N/A	Adoption Fidelity Sustainability
Ekwueme et al.[40]	33	N/A	N/A	N/A	N/A	N/A	N/A	N/A	N/A	Cost
Fiset et al.[41]	56	1	0	0	0	1	0	3	4	Acceptability
Gilkey et al.[42]	6	1	0	0	0	3	0	3	6	Acceptability Cost
Helitzer, Willging, Hathorn, and Benally[43]	51	N/A	N/A	N/A	N/A	N/A	N/A	N/A	N/A	Appropriateness
Honeycutt et al.[32]	14	N/A	N/A	N/A	N/A	N/A	N/A	N/A	N/A	Adoption Fidelity Sustainability
Hughes, Girolami, Cheadle, Harris, and Patrick[44]	18	N/A	N/A	N/A	N/A	N/A	N/A	N/A	N/A	Fidelity
Lairson et al.[30]	5	N/A	N/A	N/A	N/A	N/A	N/A	N/A	N/A	Cost

Lairson, Dicarlo, et al.[45]	0	N/A	N/A	N/A	N/A	N/A	N/A	N/A	N/A	Cost
Lairson, Chang, et al.[46]	4	N/A	N/A	N/A	N/A	N/A	N/A	N/A	N/A	Cost
C. L. Lewis, Brenner, Griffith, and Pignone[47]	41	N/A	N/A	N/A	N/A	N/A	N/A	N/A	N/A	Cost
Massett[48]	34	N/A	N/A	N/A	N/A	N/A	N/A	N/A	N/A	Appropriateness
McCormick, Steckler, and McLeroy[49]	162	N/A	N/A	N/A	N/A	N/A	N/A	N/A	N/A	Adoption Penetration
Meenan et al.[50]	3	N/A	N/A	N/A	N/A	N/A	N/A	N/A	N/A	Cost
Miller, Manne, and Palevsky[51]	19	1	4	0	4	0	0	4	12	Acceptability
Morland et al.[52]	0	N/A	N/A	N/A	N/A	N/A	N/A	N/A	N/A	Cost
Rabin et al.[53]	19	1	2	0	4	0	3	3	12	Fidelity
Rutten et al.[54]	8	1	N/A	N/A	N/A	N/A	N/A	N/A	N/A	Acceptability
Schroy, Mylvaganam, and Davidson[55]	13	1	0	0	1	0	0	3	4	Acceptability

(continued)

Table 4.3 Continued

MEASURE	NO. OF CITATIONS	NO. OF USES	INTERNAL CONSISTENCY	STRUCTURAL VALIDITY	PREDICTIVE VALIDITY	NORMS	RESPONSIVENESS	USABILITY	TOTAL SCORE	OUTCOME
Scoggins, Ramsey, Jackson, and Taylor[56]	5	N/A	N/A	N/A	N/A	N/A	N/A	N/A	N/A	Cost
Simmons et al.[57]	0	N/A	N/A	N/A	N/A	N/A	N/A	N/A	N/A	Fidelity
Steckler et al.[31]	167	1	1	0	0	4	0	4	8	Adoption Penetration
Subramanian et al.[58]	17	N/A	N/A	N/A	N/A	N/A	N/A	N/A	N/A	Cost
van Egmond, Duijts, Scholten, van der Beek, and Anema[59]	0	1	0	0	0	4	0	3	7	Acceptability

[a] The Abernethy et al.[25] measure purportedly measures both acceptability and feasibility. Given the number of uses of the Doak et al.[38] measure, we used data from a systematic review by Finnie, Felder, Linder, and Mullen[60] to inform the quality ratings.

N/A, not applicable.

Box 4.1 The Rating Process

A team of trained researchers carried out psychometric ratings of the identified measures of implementation outcomes related to the field of cancer. The method for rating these measures was developed by C. C. Lewis, Fischer, et al.[21] Studies that utilized a measure were combined into electronic PDF packets. Key phrases related to the six relevant EBA criteria (reliability, structural validity, predictive validity, norms, responsiveness, and usability) were highlighted and annotated. The process for developing these criteria is described in C. C. Lewis, Stanick, et al.[61]

Research specialists were given extensive training in the EBA criteria. Pilot packets were highlighted and reviewed by a senior researcher and project leader. When the research specialists reached adequate proficiency, they were tasked with highlighting and tagging packets independently.

After packets were highlighted, two independent raters rated packets on a 0–4 scale: "none" (0), "minimal/emerging" (1), "adequate" (2), "good" (3), or "excellent" (4). That is, the "worst score counts" methodology was employed.[62] If an instrument exhibited a "minimal" level of reliability in one study and a "good" level of reliability in another, the rater assigned a "minimal" rating for this criterion. A total score for each instrument was calculated by summing the EBA ratings for the instrument.

Important to note is that not all quantitative measures are amenable to the rating process, meaning that some of the identified measures (e.g., formulas and single-item/binary measures) would not be expected to demonstrate psychometric properties such as internal consistency or structural validity.

peer-reviewed publications. With respect to quality, evidence-based assessment (EBA) scores ranged from 4 to 15 (with a highest possible score of 24), with an average score of 8. Of these 10 measures, 1 was not suitable for rating (see Table 4.3). The most highly rated acceptability measure was the Clinician's Assessments of Practice Guidelines in Oncology (CAPGO) survey developed by Brouwers, Graham, Hanna, Cameron, and Browman,[37] which received a score of 14. This measure assesses acceptance of clinical recommendations or "draft guidelines." The measure contains six items, with an example item reading, "When applied, the DRs [draft guidelines] will produce more benefits for my patients than harms."

Appropriateness refers to the extent to which an innovation or EBI is suitable, fitting, or proper for a particular purpose or circumstance.[11] Synonyms include *applicability, compatibility, perceived fit, fitness, relevance, suitability,* and *usefulness.* The systematic review by C. C. Lewis, Fischer, et al.[21] revealed seven measures of *appropriateness,* whereas five measures were identified in the field of cancer. Of those used in cancer research, measures appeared in an average of two peer-reviewed publications. With respect to quality, only one measure was suitable for rating (see Table 4.3),

and this was the previously mentioned measure created by Brouwers and colleagues.[37] The measure assesses applicability of draft guidelines. The measure contains four items, with one example item reading, "To apply the DRs [draft guidelines] will require reorganization of services/care in my practice setting."

Feasibility refers to the extent to which an innovation or EBI is practical or possible to use.[11] Synonyms include *transferability, applicability, practicability, workability, actual fit, actual utility,* and *suitability for everyday use.* The systematic review by C. C. Lewis, Fischer, et al.[21] revealed eight measures of *feasibility,* whereas only one measure was identified in the field of cancer, and it appeared in only one peer-reviewed publication. With respect to the quality of the West Clinic Survey developed by Abernathy and colleagues,[25] the EBA score was 7. The survey assesses feasibility of e/Tablets and Patient Care Monitor (PCM). The survey contains eight items, with an example item reading, "How easy was it to use the e/Tablet computer to respond to questions?"

Adoption is the intention, initial decision, or action to try or employ an EBI.[11] Synonyms include *knowledge translation, uptake, intention to adopt, utilization,* and *initial implementation.* The systematic review by C. C. Lewis, Fischer, et al.[21] revealed 19 measures of *adoption*, whereas 5 measures were identified in the field of cancer. Of those used in cancer research, measures appeared in an average of only one peer-reviewed publication. With respect to quality, EBA scores ranged from 8 to 10, with an average score of 9. Of these 5 measures, 3 were not suitable for rating (see Table 4.3). The most highly rated adoption measure was Roger's Adoption Questionnaire used by Steckler, Goodman, McLeroy, Davis, and Koch.[31] The questionnaire assesses likeliness to adopt a tobacco prevention curriculum. The questionnaire contains nine items, with an example item reading, "The curriculum would be more effective in reducing tobacco use by students than our current curriculum practices."

Cost refers to the financial impact of an implementation effort.[11] Synonyms include *marginal cost, cost-effectiveness, cost–benefit, cost utility,* and *cost offsets.* The systematic review by C. C. Lewis, Fischer, et al.[21] revealed 8 measures of *cost*, whereas 10 measures (or formulas) were identified in the field of cancer. Of those used in cancer research, measures appeared in an average of only one peer-reviewed publication. With respect to quality, only one measure was suitable for rating, and it received a score of 6 (see Table 4.3). The only cost measure that was suitable for rating did not provide example items.

Penetration refers to the integration of a practice within a service setting and its subsystems.[11] Synonyms include *integration of practice* and *infiltration.* The systematic review by C. C. Lewis, Fischer, et al.[21] revealed four measures of *penetration*, whereas two measures were identified in the field of cancer. Of those used in cancer research, measures appeared in an average of only one peer-reviewed publication. With respect to quality, only one measure was suitable for rating, and it received a score of 8 (see Table 4.3). The most highly rated penetration measure was the Level of Success survey, also used in the previously mentioned study by Steckler and colleagues.[31] The survey assesses the level of success of a tobacco prevention curriculum. The survey contains 10 items, with one example item reading, "The tobacco prevention curriculum fulfilled most of our goals, but some people have declined to use it."

Fidelity is the degree to which an intervention was implemented as it was prescribed in the original protocol or as it was intended by the program developers. Synonyms include *delivered as intended, adherence, integrity,* and *quality of program delivery.* The systematic review by C. C. Lewis, Fischer, et al.[21] revealed zero measures of *fidelity* to an implementation strategy; that is, they did not review measures of EBI *fidelity* given that independent systematic reviews of EBI *fidelity* are available elsewhere. A total of seven measures were identified in the field of cancer. Of those used in cancer research, measures appeared in an average of only one peer-reviewed publication. With respect to quality, only one measure was suitable for rating, and it received a score of 12 (see Table 4.3). The most highly rated fidelity measure was the Pool Cool Fidelity survey developed by Rabin and colleagues.[53] The survey assesses adherence to a sun safety program for children. The survey contains 16 items, with one example item reading, "Did you take part in the Sun exposure card and UV Warning Patch Activity?"

Sustainability is the extent to which a newly implemented treatment is maintained or institutionalized within a service setting's ongoing, stable operations.[11] Synonyms include *maintenance, long-term implementation, routinization, durability, institutionalization, capacity building, (dis)continuation, incorporation, integration,* and *sustained use.* The systematic review by C. C. Lewis, Fischer, et al.[21] revealed eight measures of *sustainability*, whereas two measures were identified in the field of cancer. Of those used in cancer research, measures appeared in an average of only one peer-reviewed publication. With respect to quality, neither sustainability measure was suitable for rating, nor did either provide example items (see Table 4.3).

Although not formally rated in the quality assessment reported on previously, there is clear evidence of issues of content validity—in particular, homonymy, synonymy, and instability[63]—in the measures of the IOF variables. Homonymy, as it applies to measurement, refers to measures that purportedly assess the same construct (e.g., *acceptability*) but do so with substantively different items. For example, some *acceptability* measures include items about satisfaction with the EBI and willingness to recommend the EBI to others.[25] Other *acceptability* measures do not include such items.[42] Synonymy refers to measures that have similar items that purportedly assess different constructs. For example, some *acceptability* measures contain items about perceived benefits or harms to others that might result from the use or delivery of the EBI.[35,37,41] These items better reflect *appropriateness* (which refers to perceived applicability or suitability) than *acceptability*. Finally, instability refers to the items in a particular measure being shifted or modified over time in an unpredictable manner. For example, Beale and Lane[64] dropped an item from Beale and colleagues'[35] *acceptability* measure without explaining why. Small changes in measure content—even the addition, deletion, or substitution of a single item—can change a measure's psychometric quality. In a more dramatic example, Berg and colleagues[65] adapted Berg and Schauer's[36] *acceptability* measure by adding some items, deleting others, rewording still others, and changing the response scales from 5-point to 4-point Likert scales. These changes arguably make the two measures noncomparable; indeed, we treated the latter measure as a new measure in our environmental scan and quality analysis. Homonymy, synonymy, and instability threaten the content validity of the measure, or the extent to which a measure assesses what it intends to measure or the ability of a measure to represent all facets of a given construct. The consequences of compromised content validity are enormous and can stem from inappropriate consideration of construct synonyms beyond those reported previously. Unfortunately, use of poor measure development processes, notably the lack of construct definitions and use of theory, is the primary culprit for undermining content validity.

The IOF presents the implementation outcomes distinct from service and clinical outcomes, but it does little else to differentiate among the outcomes themselves (beyond their careful operationalization). It is possible that several of the more than 60 models, theories, or frameworks available in the field of implementation science grapple with the issue of temporal distinctions, but to our knowledge, none systematically provide guidance in this way.[66] The EPIS model is one of the few that explicitly identifies context and outcome variables as they are most relevant across different phases of an implementation effort: exploration, preparation, implementation, and sustainment.[67] This is critical because it is not always feasible or appropriate to assess all implementation outcomes in every study, and some constructs or outcomes are simply more salient at different points during an implementation process.[68] Guidance around their temporal relations with one another and with phases of the implementation process is needed.

An overview of the EPIS model is provided next, with explicit attention paid to relevant implementation outcomes within each phase of the process, as depicted in Figure 4.1.

Aarons et al.[67] proposed a four-stage timeline model for translating EBIs into public health settings. The model consists of the phases "exploration," "adoption/preparation," "implementation," and "sustainment," known collectively as "EPIS." Each phase in this model represents a benchmark during an implementation process.

The "exploration" phase is characterized as recognition of a current problem or approach to improvement,[69] and this phase marks a "typical" starting point for stakeholders who are considering EBI integration. The implementation outcomes of *acceptability*, *appropriateness*, and *feasibility* of the EBI are most salient at the phase. Indeed, these three outcomes have been identified as predictors of *adoption*.[23,61] Accordingly, identifying EBIs with high degrees of *acceptability*, *appropriateness*, and *feasibility* would optimize the "success" of the exploration phase. In this case, it may be best to consider the adoption/preparation phase as a singular event. Conversely, an EBI with suboptimal *acceptability*, *appropriateness*, and *feasibility* could emerge as the top choice (i.e., it is adopted) from the exploration phase, requiring that the work of the adoption/preparation phase be focused on EBI adaptations or modifications to enhance these three outcomes prior to formal *adoption*. *Cost* of an intervention is often a primary focus of the adoption/preparation phase. Ideally, the EBI and plans for its active implementation are budgeted out early in this phase (or in the exploration phase) to ensure success of subsequent phases. However, *cost* remains a key outcome of interest in the next phase—the active implementation phase. In addition to *cost*, the active implementation phase brings EBI *fidelity* and *penetration* to the fore. Although it is possible that the preparation phase includes an initial (small, pilot) test of the EBI implementation wherein *fidelity* and *penetration* are preliminarily evaluated, the true test of implementation "success" occurs in the implementation phase. Finally, the sustainment phase is characterized as endurance/maintenance or continued use of an EBI. There is currently no standard model of *sustainability*, but continued quality (or *fidelity*) and quantity (or *penetration*) of EBI delivery are often used to determine an EBI's *sustainability*. Valid measures of implementation outcomes would allow researchers to standardize benchmarks of success during the process and inform strategies for future implementation.

Although the focus of this chapter is on implementation outcomes and associated measures, the EPIS model also considers levels of analysis within a public health system (e.g., the "outer context" and the "inner context") for determining which factors may be worth examining as predictors, moderators, and mediators in each phase of the process. Such factors include "service environment," "inter-organizational environment," and "consumer support/advocacy" within the outer context and "intra-organizational characteristics" and "individual adopter characteristics" within the inner context. Many of these factors likely influence multiple phases of the model, whereas some may be more relevant in one more than others.[67] The model's development study focused primarily on factors relevant to the child welfare sector, but the authors assert that this implementation framework is generalizable to other health and human service sectors as well.

CHALLENGES WITH MEASURING CONTEXT AND OUTCOMES IN IMPLEMENTATION SCIENCE

We invite readers to explore a relatively recent article titled "Instrumentation Issues in Implementation Science"[68] for an in-depth analysis of critical measurement challenges. Many of the instrumentation issues that Martinez et al.[68] observed in mental and behavioral health also arise in cancer. For example, the growing number of conceptual models, theories, and frameworks guiding implementation science generates content validity issues such as synonymy, homonymy, and instability because no two models, theories, or frameworks define and operationalize implementation constructs the same way. Paradoxically, these content validity issues also arise when researchers do not use any conceptual model, framework, or theory. Both of these issues (confusion as to which framework to use to guide study measurement and complete lack of framework) are prevalent in the implementation science literature. Fortunately, recent efforts have been made toward cross-walking the existing frameworks to reveal points of overlap and distinctiveness.[70] To increase content validity and facilitate comparisons of findings across studies, it is important to specify both what the implementation outcome is and what it is not by defining it and embedding it within a theory or framework that clarifies its relationships

with other constructs. Item generation can then proceed with greater confidence of capturing the content of the construct of interest (e.g., *acceptability*) and not related constructs (e.g., *trialability* or *appropriateness*).

A second issue is that many measures of implementation outcomes, including those relevant to the field of cancer research (see Table 4.3), have questionable psychometric quality. This issue arises for two reasons: (1) Researchers often do not systematically assess the psychometric properties of the measures that they develop or use, and (2) peer-reviewed journals that publish implementation science generally do not have standards for reporting psychometric properties. To some extent, the poor state of measure development, evaluation, and reporting reflects the nascent state of implementation science as a field. At the same time, if a measure's reliability and validity are not evaluated and reported, confidence in a study's findings or interpretations is undermined because it is not clear whether the measure is assessing what it purports to evaluate. To address this issue, researchers should engage in good measurement practice by assessing key psychometric properties in every study because issues of reliability and validity are specific to the study sample, setting, and characteristics. For studies using multi-item measures, this means evaluating internal consistency and structural validity every time a measure is used. In addition, journals should require authors to report essential psychometric information in every study. Lewis and Dorsey[71] propose six minimal reporting standards for the field to consider adoption (Box 4.2). First, authors should name, define, and operationalize constructs using published models, theories, or frameworks whenever possible. Second, authors should provide a full list of items used to measure constructs. Third, authors should justify the evaluation method (e.g., self-report and observation) used to measure constructs. Fourth, authors should indicate the stage of a measure's development (e.g., needs additional evidence and unable to assess structural validity). Fifth, authors should report key measurement characteristics, such as target population, timing of measure administration, scoring procedure, and rationale for the selected scoring approach. Finally, authors should report key psychometric properties, such as internal consistency, structural validity, and criterion validity.

A third issue is that many measures, including the ones reviewed previously, are "home grown" or

Box 4.2 Recommendations for Measure Development and Validation

1. Authors should name, define, and operationalize constructs using published models, theories, or frameworks.
2. Authors should provide a full list of items used to measure constructs.
3. Authors should justify the evaluation method (e.g., self-report and observation) used to measure constructs.
4. Authors should indicate the stage of the measure's development (e.g., needs additional evidence and unable to assess structural validity).
5. Authors should report key measurement characteristics, such as target population, timing of measure administration, scoring procedure, and rationale for the selected scoring approach.
6. Authors should report key psychometric properties, such as internal consistency, structural validity, and criterion validity.
7. Measures of implementation should be pragmatic (relevant to stakeholders, feasible, responsive, and actionable).

heavily adapted for a particular study, used once, and never used again. The single-use phenomenon is not limited to implementation outcomes. Systematic reviews of measures of implementation context indicate that 34–76% of measures have been used only once.[24,72] The proliferation of "home-grown" measures, by which we mean measures created quickly by researchers for immediate use in a particular study, and heavily adapted measures, by which we mean measures whose item content has been substantially altered, occurs for several reasons. First, as noted previously, many existing measures have questionable psychometric quality. Second, no repository exists where researchers could easily find those reliable, valid measures that do exist. Third, researchers often tailor the item content of measures in order to make them more relevant or predictive for a particular intervention, population, or setting. Finally, researchers sometimes shorten measures with many items in order to reduce response burden and assess other constructs of interest. Unfortunately, "home-grown" and heavily adapted measures often have poor or unknown psychometric quality because they have not been subject to a systematic development and testing process. Moreover, they tend to be appropriate only for one-time use because they are so specific to an intervention, population, or setting that they are not relevant for use in other studies. This, in turn, limits capacity for cross-study comparisons. Addressing these measurement issues will not be easy. Development of reliable, valid, and

brief measures should be accelerated, and construction of an accessible, searchable repository of measures should be encouraged. Ideally, measures would be generic enough to use in multiple settings, with diverse populations, across interventions; at the same time, they would be at least somewhat adaptable so that researchers could tailor them without undermining their psychometric quality. While such measures are being developed, tested, and compiled, researchers should evaluate the psychometric properties of the "home-grown" measures that they develop and justify the adaptations they make to existing measures.

Finally, given that implementation science takes place in real-world settings, measures of implementation outcomes should be pragmatic. Glasgow and Riley[73] argue that pragmatic measures are relevant to stakeholders (i.e., address problems important to health care providers), feasible (i.e., brief, easy to administer, and user-friendly), responsive (i.e., sensitive to change), and actionable (i.e., capable of guiding action in real-world settings). As with psychometric quality, many measures of implementation outcomes have poor or unknown pragmatic quality. The reason is simple. To date, implementation science has focused on research, not practice. As a result, implementation scientists have emphasized psychometric quality, not pragmatic quality. However, pragmatic measures have value. Practitioners could use pragmatic measures to assess organizational needs and contexts to guide implementation strategy selection, monitor and adjust implementation processes, and evaluate implementation outcomes. If, however, measures are not feasible, actionable, relevant, and responsive, they will go unused by practitioners no matter how psychometrically strong they might be. We believe measures can be both pragmatic and psychometrically strong, but only if researchers attend to both pragmatic and psychometric properties in measure development and evaluation. Cost, length, accessibility, responsiveness, and user-friendliness should be considered in addition to reliability and validity. Researchers have only recently queried stakeholders about the pragmatic features of measures that matter most to them. Next, we describe the process of inquiry and preliminary outcomes.

EMERGING ADVANCES IN THE FIELD

Measurement is the foundation of any scientific field, yet measurement issues are among the most critical barriers to advancing implementation science. Several efforts are underway to identify existing measures that have high psychometric and pragmatic quality and to develop new measures that can inform both research and practice. For example, with funding from the National Institutes of Health, we are updating our published systematic review of implementation outcomes[21] and conducting systematic reviews of implementation context measures for 37 constructs found in the Consolidated Framework for Implementation Research.[16] For each implementation context and outcome measure, we will assess both psychometric quality and pragmatic quality and develop a graphical rating profile to facilitate head-to-head comparisons of measures. Psychometric quality will be evaluated in terms of reliability, structural validity, known-groups validity, and predictive validity. Pragmatic quality will be evaluated in terms of stakeholder-derived priorities of pragmatic features.

To inform this effort, we have established a stakeholder-informed conceptualization and operationalization of pragmatic measurement and will develop rating criteria for assessing the pragmatic quality of measures. To date, researchers, not stakeholders, have defined the features that make measures pragmatic.[73] By contrast, our work intentionally engages an international stakeholder panel that both participates in and advises every project phase. In addition to criteria identified through a systematic literature review, this project engaged stakeholders in semistructured interviews, followed by a concept mapping activity to clarify the internal structure of the construct and a Delphi activity to achieve consensus on the dimension priorities. Preliminary results from this work have revealed 47 terms with relevance to the pragmatic construct (e.g., "not wordy," "short," and "does not require an expert to answer") that were then subjected to a concept mapping activity, where stakeholders assigned the terms to clusters as well as rated their relative importance and clarity. Results from the concept mapping activity revealed that the 47 terms could be meaningfully grouped into four clusters: Acceptable ($n = 7$), Useful ($n = 13$), Compatible ($n = 8$), and Easy ($n = 19$). Furthermore, using a 10-point scale, participants rated the Useful cluster as the most important (8.07), whereas the Easy cluster was rated as the most clear (7.86). Subsequently, the term list was culled based on all existing data to reduce redundancy and enhance the ease with which stakeholders could establish consensus around term priorities in a Delphi activity in which ratings will be applied both within and across the four clusters. Finally, the resulting terms from the Delphi will be turned into objective anchors in the form of rating criteria to be applied to identify measures once test–retest reliability and known-groups validity are established. Ultimately, this work will provide the field with a rigorous, stakeholder-driven rating system for assessing the pragmatic nature of measures to inform measure development. We will use this rating system to assess the pragmatic quality of implementation outcome measures as well as implementation context measures.

In addition, we are developing reliable, valid, and pragmatic measures of three implementation outcomes: *acceptability, appropriateness*, and *feasibility*. We selected these implementation outcomes based on their importance for explaining adoption of EBIs and their applicability in a wide range of contexts. Surprisingly, none of the 60 measures of *acceptability, appropriateness*, and *feasibility* identified in systematic reviews[21,23,24] has undergone systematic development and testing. Consequently, we have an abundance of measures that have some reliability yet have largely unknown content, construct, or criterion validity. We elected to create new measures of these outcomes because addressing the definitional ambiguities and overlapping item content in existing measures would have entailed substantial adaptations such that new measures would essentially be created. Our systematic development process follows the guidelines of measurement experts and involves domain delineation, item generation, substantive validity assessment, structural validity assessment, reliability assessment, and predictive validity assessment. In addition, we will assess discriminant validity, known-groups validity, structural invariance, sensitivity to change, and other pragmatic features. Our approach involves a series of laboratory studies to assess psychometric properties under controlled conditions and field studies to gauge psychometric and pragmatic performance under "real-world" conditions. By involving implementation scientists and multiple types of stakeholders in the measurement development process, we expect our work to produce psychometrically and pragmatically strong measures of implementation outcomes that are useful for research and practice in a range of contexts.

Finally, although not specific to implementation outcomes, the Cancer Prevention and Control Research Network (CPCRN) has developed and tested measures of selected constructs from all five domains of the Consolidated Framework for Implementation Research (CFIR)[74] in order to identify factors influencing implementation of EBIs for increasing colorectal cancer screening in community health centers (CHC).[75] CPCRN investigators searched the literature for existing measures, adapted items for the health care context, pilot-tested the adapted measures in 4 CHCs, and fielded the revised measures in 78 CHCs in seven states. They psychometrically assessed the measures by conducting confirmatory factor analysis (structural validity), assessing inter-item consistency (reliability), computing scale correlations (discriminant validity), and calculating inter-rater reliability and agreement (organization-level construct reliability and validity). Their work is the first to develop reliable, valid measures of a comprehensive set of CFIR constructs. It not only lays the foundation for understanding and predicting implementation of EBIs in CHCs but also can be used to identify targets of strategies to accelerate and enhance the implementation of EBIs across the cancer control continuum in a variety of settings.

ACKNOWLEDGMENTS

Research reported in this chapter was supported by the National Institute of Mental Health of the National Institutes of Health under Award No. R01MH106510. The preparation of this manuscript was also supported, in kind, through the National Institutes of Health R13 award titled "Development and Dissemination of Rigorous Methods for Training and Implementation of Evidence-Based Behavioral Health Treatments" granted to principal investigator K. A. Comtois from 2010 to 2015. Dr. Bryan J. Weiner's time on the pilot studies supporting the parent grant was supported by the following funding: NIH CTSA at UNC UL1TR00083.

REFERENCES

1. Vidrine, J. I., Reitzel, L. R., Figueroa, P. Y., Velasquez, M. M., Mazas, C. A., Cinciripini, P. M., & Wetter, D. W. (2013). Motivation and Problem Solving (MAPS): Motivationally based skills training for treating substance use. *Cogn Behav Pract, 20*(4), 501–516. http://dx.doi.org/10.1016/j.cbpra.2011.11.001

2. Norman, G., Fayter, D., Lewis-Light, K., Chisholm, J., McHugh, K., Levine, D., ... Phillips, B. (2015). An emerging evidence base for PET-CT in the management of childhood rhabdomyosarcoma: Systematic review. *BMJ Open, 5*(1), e006030. doi:10.1136/bmjopen-2014-006030

3. Dewdney, S. B., & Mutch, D. G. (2010). Evidence-based review of the utility of radiation therapy in the treatment of endometrial cancer. *Women's Health, 6*(5), 695–703; quiz 704. doi:10.2217/whe.10.49

4. Galsky, M. D., Stensland, K. D., Moshier, E., Sfakianos, J. P., McBride, R. B., Tsao, C. K., ... Wisnivesky, J. P. (2016). Effectiveness of adjuvant chemotherapy for locally advanced bladder cancer. *J Clin Oncol, 34*(8), 825–832. doi:10.1200/JCO.2015.64.1076

5. Workman, A. D., Palmer, J. N., & Adappa, N. D. (2017). Posttreatment surveillance for sinonasal malignancy. *Curr Opin Otolaryngol Head Neck Surg, 25*(1), 86–92. doi:10.1097/MOO.0000000000000330

6. Bakitas, M., Lyons, K. D., Hegel, M. T., Balan, S., Brokaw, F. C., Seville, J., ... Ahles, T. A. (2009). Effects of a palliative care intervention on clinical outcomes in patients with advanced cancer: The Project ENABLE II randomized controlled trial. *JAMA, 302*(7), 741–749. doi:10.1001/jama.2009.1198

7. Feldstain, A., Lebel, S., & Chasen, M. R. (2016). An interdisciplinary palliative rehabilitation intervention bolstering general self-efficacy

to attenuate symptoms of depression in patients living with advanced cancer. *Support Care Cancer, 24*(1), 109–117. doi:10.1007/s00520-015-2751-4

8. Zhang, B., El-Jawahri, A., & Prigerson, H. G. (2006). Update on bereavement research: Evidence-based guidelines for the diagnosis and treatment of complicated bereavement. *J Palliat Med, 9*(5), 1188–1203. doi:10.1089/jpm.2006.9.1188

9. Berwick, D. M. (2002). A user's manual for the IOM's "Quality Chasm" report. *Health Aff, 21*(3), 80–90.

10. Proctor, E., Landsverk, J., Aarons, G., Chambers, D., Glisson, C., & Mittman, B. (2009). Implementation research in mental health services: An emerging science with conceptual, methodological, and training challenges. *Adm Policy Ment Health, 36*(1), 24–34. doi:10.1007/s10488-008-0197-4

11. Proctor, E., Silmere, H., Raghavan, R., Hovmand, P., Aarons, G., Bunger, A., . . . Hensley, M. (2011). Outcomes for implementation research: Conceptual distinctions, measurement challenges, and research agenda. *Adm Policy Ment Health, 38*(2), 65–76. doi:10.1007/s10488-010-0319-7

12. Shortell, S. M. (2004). Increasing value: A research agenda for addressing the managerial and organizational challenges facing health care delivery in the United States. *Med Care Res Rev, 61*(3 Suppl), 12S–30S. doi:10.1177/1077558704266768

13. Aarons, G. A., Ehrhart, M. G., Farahnak, L. R., & Sklar, M. (2014). Aligning leadership across systems and organizations to develop a strategic climate for evidence-based practice implementation. *Annu Rev Public Health, 35*, 255–274. doi:10.1146/annurev-publhealth-032013-182447

14. Beidas, R. S., Mychailyszyn, M. P., Edmunds, J. M., Khanna, M. S., Downey, M. M., & Kendall, P. C. (2012). Training school mental health providers to deliver cognitive–behavioral therapy. *School Ment Health, 4*(4), 197–206. doi:10.1007/s12310-012-9074-0

15. Hunter, S. B., Han, B., Slaughter, M. E., Godley, S. H., & Garner, B. R. (2015). Associations between implementation characteristics and evidence-based practice sustainment: A study of the Adolescent Community Reinforcement Approach. *Implement Sci, 10*(1), 173. doi:10.1186/s13012-015-0364-4

16. Lewis, C. C., Weiner, B. J., Stanick, C., & Fischer, S. M. (2015). Advancing implementation science through measure development and evaluation: A study protocol. *Implement Sci, 10*, 102. doi:10.1186/s13012-015-0287-0

17. Locke, J., Beidas, R. S., Marcus, S., Stahmer, A., Aarons, G. A., Lyon, A. R., . . . Mandell, D. S. (2016). A mixed methods study of individual and organizational factors that affect implementation of interventions for children with autism in public schools. *Implement Sci, 11*(1), 135. doi:10.1186/s13012-016-0501-8

18. Schreirer, M. A., & Dearing, J. W. (2011). An agenda for research on the sustainability of public health programs. *Am J Public Health, 101*(11), 2059–2067. doi:10.2105/AJPH.2011.300193

19. Swain, K., Whitley, R., McHugo, G. J., & Drake, R. E. (2010). The sustainability of evidence-based practices in routine mental health agencies. *Community Mental Health J, 46*(2), 119–129. doi:10.1007/s10597-009-9202-y

20. Rabin, B. A., Lewis, C. C., Norton, W. E., Neta, G., Chambers, D., Tobin, J. N., . . . Glasgow, R. E. (2016). Measurement resources for dissemination and implementation research in health. *Implement Sci, 11*, 42. doi:10.1186/s13012-016-0401-y

21. Lewis, C. C., Fischer, S., Weiner, B. J., Stanick, C., Kim, M., & Martinez, R. G. (2015). Outcomes for implementation science: An enhanced systematic review of instruments using evidence-based rating criteria. *Implement Sci, 10*, 155. doi:10.1186/s13012-015-0342-x

22. Rathje, H., & Bernd, H. (2010). *The Change & Transition Tools Compendium.* Retrieved from https://www.eurocontrol.int/sites/default/files/content/documents/nm/safety/safety-change-and-transition-tools-compendium-main-document-2010.pdf

23. Chor, K. H., Wisdom, J. P., Olin, S. C., Hoagwood, K. E., & Horwitz, S. M. (2015). Measures for predictors of innovation adoption. *Adm Policy Ment Health, 42*(5), 545–573. doi:10.1007/s10488-014-0551-7

24. Chaudoir, S. R., Dugan, A. G., & Barr, C. H. (2013). Measuring factors affecting implementation of health innovations: A systematic review of structural, organizational, provider, patient, and innovation level measures. *Implement Sci, 8*, 22. doi:10.1186/1748-5908-8-22

25. Abernethy, A. P., Herndon, J. E., 2nd, Wheeler, J. L., Day, J. M., Hood, L., Patwardhan, M., . . . Lyerly, H. K. (2009). Feasibility and acceptability to patients of a longitudinal system for evaluating cancer-related symptoms and quality of life: Pilot study of an e/Tablet data-collection

system in academic oncology. *J Pain Symptom Manage, 37*(6), 1027–1038. doi:10.1016/j.jpainsymman.2008.07.011

26. Allen, J. D., Torres, M. I., Tom, L. S., Rustan, S., Leyva, B., Negron, R., . . . Ospino, H. (2015). Enhancing organizational capacity to provide cancer control programs among Latino churches: Design and baseline findings of the CRUZA study. *BMC Health Serv Res, 15,* 147. doi:10.1186/s12913-015-0735-1

27. Bloch, P. (1983). The application of nuclear magnetic resonance data to radiation therapy. *Comput Radiol, 7*(3), 195–198.

28. Adelson, K. B., Qiu, Y. C., Evangelista, M., Spencer-Cisek, P., Whipple, C., & Holcombe, R. F. (2014). Implementation of electronic chemotherapy ordering: An opportunity to improve evidence-based oncology care. *J Oncol Pract, 10*(2), e113–e119. doi:10.1200/JOP.2013.001184

29. Bast, L. S., Due, P., Bendtsen, P., Ringgard, L., Wohllebe, L., Damsgaard, M. T., . . . Andersen, A. (2016). High impact of implementation on school-based smoking prevention: The X:IT study—A cluster-randomized smoking prevention trial. *Implement Sci, 11*(1), 125. doi:10.1186/s13012-016-0490-7

30. Lairson, D. R., Huo, J., Ricks, K. A., Savas, L., & Fernandez, M. E. (2013). The cost of implementing a 2-1-1 call center-based cancer control navigator program. *Eval Program Plann, 39,* 51–56. doi:10.1016/j.evalprogplan.2013.04.001

31. Steckler, A., Goodman, R. M., McLeroy, K. R., Davis, S., & Koch, G. (1992). Measuring the diffusion of innovative health promotion programs. *Am J Health Promot, 6*(3), 214–224.

32. Honeycutt, S., Carvalho, M., Glanz, K., Daniel, S. D., & Kegler, M. C. (2012). Research to reality: A process evaluation of a mini-grants program to disseminate evidence-based nutrition programs to rural churches and worksites. *J Public Health Manag Pract, 18*(5), 431–439. doi:10.1097/PHH.0b013e31822d4c69

33. Lewis, C. C., Proctor, E., & Brownson, R. C. (2018). Measurement issues in dissemination and implementation research. In R. C. Brownson, G. A. Colditz, & E. Proctor (Eds.), *Dissemination and implementation research in health: Translating science to practice* (2nd ed., pp. 229–244). New York: Oxford University Press.

34. National Cancer Institute. (2016). *Research-Tested Interventions Programs (RTIPs)*. Retrieved from http://rtips.cancer.gov/rtips

35. Beale, I. L., Marín-Bowling, V. M., Guthrie, N., & Kato, P. (2006). Young cancer patients' perceptions of a video game used to promote self care. *Glob J Health Educ Promot, 9*(1), 202–212.

36. Berg, C. J., & Schauer, G. L. (2012). Results of a feasibility and acceptability trial of an online smoking cessation program targeting young adult nondaily smokers. *J Environ Public Health, 2012,* 248541. doi:10.1155/2012/248541

37. Brouwers, M. C., Graham, I. D., Hanna, S. E., Cameron, D. A., & Browman, G. P. (2004). Clinicians' assessments of practice guidelines in oncology: The CAPGO survey. *Int J Technol Assess Health Care, 20*(4), 421–426.

38. Doak, C. C., Doak, L. G., & Root, J. H. (1996). Teaching patients with low literacy skills. *Am J Nurs, 96*(12), 16M.

39. Duffy, S. A., Ronis, D. L., Ewing, L. A., Waltje, A. H., Hall, S. V., Thomas, P. L., . . . Landstrom, G. L. (2016). Implementation of the Tobacco Tactics intervention versus usual care in Trinity Health community hospitals. *Implement Sci, 11*(1), 147. doi:10.1186/s13012-016-0511-6

40. Ekwueme, D. U., Gardner, J. G., Subramanian, S., Tangka, F. K., Bapat, B., & Richardson, L. C. (2008). Cost analysis of the National Breast and Cervical Cancer Early Detection Program: Selected states, 2003 to 2004. *Cancer, 112*(3), 626–635. doi:10.1002/cncr.23207

41. Fiset, V., O'Connor, A. M., Evans, W., Graham, I., Degrasse, C., & Logan, J. (2000). Development and evaluation of a decision aid for patients with stage IV non-small cell lung cancer. *Health Expect, 3*(2), 125–136.

42. Gilkey, M. B., Moss, J. L., Roberts, A. J., Dayton, A. M., Grimshaw, A. H., & Brewer, N. T. (2014). Comparing in-person and webinar delivery of an immunization quality improvement program: A process evaluation of the adolescent AFIX trial. *Implement Sci, 9,* 21. doi:10.1186/1748-5908-9-21

43. Helitzer, D., Willging, C., Hathorn, G., & Benally, J. (2009). Building community capacity for agricultural injury prevention in a Navajo community. *J Agric Saf Health, 15*(1), 19–35.

44. Hughes, M. C., Girolami, T. M., Cheadle, A. D., Harris, J. R., & Patrick, D. L. (2007). A lifestyle-based weight management program delivered to employees: Examination of health and economic outcomes. *J Occup Environ Med, 49*(11), 1212–1217. doi:10.1097/JOM.0b013e318159489d

45. Lairson, D. R., Dicarlo, M., Deshmuk, A. A., Fagan, H. B., Sifri, R., Katurakes, N., . . . Myers, R. E. (2014). Cost-effectiveness of a standard intervention versus a navigated intervention

on colorectal cancer screening use in primary care. *Cancer, 120*(7), 1042–1049. doi:10.1002/cncr.28535

46. Lairson, D. R., Chang, Y. C., Byrd, T. L., Lee Smith, J., Fernandez, M. E., & Wilson, K. M. (2014). Cervical cancer screening with AMIGAS: A cost-effectiveness analysis. *Am J Prev Med, 46*(6), 617–623. doi:10.1016/j.amepre.2014.01.020

47. Lewis, C. L., Brenner, A. T., Griffith, J. M., & Pignone, M. P. (2008). The uptake and effect of a mailed multi-modal colon cancer screening intervention: A pilot controlled trial. *Implement Sci, 3*, 32. doi:10.1186/1748-5908-3-32

48. Massett, H. A. (1996). Appropriateness of Hispanic print materials: A content analysis. *Health Educ Res, 11*(2), 231–242.

49. McCormick, L. K., Steckler, A. B., & McLeroy, K. R. (1995). Diffusion of innovations in schools: A study of adoption and implementation of school-based tobacco prevention curricula. *Am J Health Promot, 9*(3), 210–219.

50. Meenan, R. T., Anderson, M. L., Chubak, J., Vernon, S. W., Fuller, S., Wang, C. Y., & Green, B. B. (2015). An economic evaluation of colorectal cancer screening in primary care practice. *Am J Prev Med, 48*(6), 714–721. doi:10.1016/j.amepre.2014.12.016

51. Miller, D. L., Manne, S., & Palevsky, S. (1998). Brief report: Acceptance of behavioral interventions for children with cancer—Perceptions of parents, nurses, and community controls. *J Pediatr Psychol, 23*(4), 267–271.

52. Morland, T. B., Synnestvedt, M., Honeywell, S., Jr., Yang, F., Armstrong, K., & Guerra, C. (2017). Effect of a financial incentive for colorectal cancer screening adherence on the appropriateness of colonoscopy orders. *Am J Med Qual, 32*(3), 292–298. doi:10.1177/1062860616646848

53. Rabin, B. A., Nehl, E., Elliott, T., Deshpande, A. D., Brownson, R. C., & Glanz, K. (2010). Individual and setting level predictors of the implementation of a skin cancer prevention program: A multilevel analysis. *Implement Sci, 5*, 40. doi:10.1186/1748-5908-5-40

54. Rutten, G. M., Harting, J., Bartholomew, L. K., Schlief, A., Oostendorp, R. A., & de Vries, N. K. (2013). Evaluation of the theory-based Quality Improvement in Physical Therapy (QUIP) programme: A one-group, pre-test post-test pilot study. *BMC Health Serv Res, 13*, 194. doi:10.1186/1472-6963-13-194

55. Schroy, P. C., 3rd, Mylvaganam, S., & Davidson, P. (2014). Provider perspectives on the utility of a colorectal cancer screening decision aid for facilitating shared decision making. *Health Expect, 17*(1), 27–35. doi:10.1111/j.1369-7625.2011.00730.x

56. Scoggins, J. F., Ramsey, S. D., Jackson, J. C., & Taylor, V. M. (2010). Cost effectiveness of a program to promote screening for cervical cancer in the Vietnamese–American population. *Asian Pac J Cancer Prev, 11*(3), 717–722.

57. Simmons, R. G., Walters, S. T., Pappas, L. M., Boucher, K. M., Boonyasiriwat, W., Gammon, A., . . .Kinney, A. Y. (2014). Implementation of best practices regarding treatment fidelity in the Family Colorectal Cancer Awareness and Risk Education randomized controlled trial. *SAGE Open, 4*(4), 2158244014559021.

58. Subramanian, S., Tangka, F. K., Hoover, S., Beebe, M. C., DeGroff, A., Royalty, J., & Seeff, L. C. (2013). Costs of planning and implementing the CDC's Colorectal Cancer Screening Demonstration Program. *Cancer, 119*(Suppl 15), 2855–2862. doi:10.1002/cncr.28158

59. van Egmond, M. P., Duijts, S. F., Scholten, A. P., van der Beek, A. J., & Anema, J. R. (2016). Offering a tailored return to work program to cancer survivors with job loss: A process evaluation. *BMC Public Health, 15*, 940. doi:10.1186/s12889-016-3592-x

60. Finnie, R. K., Felder, T. M., Linder, S. K., & Mullen, P. D. (2010). Beyond reading level: A systematic review of the suitability of cancer education print and Web-based materials. *J Cancer Educ, 25*(4), 497–505. doi:10.1007/s13187-010-0075-0

61. Lewis, C. C., Stanick, C. F., Martinez, R. G., Weiner, B. J., Kim, M., Barwick, M., & Comtois, K. A. (2015). The Society for Implementation Research Collaboration Instrument Review Project: A methodology to promote rigorous evaluation. *Implement Sci, 10*(2). doi:10.1186/s13012-014-0193-x

62. Terwee, C. B., Mokkink, L. B., Knol, D. L., Ostelo, R. W., Bouter, L. M., & de Vet, H. C. (2012). Rating the methodological quality in systematic reviews of studies on measurement properties: A scoring system for the COSMIN checklist. *Qual Life Res, 21*(4), 651–657. doi:10.1007/s11136-011-9960-1

63. Gerring, J. (2001). *Social science methodology: A criterial framework.* Cambridge, UK: Cambridge University Press.

64. Beale, I. L., & Lane, V. (2010). Helping oncology nurses advise younger patients about self care: Feasibility of using animated and DVD

formats for nurse instruction. *Creat Educ, 1*(1), 51–57. doi:10.4236/ce.2010.11008

65. Berg, C. J., Stratton, E., Schauer, G. L., Lewis, M., Wang, Y., Windle, M., & Kegler, M. (2015). Perceived harm, addictiveness, and social acceptability of tobacco products and marijuana among young adults: Marijuana, hookah, and electronic cigarettes win. *Subst Use Misuse, 50*(1), 79–89. doi:10.3109/10826084.2014.958857

66. Tabak, R. G., Khoong, E. C., Chambers, D. A., & Brownson, R. C. (2012). Bridging research and practice: Models for dissemination and implementation research. *Am J Prev Med, 43*(3), 337–350. doi:10.1016/j.amepre.2012.05.024

67. Aarons, G. A., Hurlburt, M., & Horwitz, S. M. (2011). Advancing a conceptual model of evidence-based practice implementation in public service sectors. *Adm Policy Ment Health, 38*(1), 4–23. doi:10.1007/s10488-010-0327-7

68. Martinez, R. G., Lewis, C. C., & Weiner, B. J. (2014). Instrumentation issues in implementation science. *Implement Sci, 9*, 118. doi:10.1186/s13012-014-0118-8

69. Grol, R. P., Bosch, M. C., Hulscher, M. E., Eccles, M. P., & Wensing, M. (2007). Planning and studying improvement in patient care: The use of theoretical perspectives. *Milbank Q, 85*(1), 93–138. doi:10.1111/j.1468-0009.2007.00478.x

70. Center for Research in Implementation Science and Prevention. (n.d.). *Dissemination & implementation models in health research & practice*. Retrieved from http://www.dissemination-implementation.org/index.aspx

71. Lewis, C. C., & Dorsey, C. N. (*under review*). Advancing implementation science measurement. In R. Mildon, A. Shlonsky, & B. Albers (Eds.). *Implementation science version 2.0*. Springer.

72. Weiner, B. J., Amick, H., & Lee, S. Y. (2008). Conceptualization and measurement of organizational readiness for change: A review of the literature in health services research and other fields. *Med Care Res Rev, 65*(4), 379–436. doi:10.1177/1077558708317802

73. Glasgow, R. E., & Riley, W. T. (2013). Pragmatic measures: What they are and why we need them. *Am J Prev Med, 45*(2), 237–243. doi:10.1016/j.amepre.2013.03.010

74. Damschroder, L. J., Aron, D. C., Keith, R. E., Kirsh, S. R., Alexander, J. A., & Lowery, J. C. (2009). Fostering implementation of health services research findings into practice: A consolidated framework for advancing implementation science. *Implement Sci, 4*, 50. doi:10.1186/1748-5908-4-50

75. Fernandez, M. E., Savas, L. S., Wilson, K. M., Byrd, T. L., Atkinson, J., Torres-Vigil, I., & Vernon, S. W. (2015). Colorectal cancer screening among Latinos in three communities on the Texas–Mexico border. *Health Educ Behav, 42*(1), 16–25. doi:10.1177/1090198114529592

5

STUDY DESIGN, DATA COLLECTION, AND ANALYSIS IN IMPLEMENTATION SCIENCE

Marisa Sklar, Joanna C. Moullin, and Gregory A. Aarons

INTRODUCTION

Implementing interventions with demonstrated effectiveness is a critical component of improved patient health and experience at a reduced cost across the cancer control continuum. The field of implementation science, often characterized as dissemination and implementation research, intends to improve the adoption, delivery, and sustainment of effective, appropriate, and evidence-based interventions by providers, clinics, organizations, communities, and systems of care. implementation science represents a later stage of research in the traditional translation pipeline.[1-3] Unlike basic research and effectiveness and efficacy studies, implementation science aims to address different questions. Whereas basic research informs the development of clinical interventions, and efficacy and effectiveness trials are designed to test whether a new intervention produces effects, implementation science is designed to test approaches and strategies for successful utilization of evidence-based interventions in real-world service settings. Because there are different purposes of basic, efficacy, effectiveness, and implementation science, different research designs are often employed.

Traditionally, basic, efficacy, and effectiveness research have placed greatest emphasis on internal validity, the extent to which the intervention produces an effect. To strengthen the validity of causal inference, researchers have relied heavily on the randomized controlled trial (RCT). This RCT research design involves randomization at an individual level to different intervention conditions. In comparison, implementation science often emphasizes external validity, or the generalizability of a causal inference in a variety of real-world settings.[4-8] Consequently, the RCT research design is not often feasible, appropriate, nor useful for implementation science.[9] Alternative designs to the RCT are often used in implementation science to facilitate adoption, adaptation, delivery, and sustainment of an intervention in a variety of real-world service settings.

This chapter discusses study designs, data collection, and analytic techniques appropriate for implementation science. There exists considerable variability in methodological approaches for implementation science. Implementation often involves multilevel contextual factors (e.g., perceived need for change, organizational readiness for change, provider knowledge, sociopolitical context, funding, patient and/or client advocacy, and interorganizational networks) over time.[10] With great variability in multilevel and multiphasic factors, approaches for implementation science require an effort to balance methodological flexibility and rigor.

To shape this chapter's presentation of implementation science methodology, the National Institutes of Health (NIH) RePORTER database was reviewed for currently funded implementation studies focused on the cancer control continuum. Specifically, active projects (fiscal year 2017) funded by the National Cancer Institute (NCI) and reviewed by the NIH Dissemination and Implementation Research in Health (DIRH) study section were appraised with regard to study design, data collection, and analysis. Currently, funded studies span the length of the translational phases, including comparative effectiveness, health intervention/program adaptation, diffusion and/or dissemination investigation, as well as a range of implementation studies, such as context assessment and strategy development and/or testing. The majority of studies detail hybrid experimental designs in order to assess both clinical and implementation outcomes. The projects predominantly include both qualitative and quantitative aspects, although true mixed method data analyses appear rare.

This chapter reviews methodological approaches for implementation science that are frequently used as evidenced in the NIH RePORTER database review. Additional methodological approaches and considerations for implementation science are presented. At the close of this chapter, gaps in the field of implementation science, along with future directions, are discussed.

STUDY DESIGN

A number of study designs are appropriate for implementation science. Our discussion of implementation science study design targets use of experimental, quasi-experimental/observational, and alternative randomized designs. Box 5.1 provides a summary of study designs commonly used in implementation science. A recently introduced study design that simultaneously assesses clinical effectiveness and implementation, the effectiveness–implementation hybrid design, is also discussed. Hybrid designs were proposed in 15 of the 27 current NCI-funded projects that were reviewed in the DIRH study section. Another notable feature of implementation science is the importance of collaboration with relevant stakeholders. Specific designs for collaboration, such as community academic partnerships, are introduced.

Experimental Design

Experimental designs wherein internal validity is prioritized and often involves randomization still dominate NCI-funded implementation science. Often considered the "gold standard" of experimental designs, the RCT represents the modal research design, particularly with regard to basic research conducted in laboratory settings.[11] This design has clear dominance in strengthening causal inference, that a given intervention has caused an observed response. However, establishing internal validity becomes more difficult when complications arise. For example, experiments conducted over repeated sessions may involve attrition, or staff/employee turnover. As a result, researchers must consider threats to internal validity that can present in their particular research context.

The most common technique for limiting potential threats to causal inference is randomization. Randomization is used to equate the intervention and control conditions at baseline, prior to any delivery of intervention. In randomization, participants are assigned to intervention conditions using a method that gives every participant an equal chance of being assigned to the intervention and control conditions. Although randomization is relatively straightforward in laboratory settings, implementation science settings present more nuanced randomization challenges.

One challenge for randomization in implementation science involves the unit of observation. In contrast to basic, efficacy, and effectiveness research wherein a intervention is often tested for its effect on individual participants, implementation science tests strategies that influence adoption, uptake, and sustainment of a intervention in one or more service settings. Consequently, randomization in implementation science often occurs at the level of the service setting. Physicians, clinics, communities, and care

Box 5.1 Summary of Study Designs for Implementation Science

Experimental design: Prioritizes internal validity.

Randomized controlled trial (RCT): Randomization is used to equate intervention and control conditions at baseline. Randomization can be a challenge in implementation science due to higher level units of observation, attrition over repeated sessions, contamination, and staff/employee turnover. Having adequate statistical power for an RCT is a major challenge for implementation science.

Cluster randomized trial: Randomization occurs at the group, rather than individual, level. Randomization at a higher unit can threaten internal validity due to fewer numbers of units to randomize.

Quasi-experimental and/or observational design: Prioritizes external validity. Often used when randomization is not feasible, appropriate, or helpful.

Controlled before and after study: Intervention and control groups are assigned in a nonrandomized manner and include the measurement of main outcomes during baseline period. Pre- and post-intervention periods for intervention and control sites should be equivalent.

Regression discontinuity: One of most rigorous alternatives to RCT. Intervention groups are assigned on the basis of whether they exceed or are below a cut-point on a quantitative measure.

Interrupted time series: An excellent alternative for producing high-quality causal inference. Measurements of the outcome variable are collected at equally spaced intervals over a long period of time. Changes in level and slope that occur as a function of the introduction of the intervention can indicate an effect.

Alternative randomized design: Increase strength of external validity while maintaining strength of internal validity.

Effectiveness–implementation hybrid study design: There are three types of hybrid designs, all placing a dual emphasis on intervention effectiveness and implementation outcomes.

Roll-out design (stepped wedge): All units start in a usual practice setting, although the cross over to a new intervention condition at randomly determined time intervals. This results in the ability to make both between-unit and within-unit comparisons as units are assigned to the new intervention condition.

Cumulative trial design: Outcomes from replicate cohorts or related trials are combined. The intervention is improved through repeated trials while using cumulative data to conduct an overall evaluation of the intervention. The combination of trial data also increases statistical power.

Randomized encouragement trial and randomized consent design: Strengthens external validity by offering the option to adhere to a randomly assigned condition or switch to a preferred condition with the intention of preventing non-adherence.

Randomized factorial design: Investigates the combination of two or more interventions at a time, with each experimental factor having two or more levels. Main and interaction effects are estimated.

organizations may be randomized in implementation science, rather than randomization occurring at an individual patient level. Randomization at a higher unit level can pose a threat to internal validity due to having fewer numbers of units to randomize, reducing the likelihood of randomization truly equating intervention and control groups. Randomization that occurs at the group, rather than individual, level represents a cluster randomized trial, a commonly used design in implementation science that is useful in testing the effects of implementation strategies.[12,13] Cluster randomized controlled trials were frequently proposed in currently funded NCI studies in the DIRH study section. For example, one study investigating the implementation of tobacco use treatment guidelines[14] involved randomization of worksites to one of three intervention arms. These intervention arms were different implementation strategies. All conditions received current best practices, in addition to one of the following: (1) staff training, (2) provider performance feedback, or (3) provider performance feedback plus pay for performance. In another example, 14 Black churches were randomized to low level of technical assistance versus high community autonomy implementation strategy to implement an early cancer detection intervention. The number of intervention arms (implementation strategies) in included studies of the NIH RePORTER database varied between two, three and four.

If similar teams of physicians exist and work independently within each organization, an efficient design to study implementation could involve random assignment of teams within each organization into intervention and control conditions such that a comparison can be made between implementation strategies within each organization.[15] However, implementation often occurs within complex, multilevel contexts. If two implementation conditions are tested in the same site, organization, community, or service system, there is a potential for contamination. Contamination occurs when an implementation strategy leaks from a designated intervention condition into a non-assigned intervention condition. For example, if two groups of physicians are each assigned to separate implementation strategy conditions, leakage can occur when these two groups meet with each other and share experiences regarding implementation techniques. In addition, if a research design aims to test system-level policies on implementation, a design that randomizes small subunits within the system would not be able to test a systems-level approach.[16]

Additional challenges exist with regard to randomized experiments in implementation science. An inherent assumption for randomized experiments is the stable unit treatment value assumption (SUTVA).[11] This assumption has the following two parts: (1) The randomization should not impact the participants' response to experimental or control intervention condition, and (2) the response of the participants should not be impacted by the interventions assigned to other units. If a service setting is assigned a particular implementation strategy

via randomization rather than via beliefs, if it is particularly well suited for a particular implementation strategy, or if it believes it has earned assignment to a particular implementation strategy for meritorious achievements, might the response to implementation strategy differ? Some social psychological theorists would predict differences in motivation as a result.[17] In addition, knowledge of other intervention conditions can change the participants' level of motivation, particularly for those randomized to control conditions. For example, a service setting that is randomized to an implementation-as-usual control condition with full knowledge that another service setting has been assigned to a promising implementation strategy might experience resentful demoralization resulting in poorer outcomes in the control group than normal.[11]

Breakdown of randomization also presents as a challenge for experimental designs. For a randomized experiment to yield an unbiased estimate of the causal effect, random assignment of participants to intervention and control conditions must be appropriately carried out. Studies of large-scale randomized field experiments have noted that breakdowns of randomization occur with some frequency. Problems occur more frequently when individuals responsible for carrying out an implementation strategy are allowed to assign participants to intervention conditions and when monitoring of the maintenance of the intervention assignment is poor. For example, a breakdown may occur when multiple clinics within a single service system are to be randomized to different implementation conditions and the centralized, service system leaders are conducting the randomization without sufficient monitoring.

A major challenge that presents for experimental designs concerns statistical power. For a randomized trial to be worth performing, it must have adequate statistical power to detect differences between the intervention and control conditions. However, for many years this design has continued to be used despite inadequate power,[18] and this issue pervades currently funded implementation studies. Only one study in the NIH RePORTER database funded by NCI and reviewed in the DIRH study section details the statistical power calculation.[19] Yet even this study conducts statistical power calculation on effectiveness rather than implementation outcomes. The study details a cluster RCT of 20 community coalitions in four different implementation conditions, with each coalition partnering with three different settings, resulting in five potential clusters per condition. Statistical power calculation is based on the number of participants per community coalition ($n = 3,600$) and per study arm ($n = 1,800$) to increase screening rates. Following Cohen's[20] convention for power, in a randomized experiment with an equal number of participants in intervention and control groups, 52 total participants would be needed to detect a large effect (26 in each arm), 126 participants would be needed to detect a moderate effect (63 in each arm), and 786 participants would be needed to detect a small effect (393 in each arm) (at $\alpha = .05$ and power $= .80$). When designing experiments, several techniques can be used to increase power, such as increasing sample size, including stronger interventions, maintaining fidelity of implementation (fidelity of implementation strategy and/ or clinical intervention), using reliable measures, maximizing participant uniformity, minimizing participant attrition, and adding covariates measured at pretest that are related to the dependent variable of interest. However, practice issues often serve as a barrier to increasing power with these techniques in implementation science. Cost, limited availability of resources, or limited availability of certain special participant populations can prevent one from increasing power with these techniques.

Quasi-Experimental and/or Observational Design

implementation science study designs can be quasi-experimental and/or observational. In contrast to experimental designs, namely the RCT, quasi-experimental and/or observational designs provide a more convincing basis for generalization of causal inferences found in basic, efficacy, and effectiveness research. Quasi-experimental and/or observational designs prioritize external validity and can be used in situations in which randomization is not feasible, appropriate, or helpful. In implementation science, randomization may be precluded by ethical, legal, practical, or policy concerns. In some cases, quasi-experimental and/or observational designs using survey or interview data collection methods may provide useful information on the implementation context. For example, one current NCI-funded study that was reviewed by the DIRH study section surveyed 72 Federally Qualified Health Centers and Rural Health Clinics that were implementing patient navigation to assist women

after they receive abnormal mammograms. The investigators plan to assess the level of implementation as well as organizational constructs thought to influence implementation with the aim of using this information, together with interview data, in a latent content analysis approach to understand how and why implementation is successful in some but not all organizations. In many cases, it is possible to develop alternative quasi-experimental designs that share many of the strengths of randomized experiment with regard to causal inference. Many of these designs involve manipulation of the independent variable, pre- and post-test measurement, and design or statistical controls that attempt to address threats to internal validity. Three types of quasi-experimental and/or observational designs often used in implementation science are the controlled before and after study, interrupted time series, and regression discontinuity designs.

Controlled before and after study designs involve intervention and control groups that are assigned in a non-randomized manner and include the measurement of main outcomes during a baseline period. To improve scientific rigor in controlled before and after study designs, pre- and post-intervention periods for study and control sites should be equivalent, and a control site should be chosen appropriately such that sites are comparable with respect to characteristics, level of care, setting, and so on. In addition, although these designs require the use of at least two sites, it is not uncommon to include more.

Regression discontinuity design is one of the most rigorous alternatives to the randomized experiment. This design can be used when interventions are assigned on the basis of some quantitative measure. For example, clinics could be assigned to intervention and control implementation strategy conditions based on the proportion of patients appropriately screened for cancer conditions (i.e., mammogram and colonoscopy) during a specified quarter of the year. Clinics that have a proportion below .80 screened within a fall quarter may be assigned to a tailored implementation strategy, whereas clinics who have a proportion of .70 or above within a fall quarter may be assigned to an implementation-as-usual control condition. The outcome of interest could be proportion of patients appropriately screened in the winter quarter as a function of implementation strategy condition. The central features of regression discontinuity designs are that the participants are assigned to intervention or control conditions solely on the basis of

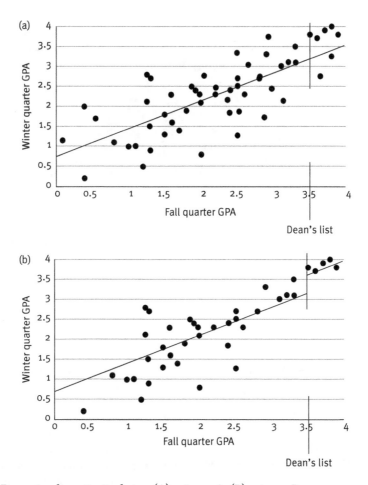

FIGURE 5.1   Regression discontinuity design: (A) outcome A; (B) outcome B.

Source: Adapted with permission from West et al.[11]

whether they exceed or are below a cut-point on a quantitative assignment variable and that an outcome hypothesized to be affected by the intervention is measured following intervention. Figure 5.1 provides a graphical representation of a regression discontinuity design wherein students with a grade point average (GPA) of 3.5 in the fall quarter are assigned to the dean's list.[11] In outcome A, the dean's list assignment has no effect on winter quarter GPA. In outcome B, the dean's list assignment results in an elevated regression line. The discontinuity in the two regression lines can be interpreted as an intervention effect.

The interrupted time series design is another quasi-experimental design with excellent scientific rigor for producing high-quality causal inference. In simple interrupted time series designs, measurements of the outcome variable are collected at equally spaced intervals (i.e., daily, monthly, or annually) over a long period of time. An intervention is introduced at a specified point in time and is expected to affect the outcome variable measured in the series. Changes in the level and slope of the series that occur as a function of the introduction of the intervention can indicate an effect. This study design was adopted in a current NCI-funded study reviewed by the DIRH study section, wherein investigators planned to use segmented regression analysis of cross-sectional interrupted time series data of the two interventions being tested before and after implementation. In this case, the design targeted the clinical interventions as a comparative effectiveness study rather than testing implementation strategies; however, additional data on implementation were gathered through surveys.

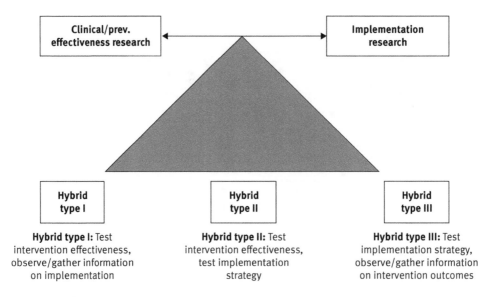

FIGURE 5.2   Effectiveness–implementation hybrid designs.

Source: Adapted with permission from Curran et al.[21]

Alternative Randomized Design

To address concerns regarding generalizability while simultaneously testing an intervention/treatment effect, many alternative randomized designs have been utilized. These designs attempt to increase the strength of external validity (compared to that of the traditional RCT) while maintaining the strength of internal validity.

Traditionally, implementation science occurs as the final stage of the translational research pipeline. More recently, effectiveness–implementation hybrid study designs have been introduced as an alternative to the sequential test from basic science to efficacy and effectiveness research and then to implementation.[21] There are three types of hybrid designs, all placing a dual emphasis on clinical effectiveness and implementation. Figure 5.2 provides a visual representation of these designs. Type 1 hybrid designs place greater emphasis on clinical effectiveness by testing the effects of a clinical intervention on relevant outcomes while simultaneously collecting information on implementation. Type 3 hybrid designs place greater emphasis on implementation by testing an implementation strategy while collecting information on the clinical intervention's impact on relevant outcomes. Type 2 hybrid designs place equal emphasis on clinical effectiveness and implementation through the dual testing of clinical intervention and implementation strategies. Use

of a hybrid design has the potential for more rapid translation of research findings into routine practice.

Roll-out designs, such as the stepped wedge design, have also been used in implementation science as an alternative randomized design. In a simple roll-out implementation science design, all units start in a usual practice setting. At randomly determined time intervals, units cross over to a new intervention condition (which is often the assignment of an alternative implementation strategy). As a result, at each time interval, there is a between-unit comparison of those units that are assigned to the new implementation strategy and those units that remain as a usual practice setting. In addition, a within-unit comparison can be made as the units change from a usual practice setting to a new implementation strategy at some randomly assigned time. One study identified from the NIH RePORTER database of currently NCI-funded studies reviewed in the DIRH study section proposed to conduct a randomized controlled pragmatic trial with a stepped wedge design. This study aims to compare simple audit and feedback strategy versus a tailored multicomponent intervention to improve the implementation of facility-level optimization of computed tomography radiation dose.

Cumulative trial designs are also used in implementation science as an alternative randomized design wherein outcomes from replicate cohorts or related trials are combined. In this design, an intervention is continuously improved through repeated trials while using the cumulative data to conduct an overall evaluation of the intervention.[22] For example, a strategic plan for these trials might be twofold: (1) to assess the relationship between a particular intervention and hypothesized mediators of an intervention's effect, such as implementation outcomes, and early proximal outcomes; and (2) to then assess the intervention's effect on more distal outcomes of interest. The cumulative sequence of trials aims to improve quality over time by using the results between trials to refine such interventions. The cumulative sequence of trials also aims to improve evaluation of intervention impact by increasing statistical power through the combination of trial data.

Alternative designs such as the randomized encouragement trial and the randomized consent design attempt to strengthen external validity by offering a set of strategies for addressing participant preference. In such designs, participants are randomized to condition but are then offered the option to adhere to their assigned condition or switch to a more preferred condition. The intention is to prevent non-adherence to intervention condition by allowing participants to choose according to protocol. In Zelen's[23] original proposal, two types of randomized consent designs were defined. In the single consent randomized design, only study participants randomized to the experimental condition are asked to consent to the experimental condition or to the standard condition, whereas participants randomized to the standard condition are not asked for their consent and are expected to adhere. In the double consent randomized design, participants in each condition are asked to consent to the randomly assigned condition or to the alternative. Duan et al.'s[24,25] extension of this design, the randomized encouragement trial, includes encouragement strategies for participants randomized to the experimental condition as a method for formalizing adherence strategies.

The randomized factorial design represents an alternative randomized trial. Factorial designs for implementation investigate the combination of two or more implementation strategies at a time. Each experimental factor, or arm, has two or more levels. For example, one experimental factor representing an implementation strategy that is commonly used could be consultation type, with remote and in-person consultation as distinct levels. Another experimental factor could be feedback timing, with monthly and as-needed as two distinct levels. Such a design would be classified as a 2×2 factorial implementation design, with participants (physicians, clinics, organizations, etc.) randomly assigned to one of the four conditions. Main effects of each factor, as well as the interactions between factors, can be estimated. Sequential multiple assignment randomized trial (SMART) designs serve as a specific type of factorial design, and another alternative randomized design that can accommodate participant preferences.[26,27] SMART designs are clinical trials that experimentally examine strategy choices and allow for multiple comparison options. For example, Kilbourne et al.'s[28] trial used SMART to test the Replicating Effectiveness Programs (REP) strategy for promoting implementation of evidence-based health care interventions. In this trial, clinics that did not respond to REP were randomized to receive additional support from an external facilitator or both an external and an internal facilitator. Clinics that were randomized to receive an external facilitator only and were still unresponsive to REP were randomized again to continue with only an external facilitator or both an external and an internal facilitator.

Stakeholder Involvement

Stakeholder involvement can be a useful methodological consideration in facilitating implementation, and it is often explicitly targeted in implementation science such as through the Community-Based Participatory Research, Community–Academic Partnership designs, and intervention mapping. One barrier to the implementation of evidence-based interventions in practice is the "poor links between those who carry out research and those who provide services."[29,p.143] Collaborative partnerships between researchers and practitioners have potential to close this gap between research on health services and actual practice of such services.[30] Methodologies for stakeholder selection can include network analyses and community consensus. Four fundamental assumptions exist regarding the conduct of such collaborative research:[31]

1. It is distinguished from other forms of research by its emphasis on developing and managing relationships between university-based researchers and community collaborators and by its focus on achieving social change through community empowerment.

2. Genuine partnerships require a willingness of all stakeholders to learn from one another.

3. There must be a commitment to training community members in research.

4. The knowledge and other products gained from research activities should benefit all partners.

Additional criteria for determining the success of projects undertaken by such partnerships include (but are not limited to) the presence of clear goals that are jointly defined by all partners; that all partners are engaged in all levels of activity, including planning and execution; and that the partnership includes ongoing reflective evaluation, including evaluation of the project and the partnership as well as an assessment by all partners.[32] A recently published systematic review of research–practice partnerships found a growing emphasis on using partnerships in the past several years that spans multiple disciplines, research areas, and involves a variety of community populations.[33] Successful research–practice partnerships conduct research that is valid and reliable, relevant to the needs of policymakers and practitioners, and critical to effectively translating research into practice. Collaboration and community involvement are often considered to be desirable qualities in research studies, particularly for facilitating implementation effectiveness and stakeholder engagement. A number of studies in the NIH RePORTER database funded by NCI reviewed in the DIRH study section planned to incorporate working with stakeholders. Stakeholder involvement ranged from conducting focus groups and/or interviews for the tailoring of both clinical interventions and implementation strategies to more comprehensive community-based participatory research projects wherein communities were fully integrated throughout the research process, including involvement in intervention mapping methodology in some studies.

DATA COLLECTION

The types of data collected in implementation studies emulate efficacy and effectiveness research, although a greater emphasis is placed on mixed methods that combine both quantitative and qualitative data. Following a brief introduction to considerations for data collection in implementation science, quantitative, qualitative, and mixed methods and sampling are discussed.

One critical feature of implementation science is that the data collected incorporate data on the implementation process, influences, and/or outcomes, either with or without the collection of clinical outcomes (see the previous discussion on hybrid designs). Implementation outcomes serve as intermediate outcomes to health outcomes.[34] For example, "reach" refers to the percentage of an eligible population who receive the intervention being implemented. Reach is therefore both an implementation outcome and a clinical process measure or output and necessary to determine the impact of a clinical intervention.[34,35] Moreover, as implementation researchers investigate implementation strategies, the direct outcomes of the implementation strategies should be collected and analyzed. (For further discussion, see Chapter 4, this volume.)

A second data collection issue for implementation science is that implementation data are frequently multilevel (e.g., individual, team, organization, local setting, and system). All contextual levels that have potential to influence the implementation effort should be determined,[36] and subsequently the referent level of the data to be collected should be carefully decided. For instance, the implementation of a clinical guideline may involve data collection from individuals such as physicians, nurses, and patients to gather information about their attitudes toward the guideline. The data collected from these individuals, however, may also concern the functioning of their team, the climate of their organization, their perceptions of the health system, and so on. The nested structure of data is discussed further in the section titled Data Analysis.

The third facet of implementation science that influences data collection is that implementation is a multistage process. Implementation is a complex process rather than a single event.[10] In efficacy and effectiveness studies, data on the implementation and clinical intervention processes are often not collected due to a focus on outcomes.[37] This leads to a lack of knowledge about the mechanism of action of the intervention and generalizability of findings. Implementation data are time-dependent, and collection ideally should involve repeated measures over time.[38]

Quantitative

The purpose of quantitative data is enumeration. To ensure rigor of findings using quantitative data, an appropriate study design and appropriate measurement tools must be selected. In addition, for inferences to be made and hypotheses tested, sampling and sample size are crucial. After collection, quantitative data are managed in a database and analyzed using various statistical methods as described later in the section titled Data Analysis.

QUANTITATIVE APPROACHES

Based on our review of currently funded NCI projects reviewed by the DIRH study section, surveys are the most common primary data collection method for implementation science. Quantitative surveys typically consist of closed-ended questions and rating scales with limited response options.[39] Surveys may include questions completed by respondents about themselves or their actions (self-report) or about their perceptions of a different entity or phenomenon, such as the leadership, culture, or climate of the organization in which they work.[40] Surveys continue to be distributed in paper form, but they are also often developed and administered via internet programs such as Qualtrics and SurveyMonkey. Other digital survey management methods include the use of kiosks, tablets, text message, or computer-assisted telephone interviewing. A further method for quantitative data collection is ecological momentary assessment (EMA), which allows collection of data in real time rather than retrospective responses. EMA holds potential for fidelity monitoring and in dynamic adaptation processes of clinical innovations and/or implementation strategies.[41]

Technological advances have led to a burgeoning array of new data collection options—for example, abstraction from large databases, including electronic health records and all-payer databases. Digital health technologies, such as mobile phone apps and wearables, also facilitate the collection of quantitative data.

QUANTITATIVE SAMPLING AND SAMPLE SELECTION

As with all data collection methodologies, sampling is an important consideration for quantitative data collection. The principal issue of sampling for quantitative data is to ensure sufficient sample size for power analyses (accounting for effect size and the nested structure of data). Representative probability samples such as random and stratified are generally desirable for quantitative data. For further discussion, see the section titled Mixed Methods.

Qualitative

It is widely acknowledged that strong evidence of a clinical intervention's effectiveness will not automatically lead to adoption and implementation. The dissemination, adoption, implementation, and sustainment of clinical interventions constitute a long, complex process.[10] Understanding the complexities and nuances of contextual differences that influence the implementation process is crucial to implementation science and consequently the rate and spread of clinical interventions into routine practice. Qualitative data have significant advantages with regard to evoking responses that are meaningful and culturally salient to participants, unanticipated by the researcher, rich and explanatory in nature. As such, throughout the implementation process, qualitative methods are valuable to develop a profound understanding of the context, perspectives of the different players, and the unique barriers and enablers to each implementation effort.[42] Furthermore, in the early stages of implementation science, observational studies can illicit crucial exploratory information that may aid in understanding the need and demand for a clinical intervention, and such data may be helpful in hypothesis generation.[42] As the implementation process continues, qualitative data provide information on the complexity of implementing the changes and explanations for success or failure.

Many currently NCI-funded studies in the DIRH study section are designed in phases. The first phase often involves a qualitative study, followed by an experimental quantitative or mixed methods study. In these instances, projects utilize qualitative data to gain information to develop hypotheses, adapt interventions to be more contextually appropriate, or tailor an implementation strategy based on the context. For example, one participatory action research proposal is to conduct focus groups with stakeholders established from a community consensus initially to develop a screening intervention. An interrupted time series study will be utilized to study the implementation of the developed intervention, monitored and evaluated iteratively in both pre- and post-implementation phases using mixed methodologies.[43]

Interestingly, few traditional observational qualitative studies are currently being conducted. This may indicate a move away from case studies focusing on factors influencing implementation and toward experimental studies investigating implementation strategies.[44]

QUALITATIVE APPROACHES

Qualitative data collection approaches in implementation science mimic the data collection procedure in efficacy and effectiveness research: Define the research question; select a study design suitable to answer the research question; determine the participants (sampling); ascertain where, when, and how data will be collected; analyze the data; and generate findings.

As per quantitative methods, it is necessary to ensure scientific rigor in the data collection and later during data analysis. The study design should be chosen to answer the research question by following an appropriate qualitative approach—that is, ethnography, phenomenology, narrative, grounded theory, and case study.[45]

Data collection methods include direct observation; participant (indirect) observation; and elicitation techniques such as focus groups, unstructured, semistructured, and structured interviews, and open-ended questions on surveys. Qualitative data may involve audio, object, video, and text, where text may be the object of analysis or the proxy for experiences collected from observation and elicitation.[46]

Qualitative approaches yield rich information but are often costly in terms of the time required to collect and analyze the data. Data for fidelity monitoring and evaluation may be collected quantitatively by self-reported questionnaires or clinical documents or through qualitative data collection using interviews or direct observation (including video and audio recordings). Although quantitative data collection holds advantages, it is important to consider when qualitative data should be utilized because prior studies have shown that self-report of fidelity may not converge with objective rater coding of implementation or clinical process.[47] However, recent developments in computer automated coding of fidelity to evidence-based practices (e.g., motivational interviewing[48]) hold promise to make effective and efficient coding of fidelity a cost-effective reality.[49]

QUALITATIVE SAMPLING AND SAMPLE SELECTION

Ideally, to identify an appropriate sample that is representative, sampling should be determined by research objective, characteristics of the study population (e.g., size and diversity), and unit of analysis. In addition, triangulation of viewpoints across roles related to the phenomena is encouraged (e.g., interviews from patients, nurses, physicians, and those who work in management). Qualitative studies usually employ a form of non-probability/non-representative sampling, such as quota, purposeful (including deviant case, criterion, and maximum variation), or convenience. The snowball method, stakeholder analyses, and network analyses may be used gather a purposive sample. Data collection is often an iterative process between collection and analysis until "saturation" is achieved.[42] Data saturation is a concept to ensure validity; it occurs when no additional codes are derived from the data and thus no further sampling or data collection is required. The following section provides a more detailed discussion.

Mixed Methods

Mixed method research involves the integration of qualitative and quantitative method philosophies, designs, strategies, analytic approaches, and interpretations.[50-52] Mixed method research is increasingly critical for implementation science in health and allied health settings[53-57] and in implementation science in cancer prevention and treatment.[58] Indeed, the use of mixed methods has been strongly recommended "to enhance the value of dissemination and implementation research for end users" (p. 49).[59]

In implementation science, mixed method designs are being utilized for a number of purposes, but they have particular strength with regard to contextualizing and understanding nuance in the implementation process; identifying and understanding facilitators and barriers to implementation; understanding the process and outcomes of implementation; and assessing feasibility, acceptability, and utility of novel implementation strategies.[55,60-62] In cancer research, mixed methods have been used for studies on patient-reported outcome assessment,[63] radical treatment for prostate cancer,[64] standards of care in pediatric cancer,[65] web-based programs for adolescent cancer survivors,[66] and understanding the implementation of cancer networks.[67] Although there are calls for increased use of mixed methods, many studies with qualitative and quantitative components lack effective "mixing" of design, analytic strategies, results, and reporting from these potentially complementary methods.

MIXED METHOD APPROACHES

Mixed method research designs encompass collecting, analyzing, and integrating quantitative and qualitative data and their analyses and interpretations. The use of mixed methods provides a more comprehensive, more detailed, and richer understanding of research issues compared to either approach used alone.[61,68,69] In implementation studies, mixed method designs can be used to explore and obtain depth of understanding not possible with one approach and data source alone. For example, one can explore the reasons for success or failure to attain important implementation outcomes such as model fidelity or the reach of the intervention to service providers or the appropriate clinical population. Mixed methods can also be used to identify strategies for facilitating implementation. For example, conceptual models and their components can be assessed through formative and confirmatory evaluation,[10,57,70,71] and implementation approaches can be tested and evaluated.[72] Quantitative methods may be best used to test and confirm hypotheses based on an existing conceptual model, whereas qualitative data can increase breadth of understanding of predictors and quantitative outcomes.[68,73] Quantitative data can also be used for purposes such as identifying and selecting appropriate samples for qualitative data collection.[74]

MIXED METHOD FUNCTIONS

Mixed method approaches are characterized by several functions (also known as "component features"). The functions of mixed methods depend on whether the two methods are being used to answer the same question, to answer related questions, or to answer different questions. Designs can emphasize quantitative or qualitative methods as equal or one as a primary method (indicated by abbreviations in capital letters to indicate quantitative ["QUAN"] or qualitative ["QUAL"] approaches) with the other being secondary (indicated by abbreviations in lowercase letters—"quan"

and "qual"). The sequencing of methods is another design element. Methods can be concurrent or sequential with regard to data collection, analysis, interpretation, and reporting. Sequencing can be indicated by one preceding the other with an arrow in between (e.g., "qual → quant" or "quant → qual") or concurrent methods indicated by a plus sign (e.g., "qual + quant"). For both emphasis and sequencing, the previously mentioned indicators can be used with capital letters (e.g., "QUANT → qual" to indicate emphasis on primary quantitative methods that precede qualitative methods).

Qualitative and quantitative data can be integrated through "triangulation"—a process for strategically utilizing multiple methods together—in order to examine convergence, expansion, and complementarity of qualitative and quantitative methods.[68,73] Convergence is used to determine if qualitative and quantitative results provide the same answer to the same question. For example, does interview or observational data concur with quantitative data regarding factors influencing adoption of cancer screening? Complementarity is used to answer related questions for the purpose of evaluation or elaboration. For example, an implementation strategy for sun protection may be preferred, and qualitative methods can elaborate on conditions under which the strategy may be more applicable. Expansion is used to examine whether or not unanticipated findings produced by one data set can be explained by another. For example, survey data that suggest reasons for use of a cancer prevention strategy can be further expanded on or explained by qualitative data in order to understand nuance in patient preference and adoption.

MIXED METHOD SAMPLING AND SAMPLE SELECTION

A number of sampling approaches can be used in mixed method research. Common approaches to sampling for mixed method research include probability sampling, purposive sampling, convenience sampling, and mixed methods sampling.[75] We briefly describe each here, and we refer the reader to the taxonomy described by Teddlie and Yu[75] for a more detailed description of the issues and choices.

Probability sampling is typically used to promote the representativeness of a sample so that inferences can be made to a larger heterogeneous population.[76] Probability sampling can be random (i.e., individuals from a population), stratified (i.e., from target subgroups to ensure representativeness), or cluster (i.e., from groups of people in units such as neighborhoods or regions). The particular approach to probability sampling depends on the goals of the study and the population to which inferences are to be made.

Purposive sampling may be utilized to identify and select specific groups of interest. One approach to purposive sampling is maximum variation sampling, in which the goal is to select participants with divergent perspectives, such as those with the most positive or negative views on a topic, issue, or experience.[74,77]

Convenience sampling involves utilizing samples of people who are readily available and willing to participate. However, there are drawbacks to this approach in that such participants may not be representative of populations of interest or may not be comparable to those who avoid or refuse participation.[76]

Mixed methods sampling can involve probability sampling and purposive sampling.[75] It also includes consideration of whether quantitative and qualitative aspects of a study are sequential or concurrent and considers the multiple levels of interest in a study (e.g., system, organizations, team, clinician, and patient). As such, mixed methods sampling has a high degree of utility for studies across implementation phases of exploration, preparation, implementation, and sustainment and across the outer context (e.g., state health system) and inner context (e.g., clinic).[10]

DATA ANALYSIS

In many ways, considerations for data analyses in implementation science are similar to those of efficacy and/or effectiveness trials. Data are similarly managed and cleaned, and the data analytic technique utilized should complement the research design and be appropriate for the type of quantitative, qualitative, and/or mixed data collected. Although many similarities exist between data analyses for implementation science and efficacy/effectiveness research, there are some considerations more heavily present in implementation science. For example, alternatives to the traditional RCT are often used in implementation science. Techniques for enhancing the rigor of non-randomized designs with regard to internal validity can be employed, such as propensity score analysis and sensitivity analysis. To demonstrate the connection between implementation and effectiveness outcomes, mediation, moderation,

and path analysis are often employed. Finally, nested, multilevel designs are common in implementation science. As such, statistics for assessing the nested nature of data are often assessed, and data analytic techniques must take into account the nested data structure when present. In this section, we discuss in greater detail some of the previously mentioned challenges that often present in implementation science.

Statistical Considerations for Non-Randomized Controlled Trials

As discussed previously, implementation science often employs a quasi-experimental or alternative randomized design. A primary concern when utilizing designs other than the RCT is non-equivalence between intervention conditions. For example, when utilizing a randomized consent design, it is possible that participants who elect to opt out of their originally assigned intervention condition for some alternative are inherently different in some way from those who consent to their originally assigned intervention condition. The differing characteristics between groups or unobserved, hidden variables[11] can cause misleading inferences regarding post-intervention group differences. For this reason, causal inference is weakened in quasi-experimental and alternative randomized designs.

Several statistical precautions are often taken in implementation science to prevent inaccurate inferences due to differences between groups. One such technique is covariate analysis. Analysis of covariance adjusts post-intervention scores for the measured pre-intervention scores. Typically, adjustment is made only for the linear effect of pre-intervention scores on the post-test scores. No adjustment is made for variables that are not included in the analysis, nor is the proper adjustment made for variables that are measured with error. Analysis of covariance with correction for unreliability is a technique that adjusts the post-intervention scores based on an estimate for what the post-intervention scores would have been if they were measured without error, and it is typically performed using structural equation modeling programs.

Propensity score analysis is another, rigorous, technique for assessing intervention effect in the absence of random assignment.[78] Introduced in 1983, propensity score analysis is slowly gaining attention as a promising technique for research. The number of yearly published papers that use propensity score analyses is increasing exponentially.[79] In the absence of an RTC, wherein covariates are accounted for by the process of randomization, propensity score analysis provides a promising mechanism by which one can assess causality while reducing confounding variables. Although there are four methods of using estimated propensity scores to assess intervention effects, all attempt to balance covariates, reducing/eliminating the effects of confounding variables. Rosenbaum and Rubin's iterative approach[80] to specifying a propensity score model specifies the probability of having been selected for the intervention group using baseline, pre-intervention, characteristics. Next, the comparability of intervention and comparison groups is assessed, and model specification is repeated until the distribution of observed baseline covariates is similar between intervention and comparison group participants.

Sensitivity analyses are often used with propensity score analysis or other matched group designs. Sensitivity analyses give an indication of the magnitude of bias due to hidden variables that would be necessary for eliminating the appearance of an intervention effect.

Moderation, Mediation, and Path Analysis

Studies that assess moderation and/or mediation are prevalent in implementation science. Moderation occurs when the effect of an independent variable on a dependent variable varies in accordance with a third variable, a *moderator*.[81] For example, in community-based participatory research that aims to improve rates of colorectal cancer screening, the effect of partnership functioning on screening rates might be moderated by attitudes about screening. Mediation indicates that the effect of an independent variable on a dependent variable is facilitated through a third variable, called a *mediator*. In path analysis, mediation refers to an indirect effect of an independent variable on a dependent variable that passes through a mediator variable.[82] For example, the effect of partnership functioning on colorectal cancer screening rates might be mediated by sustainability of partnership infrastructure. When hypothesizing causal connections, researchers may be interested in assessing the presence, strength, and significance of moderator and indirect effects. Path analysis is an extension of multiple regression that aims to provide estimates of the

magnitude and significance of hypothesized causal connections between sets of variables, and it may be completed using structural equation modeling software or standard least-squares or maximum likelihood regression routines.[83]

NESTED STUDY DESIGNS AND DATA

Nested, multilevel designs are common in implementation science. For example, the implementation of a clinical guideline may involve data collection from individuals such as physicians, nurses, and patients to gather information about their attitudes toward the guideline. The data collected from these individuals, however, may also concern the functioning of their team, the climate of their organization, their perceptions of the health system, and so on. In addition, implementation often occurs across multiple stages or phases across time. As such, data may be collected repeatedly, at several time points, across time.[84] Such designs involve nested, multilevel data, wherein repeated assessments (level 1) might be nested within individual participants (level 2), and participants might be nested within teams/organizations (level 3). Statistics for assessing the nested nature of data are often assessed in implementation science, and data analytic techniques must take into account the nested data structure when present.

Statistics commonly used in implementation science for assessing the nested nature of data include the intraclass correlation coefficient (ICC) and within-group agreement (r_{wg} and $r_{wg(j)}$). The ICC provides an index of the degree of non-independence due to grouped observations. It indicates the extent to which observations are more similar within groups than between groups and also the extent to which the test of the between-group effect is substantially biased if this non-independence is ignored.[85] The ICC can theoretically range from 0 to 1, although in practice the ICC can take on small negative values due to sampling errors (in such cases, the ICC is assigned a value of 0). To the extent that the ICC exceeds 0, the standard errors of the regression coefficients will be too small. When clustering is ignored, significance tests of regression coefficients will be too liberal, and the null hypothesis will be rejected when it is true at rates far exceeding the stated value (e.g., $\alpha = .05$).

The r_{wg} and $r_{wg(j)}$ are other statistics often used in implementation science for assessing the nested nature of data. First described by L. R. James et al. in 1984,[86] r_{wg} was proposed as a measure of interrater agreement. The $r_{wg(j)}$ is a later iteration of this statistic and is typically used to determine the appropriateness of aggregating data to higher levels of analysis. Unlike the ICC statistics, the r_{wg} and $r_{wg(j)}$ are calculated separately for each group and represent the within-group agreement coefficient for mean scores based on the number of items, the mean of the observed variances of the items, and the expected variance of a hypothesized null distribution.

There are strengths and limitations to the ICC and r_{wg} and $r_{wg(j)}$ statistics. Readers are encouraged to review Castro's[87] discussion for more information.

Assuming the data structure is indeed nested, and statistics indicate the appropriateness of aggregating data to higher levels of analysis, implementation researchers often utilize multilevel modeling and/or multilevel structural equation modeling for assessing quantitative data. Multilevel modeling and/or multilevel structural equation modeling should be utilized in designs wherein observations are nested within a higher level unit.[84,88] For a thorough discussion of multilevel modeling, see Raudenbush and Byrk[88] and Snijders and Bosker.[89]

As discussed previously, implementation researchers are often interested in determining mediating effects. In nested study designs, multilevel modeling and multilevel structural equation modeling can be used for testing mediation hypotheses when the data are hierarchically organized. Recommended procedures for testing multilevel mediation have been developed almost exclusively within the standard multilevel modeling paradigm. However, the multilevel modeling paradigm poses some limitations with regard to unbiased estimation of between- and within-group effects and estimation of upper level dependent variables. As a result, multilevel structural equation modeling has been proposed more recently as a comprehensive alternative for examining mediation effects in multilevel data.[90]

DISCUSSION

This chapter has provided a brief introduction to study design, data collection, and data analytic techniques employed in implementation science. In addition, based on the NIH RePORTER database, active NCI-funded implementation studies targeting the cancer control continuum were reviewed and discussed throughout this chapter as an exploration of the current state of the field.

The currently funded studies reviewed in NIH RePORTER span the translational phases of research, including comparative effectiveness, health intervention/program adaptation, and diffusion and/or dissemination investigation, as well as a range of implementation studies, such as context assessment and strategy development and/or testing. A review of these studies with regard to study design, data collection, and data analytic techniques revealed that an overwhelming majority utilize effectiveness–implementation hybrid study designs in order to simultaneously assess both clinical and implementation outcomes. The projects predominantly include both qualitative and quantitative aspects, although true mixed method data analytic techniques appear less frequently.

Randomized controlled trials and cluster randomized controlled trials were frequently proposed in currently funded NCI studies in the DIRH study section. For example, one study randomized worksites to one of three intervention arms, each representing a different implementation strategy. Although randomized study designs are the "gold standard" for strengthening internal validity, the RCT research design is not often feasible, appropriate, nor useful for implementation science. The greatest challenge that presents for experimental designs in implementation science concerns statistical power. For a randomized trial to be worth performing, it must have adequate statistical power to detect differences between the intervention and control conditions. Only one study in the NIH RePORTER database funded by NCI and reviewed in the DIRH study section detailed the statistical power calculation, and this study's power calculation targeted effectiveness rather than implementation outcomes. For many years, the RCT design has continued to be used despite inadequate power.

When the RCT research design is not feasible, appropriate, nor useful for implementation science, other designs can be used. This chapter briefly discussed two very powerful quasi-experimental designs that can be use when conducting implementation science: the regression discontinuity design and the interrupted time-series design. In addition, many alternative randomized designs, such as the stepped wedge design and the cumulative trial design, provide great promise as rigorous study design alternatives to the RCT. The use of such quasi-experimental and alternative randomized designs supports stronger generalizability without sacrificing causal inference. The future of implementation science could benefit from researchers' greater consideration and utilization of these approaches.

The field of implementation science is also more frequently acknowledging the benefit of utilizing mixed, qualitative, and qualitative methodologies. Although currently funded implementation trials often involve the collection of both qualitative and quantitative data, the field of implementation science can benefit from greater attention to the integration of these data. Merely collecting both qualitative and quantitative data without truly integrating the data will limit the depth and breadth of understanding gleaned from an evaluation. Researchers conducting mixed methods implementation science are strongly encouraged to consider the ways in which their data can be integrated to more appropriately examine convergence, expansion, and complementarity of qualitative and quantitative methods.

The field of implementation science is also acknowledging the appropriateness of collecting, analyzing, and interpreting hierarchical, multilevel data. The use of techniques for analyzing multilevel data is rapidly increasing. As briefly discussed in this chapter, path analysis is often utilized in implementation science, particularly with regard to better understanding mediating factors. In nested study designs, multilevel structural equation modeling has been proposed as a more thorough alternative to multilevel modeling for examining mediation effects. Although many similarities exist between data analyses for implementation science and efficacy/effectiveness research, there are some considerations more heavily present in implementation science. Researchers conducting implementation trials are urged to consider the multilevel, and multiphasic, nature of their data and ensure the data analytic technique utilized complements the research design and type of data collected.

SUMMARY

There exists considerable variability in methodological approaches for implementation science. In this chapter, we discussed study designs, data collection, and analytic techniques appropriate for implementation science. Although space limitations preclude a thorough discussion of these designs and

techniques, we hope this introduction can serve as a springboard for the consideration of appropriate, flexible, and rigorous methodology for addressing the multilevel and multiphasic contexts intrinsic to implementation science.

REFERENCES

1. National Research Council and Institute of Medicine. *Preventing Mental, Emotional, and Behavioral Disorders Among Young People: Progress and Possibilities*. Washington, DC: National Academies Press; 2009.
2. Zerhouni E. The NIH roadmap. *Science*. 2003;302(5642):63–72.
3. Westfall J, Mold J, Fagnan L. Practice-based research—"Blue highways" on the NIH roadmap. *JAMA*. 2007;297(4):403–406.
4. Campbell DT. Factors relevant to the validity of experiments in social settings. *Psychol Bull*. 1957;54(4):297–312.
5. Campbell DT. Relabeling internal and external validity for applied social scientists. In: Trochim WMK, ed. *Advances in Quasi-Experimental Design and Analysis*. San Francisco, CA: Jossey–Bass; 1986.
6. Campbell DT, Stanley JC. *Experimental and Quasi-Experimental Designs for Research*. Boston, MA: Houghton Mifflin; 1963.
7. Cook TD, Campbell DT. *Quasi-Experimentation: Design & Analysis Issues for Field Settings*. Boston, MA: Houghton Mifflin; 1979.
8. Shadish WR, Cook TD, Campbell DT. *Experimental and Quasi-Experimental Design for Generalized Causal Inference*. Boston, MA: Houghton Mifflin; 2002.
9. Berwick D. The science of improvement. *JAMA*. 2008;299(10):1182–1184.
10. Aarons GA, Hurlburt M, Horwitz SM. Advancing a conceptual model of evidence-based practice implementation in public service sectors. *Adm Policy Ment Health*. 2011;38(1):4–23.
11. West SG, Biesanz JC, Pitts SC. Causal inference and generalization in field settings: Experimental and quasi-experimental designs. In: Reis HT, Judd CM, eds. *Handbook of Research Methods in Social and Personality Psychology*. New York: Cambridge University Press; 2000:40–84.
12. Murray DM. *Design and Analysis of Group-Randomized Trials*. New York: Oxford University Press; 1998.
13. Raudenbush SW. Statistical analysis and optimal design for cluster randomized trials. *Psychol Methods*. 1997;2(2):173–185.

14. Ostroff JS, Li Y, Shelley DR. Dentists United to Extinguish Tobacco (DUET): A study protocol for a cluster randomized, controlled trial for enhancing implementation of clinical practice guidelines for treating tobacco dependence in dental care settings. *Implement Sci.* 2014;9:25.

15. Brown CH, Liao J. Principles for designing randomized preventive trials in mental health: An emerging developmental epidemiology paradigm. *Am J Community Psychol.* 1999;27:673–710.

16. Brown CH, Curran G, Palinkas L, et al. An overview of research and evaluation designs for dissemination and implementation. *Annu Rev Public Health.* 2017;38:1–22.

17. Weiner B. *Achievement Motivation and Attribution Theory.* Morristown, NJ: General Learning Press; 1974.

18. Rossi JS. Statistical power of psychological research: What have we gained in 20 years? *J Consult Clin Psychol.* 1990;58(5):646–656.

19. Smith SA, Blumenthal DS. Efficacy to effectiveness transition of an Educational Program to Increase Colorectal Cancer Screening (EPICS): Study protocol of a cluster randomized controlled trial. *Implement Sci.* 2013;8:86.

20. Cohen J. *Statistical Power Analysis for the Behavioral Sciences.* Hillsdale, NJ: Erlbaum; 1988.

21. Curran GM, Bauer M, Mittman B, Pyne JM, Stetler C. Effectiveness–implementation hybrid designs: Combining elements of clinical effectiveness and implementation research to enhance public health impact. *Med Care.* 2012;50(3):217–226.

22. Brown CH, Ten Have TR, Jo B, et al. Adaptive designs for randomized trials in public health. *Annu Rev Public Health.* 2009;30:1–25.

23. Zelen M. A new design for randomized clinical trials. *N Engl J Med.* 1979;300:1242–1246.

24. Duan N, Wells KB, Braslow JT, Weisz JR. Randomized encouragement trial: A paradigm for public health intervention evaluation. Unpublished manuscript; n.d.

25. Wells K. The design of partners in care: Evaluating the cost-effectiveness of improving care for depression in primary care. *Soc Psychiatry Psychiatr Epidemiol.* 1999;34:20–29.

26. Lavori P, Dawson R, Rush A. Flexible treatment strategies in chronic disease: Clinical and research implications. *Biol Psychiatry.* 2000;48(6):605–614.

27. Lavori P, Rush A, Wisniewski S, et al. Strengthening clinical effectiveness trials: Equipoise-stratified randomization. *Biol Psychiatry.* 2001;50(10):792–801.

28. Kilbourne AM, Almirall D, Eisenberg D, et al. Protocol: Adaptive Implementation of Effective Programs Trial (ADEPT): Cluster randomized SMART trial comparing a standard versus enhanced implementation strategy to improve outcomes of a mood disorders program. *Implement Sci.* 2014;9:132.

29. Barratt M. Organizational support for evidence-based practice within child and family social work: A collaborative study. *Child Family Social Work.* 2003;8:143–150.

30. Garland AF, Plemmons D, Koontz L. Research–practice partnership in mental health: Lessons from participants. *Adm Policy Ment Health.* 2006;33:517–528.

31. Israel BA, Schulz AJ, Parker EA, Becker AB. Review of community-based research: Assessing partnership approaches to improve public health. *Annu Rev Public Health.* 1998;19:173–202.

32. Minkler M, Wallerstein N. *Community-Based Participatory Research for Health.* San Francisco, CA: Jossey-Bass; 2003.

33. Drahota A, Meza R, Brikho G, et al. Community–academic partnerships: A systematic review of the state of the literature and recommendations for future research. *Milbank Q.* 2016;94(1):163–214.

34. Proctor EK, Silmere H, Raghavan R, et al. Outcomes for implementation research: Conceptual distinctions, measurement challenges, and research agenda. *Adm Policy Ment Health.* 2011;38(2):65–76.

35. Glasgow RE, Klesges LM, Dzewaltowski DA, Estabrooks PA, Vogt TM. Evaluating the impact of health promotion programs: Using the RE-AIM framework to form summary measures for decision making involving complex issues. *Health Educ Res.* 2006;21(5):688–694.

36. Aarons GA, Green AE, Trott E, et al. The roles of system and organizational leadership in system-wide evidence-based intervention sustainment: A mixed-method study. *Adm Policy Ment Health.* 2016;43(6):991–1008.

37. Balasubramanian BA, Cohen DJ, Davis MM, et al. Learning evaluation: Blending quality improvement and implementation research methods to study healthcare innovations. *Implement Sci.* 2015;10(1):31.

38. Haynes A, Brennan S, Carter S, et al. Protocol for the process evaluation of a complex intervention designed to increase the use of research in health policy and program organisations (the SPIRIT study). *Implement Sci.* 2014;9(1):113.

39. Southam-Gerow M, Dorsey S. Qualitative and mixed methods research in dissemination and implementation science: Introduction to the special issue. *J Clin Child Adolesc Psychol*. 2014;43(6):845–859.

40. Aarons GA, Ehrhart MG, Farahnak LR, Sklar M. Aligning leadership across systems and organizations to develop a strategic climate for evidence-based practice implementation. *Annu Rev Public Health*. 2014;35:255–274.

41. Chaffin M, Hecht D, Bard D, Silovsky J, Beasley WH. A statewide trial of the SafeCare home-based services model with parents in Child Protective Services. *Pediatrics*. 2012;129(3):509–515.

42. Palinkas LA. Qualitative and mixed methods in mental health services and implementation research. *J Clin Child Adolesc Psychol*. 2014;43(6):851–861.

43. National Cancer Institute. Grant 1R01CA190366-01A1 NCI: Translating molecular diagnostics for cervical cancer prevention into practice. 2016. https://maps.cancer.gov/overview/DCCPSGrants/abstract.jsp?applId=9028945&term=CA190366

44. Neta G, Sanchez MA, Chambers DA, et al. Implementation science in cancer prevention and control: A decade of grant funding by the National Cancer Institute and future directions. *Implement Sci*. 2015;10:4.

45. Urquhart R, Porter GA, Sargeant J, Jackson L, Grunfeld E. Multi-level factors influence the implementation and use of complex innovations in cancer care: A multiple case study of synoptic reporting. *Implement Sci*. 2014;9:121.

46. Guest G, Namey E, Mitchell M. Qualitative research: Defining and designing. In: *Collecting Qualitative Data: A Field Manual for Applied Research*. Thousand Oaks, CA: Sage; 2013:1–40.

47. Hurlburt MS, Garland AF, Nguyen K, Brookman-Frazee L. Child and family therapy process: Concordance of therapist and observational perspectives. *Adm Policy Ment Health*. 2010;37(3):230–244.

48. Ream E, Gargaro G, Barsevick A, Richardson A. Management of cancer-related fatigue during chemotherapy through telephone motivational interviewing: Modeling and randomized exploratory trial. *Patient Educ Couns*. 2015;98(2):199–206.

49. Atkins DC, Steyvers M, Imel ZE, Smyth P. Scaling up the evaluation of psychotherapy: Evaluating motivational interviewing fidelity via statistical text classification. *Implement Sci*. 2014;9(1):1.

50. Greene JC. Toward a methodology of mixed methods social inquiry. *Res Schools*. 2006;13(1):93–98.

51. Johnson RB, Onwuegbuzie JA, Turner LA. Toward a definition of mixed methods research. *J Mixed Methods Res*. 2007;1(2):112–133.

52. Tashakkori A, Teddlie C. Issues and dilemmas in teaching research methods courses in social and behavioural sciences: US perspective. *Int J Soc Res Methodol*. 2003;6(1):61–77.

53. Demakis JG, McQueen L, Kizer KW, Feussner JR. Quality Enhancement Research Initiative (QUERI): A collaboration between research and clinical practice. *Med Care*. 2000;38:17–25.

54. Greenhalgh T, Stramer K, Bratan T, et al. Adoption and non-adoption of a shared electronic summary record in England: A mixed-method case study. *Br Med J*. 2010;340:c3111.

55. Palinkas LA, Aarons GA, Horwitz S, Chamberlain P, Hurlburt M, Landsverk J. Mixed method designs in implementation research. *Adm Policy Ment Health*. 2011;38(1):44–53.

56. Soh KL, Davidson PM, Gavin L, et al. Factors to drive clinical practice improvement in a Malaysian intensive care unit: Assessment of organisational readiness using a mixed method approach. *Int J Multiple Res Approach*. 2011;5(1):104–121.

57. Stetler CB, Legro MW, Rycroft-Malone J, et al. Role of "external facilitation" in implementation of research findings: A qualitative evaluation of facilitation experiences in the Veterans Health Administration. *Implement Sci*. 2006;1:23.

58. Rabin BA, Glasgow RE. An implementation science perspective on psychological science and cancer: What is known and opportunities for research, policy, and practice. *Am Psychol*. 2015;70(2):211.

59. Neta G, Glasgow RE, Carpenter CR, et al. A framework for enhancing the value of research for dissemination and implementation. *Am J Public Health*. 2014;105(1):49–57.

60. Palinkas LA, Horwitz SM, Chamberlain P, Hurlburt MS, Landsverk J. Mixed-methods designs in mental health services research: A review. *Psychiatr Serv*. 2011;62:255–263.

61. Waitzkin H, Schillaci M, Willging CE. Multimethod evaluation of health policy change: An application to Medicaid managed care in a rural state. *Health Serv Res*. 2008;43(4):1325–1347.

62. Aarons GA, Ehrhart MG, Farahnak LR, Hurlburt MS. Leadership and Organizational Change for Implementation (LOCI): A randomized mixed method pilot study of a leadership

and organization development intervention for evidence-based practice implementation. *Implement Sci.* 2015;10(1):11.

63. Schmidt H, Merkel D, Koehler M, et al. PRO-ONKO: Selection of patient-reported outcome assessments for the clinical use in cancer patients—A mixed-method multicenter cross-sectional exploratory study. *Support Care Cancer.* 2015;24(6):2503–2512.

64. Taylor S, Demeyin W, Muls A, et al. Improving the well-being of men by Evaluating and Addressing the Gastrointestinal Late Effects (EAGLE) of radical treatment for prostate cancer: Study protocol for a mixed-method implementation project. *BMJ Open.* 2016;6(10):e011773.

65. Wiener L, Kazak AE, Noll RB, Patenaude AF, Kupst MJ. Standards for the psychosocial care of children with cancer and their families: An introduction to the special issue. *Pediatr Blood Cancer.* 2015;62(S5):S419–S424.

66. Johnson-Turbes A, Schlueter D, Moore AR, Buchanan ND, Fairley TL. Evaluation of a web-based program for African American young breast cancer survivors. *Am J Prev Med.* 2015;49(6):S543–S549.

67. Tremblay D, Touati N, Roberge D, et al. Understanding cancer networks better to implement them more effectively: A mixed methods multi-case study. *Implement Sci.* 2016;11:39.

68. Creswell JW, Plano Clark VL. *Designing and Conducting Mixed Methods Research.* 2nd ed. Thousand Oaks, CA: Sage; 2011.

69. Robins CS, Ware NC, dosReis S, Willging CE, Chung JY, Lewis-Fernández R. Dialogues on mixed-methods and mental health services research: Anticipating challenges, building solutions. *Psychiatr Serv.* 2008;59(7):727–731.

70. Mendel P, Meredith L, Schoenbaum M, Sherbourne C, Wells K. Interventions in organizational and community context: A framework for building evidence on dissemination and implementation in health services research. *Adm Policy Ment Health.* 2008;35(1–2):21–37.

71. Damschroder L, Hall CS, Gillon L, et al. The Consolidated Framework for Implementation Research (CFIR): Progress to date, tools and resources, and plans for the future. *Implement Sci.* 2015;10(Suppl 1):A12.

72. Glisson C, Schoenwald SK, Hemmelgarn A, et al. Randomized trial of MST and ARC in a two-level evidence-based treatment implementation strategy. *J Consult Clin Psychol.* 2010;78(4):537–550.

73. Teddlie C, Tashakkori A. Major issues and controversies in the use of mixed methods in the social and behavioral sciences. In: Teddlie C, Tashakkori A, eds. *Handbook of Mixed Methods in Social and Behavioral Research.* Thousand Oaks, CA: Sage; 2003:3–50.

74. Aarons GA, Palinkas LA. Implementation of evidence-based practice in child welfare: Service provider perspectives. *Adm Policy Ment Health.* 2007;34(4):411–419.

75. Teddlie C, Yu F. Mixed methods sampling: A typology with examples. *J Mixed Methods Res.* 2007;1(1):77–100.

76. Babbie E. *The Practice of Social Research.* 12th ed. Belmont, CA: Wadsworth; 2010.

77. Palinkas LA, Horwitz SM, Green CA, Wisdom JP, Duan N, Hoagwood K. Purposeful sampling for qualitative data collection and analysis in mixed method implementation research. *Adm Policy Ment Health.* 2015;42(5):533–544.

78. Rosenbaum PR, Rubin DB. The central role of the propensity score in observational studies for causal effects. *Biometrika.* 1983;70:41–55.

79. Pruzek RM. Introduction to the special issue on propensity score methods in behavioral research. *Multivariate Behav Res.* 2011;46:389–398.

80. Rosenbaum PR, Rubin DB. Constructing a control group using multivariate matched sampling methods that incorporate the propensity score. *Am Stat.* 1985;39:33–38.

81. Baron RM, Kenny DA. The moderator–mediator variable distinction in social psychological research: Conceptual, strategic, and statistical considerations. *J Pers Soc Psychol.* 1986;51(6):1173–1182.

82. Shrout PE, Bolger N. Mediation in experimental and nonexperimental studies: New procedures and recommendations. *Psychol Methods.* 2002;7:422–445.

83. Preacher KJ, Rucker DD, Hayes AF. Addressing moderated mediation hypotheses: Theory, methods, and prescriptions. *Multivariate Behav Res.* 2007;42(1):185–227.

84. Gibbons RD, Hedeker D, Elkin I, et al. Some conceptual and statistical issues in analysis of longitudinal psychiatric data: Application to the NIMH Treatment of Depression Collaborative Research Program dataset. *Arch Gen Psychiatry.* 1993;50(9):739–750.

85. Judd CM, McClelland GH, Ryan CS. *Data Analysis: A Model Comparison Approach.* 2nd ed. New York: Routledge; 2009.

86. James LR, Demaree RG, Wolf G. Estimating within-group interrater reliability with and without response bias. *J Appl Psychol.* 1984;69(1):85–98.

87. Castro SL. Data analytic methods for the analysis of multilevel questions: A comparison of intraclass correlation coefficients, rwg(j), hierarchical linear modeling, within- and between-analysis, and random group resampling. *Leadership Quart.* 2002;13:69–93.

88. Raudenbush SW, Bryk AS. *Hierarchical Linear Models: Applications and Data Analysis Methods.* Thousand Oaks, CA: Sage; 2002.

89. Snijders T, Bosker R. *Multilevel Analysis: An Introduction to Basic and Advanced Multilevel Modeling.* London: Sage; 1999.

90. Preacher KJ, Zyphur MJ, Zhang Z. A general multilevel SEM framework for assessing multilevel mediation. *Psychol Methods.* 2010;15 (3):209–233.

6

IMPLEMENTATION STRATEGIES

Byron J. Powell, Krystal G. Garcia, and Maria E. Fernandez

INTRODUCTION

Persistent gaps in the quality of health care, including the prevention of and care for cancer,[1-4] have led to the prioritization of implementation science,[5-7] which promises to improve the quality of care by generating an understanding of both the strategies that can be used to move effective cancer control practices into routine care and the factors that influence relevant stakeholders' behavior.[8] This chapter conveys the state of the science with respect to implementation strategies. It tackles the foundational issue of defining implementation strategies, presents a range of taxonomies that can be used to construct multifaceted and multilevel strategies, describes guidelines for reporting and specifying strategies in published work to ensure that they can be replicated in research and practice, discusses the state of the evidence, and provides some thoughts about how to effectively develop and apply implementation strategies in a way that will address the specific needs of particular contexts. The chapter concludes by presenting some research priorities for implementation strategies.

FOUNDATIONAL DEFINITIONS AND EXAMPLES OF IMPLEMENTATION STRATEGIES

Like many new fields, implementation science is beset by the challenge of reaching consensus on the core terms and definitions that will serve to promote clarity and consistency in scientific discourse. It has been deemed a "Tower of Babel," with 100 terms used to describe the field.[9] The field is also challenged by homonymy (i.e., the same term having multiple meanings), synonymy (i.e., different terms having the same meanings), and instability (i.e., terms shifting unpredictably over time).[10,11] Although widespread consensus on key terms and definitions may be desirable, it is clear that this worthy objective has yet to be achieved.

Table 6.1. Various Terms and Definitions Related to Implementation Strategies

REFERENCE	TERM	DEFINITION
Powell et al.[15]	Implementation strategy	A systematic intervention process to adopt and integrate evidence-based health innovations into usual care.
Curran et al.[16]	Implementation intervention	A method or technique to enhance adoption of a "clinical" intervention. Examples include an electronic clinical reminder, audit/feedback, and interactive education.
	Implementation strategy	A "bundle" of interventions. Many implementation studies test such bundles of interventions.
Mazza et al.[17]	Implementation strategy	A purposeful procedure to achieve clinical practice compliance with a guideline recommendation.
Proctor et al.[18]	Implementation strategy	Methods or techniques used to enhance the adoption, implementation, and sustainability of clinical program or practice.
Bartholomew Eldridge et al.[19]	Implementation interventions	Theory and evidence-based methods and practical applications to increase program use (adoption, implementation, and/or maintenance).
Michie et al.[20]	Behavior change techniques	Observable, replicable, and irreducible component of an intervention designed to alter or redirect causal processes that regulate behavior; that is, a technique is proposed to be an "active ingredient."
Kok et al.[21]	Behavior change methods	General techniques or processes that have been shown to be able to change one or more determinants of behavior of members of the at-risk group or of environmental decisions-makers.

Thus, it is critical across the field of implementation science that key constructs be carefully named, defined, and described in enough detail to be useful to stakeholders. Table 6.1 demonstrates a number of terms and definitions that have been used to describe implementation strategies (and related concepts). This table is not intended to be exhaustive. Other terms could be added, including knowledge translation interventions,[12] interventions to increase the impact of research,[13] and methods for implementing change.[14] However, what these terms have in common is that they all constitute what might be described as "the how" of implementation.

The last two definitions in Table 6.1 refer to the theoretical methods or techniques that are often contained within implementation strategies or interventions. They represent the mechanisms of change and are often selected because they cause change in specific determinants of implementation. Bartholomew Eldridge et al.[19] and Kok et al.[21] argue that all strategies must contain methods of change.

This chapter relies on a variant of the definition proposed by Proctor et al.,[18] defining implementation strategies as methods or techniques used to enhance the adoption, implementation, sustainment, and scale-up of a program or practice. This definition includes the key concept of scale-up,[22,23] and it also broadens the definition to include nonclinical programs and practices (e.g., preventive and other community-based interventions). Implementation strategies can be further differentiated as discrete, multifaceted, or blended.[11,15]

Discrete implementation strategies involve one action or process, such as educational meetings,[24] computerized reminders,[25] or audit and feedback.[26]

More often, overcoming the many barriers to effective implementation requires the use of *multifaceted* implementation strategies that combine two or more discrete strategies.[27–29] Rabin et al.[27] give several examples of multifaceted implementation strategies to integrate cancer prevention programs in community-based settings, such as Coleman et al.'s[30] use of educational meetings, technical assistance, financial support, provision of materials, and coalition building to integrate a health promotion intervention in low-income schools. The implementation of the CATCH (Coordinated Approach to Child Health) program[31] provides another example of a multifaceted implementation strategy. CATCH is an effective school-based program that aims to prevent chronic disease by promoting healthy eating and physical activity among young schoolchildren and their families. It includes school and home curricula, instructor and food personnel training, physical education tools for instructors, school coordination kits, and community engagement. Implementation strategies were informed by theoretical constructs from social cognitive theory,[32] social marketing,[33] and diffusion of innovations theory.[34,35] Messages and strategies focused on attributes of CATCH consistent with diffusion of innovations theory, including relative advantage, compatibility, complexity, trialability, and observability.[34,35] For example, messages emphasized that CATCH was one of the most innovative, reasonably priced programs that resulted in demonstrated positive behavioral changes (relative advantage); it was compatible with the needs of teachers, as well as with the national guidelines for school meal menus; and it was designed with minimal complexity to facilitate integration into the classroom curriculum and activities. Presentations, training videos, video testimonials from implementing schools, and hands-on training sessions throughout the state gave the CATCH program observability, allowing potential adopters to see how the various program components worked.[36] CATCH was disseminated through various media channels, including training and recruitment videos; brochures; cover letters; and a website detailing the attributes of the program, testimonials from other adopters, successful implementation stories, and the ease of use. The careful development of implementation strategies informed by theory contributed to successful dissemination. Currently, CATCH is well recognized in the Texas public school system and is used in its various formats within 8,500 schools throughout the United States and overseas.

Finally, *blended* implementation strategies are composed of multiple strategies that have been protocolized or branded. For example, the Availability, Responsiveness, and Continuity (ARC) organizational implementation strategy[37] is intended to enhance implementation by improving organizational culture and climate,[38] and the recently developed Leadership and Organizational Change Intervention[39] is intended to improve implementation by facilitating the development of more effective implementation leadership.[40]

Discrete, multifaceted, and blended strategies can focus on a single level (e.g., patient,[41] provider,[42] organizational,[43] and policy and financing[44]) or on multiple levels. For example, in attempting to implement survivorship care plans (SCPs) in a comprehensive cancer center, Garcia et al.[45] utilized a strategy that primarily targeted the organizational level. They focused on the first two phases of the Quality Implementation Framework,[46] which included considering the host setting and creating a structure for implementation. In Phase 1, they conducted an assessment of clinic needs, provider needs, resources, and readiness; the fit of different care delivery models; and whether SCP templates needed to be adapted. In Phase 2, they developed customized SCP templates and delivery models.

TAXONOMIES OF IMPLEMENTATION STRATEGIES

A number of taxonomies have been developed to describe and organize the types of implementation strategies that can be used by clinicians, public health practitioners, and other stakeholders to integrate effective practices into routine clinical care and community-based cancer control.[11,13,15,17,20,21,47] The first and most widely used taxonomy was developed by the Cochrane Collaboration's Effective Practice and Organization of Care (EPOC) group to facilitate the coding of implementation strategies in systematic reviews.[47] The EPOC's Data Collection

Checklist (or the EPOC taxonomy)[47] was generated primarily from implementation science literature focusing on clinical settings, and it includes four broad categories: professional interventions, financial interventions, organizational interventions, and regulatory interventions. Additional taxonomies have further refined and expanded the EPOC taxonomy. For example, Mazza and colleagues[17] refined EPOC so that it better captured the nature and content of guideline implementation strategies. Powell et al.[15] attempted to advance clarity by developing a consolidated compilation of discrete implementation strategies, carefully defining included strategies, and providing referenced examples. They did so by conducting a structured literature review that included (1) a review of known documents (e.g., the EPOC taxonomy[47]), (2) a distillation of blended implementation strategies (e.g., ARC[37]), (3) a database search, and (4) additional sources suggested by members of the *Implementation Science* editorial board. Ultimately, this process resulted in a compilation of 68 discrete implementation strategies that focused on enhancing implementation by planning, educating, financing, restructuring, managing quality, and attending to the policy context. This compilation has since been refined through the Expert Recommendations for Implementing Change (ERIC) study,[48] which sought to develop wider consensus on the strategy terms and definitions by engaging 71 experts in implementation and clinical practice in a modified Delphi process. This resulted in a refined compilation of 73 discrete implementation strategies.[11] Expert panelists then participated in a concept mapping[49] exercise that yielded ratings for each strategy's "importance" and "feasibility" as well as nine empirically derived categories.[50] The compilation is shown in its entirety in Box 6.1.

At a more granular level, authors have highlighted the use of taxonomies of behavior change techniques and methods for both the development of interventions and implementation strategies.[20,21,51] Michie and colleagues[20] have developed a taxonomy of 93 behavior change techniques (e.g., negative reinforcement, material reward, and exposure) that are clustered in 16 different groups (e.g., scheduled consequences, reward and threat, and repetition and substitution). Bartholomew Eldridge et al.[19] and Kok et al.[21] describe the behavior change methods that are drawn from the intervention mapping approach to developing public health interventions and implementation strategies.[19] These methods target determinants at multiple levels of influence, including the individual, interpersonal, organizational, community, and societal levels. For example, personal determinants include knowledge; awareness; habitual, automatic, and impulsive behaviors; attitudes, beliefs, and outcome expectations; social influence; and skills, capability, and self-efficacy. Bartholomew Eldridge et al. also describe methods for addressing environmental conditions, including public stigma, social norms, social support and social networks, organizations, communities, and policies. Helpful tables of these methods are provided in Chapter 8 of the textbook by Bartholomew Eldridge et al.[19] and as a supplementary file in Kok et al.[21] Behavior change techniques and methods, then, are contained within implementation strategies because they are rooted in the basic science of behavior change and may provide nuance and theoretical grounding to inform the development of strategies.

Although taxonomies of implementation strategies and behavior change techniques are not typically explicitly linked in the published literature, there are examples of how behavior change techniques have been used to enhance the description of implementation strategies. For example, Aarons et al.[39] used Michie et al.'s[20] behavior change techniques to provide further description of their Leadership and Organizational Change Intervention (see Additional File 2 of Aarons et al.[39]). Intervention Mapping[19] also explicitly links behavior change methods and implementation strategies through a step-by-step approach to developing (often) multifaceted, multilevel implementation strategies (step 5 of Intervention Mapping, Planning an Implementation Intervention). This process includes the detailed identification of implementers (i.e., those responsible for adopting, implementing, and maintaining new practices, programs, or other innovations), implementation behaviors (performance objectives), and determinants of these implementation behaviors. The Intervention Mapping planning framework then guides the selection of behavior change methods and implementation strategies containing these methods that are most likely to influence implementation. Several authors have used Intervention Mapping processes to identify determinants of implementation for physical activity and obesity prevention[52–55] and cancer screening interventions.[56,57] To enhance implementation of a lay health worker-delivered program to increase breast and cervical cancer screening among

Box 6.1 Expert Recommendations for Implementing Change (ERIC) Compilation of Implementation Strategies

Use Evaluative and Iterative Strategies

Assess for readiness and identify barriers and facilitators
Assess various aspects of an organization to determine its degree of readiness to implement, barriers that may impede implementation, and strengths that can be used in the implementation effort.

Audit and provide feedback
Collect and summarize clinical performance data over a specified time period, and give it to clinicians and administrators to monitor, evaluate, and modify provider behavior.

Conduct cyclical small tests of change
Implement changes in a cyclical fashion using small tests of change before taking changes system-wide. Tests of change benefit from systematic measurement, and results of the tests of change are studied for insights on how to do better. This process continues serially over time, and refinement is added with each cycle.

Conduct local needs assessment
Collect and analyze data related to the need for the innovation.

Develop a formal implementation blueprint
Develop a formal implementation blueprint that includes all goals and strategies. The blueprint should include (1) aim/purpose of the implementation, (2) scope of the change (e.g., what organizational units are affected), (3) time frame and milestones, and (4) appropriate performance/progress measures. Use and update this plan to guide the implementation effort over time.

Develop and implement tools for quality monitoring
Develop, test, and introduce into quality-monitoring systems the right input—the appropriate language, protocols, algorithms, standards, and measures (of processes, patient/consumer outcomes, and implementation outcomes) that are often specific to the innovation being implemented.

Develop and organize quality monitoring systems
Develop and organize systems and procedures that monitor clinical processes and/or outcomes for the purpose of quality assurance and improvement.

Obtain and use patients/consumers and family feedback
Develop strategies to increase patient/consumer and family feedback on the implementation effort.

Purposely re-examine the implementation
Monitor progress and adjust clinical practices and implementation strategies to continuously improve the quality of care.

Stage implementation scale-up
Phase implementation efforts by starting with small pilots or demonstration projects and gradually moving to a system-wide rollout.

Provide Interactive Assistance

Centralize technical assistance
Develop and use a centralized system to deliver technical assistance focused on implementation issues.

Facilitation
Provide interactive problem-solving and support within the context of a recognized need for improvement and a supportive interpersonal relationship.

Provide clinical supervision
Provide clinicians with ongoing supervision focusing on the innovation. Provide training for clinical supervisors who will supervise clinicians who provide the innovation.

Provide local technical assistance
Develop and use a system to deliver technical assistance focused on implementation issues using local personnel.

Adapt and Tailor to Context

Promote adaptability
Identify the ways a clinical innovation can be tailored to meet local needs and clarify which elements of the innovation must be maintained to preserve fidelity.

Tailor strategies
Tailor the implementation strategies to address barriers and leverage facilitators that were identified through earlier data collection.

Use data experts
Involve, hire, and/or consult experts to inform management on the use of data generated by implementation efforts.

Use data warehousing techniques
Integrate clinical records across facilities and organizations to facilitate implementation across systems.

Develop Stakeholder Interrelationships

Build a coalition
Recruit and cultivate relationships with partners in the implementation effort.

Capture and share local knowledge
Capture local knowledge from implementation sites on how implementers and clinicians made something work in their setting and then share it with other sites.

Conduct local consensus discussions
Include local providers and other stakeholders in discussions that address whether the chosen problem is important and whether the clinical innovation to address it is appropriate.

Develop academic partnerships
Partner with a university or academic unit for the purposes of shared training and bringing research skills to an implementation project.

Identify and prepare champions
Identify and prepare individuals who dedicate themselves to supporting, marketing, and driving through an implementation, overcoming indifference or resistance that the intervention may provoke in an organization.

Develop an implementation glossary
Develop and distribute a list of terms describing the innovation, implementation, and the stakeholders in the organizational change.

Identify early adopters
Identify early adopters at the local site to learn from their experiences with the practice innovation.

Inform local opinion leaders
Inform providers identified by colleagues as opinion leaders or "educationally influential" about the clinical innovation in the hope that they will influence colleagues to adopt it.

Involve executive boards
Involve existing governing structures (e.g., boards of directors and medical staff boards of governance) in the implementation effort, including the review of data on implementation processes.

Model and simulate change
Model or simulate the change that will be implemented prior to implementation.

Obtain formal commitments
Obtain written commitments from key partners that state what they will do to implement the innovation.

Organize clinician implementation team meetings
Develop and support teams of clinicians who are implementing the innovation and give them protected time to reflect on the implementation effort, share lessons learned, and support one another's learning.

Promote network weaving
Identify and build on existing high-quality working relationships and networks within and outside the organization, organizational units, teams, and so on to promote information sharing, collaborative problem-solving, and a shared vision/goal related to implementing the innovation.

Recruit, designate, and train for leadership
Recruit, designate, and train leaders for the change effort.

Use advisory boards and work groups
Create and engage a formal group of multiple kinds of stakeholders to provide input and advice on implementation efforts and to elicit recommendations for improvements.

Use an implementation advisor
Seek guidance from experts in implementation.

Visit other sites
Visit sites where a similar implementation effort has been considered successful.

Train and Educate Stakeholders

Conduct educational meetings
Hold meetings targeted toward different stakeholder groups (e.g., providers, administrators, other organizational stakeholders, and community, patient/consumer, and family stakeholders) to teach them about the clinical innovation.

Conduct educational outreach visits
Have a trained person meet with providers in their practice settings to educate providers about the clinical innovation with the intent of changing the providers' practice.

Conduct ongoing training
Plan for and conduct training in the clinical innovation in an ongoing manner.

Create a learning collaborative
Facilitate the formation of groups of providers or provider organizations, and foster a collaborative learning environment to improve implementation of the clinical innovation.

Develop educational materials
Develop and format manuals, toolkits, and other supporting materials in ways that make it easier for stakeholders to learn about the innovation and for clinicians to learn how to deliver the clinical innovation.

Distribute educational materials
Distribute educational materials (including guidelines, manuals, and toolkits) in person, by mail, and/or electronically.

Make training dynamic
Vary the information delivery methods to cater to different learning styles and work contexts, and shape the training in the innovation to be interactive.

Provide ongoing consultation
Provide ongoing consultation with one or more experts in the strategies used to support implementing the innovation.

Shadow other experts
Provide ways for key individuals to directly observe experienced people engage with or use the targeted practice change/innovation.

Use train-the-trainer strategies
Train designated clinicians or organizations to train others in the clinical innovation.

Work with educational institutions
Encourage educational institutions to train clinicians in the innovation.

Support Clinicians

Create new clinical teams
Change who serves on the clinical team, adding different disciplines and different skills to make it more likely that the clinical innovation is delivered (or is more successfully delivered).

Develop resource-sharing agreements
Develop partnerships with organizations that have resources needed to implement the innovation.

Facilitate relay of clinical data to providers
Provide as close to real-time data as possible about key measures of process/outcomes using integrated modes/channels of communication in a way that promotes use of the targeted innovation.

Remind clinicians
Develop reminder systems designed to help clinicians recall information and/or prompt them to use the clinical innovation.

Revise professional roles
Shift and revise roles among professionals who provide care, and redesign job characteristics.

Engage Consumers

Increase demand
Attempt to influence the market for the clinical innovation to increase competition intensity and to increase the maturity of the market for the clinical innovation.

Intervene with patients/consumers to enhance uptake and adherence
Develop strategies with patients to encourage and problem-solve around adherence.

Involve patients/consumers and family members
Engage or include patients/consumers and families in the implementation effort.

Prepare patients/consumers to be active participants
Prepare patients/consumers to be active in their care; to ask questions; and specifically to inquire about care guidelines, the evidence behind clinical decisions, or about available evidence-supported treatments.

Use mass media
Use media to reach large numbers of people to spread the word about the clinical innovation.

Utilize Financial Strategies

Access new funding
Access new or existing money to facilitate the implementation.

Alter incentive/allowance structures
Work to incentivize the adoption and implementation of the clinical innovation.

Alter patient/consumer fees
Create fee structures in which patients/consumers pay less for preferred treatments (the clinical innovation) and more for less-preferred treatments.

Develop disincentives
Provide financial disincentives for failure to implement or use the clinical innovations.

Fund and contract for the clinical innovation
Governments and other payers of services issue requests for proposals to deliver the innovation, use contracting processes to motivate providers to deliver the clinical innovation, and develop new funding formulas that make it more likely that providers will deliver the innovation.

Make billing easier
Make it easier to bill for the clinical innovation.

Place innovation on fee-for-service lists/formularies
Work to place the clinical innovation on lists of actions for which providers can be reimbursed (e.g., a drug is placed on a formulary, and a procedure is now reimbursable).

Use capitated payments
Pay providers or care systems a set amount per patient/consumer for delivering clinical care.

Use other payment schemes
Introduce payment approaches (in a catch-all category).

Change Infrastructure

Change accreditation or membership requirements
Strive to alter accreditation standards so that they require or encourage use of the clinical innovation. Work to alter membership organization requirements so that those who want to affiliate with the organization are encouraged or required to use the clinical innovation.

Change liability laws
Participate in liability reform efforts that make clinicians more willing to deliver the clinical innovation.

Change physical structure and equipment
Evaluate current configurations and adapt, as needed, the physical structure and/or equipment (e.g., changing the layout of a room and adding equipment) to best accommodate the targeted innovation.

Change records systems
Change records systems to allow better assessment of implementation or clinical outcomes.

Change service sites
Change the location of clinical service sites to increase access.

Create or change credentialing and/or licensure standards
Create an organization that certifies clinicians in the innovation, or encourage an existing organization to do so. Change governmental professional certification or licensure requirements to include delivering the innovation. Work to alter continuing education requirements to shape professional practice toward the innovation.

Mandate change
Have leadership declare the priority of the innovation and its determination to have it implemented.

Start a dissemination organization
Identify or start a separate organization that is responsible for disseminating the clinical innovation. It could be a for-profit or non-profit organization.

Source: This box draws on definitions and clusters of implementation strategies that were developed through the ERIC project.[48] Specifically, it draws on the specific definitions established by Powell et al.[11] and the categories developed by Waltz et al.[50] Additional File 6 of Powell et al.[11] and Table 3 of Powell et al.[15] provide additional material that clarifies and provides exemplars of these strategies.

farmworkers in the Lower Rio Grande Valley, Fernández et al.[56,57] used a systematic approach that included community participatory methods and intervention mapping to plan implementation strategies that addressed factors influencing program adoption and implementation. Community clinic leaders, outreach coordinators, and lay health workers were identified as the primary program implementers. The team subsequently delineated specific adoption and implementation performance objectives, determinants, and theoretical methods and created specific implementation strategies and materials. This process led to the creation of a packaged dissemination kit that included a program manual for clinic decision-makers and outreach coordinators, a curriculum for training lay health workers, and detailed instructions for the delivery and evaluation of the program.

These taxonomies of implementation strategies and behavior change techniques can be useful in several ways. First, stakeholders can use these taxonomies to identify potentially useful implementation strategies because they may highlight strategies not previously considered. Second, the taxonomies highlight areas in which further development is needed. For example, the taxonomies of Powell et al.[11,15] highlight relatively few strategies that address the "policy ecology" or outer setting, signaling the need for more strategy development and testing in that area. Third, stakeholders can use the taxonomies to help them build multifaceted and (if appropriate) multilevel implementation strategies to be tested through formal studies or to be used in practice. Fourth, the taxonomies can be used to document implementation strategy use prospectively (e.g., in ongoing implementation studies or practice efforts) or retrospectively (using qualitative interview data, published descriptions of implementation efforts, etc.).[58] Finally, these taxonomies may be useful in moving us toward better description of implementation strategies, and they may aid in efforts to assess fidelity to core components of implementation strategies—a recognized gap in the field.[59]

REPORTING GUIDELINES FOR IMPLEMENTATION STRATEGIES

The poor reporting of implementation strategies in the published literature limits the development of a robust evidence base for implementation strategies

and our ability to obtain clear guidance about how to apply them in cancer control research and practice.[60] Problems with reporting include inconsistent labeling; lack of operational definitions; poor description and the absence of manuals to guide their use; and lack of a clear theoretical, empirical, or pragmatic justification for how the strategies were developed and applied.[18] This makes it difficult to interpret the results of studies evaluating the impact of implementation strategies, precludes replication in both research and practice, and limits our ability to synthesize results across studies through systematic reviews and meta-analyses.[18,60] Findings from systematic reviews illustrate this problem, although scores more articulate the same point. Brouwers and colleagues' (p. 11)[61] systematic review of strategies to increase cancer screening rates noted that poor reporting and "lack of precision and consistency in defining operational elements" limited their ability to identify effective strategies. Nadeem and colleagues' (p. 355)[62] systematic review of learning collaboratives concluded that "reporting on specific components of the collaborative was imprecise across articles, rendering it impossible to identify active quality improvement collaborative ingredients linked to improved care." Brouwers et al.[63] reviewed systematic reviews of cancer control implementation strategies and found that "the approach to KT [knowledge translation] in cancer control appears patchy and unsystematic" and may be due to "the failure of the research community to consistently embrace high-quality research paradigms and standards, and the inability to create a common language and taxonomy in the field" (p. 11). Other issues the authors mention are that the primary cancer control studies that support the systematic reviews they included "often fail to adequately describe all aspects of the KT intervention under investigation and (where relevant) the control group," making it difficult to synthesize results, and "measures of intervention fidelity (or adherence to intervention), relevant clinical end points, and valid patient-centered outcomes are often lacking" (p. 11). Word limits for many journals have been cited as one reason for the poor description of implementation strategies; however, that claim has limited validity at a time when many journals are open access, have liberal word limits, and allow additional files that would allow detailed description of implementation strategies or the inclusion of manuals to guide their use. Nevertheless, concerns about reporting quality have persisted.[18,60,64]

There are a number of useful frameworks to guide the design and description of cancer control interventions.[65] In 2009, a prominent editorial[60] in the journal *Implementation Science* advocated for the use of the Workgroup for Intervention Development and Evaluation Research (WIDER) recommendations,[66] which urge authors to (1) provide detailed descriptions of interventions (and implementation strategies) in published papers, (2) clarify assumed change processes and design principles, (3) provide access to manuals and protocols that provide information about the clinical interventions or implementation strategies, and (4) give detailed descriptions of active control conditions. Those applying the WIDER recommendations to their work may benefit from a published checklist that describes each criterion in detail.[67]

Proctor and colleagues[18] proposed recommendations for specifying and reporting implementation strategies. They suggest that researchers should name and define implementation strategies in ways that are consistent with the published literature (ideally drawing from the many published frameworks that guide the development, description, and reporting of implementation strategies,[65] such as the taxonomies of implementation strategies and behavior change techniques that we described previously[11,15,17,20,21,47]) and carefully operationalize the strategy by specifying the following elements:

Actor(s): Specify who actually delivers the implementation strategy. This could include payers, administrators, intervention developers, outside consultants, personnel within an organization charged with being "implementers," providers/clinicians/support staff, clients/patients/consumers, or community stakeholders.

Action(s): Clearly describe the specific actions, steps, and processes that need to be enacted.

Action target(s): Identify the specific mechanisms that are targeted. It may be helpful to draw upon theoretical frameworks that detail an array of implementation determinants that could be addressed.[68,69]

Temporality: Clearly describe factors related to the timing or sequencing of implementation strategies, which could include information about the stage (e.g., exploration, preparation, implementation, or sustainment) in which the strategy is most helpful or how a specific discrete strategy fits within a multifaceted strategy in terms of timing.

For example, Lyon et al.[70] suggest that strategies to boost providers' motivation to learn new treatments may need to precede other common implementation strategies such as training and supervision.

Dose: Describe any details about the dose or intensity of the implementation strategy, such as time spent with an external facilitator,[71] the time and intensity of training,[72] or the frequency of audit and feedback.[26]

Implementation outcome(s): Identify which implementation outcome(s) is likely to be affected by each strategy, such as acceptability, appropriateness, feasibility, adoption, fidelity, cost, penetration, and sustainment.[73] Certain strategies may target one or more of these implementation outcomes (or other outcomes not identified).

Justification: Suggest the theoretical, empirical, or pragmatic justification for the application of specific implementation strategies (including discrete strategy components of multifaceted strategies).

Specifying implementation strategies in this way has the potential to increase our understanding of not only which strategies are most effective but also, more important, the processes and mechanisms by which they exert their effects.[29] Practical examples of reporting implementation strategies using the Proctor et al.[18] guidelines are beginning to emerge. Bunger et al.[74] use these guidelines to report key components of a learning collaborative intended to increase the use of trauma-focused cognitive–behavioral therapy. Similarly, Gold et al.[75] use the guidelines to report a strategy to implement a diabetes quality improvement intervention within community health centers. Both of these examples focus on applying the reporting guidelines retrospectively; however, a recent example by Bunger and colleagues[58] demonstrates how elements of these guidelines can be used to prospectively track implementation strategy use in quality improvement, research, or other applied implementation efforts.

Additional frameworks and reporting guidelines intended to improve the design, delivery, and reporting of implementation strategies have been developed,[65] and Adeyose et al.[76] discuss the importance of these types of reporting guidelines in relation to cancer control. These reporting guidelines include the Simplified Framework[77] (and its extension AIMD [Aims, Ingredients, Mechanism, Delivery][78]), Standards for Reporting Implementation Studies (StaRI),[79] and the Template for Intervention Description and Replication (TIDieR) checklist.[80] There is no evidence that suggests which of these guidelines would best suit the needs of a given study. In fact, leaders in the field have called for not a single guideline but, rather, a suite of guidelines for different types of implementation science.[81] The use of *any* of the existing guidelines to improve reporting would enhance the clarity of implementation strategies, moving us closer to developing a generalizable body of knowledge and ensuring that strategies can be replicated in research and practice.

EVIDENCE BASE FOR IMPLEMENTATION STRATEGIES

The evidence base for implementation strategies is developing, with an increasing number of rigorous studies demonstrating the effectiveness of implementation strategies. There are also a number of resources that synthesize and compile the evidence for implementation strategies. The Cochrane Collaboration's EPOC group has been a leader in this regard, with 94 systematic reviews (either published or in protocol phase) that summarize evidence for different implementation strategies, such as educational meetings,[24] audit and feedback,[26] printed educational materials,[82] and local opinion leaders,[83] and also implementation strategies that are tailored to address identified barriers and facilitators.[84] The number of rigorous trials and effect sizes for some of the key EPOC reviews are shown in Table 6.2. In addition to EPOC,[86] two online databases—Health Systems Evidence[87] and Rx for Change[88]—catalog evidence for implementation strategies, and both provide relevant stakeholders access to high-quality systematic reviews and meta-analyses.

In considering the historical patterns of research on implementation strategies, Mittman[29] notes that the field initially followed the tradition of "empirical treatment," as single-component, narrowly focused strategies found to be effective in earlier studies were selected in subsequent studies despite differences between the clinical problems and contexts in which they were deployed. This was based in part on the assumption that "magic bullets"—strategies that were effective independent of the implementation problems being addressed—would be found.[29] However, this approach was ultimately not successful, as systematic reviews of rigorous trials demonstrated that there were in fact

"no magic bullets."[91] This has led to a recognition that implementation strategies should be selected based on the identification of causes of quality and implementation gaps and an assessment of barriers and facilitators to practice change.[29] Ideally, this process would be driven by theory, evidence, stakeholder involvement, and a robust understanding of the context of implementation.[92] Moreover, the myriad of barriers at multiple levels and phases of implementation may necessitate the use of multifaceted implementation strategies and/or strategies that are specifically tailored to overcome context-specific barriers.[28,29,63,84,92-94]

Although the use of multifaceted and tailored implementation strategies is intuitive and has considerable face validity, the evidence has been mixed.[84,95,96] A recent review of 25 systematic reviews (only 3 of which contributed to the statistical comparison between single and multicomponent implementation strategies) concluded that there is "no compelling evidence that multifaceted interventions are more effective than single-component interventions." Grimshaw et al.[85] provide one possible explanation for this, emphasizing that the general lack of an a priori rationale for the selection of the components (i.e., discrete strategies) in multifaceted implementation strategies makes it difficult to determine how these decisions were made. It could be that they were made thoughtfully in an effort to address theoretically or empirically derived change mechanisms and prospectively identified barriers, or they may simply be the manifestation of a "kitchen sink" approach. A complementary perspective is provided by Wensing and colleagues,[97] who acknowledge that what we may consider a discrete strategy and a multifaceted strategy is problematic. For instance, a discrete strategy such as outreach visits may include instruction, motivation, planning of improvement, and technical assistance; thus, it may not be accurate to characterize it as a single intervention or discrete strategy. Conversely, a multifaceted strategy such as professional education may include lectures and educational materials that solely target provider knowledge. Wensing et al.[97] propose that multifaceted interventions that truly target multiple implementation barriers could be more effective than single interventions. Despite concluding that there is a lack of strong evidence for the superiority of multifaceted implementation strategies, Squires et al.[95] underscore that they are not suggesting multifaceted strategies are not useful but, rather, that in some cases single or less complex multifaceted

Table 6.2. Evidence for Common Implementation Strategies

META-ANALYSES	NO. OF STUDIES/ INDIVIDUALS	EFFECT SIZES
Printed educational materials[89]	14 RCTs and 31 ITS	Median absolute improvement of 2.0% (range, 0–11%)
Educational meetings[24]	81 RCTs (involving more than 11,000 health professionals)	Median absolute improvement in care of 6.0% (interquartile range, 1.8–15.3%)
Educational outreach[90]	69 RCTs (involving more than 15,000 health professionals)	Median absolute improvements in Prescribing behaviors (17 comparisons) of 4.8% (interquartile range, 3.0–6.5%) Other behaviors (17 comparisons) of 6.0% (interquartile range, 3.6–16.0%)
Local opinion leaders[83]	18 RCTs (involving more than 296 hospitals and 318 primary care physicians)	Median absolute improvement of care of 12% across studies (interquartile range, 6.0–14.5%)
Audit and feedback[26]	140 RCTs	Median absolute improvement of 4.3% (interquartile range, 0.5–16%)
Computerized reminders[25]	28 RCTs	Median absolute improvement of care 4.2% (interquartile range, 0.8–18.8%)
Tailored implementation strategies[84]	32 RCTs	Meta-regression using 15 randomized trials. Pooled odds ratio of 1.56 (95% CI, 1.27–1.93, $p < .001$)

Note: CI, confidence interval; ITS, interrupted time series; RCTs, randomized controlled trials.

Source: Table updated from Grimshaw et al.,[85] and draws upon Cochrane Reviews from the Effective Practice and Organization of Care (EPOC) group.[86]

strategies that are tailored to overcome the barriers and enhance facilitators of behavior change may be most appropriate.

A systematic review of 32 studies testing implementation strategies that were tailored to overcome identified determinants (barriers and facilitators) of practice concluded that tailored approaches to implementation can be effective; however, the methods used to identify and prioritize barriers to change and to select implementation strategies to address them are not well established.[84] The lack of systematic methods to guide this process is problematic, as evidenced by a review of 20 studies that found that implementation strategies were often poorly conceived, with mismatches between strategies and determinants (e.g., barriers were identified at the team or organizational level, but strategies were primarily educational and not focused on core structures and processes at those levels).[98] An ambitious multinational program of research was undertaken to improve the methods of tailoring implementation strategies;[94] however, the findings have not been overly positive.[96] Questions about the best methods to develop tailored implementation strategies that effectively address barriers to change remain. One key finding is that barriers can be identified prospectively, but it is difficult to prioritize them and know which barriers will be most salient to implementation and clinical processes. Moreover, barriers emerged throughout the course of implementation, suggesting that ongoing identification of barriers may be necessary. In cancer control, these barriers might be related to the complexities of the cancer field, including unique diagnoses, various types of providers and settings, the risk of some of the available care or treatment options, and variation in patient decision-making preferences.[63] Similarly, it may be that strategies need to be adjusted adaptively throughout the different phases of implementation.[96,99] Specific methods that may be helpful in increasing the rigor of the selection and tailoring process have been proposed, including intervention mapping, concept mapping, conjoint analysis, and system dynamics modeling.[92] However, empirical tests of these methods are required to determine whether they improve implementation and clinical outcomes by better integrating evidence, theory, and stakeholder involvement in the selection and tailoring process.

Overall, the effect sizes for most implementation strategies are modest,[85] and several factors continue to limit our ability to understand how, when, where, and why implementation strategies are effective. These factors include a lack of definition and clear reporting of implementation strategies;[18,60,64] the poor integration of theory to justify the design of implementation strategies;[100–102] and the difficulty of assessing the effects of implementation strategies that are essentially "context-dependent, time-varying, adaptable complex social interventions."[103]

FUTURE DIRECTIONS FOR RESEARCH ON IMPLEMENTATION STRATEGIES

There is a need for more and better comparative effectiveness research on implementation strategies,[6,7,81,104] a greater focus on processes and mechanisms of change, increased use of economic evaluation of implementation strategies, and an increased focus on the quality of reporting in implementation science involving implementation strategies.

Comparative Effectiveness Research

Comparative effectiveness research could focus on the identification, development, and testing of discrete, multifaceted, blended, and tailored implementation strategies. First, although a number of discrete implementation strategies have been identified[11,15,17,47] and tested,[86] there are still substantial gaps in our understanding about how to optimize these strategies. For example, although there have been more than 140 randomized trials on audit and feedback, Ivers and colleagues[105] conclude that there are still gaps in our understanding of when it will work best and why and also how to design reliable and effective audit and feedback strategies across different settings and providers. Indeed, although it is classified as a discrete implementation strategy, audit and feedback is an excellent example of how complex these interventions can be and the difficulty of studying them in real-world settings. The ICeBERG group[106] provocatively points to the fact that even varying five modifiable elements of audit and feedback (content, intensity, method of delivery, duration, and context) produces 288 potential combinations. These variations matter,[107] and there is a need for further tests of audit and feedback and other discrete implementation strategies that include clearly described components that are theoretically and empirically derived. The results of these studies could inform not only the use of single-component implementation strategies but also their inclusion in multifaceted and blended implementation strategies.

Second, there is a need for further tests of multifaceted and blended implementation strategies.[95] These strategies could be compared to either discrete/single-component implementation strategies or multifaceted or blended strategies of varying complexity and intensity. However, as noted previously, these studies should involve multifaceted strategies with well-defined components that are theoretically aligned with existing quality gaps and implementation barriers. We should be increasingly wary of "kitchen sink" components without clear rationales based on theory, evidence, and stakeholder engagement.

Third, there is a need for further tests of implementation strategies that are prospectively tailored to address barriers to implementation.[84] Although the findings regarding the effectiveness of tailored approaches have been mixed thus far,[84,96] there is substantial room for methodological development and innovation with regard to when, where, and how implementation strategies need to be tailored. When to assess barriers to implementation is an open question. Assessing barriers prior to implementation is advisable and is central to many process models of implementation;[108,109] however, these models also stress that implementation is an iterative process and that stakeholders may need to cycle through the processes multiple times. Barriers may need to be assessed and addressed throughout the implementation process, which makes it difficult to completely specify implementation strategies a priori. Just as with clinical treatments, the appropriate balance between fidelity and flexibility will need to be scrutinized. Ultimately, the field may be better off developing and testing protocols that represent generalizable processes for selecting and tailoring implementation strategies than testing rigid, setting-specific strategies.[92,110-114] Testing approaches that involve the flexible use of implementation strategies over the course of an implementation project increase the importance of carefully specifying and tracking the implementation strategies used.[18,58,60] Only then will we have an accurate picture of the frequency and intensity of strategy use that is needed to ensure that implementation is successful. There are also open questions about where or at which level to tailor implementation efforts (e.g., at a regional, local, organizational, team, or individual level), with more intense and personal tailoring obviously associated with higher costs.[94] Finally, there are questions about how to tailor implementation strategies effectively.[84,92,96] This includes questions about how the increasing number of frameworks and theories can be readily applied to the tailoring process, how to effectively and efficiently identify and prioritize barriers, and how to link discrete strategies and behavior change techniques to address them over the course of implementation.[92,96,115,116] The Tailoring Interventions for Chronic Disease project[94,96] and other innovative National Institutes of Health (NIH)-funded research[117] are addressing some of these questions. Further work to explore how strategies can be appropriately matched to contextual needs is warranted. This work could involve comparative tests between tailored and non-tailored multifaceted implementation strategies,[117] as well as tests of established and innovative methods that could inform the identification, selection, and tailoring of implementation strategies.[92]

Increased Focus on Mechanisms of Change in Implementation Science

Studies of implementation strategies should increasingly focus on establishing the processes and mechanisms by which strategies exert their effects rather than simply establishing whether or not they were effective.[7,29,118] The most recent program announcement for dissemination and implementation research proposals issued by NIH provides the following guidance:[7]

> Wherever possible, studies of dissemination or implementation strategies should build knowledge both on the overall effectiveness of the strategies, as well as "how and why" they work. Data on mechanisms of action, moderators, and mediators of dissemination and implementation strategies will greatly aid decision-making on which strategies work for which interventions, in which settings, and for which populations.

Williams[118] emphasizes that we need more trials that test a wider range of multilevel mediators of implementation strategies, stronger theoretical links between strategies and hypothesized mediators, improved design and analysis of multilevel mediation models in randomized trials, and an increasing eye toward identifying the specific implementation strategies and behavior change techniques that contribute most to improvement. Drawing upon existing theories and frameworks,[68,69,119,120] rigorous research designs,[121] and methods that capture the complexity of implementation, such as systems science[92,122-124] and mixed methods approaches,[125,126] will go a long way in helping us sharpen our understanding of how implementation strategies engage hypothesized mediators.

Economic Evaluation of Implementation Strategies

Few studies have included an economic evaluation of implementation strategies to determine whether the added costs actually pay off in the form of improved implementation and clinical outcomes.[127,128] It is critical that comparative effectiveness tests involving implementation strategies begin to add these analyses, and it is particularly pertinent as we consider whether complex multifaceted strategies are superior to single-component or less complex multifaceted studies[95] or whether intensive tailoring is superior to more standard multifaceted strategies.[94,96]

Improving the Quality of Reporting in Implementation Science

Finally, the problem of poor reporting in implementation science, and specifically reporting the details of implementation strategies, is long-standing. Although there is not widespread consensus on the most appropriate reporting guidelines to use, there are many that would dramatically improve reporting if they were used routinely. Thus, researchers should use these guidelines as they report their work, and journal editors and grant reviewers should point scholars to them routinely, as *Implementation Science* has done in a recent editorial.[64] Failing to improve the quality of reporting will mean that other advances in this area are for naught because we cannot benefit from knowledge of implementation strategies that we cannot replicate in science and practice.

SUMMARY

The field of implementation science has come a long way in a short period of time. We have developed a much more robust and nuanced understanding of implementation strategies, and implementation stakeholders have several helpful resources that can inform the selection and tailoring of implementation strategies, including established taxonomies of implementation strategies[11,15,17,47] and behavior change techniques,[20,21] repositories of systematic reviews and meta-analyses,[86-88] reporting guidelines,[18,65-67,79,80] and potential methods for selecting and tailoring implementation strategies.[92,96] Further comparative effectiveness research and methodological development are needed to ensure that unanswered questions are addressed and that the knowledge we gain through our research and scholarship is translated into real-world cancer control practice for clinicians and public health practitioners. It is hoped that an increasing focus on mechanisms of implementation will lead us to a better understanding of when, where, why, and how implementation strategies exert their effects.[29,118]

REFERENCES

1. McGlynn EA, Asch SM, Adams J, et al. The quality of health care delivered to adults in the United States. *N Engl J Med.* 2003;348(26):2635–2645.
2. Institute of Medicine. *Crossing the Quality Chasm: A New Health System for the 21st Century.* Washington, DC: National Academies Press; 2001.
3. Levine DM, Linder JA, Landon BE. The quality of outpatient care delivered to adults in the United States, 2002 to 2013. *JAMA Intern Med.* 2016;176(12):1778–1790. doi:10.1001/jamainternmed.2016.6217
4. Bryant J, Boyes A, Jones K, Sanson-Fisher R, Carey M, Fry R. Examining and addressing evidence-practice gaps in cancer care: A systematic review. *Implement Sci.* 2014;9(37):1–7. doi:10.1186/1748-5908-9-37
5. Institute of Medicine. *The State of Quality Improvement and Implementation Research: Workshop Summary.* Washington, DC: National Academies Press; 2007.
6. Institute of Medicine. *Initial National Priorities for Comparative Effectiveness Research.* Washington, DC: National Academies Press; 2009.
7. National Institutes of Health. *Dissemination and Implementation Research in Health (R01).* Bethesda, MD: National Institutes of Health; 2016. https://grants.nih.gov/grants/guide/pa-files/PAR-16-238.html
8. Eccles MP, Mittman BS. Welcome to implementation science. *Implement Sci.* 2006;1(1):1–3. doi:10.1186/1748-5908-1-1
9. McKibbon KA, Lokker C, Wilczynski NL, et al. A cross-sectional study of the number and frequency of terms used to refer to knowledge translation in a body of health literature in 2006: A Tower of Babel? *Implement Sci.* 2010;5(16):1–11. doi:10.1186/1748-5908-5-16
10. Gerring J. *Social Science Methodology: A Criterial Framework.* Cambridge, UK: Cambridge University Press; 2001.
11. Powell BJ, Waltz TJ, Chinman MJ, et al. A refined compilation of implementation strategies: Results from the Expert Recommendations for Implementing Change (ERIC) project. *Implement Sci.* 2015;10(21):1–14. doi:10.1186/s13012-015-0209-1
12. Straus S, Tetroe J, Graham ID, eds. *Knowledge Translation in Health Care: Moving from Evidence to Practice.* 2nd ed. Chichester, UK: Wiley; 2013.
13. Walter I, Nutley S, Davies H. *Developing a Taxonomy of Interventions Used to Increase the Impact of Research.* St. Andrews, UK: Research Unit for Research Utilisation, Department of Management, University of St. Andrews; 2003.
14. Leeman J, Baernholdt M, Sandelowski M. Developing a theory-based taxonomy of methods for implementing change in practice. *J Adv Nurs.* 2007;58(2):191–200.
15. Powell BJ, McMillen JC, Proctor EK, et al. A compilation of strategies for implementing clinical innovations in health and mental health.

Med Care Res Rev. 2012;69(2):123–157. doi:10.1177/1077558711430690

16. Curran GM, Bauer M, Mittman B, Pyne JM, Stetler C. Effectiveness–implementation hybrid designs: Combining elements of clinical effectiveness and implementation research to enhance public health impact. *Med Care.* 2012;50(3):217–226. doi:10.1097/MLR.0b013e3182408812

17. Mazza D, Bairstow P, Buchan H, et al. Refining a taxonomy for guideline implementation: Results of an exercise in abstract classification. *Implement Sci.* 2013;8(32):1–10. doi:10.1186/1748-5908-8-32

18. Proctor EK, Powell BJ, McMillen JC. Implementation strategies: Recommendations for specifying and reporting. *Implement Sci.* 2013;8(139):1–11. doi:10.1186/1748-5908-8-139

19. Bartholomew Eldridge LK, Markham CM, Ruiter RAC, Fernández ME, Kok G, Parcel GS. *Planning Health Promotion Programs: An Intervention Mapping Approach.* 4th ed. San Francisco, CA: Jossey-Bass; 2016.

20. Michie S, Richardson M, Johnston M, et al. The behavior change technique taxonomy (v1) of 93 hierarchically clustered techniques: Building an international consensus for the reporting of behavior change interventions. *Ann Behav Med.* 2013;46(1):81–95. doi:10.1007/s12160-013-9486-6

21. Kok G, Gottlieb NH, Peters GY, et al. A taxonomy of behaviour change methods: An intervention mapping approach. *Health Psychol Rev.* 2016;10(3):297–312. doi:10.1080/17437199.2015.1077155

22. Norton WE, Mittman BS. *Scaling-Up Health Promotion/Disease Prevention Programs in Community Settings: Barriers, Facilitators, and Initial Recommendations.* West Hartford, CT: The Donaghue Foundation; 2010. www.donaghue.org

23. Milat AJ, Bauman A, Redman S. Narrative review of models and success factors for scaling up public health interventions. *Implement Sci.* 2015;10(113):1–11. doi:10.1186/s13012-015-0301-6

24. Forsetlund L, Bjørndal A, Rashidian A, et al. Continuing education meetings and workshops: Effects on professional practice and health care outcomes. *Cochrane Database Syst Rev.* 2009;2009(2):CD003030. doi:10.1002/14651858.CD003030.pub2

25. Shojania KG, Jennings A, Mayhew A, Ramsay CR, Eccles MP, Grimshaw JM. The effects of on-screen, point of care computer reminders on processes and outcomes of care. *Cochrane Database Syst Rev.* 2009;2009(3):CD001096. doi:10.1002/14651858.CD001096.pub2

26. Ivers N, Jamtvedt G, Flottorp S, et al. Audit and feedback: Effects on professional practice and healthcare outcomes. *Cochrane Database Syst Rev.* 2012; 2012(6):CD000259. doi:10.1002/14651858.CD000259.pub3

27. Rabin BA, Glasgow RE, Kerner JF, Klump MP, Brownson RC. Dissemination and implementation research on community-based cancer prevention: A systematic review. *Am J Prev Med.* 2010;38(4):443–456.

28. Aarons GA, Hurlburt M, Horwitz SM. Advancing a conceptual model of evidence-based practice implementation in public service sectors. *Adm Policy Ment Health Ment Health Serv Res.* 2011;38:4–23. doi:10.1007/s10488-010-0327-7

29. Mittman BS. Implementation science in health care. In: Brownson RC, Colditz GA, Proctor EK, eds. *Dissemination and Implementation Research in Health: Translating Science to Practice.* New York, NY: Oxford University Press; 2012:400–418.

30. Coleman KJ, Tiller CL, Sanchez J, et al. Prevention of the epidemic increase in child risk of overweight in low-income schools: The El Paso coordinated approach to child health. *Arch Pediatr Adolesc Med.* 159:217–224.

31. CATCH (Coordinated Approach to Child Health). https://catchinfo.org. 2016.

32. Bandura A. *Social Foundation of Thought and Action: A Social Cognitive Theory.* New York, NY: Prentice-Hall; 1986.

33. Sigel M, Doner L. *Marketing Public Health: Strategies to Promote Social Change.* Gaithersburg, MD: Aspen; 2004.

34. Rogers EM. Lessons for guidelines from the diffusion of innovations. *Jt Comm J Qual Improv.* 1995;21(7):324–328.

35. Rogers EM. *Diffusion of Innovations.* 5th ed. New York, NY: Free Press; 2003.

36. Hoelscher DM, Kelder SH, Murray N, Cribb PW, Conroy J, Parcel GS. Dissemination and adoption of the Child and Adolescent Trial for Cardiovascular Health (CATCH): A case study in Texas. *J Public Health Manag Pract.* 2001;7(2):90–100.

37. Glisson C, Schoenwald S, Hemmelgarn A, et al. Randomized trial of MST and ARC in a two-level evidence-based treatment implementation strategy. *J Consult Clin Psychol.* 2010;78(4):537–550. doi:10.1037/a0019160

38. Glisson C, Landsverk J, Schoenwald S, et al. Assessing the organizational social context (OSC) of mental health services: Implications for research and practice. *Adm Policy Ment Health Ment Health Serv Res.* 2008;35(1–2):98–113. doi:10.1007/s10488-007-0148-5

39. Aarons GA, Ehrhart MG, Farahnak LR, Hurlburt MS. Leadership and Organizational Change for Implementation (LOCI): A randomized mixed method pilot study of a leadership and organization development intervention for evidence-based practice implementation. *Implement Sci.* 2015;10(11):1–12. doi:10.1186/s13012-014-0192-y

40. Aarons GA, Ehrhart MG, Farahnak LR. The Implementation Leadership Scale (ILS): Development of a brief measure of unit level implementation leadership. *Implement Sci.* 2014;9(45):1–10. doi:10.1186/1748-5908-9-45

41. Gagliardi AR, Légaré F, Brouwers MC, Webster F, Badley E, Straus S. Patient-mediated knowledge translation (PKT) interventions for clinical encounters: A systematic review. *Implement Sci.* 2016;11(1):1–13. doi:10.1186/s13012-016-0389-3

42. Flanagan ME, Ramanujam R, Doebbeling BN. The effect of provider- and workflow-focused strategies for guideline implementation on provider acceptance. *Implement Sci.* 2009;4(71):1–10.

43. Wensing M, Laurant M, Ouwens M, Wollersheim H. Organizational implementation strategies for change. In: Grol R, Wensing M, Eccles M, Davis D, eds. *Improving Patient Care: The Implementation of Change in Health Care.* 2nd ed. Chichester, UK: Wiley-Blackwell; 2013:240–253.

44. Wensing M, Eccles M, Grol R. Economic and policy strategies for implementation of change. In: Grol R, Wensing M, Eccles M, Davis D, eds. *Improving Patient Care: The Implementation of Change in Health Care.* 2nd ed. Chichester, UK: Wiley-Blackwell; 2013:269–277.

45. Garcia SF, Kircher SM, Oden M, Mckoy JM, Pearman T, Penedo FJ. Survivorship care planning in a comprehensive cancer center using an implementation framework. *J Community Support Oncol.* 2016;14(5):192–199. doi:10.12788/jcso.0255.192

46. Meyers DC, Durlak JA, Wandersman A. The Quality Implementation Framework: A synthesis of critical steps in the implementation process. *Am J Community Psychol.* 2012;50:462–480. doi:10.1007/s10464-012-9522-x

47. Cochrane Effective Practice and Organisation of Care Group. Data collection checklist. 2002:1–30. http://epoc.cochrane.org/sites/epoc.cochrane.org/files/uploads/datacollectionchecklist.pdf

48. Waltz TJ, Powell BJ, Chinman MJ, et al. Expert Recommendations for Implementing Change (ERIC): Protocol for a mixed methods study. *Implement Sci.* 2014;9(39):1–12. doi:10.1186/1748-5908-9-39

49. Kane M, Trochim WMK. *Concept Mapping for Planning and Evaluation.* Thousand Oaks, CA: Sage; 2007.

50. Waltz TJ, Powell BJ, Matthieu MM, et al. Use of concept mapping to characterize relationships among implementation strategies and assess their feasibility and importance: Results from the Expert Recommendations for Implementing Change (ERIC) study. *Implement Sci.* 2015;10(109):1–8. doi:10.1186/s13012-015-0295-0

51. Abraham C, Michie S. A taxonomy of behavior change techniques used in interventions. *Health Psychol.* 2008;27(3):379–387.

52. van Nassau F, Singh AS, van Mechelen W, Paulussen TG, Brug J, Chinapaw MJM. Exploring facilitating factors and barriers to the nationwide dissemination of a Dutch school-based obesity prevention program "DOiT": A study protocol. *BMC Public Health.* 2013;13(1201):1–11. doi:10.1186/1471-2458-13-1201

53. Verloigne M, Ahrens W, De Henauw S, et al. Process evaluation of the IDEFICS school intervention: Putting the evaluation of the effect on children's objectively measured physical activity and sedentary time in context. *Obes Rev.* 2015;16(S2):89–102. doi:10.1111/obr.12353

54. Schijndel-Speet M, Evenhuis HM, Wijck R, Echteld MA. Implementation of a group-based physical activity programme for ageing adults with ID: A process evaluation. *J Eval Clin Pract.* 2014;20(4):401–407. doi:10.1111/jep.12145

55. Peels DA, Bolman C, Golsteijn RHJ, et al. Differences in reach and attrition between web-based and print-delivered tailored interventions among adults over 50 years of age: Clustered randomized trial. *J Med Internet Res.* 2012;14(6):e179. doi:10.2196/jmir.2229

56. Fernández ME, Gonzales A, Tortolero-Luna G, Williams J, Saavedra-Embesi M, Vernon S. Effectiveness of Cultivando La Salud: A breast and cervical cancer screening education program for low income Hispanic women living in

farmworker communities. *Am J Public Health.* 2009;99(5):936–943.

57. Fernández, ME, Gonzales A, Tortolero-Luna G, Partida S, Bartholomew LK. Using intervention mapping to develop a breast and cervical cancer screening program for Hispanic farmworkers: Cultivando la Salud. *Health Promot Pract.* 2005;6(4):394–404. doi:10.1177/1524839905278810

58. Bunger AC, Powell BJ, Robertson HA, MacDowell H, Birken SA, Shea C. Tracking implementation strategies: A description of a practical approach and early findings. *Health Res Policy Syst.* 2017;15(15):1–12. doi:10.1186/s12961-017-0175-y

59. Slaughter SE, Hill JN, Snelgrove-Clarke E. What is the extent and quality of documentation and reporting of fidelity to implementation strategies: A scoping review. *Implement Sci.* 2015;10(129):1–12. doi:10.1186/s13012-015-0320-3

60. Michie S, Fixsen DL, Grimshaw JM, Eccles MP. Specifying and reporting complex behaviour change interventions: The need for a scientific method. *Implement Sci.* 2009;4(40):1–6. doi:10.1186/1748-5908-4-40

61. Brouwers MC, De Vito C, Bahirathan L, et al. What implementation interventions increase cancer screening rates? A systematic review. *Implement Sci.* 2011;6(111):1–17. doi:10.1186/1748-5908-6-111

62. Nadeem E, Olin S, Hoagwood KE, Horwitz SM. Understanding the components of quality improvement collaboratives: A systematic literature review. *Milbank Q.* 2013;91(2):354–394. doi:10.1111/milq.12016

63. Brouwers MC, Garcia K, Makarski J, Daraz L; Evidence Expert Panel, KT for Cancer Control in Canada Project Research Team. The landscape of knowledge translation interventions in cancer control: What do we know and where to next? A review of systematic reviews. *Implement Sci.* 2011;6(130):1–15. doi:10.1186/1748-5908-6-130

64. Wilson PM, Sales A, Wensing M, et al. Enhancing the reporting of implementation research. *Implement Sci.* 2017;12(13):1–5. doi:10.1186/s13012-017-0546-3

65. Lokker C, McKibbon KA, Colquhoun H, Hempel S. A scoping review of classification schemes of interventions to promote and integrate evidence into practice in healthcare. *Implement Sci.* 2015;10(27):1–12. doi:10.1186/s13012-015-0220-6

66. Workgroup for Intervention Development and Evaluation Research. WIDER recommendations to improve reporting of the content of behaviour change interventions. 2008. http://interventiondesign.co.uk/wp-content/uploads/2009/02/wider-recommendations.pdf

67. Albrecht L, Archibald M, Arseneau D, Scott SD. Development of a checklist to assess the quality of reporting of knowledge translation interventions using the Workgroup for Intervention Development and Evaluation Research (WIDER) recommendations. *Implement Sci.* 2013;8(52):1–5. doi:10.1186/1748-5908-8-52

68. Nilsen P. Making sense of implementation theories, models and frameworks. *Implement Sci.* 2015;10(53):1–13. doi:10.1186/s13012-015-0242-0

69. Tabak RG, Khoong EC, Chambers DA, Brownson RC. Bridging research and practice: Models for dissemination and implementation research. *Am J Prev Med.* 2012;43(3):337–350. doi:10.1016/j.amepre.2012.05.024

70. Lyon AR, Wiltsey Stirman S, Kerns SEU, Burns EJ. Developing the mental health workforce: Review and application of training approaches from multiple disciplines. *Adm Policy Ment Health.* 2011;38:238–253. doi:10.1007/s10488-010-0331-y

71. Kauth MR, Sullivan G, Blevins D, et al. Employing external facilitation to implement cognitive behavioral therapy in VA clinics: A pilot study. *Implement Sci.* 2010;5(75):1–11. doi:10.1186/1748-5908-5-75

72. Herschell AD, Kolko DJ, Baumann BL, Davis AC. The role of therapist training in the implementation of psychosocial treatments: A review and critique with recommendations. *Clin Psychol Rev.* 2010;30:448–466. doi:10.1016/j.cpr.2010.02.005

73. Proctor EK, Silmere H, Raghavan R, et al. Outcomes for implementation research: Conceptual distinctions, measurement challenges, and research agenda. *Adm Policy Ment Health Ment Health Serv Res.* 2011;38(2):65–76. doi:10.1007/s10488-010-0319-7

74. Bunger AC, Hanson RF, Doogan NJ, Powell BJ, Cao Y, Dunn J. Can learning collaboratives support implementation by rewiring professional networks? *Adm Policy Ment Health Ment Health Serv Res.* 2016;43(1):79–92. doi:10.1007/s10488-014-0621-x

75. Gold R, Bunce AE, Cohen DJ, et al. Reporting on the strategies needed to implement proven interventions: An example from a "real world" cross-setting implementation study. *Mayo Clin Proc.* 2016. doi:10.1016/j.mayocp.2016.03.014

76. Adesoye T, Greenberg CC, Neuman HB. Optimizing cancer care delivery through implementation science. *Front Oncol.* 2016;6(1):1–8. doi:10.3389/fonc.2016.00001

77. Colquhoun H, Leeman J, Michie S, et al. Towards a common terminology: A simplified framework of interventions to promote and integrate evidence into health practices, systems, and policies. *Implement Sci.* 2014;9(51):1–6. doi:10.1186/1748-5908-9-51

78. Bragge P, Grimshaw JM, Lokker C, Colquhoun H; The AIMD Writing/Working Group. AIMD—A validated, simplified framework of interventions to promote and integrate evidence into health practices, systems, and policies. *BMC Med Res Methodol.* 2017;17(38):1–11. doi:10.1186/s12874-017-0314-8

79. Pinnock H, Epiphaniou E, Sheikh A, et al. Developing standards for reporting implementation studies of complex interventions (StaRI): A systematic review and e-Delphi. *Implement Sci.* 2015;10(42):1–9. doi:10.1186/s13012-015-0235-z

80. Hoffman TC, Glasziou PP, Boutron I, et al. Better reporting of interventions: Template for Intervention Description and Replication (TIDieR) checklist and guide. *BMJ.* 2014;348:g1687. doi:10.1136/bmj.g1687

81. Eccles MP, Armstrong D, Baker R, et al. An implementation research agenda. *Implement Sci.* 2009;4(18):1–7. doi:10.1186/1748-5908-4-18

82. Farmer AP, Légaré F, Turcot L, et al. Printed educational materials: Effects on professional practice and health care outcomes. *Cochrane Database Syst Rev.* 2011;2011(3):CD004398. doi:10.1002/14651858.CD004398.pub2.

83. Flodgren G, Parmelli E, Doumit G, et al. Local opinion leaders: Effects on professional practice and health care outcomes. *Cochrane Database Syst Rev.* 2011;2011(8):CD000125. doi:10.1002/14651858.CD000125.pub4

84. Baker R, Comosso-Stefinovic J, Gillies C, et al. Tailored interventions to address determinants of practice. *Cochrane Database Syst Rev.* 2015;2015(4):CD005470. doi:10.1002/14651858.CD005470.pub3

85. Grimshaw JM, Eccles MP, Lavis JN, Hill SJ, Squires JE. Knowledge translation of research findings. *Implement Sci.* 2012;7:50. doi:10.1186/1748-5908-7-50

86. Cochrane Collaboration. Cochrane Effective Practice and Organisation of Care Group. April 15, 2013. http://epoc.cochrane.org. Accessed April 15, 2013.

87. McMaster University. Health systems evidence. 2012. https://www.mcmasterhealthforum.org/healthsystemsevidence-en. Accessed July 1, 2012.

88. Canadian Agency for Drugs and Technologies in Health. Rx for Change interventions database. 2011. https://www.cadth.ca/rx-change. Accessed February 8, 2017.

89. Giguère A, Légaré F, Grimshaw J, et al. Printed educational materials: Effects on professional practice and healthcare outcomes. *Cochrane Database Syst Rev.* 2012;2012(10):CD004398. doi:10.1002/14651858.CD004398.pub3

90. O'Brien MA, Rogers S, Jamtvedt G, et al. Educational outreach visits: Effects on professional practice and health care outcomes. *Cochrane Database Syst Rev.* 2007;2007(4):CD000409. doi:10.1002/14651858.CD000409.pub2

91. Oxman AD, Thomson MA, Davis DA, Haynes B. No magic bullets: A systematic review of 102 trials of interventions to improve professional practice. *Can Med Assoc J.* 1995;153(10):1424–1431.

92. Powell BJ, Beidas RS, Lewis CC, et al. Methods to improve the selection and tailoring of implementation strategies. *J Behav Health Serv Res.* 2017;44(2):177–194. doi:10.1007/s11414-015-9475-6

93. Weiner BJ, Lewis MA, Clauser SB, Stitzenberg KB. In search of synergy: Strategies for combining interventions at multiple levels. *JNCI Monogr.* 2012;44:34–41. doi:10.1093/jncimonographs/lgs001

94. Wensing M, Oxman A, Baker R, et al. Tailored Implementation for Chronic Diseases (TICD): A project protocol. *Implement Sci.* 2011;6(103):1–8. doi:10.1186/1748-5908-6-103

95. Squires JE, Sullivan K, Eccles MP, Worswick J, Grimshaw JM. Are multifaceted interventions more effective than single component interventions in changing healthcare professionals' behaviours? An overview of systematic reviews. *Implement Sci.* 2014;6(9):152. doi:10.1186/s13012-014-0152-6

96. Wensing M. The Tailored Implementation in Chronic Diseases (TICD) project: Introduction and main findings. *Implement Sci.* 2017;12(5):1–4. doi:10.1186/s13012-016-0536-x

97. Wensing M, Bosch M, Grol R. Selecting, tailoring, and implementing knowledge translation interventions. In: Straus S, Tetroe J, Graham ID, eds. *Knowledge Translation in Health Care: Moving from Evidence to Practice.* Oxford, UK: Wiley-Blackwell; 2009:94–113.

98. Bosch M, van der Weijden T, Wensing M, Grol R. Tailoring quality improvement interventions to identified barriers: A multiple case analysis. *J Eval Clin Pract.* 2007;13:161–168. doi:10.1111/j.1365-2753.2006.00660.x

99. Chambers DA, Glasgow RE, Stange KC. The dynamic sustainability framework: Addressing the paradox of sustainment amid ongoing change. *Implement Sci.* 2013;8(117):1–11. doi:10.1186/1748-5908-8-117

100. Davies P, Walker AE, Grimshaw JM. A systematic review of the use of theory in the design of guideline dissemination and implementation strategies and interpretation of the results of rigorous evaluations. *Implement Sci.* 2010;5(14):1–6. doi:10.1186/1748-5908-5-14

101. Colquhoun HL, Brehaut JC, Sales A, et al. A systematic review of the use of theory in randomized controlled trials of audit and feedback. *Implement Sci.* 2013;8(66):1–8. doi:10.1186/1748-5908-8-66

102. Powell BJ, Proctor EK, Glass JE. A systematic review of strategies for implementing empirically supported mental health interventions. *Res Soc Work Pract.* 2014;24(2):192–212. doi:10.1177/1049731513505778

103. Lee ML, Mittman BS. Quantitative approaches for studying context-dependent, time-varying, adaptable complex social interventions. Los Angeles, CA; 2012.

104. Newman K, Van Eerd D, Powell BJ, et al. Identifying priorities in knowledge translation from the perspective of trainees: Results from an online survey. *Implement Sci.* 2015;10(92):1–4. doi:10.1186/s13012-015-0282-5

105. Ivers NM, Sales A, Colquhoun H, et al. No more "business as usual" with audit and feedback interventions: Towards an agenda for a reinvigorated intervention. *Implement Sci.* 2014;9(14):1–8. doi:10.1186/1748-5908-9-14

106. The Improved Clinical Effectiveness through Behavioural Research Group (ICEBeRG). Designing theoretically-informed implementation interventions. *Implement Sci.* 2006;1(4):1–8. doi:10.1186/1748-5908-1-4

107. Hysong SJ. Audit and feedback features impact effectiveness on care quality. *Med Care.* 2009;47(3):1–8.

108. Graham ID, Logan J, Harrison MB, et al. Lost in knowledge translation: Time for a map? *J Contin Educ Health Prof.* 2006;26(1):13–24. doi:10.1002/chp.47

109. Grol R, Wensing M. Effective implementation: A model. In: Grol R, Wensing M, Eccles M, eds. *Improving Patient Care: The Implementation of Change in Clinical Practice.* Edinburgh, UK: Elsevier; 2005:41–57.

110. Aarons GA, Green AE, Palinkas LA, et al. Dynamic adaptation process to implement an evidence-based child maltreatment intervention. *Implement Sci.* 2012;7(32):1–9. doi:10.1186/1748-5908-7-32

111. Glisson C, Hemmelgarn A, Green P, Williams NJ. Randomized trial of the Availability, Responsiveness and Continuity (ARC) organizational intervention for improving youth outcomes in community mental health programs. *J Am Acad Child Adolesc Psychiatry.* 2013;52(5):493–500. doi:10.1016/j.jaac.2013.02.005

112. Hurlburt M, Aarons GA, Fettes D, Willging C, Gunderson L, Chaffin MJ. Interagency collaborative team model for capacity building to scale-up evidence-based practice. *Child Youth Serv Rev.* 2014;39:160–168. doi:10.1016/j.childyouth.2013.10.005

113. Meyers DC, Katz J, Chien V, Wandersman A, Scaccia JP, Wright A. Practical implementation science: Developing and piloting the quality implementation tool. *Am J Community Psychol.* 2012;50:481–496. doi:10.1007/s10464-012-9521-y

114. Pipkin S, Sterrett EM, Antle B, Christensen DN. Washington state's adoption of a child welfare practice model: An illustration of the Getting to Outcomes implementation framework. *Child Youth Serv Rev.* 2013;35(12):1923–1932. doi:10.1016/j.childyouth.2013.09.017

115. Flottorp SA, Oxman AD, Krause J, et al. A checklist for identifying determinants of practice: A systematic review and synthesis of frameworks and taxonomies of factors that prevent or enable improvements in healthcare professional practice. *Implement Sci.* 2013;8(35):1–11. doi:10.1186/1748-5908-8-35

116. Krause J, Van Lieshout J, Klomp R, et al. Identifying determinants of care for tailoring implementation in chronic diseases: An

evaluation of different methods. *Implement Sci.* 2014;9:102. doi:10.1186/s13012-014-0102-3

117. Lewis CC, Scott K, Marti CN, et al. Implementing measurement-based care (iMBC) for depression in community mental health: A dynamic cluster randomized trial study protocol. *Implement Sci.* 2015;10:127. doi:10.1186/s13012-015-0313-2

118. Williams NJ. Multilevel mechanisms of implementation strategies in mental health: Integrating theory, research, and practice. *Adm Policy Ment Health Ment Health Serv Res.* 2016;43(5):783–798. doi:10.1007/s10488-015-0693-2

119. Wilson PM, Petticrew M, Calnan MW, Nazareth I. Disseminating research findings: What should researchers do? A systematic scoping review of conceptual frameworks. *Implement Sci.* 2010;5:91. doi:10.1186/1748-5908-5-91

120. Grol R, Bosch MC, Hulscher MEJL, Eccles MP, Wensing M. Planning and studying improvement in patient care: The use of theoretical perspectives. *Milbank Q.* 2007;85(1):93–138. doi:10.1111/j.1468-0009.2007.00478.x

121. Brown CH, Curran G, Palinkas LA, et al. An overview of research and evaluation designs for dissemination and implementation. *Annu Rev Public Health.* 2017;38:1–22. doi:10.1146/annurev-publhealth-031816-044215

122. Burke JG, Lich KH, Neal JW, Meissner HI, Yonas M, Mabry PL. Enhancing dissemination and implementation research using systems science methods. *Int J Behav Med.* 2015;22(3):283–291. doi:10.1007/s12529-014-9417-3

123. Zimmerman L, Lounsbury D, Rosen C, Kimerling R, Trafton J, Lindley S. Participatory system dynamics modeling: Increasing engagement and precision to improve implementation planning in systems. *Adm Policy Ment Health Ment Health Serv Res.* 2016;43:834–849. doi:10.1007/s10488-016-0754-1

124. Hovmand PS. *Community Based System Dynamics.* New York, NY: Springer; 2014.

125. Palinkas LA, Aarons GA, Horwitz S, Chamberlain P, Hurlburt M, Landsverk J. Mixed methods designs in implementation research. *Adm Policy Ment Health Ment Health Serv Res.* 2011;38:44–53. doi:10.1007/s10488-010-0314-z

126. Alexander JA, Hearld LR. Methods and metrics challenges of delivery-systems research. *Implement Sci.* 2012;7:15. doi:10.1186/1748-5908-7-15

127. Vale L, Thomas R, MacLennan G, Grimshaw J. Systematic review of economic evaluations and cost analyses of guideline implementation strategies. *Eur J Health Econ.* 2007;8:111–121. doi:10.1007/s10198-007-0043-8

128. Raghavan R. The role of economic evaluation in dissemination and implementation research. In: Brownson RC, Colditz GA, Proctor EK, eds. *Dissemination and Implementation Research in Health: Translating Science to Practice.* New York, NY: Oxford University Press; 2012:94–113.

SECTION II

IMPLEMENTATION CASE STUDIES IN CANCER PREVENTION AND CONTROL

7

CANCER PREVENTION AND PUBLIC HEALTH PROMOTION

OVERVIEW OF CASE STUDIES

Lisa M. Klesges

AS PUBLIC health and prevention professions focus on emerging research at the nexus of social determinants of health and multisector population strategies, implementation methods provide a vehicle to accelerate improvements in cancer outcomes. In this chapter, four case studies[1-4] offer practical examples of implementation approaches that can accelerate evidence-based cancer prevention. The applied knowledge from the cases adds to our understanding that culture, context, politics, and partnership are key elements in driving health improvement, and although not always well understood or easily measured, they remind us that cancer prevention and care delivery exist within a complex system. In considering transformations in health care, moving from a linear and deconstructed model of delivery to one that crossed disciplinary boundaries to consider complex adaptive models that could drive better outcomes[5] was key to improvements. Understanding context and complexity continues to be a key consideration for implementing cancer prevention and control

interventions into existing multisector social systems, be they health care, community, or statewide systems.

LEARNING SYSTEMS FOR PUBLIC HEALTH IMPLEMENTATION

The four cases[1-4] in this chapter traverse the cancer continuum, with examples ranging from accelerating uptake of prevention interventions (human papillomavirus [HPV] vaccination) to early detection screening interventions for breast, cervical, and colorectal cancer and promoting tobacco control policies. Several shared viewpoints in their approaches to implementation science can also be highlighted. The first tenet is recognition of the need for expedient progress—that new evidence can bring about more equitable and improved population health outcomes. Another is broad engagement of partners and community sectors, which allows a larger base of experience, greater resources, and a deeper understanding of what is valued in the social context of local communities or state politics. Finally, they all emphasize the great importance of having access to evidence and having skilled leadership in evidence-based decision-making. Although not explicitly named by the authors as such, these elements come together as key aspects of a "learning implementation system" for population health improvement[6,7] that relies on rapid and expedient decisions, a broad engagement of stakeholders to build a use perspective, evaluation of needed skills for additional learning, and the generation of practice-based evidence.

Illustrations of this learning systems perspective are found in all four cases presented in this chapter. Vanderpool et al.[3] describe clinical delivery improvement processes, social marketing, behavioral economics using "push and pull" levers, and policies to improve availability and access with multisector partnerships with pharmacy systems to increase HPV vaccination rates. Combs et al.[4] illustrate how systems models can be considered and adapted for use in the context of other community needs and preferences to enact retail tobacco policies. Allen et al.[1] consider how local public health systems can be strategically restructured to incorporate improvement strategies and evidence-based decision-making for cancer control programs. Kohler et al.[2] focus on evidence-based approaches and communications that drive structural policy changes to improve social determinants and disparities in health outcomes. In addition, although each case study is highly instructive in its own application, these common strategies and intervention features can also be assembled into aspects of a learning system framework.

Creating an Environment of Learning

Given that perceived lack of relevance is a primary concern among the practice community for not implementing evidence-based programs, participatory approaches are critical to uptake and long-term sustainability of improvements.[6,8] The case studies all embrace an environment of engagement and participatory learning, with applications varying from community-based participatory methods[2] to social marketing,[3] process improvement,[1] quality improvement,[3] and community improvement,[2,4] but all share features of collaborative, team-based, and problem-solving approaches that develop trust and promote

the uptake of new processes and practices. Along with helpful "lessons learned" in building a learning environment described in each case, the examples provide valuable practice-based evidence of relevance to the local health system and community.

Building Capacity for Implementation

Various methods are described in the four cases, but all seek to build capacity in their local context to enhance the skills of community partners, engaged citizens, decision-makers, and other stakeholders. For example, Combs et al.[4] used policy case studies to help communities identify local problems and connect to tested policies; Vanderpool et al.[3] provided expert advice, education, and training to establish new skills among health care delivery agents, patients, and families; Kohler et al.[2] focused on improving communication skills and knowledge needed to influence local politicians; and Allen et al.[1] utilized facilitators from the study team to lead group training of program managers with long-term plans to sustain the capacity building through embedded technical assistance and performance evaluations. University partnerships in each case supported implementation in localized contexts that were responsive to community needs.

Academic partnerships and education of a public health workforce as described in the current case examples resonate with recent calls for transforming the nation's health professions training.[9,10] Based on an interactive competency-driven system of education and participatory action, Frenk et al.[9] promote transformed training that builds deeper capacity in the workforce and connects with local health issues, producing shared efforts that positively effect more equitable health outcomes. The current case examples[1-4] are representative of the great potential in transformed academic partnerships and improved local capacity for implementing health improvements.

Research Evidence and Evidence-Based Decision-Making

Important shortcomings of our current research and evaluation approaches to implement evidence are described across the four cases, with authors noting the need for more timely local data and "data liberation" from existing sources to support the flow of community information for needs assessments and action decisions. The authors also note the need for a body of generalizable evidence with adequate contextual information to judge its relevance to a local context. These challenges highlight the urgency and pace of change needed to address cancer control implementation science challenges.

New design approaches are needed to create implementation evidence that cannot be provided by traditional clinical research designs.[6-8] As one illustration, Peek et al.[11] note opportunities to increase the value, timeliness, and applicability of evidence and offer a standard of evidence (the five R's) that provides more relevant and rapid research for evolving clinical and community health decisions. Combs et al.[4] note emerging opportunities to consider systems science approaches to build context-rich evidence in implementation science. Systems models could provide a means to evaluate the effectiveness of cancer control strategies considering the complex environment that often surrounds their implementation in state and local policy, public health departments, and communities.[4] Advancing the cancer implementation field requires continued renewal of the research enterprise to discover new methods, improving the fit of evidence to more fully inform practices and policies.

SUMMARY

The case examples included in this chapter are applauded for offering promising approaches that can improve capacity, speed up discovery, and support more timely implementation of evidence-based strategies that address local cancer control issues. They highlight that much has been accomplished in improving our understanding of implementation of cancer control strategies within a local complex community system of public health. However, as noted in the cases, much remains to be done to fully realize progress in evidence-based solutions to equitable population-level cancer outcomes. Our challenge is to continue to seek solutions that fit the scale of our problems.

REFERENCES

1. Allen PM, Ahrendt LJ, Hump KA, Brownson RC. Cancer prevention through scaling up the process of evidence-based decision making in a state health department. In: Chambers D, Vinson CA, Norton WE, eds. *Optimizing the Cancer Control Continuum: Advancing Implementation Research.* New York: Oxford University Press; 2018.

2. Kohler RE, Ramanadhan S, Viswanath K. Intervening on the information environment to address cancer disparities: A case study. In: Chambers D, Vinson CA, Norton WE, eds. *Optimizing the Cancer Control Continuum: Advancing Implementation Research.* New York: Oxford University Press; 2018.

3. Vanderpool RC, Brandt HM, Pilar MR. Case study: Human papillomavirus vaccination. In: Chambers D, Vinson CA, Norton WE, eds. *Optimizing the Cancer Control Continuum: Advancing Implementation Research.* New York: Oxford University Press; 2018.

4. Combs TB, Brossart L, Ribisl KN, Luke DA. Case study: Dissemination & implementation research in retail tobacco control policy. In: Chambers D, Vinson CA, Norton WE, eds. *Optimizing the Cancer Control Continuum: Advancing Implementation Research.* New York: Oxford University Press; 2018.

5. Batalden P, Mohr J. Building knowledge of health care as a system. *Qual Manage Health Care.* 1997;5(3):1–12.

6. Glasgow RE, Chambers D. Developing robust, sustainable, implementation systems using rigorous, rapid and relevant science. *Clin Transl Sci.* 2012;5(1):48–55.

7. Mays GP, Hogg RA, Castellanos-Cruz DM, Hoover AG, Fowler LC. Engaging public health settings in research implementation and translation activities: Evidence from practice-based research networks. *Am J Prev Med.* 2013;45(6):752–762.

8. Green LW. Making research relevant: If it is an evidence-based practice, where's the practice-based evidence? *Fam Pract.* 2008;25(Suppl 1):i20–i24.

9. Frenk J, Chen L, Bhutta ZA, et al. Health professionals for a new century: Transforming education to strengthen health systems in an interdependent world. *Lancet.* 2010;376(9756):1923–1958.

10. Petersen DJ, Weist EM. Framing the future by mastering the New Public Health. *J Public Health Manage Pract.* 2014;20(4):371–374.

11. Peek CJ, Glasgow RE, Stange KC, Klesges LM, Purcell EP, Kessler RS. The 5 R's: An emerging bold standard for conducting relevant research in a changing world. *Ann Fam Med.* 2014;12(5):447–455.

Case Study 7A

IMPLEMENTATION STRATEGIES FOR INCREASING RATES OF HUMAN PAPILLOMAVIRUS VACCINATION

Robin C. Vanderpool, Heather M. Brandt, and Meagan R. Pilar

HUMAN PAPILLOMAVIRUS (HPV) is the most common sexually transmitted infection (STI) in the United States;[1] an estimated 80% of women and men will acquire the virus by their mid-forties.[2] Surveillance data suggest almost 40,000 cases of cancer annually are caused by oncogenic HPV.[3] HPV-related disease costs $8 billion annually, resulting in medical procedures that are expensive, invasive, and often detrimental to patients' quality of life.[4]

In 2006, the US Food and Drug Administration approved the first HPV vaccine covering four virus types (HPV4) for use among females aged 9–26 years.[5] Currently, the Centers for Disease Control and Prevention's Advisory Committee on Immunization Practices (ACIP) recommends routine vaccination with a vaccine covering nine virus types (HPV9) for males and females with specific dosing recommendations based on age and health status.[6] Under current guidelines, 11- and 12-year-olds are the priority age group for HPV vaccination given their higher immune response compared to older adolescents. In addition, the earlier age

recommendation ensures that children are protected before ever being exposed to the virus. Moreover, this age group may be given the opportunity to receive HPV vaccination at the same time as tetanus–diphtheria–pertussis and meningococcal conjugate immunizations.[1]

Despite the significant cancer burden associated with HPV and the advent of a safe and effective preventive vaccine, HPV vaccination rates remain well below national *Healthy People 2020* goals of 80% coverage for adolescent females and males aged 13–17 years.[7] Nationally, in 2015, 63% of adolescent girls had received dose 1 of the vaccine, and only 42% completed the three-dose series.[8] Similarly, only 50% of adolescent boys received dose 1 of the vaccine in 2015, and only 28% completed the full series. Moreover, there is incongruence of HPV vaccination coverage in geographic regions with high HPV-associated disease.[8]

Health agencies recognize that uptake and completion of the full HPV vaccine series remains a public health challenge,[9] despite its recommendation as a part of the adolescent immunization platform, coverage by most health insurance programs, and inclusion in the Vaccines for Children (VFC) program.[10] However, in the United States, HPV vaccination policies vary by state,[11] resulting in smaller-scale HPV vaccination initiatives led by community, state, and national stakeholders. Moreover, segments of the population experience significant gaps in knowledge about the vaccine,[12] and existing research has also showcased the polemic atmosphere around the vaccine due to varied moral, religious, political, medical, gendered, and sociocultural beliefs.[13,14] Low vaccination rates are also influenced by the 6-month multidose schedule,[15] lack of consistent and strong recommendations from health care providers,[16] and limited school-entry HPV vaccine policies.[11]

Due to the unique issues surrounding HPV vaccination, implementation strategies recommended by The Community Guide to improve access to vaccinations, increase community demand, and encourage providers and health care systems to administer vaccines[17] have not translated as well to the HPV vaccination context compared to other immunizations. However, several studies have found that combining patient-focused, provider-level, and community-based interventions adapted from The Community Guide—with a focus on addressing specific HPV vaccination challenges—results in increased rates of HPV vaccination initiation and completion.[18,19] Unfortunately, however, many of these interventions are inconsistent in their results and limited in their impact.[20,21] In addition, to date, only six HPV vaccination interventions have qualified for inclusion in the National Cancer Institute's (NCI) Research-Tested Intervention Programs (RTIPs) database on Cancer Control P.L.A.N.E.T.[22]

Despite the limited success and challenges described previously, HPV vaccination advocates have remained steadfast and innovative in their work. Notably, implementation strategies have required a partnership-based approach, utilizing local/state/national collaborations, including the American Cancer Society's National HPV Vaccination Roundtable,[23] the National Association of County and City Health Officials,[24] and local community–clinical linkages, among other initiatives. In addition, strategies have included intensive provider assessment and educational efforts,[20,25] innovative patient reminder/recall protocols,[25] strategic use of immunization information systems, health communication campaigns for both the public and providers,[26,27] testimonials from survivors of HPV-related cancers,[23] school-based immunization programs,[21,25] provision of technical assistance to public health partners, delivery of HPV vaccination in alternative settings,[25,28] and combination approaches.[19–21,25] Specifically, we have chosen to briefly discuss three project examples that have applied varying implementation strategies in practice and highlight the need for optimized implementation across multiple levels.

Developed by the University of Kentucky Rural Cancer Prevention Center, "1-2-3 Pap" was the first HPV vaccination intervention posted to NCI's RTIPs database. The health communication project capitalized on community partnerships and multiple implementation strategies to increase HPV vaccination rates among young adult women in Appalachian Kentucky, including increasing community demand through a social marketing campaign, incentivizing vaccine uptake, reducing out-of-pocket costs, providing immunizations in community settings (e.g., Walmart stores and local festivals), establishing a reminder system for subsequent doses, and using an immunization tracking system.[28] Details of the 1-2-3 Pap efficacy study are published elsewhere, but in brief, women who were randomized to the intervention arm (1-2-3 Pap video + reminder phone calls) were almost 2.5 times more likely to complete the vaccination series compared to women in the control arm (reminder phone calls only).[28] The program was originally designed to be amenable to future dissemination efforts and has been adapted for use in Kentucky (the entire state), West Virginia, and North Carolina.[29] Specifically, the method of delivery has also been adapted to include dissemination of DVDs to health care providers, video posting on organizational websites, television loops in waiting rooms, and via laptop or tablet in clinic exam rooms. As with many evidence-based interventions, future challenges to disseminating and implementing 1-2-3 Pap include the fact that it is now dated given it was originally developed in 2010. Groups wanting to adapt and implement 1-2-3 Pap would need to reshoot the video with information regarding the new dosing schedule as well as with age-, sex-, and ethnic/racial-appropriate actors to increase its generalizability—all the while monitoring implementation outcomes such as fidelity to the original program, cost, and acceptability among new audiences.

Another example of implementation science occurred at a Federally Qualified Health Center (FQHC) in the southeastern United States that

Table 7A.1. Levels of Influence

LEVEL OF INFLUENCE	PRIORITY IMPLEMENTATION SCIENCE THEMES IN HPV VACCINATION
Intrapersonal	• Informed and activated vaccine decision-maker (patient/parent) • Informed and activated providers and pharmacists • Incentives for providers and vaccine decision-makers • Engaging high-risk populations such as HIV-positive youth and young adults and LGBTQ populations
Interpersonal	• Patient–provider communication and shared decision-making related to the HPV vaccination, including vaccine safety, dispelling myths, and cancer-prevention messages • Patient-trusted source communication of accurate information, especially dispelling myths
Organizational	• Clinic and pharmacy champions to advocate, promote, and encourage HPV vaccination among parents/patients, their peers, and other staff members • Provider assessment and feedback • Client reminder/recall systems implemented by providers and/or insurers to ensure completion of HPV vaccine doses 2 and/or 3 • Provider reminders for offering HPV vaccination to age-eligible adolescents and young adults • Clinic and pharmacy participation in the VFC program • Strategic use of immunization information systems by providers, pharmacists, and insurers • Organizational characteristics supportive of HPV vaccination promotion and service delivery
Community	• Supportive social norms, including appreciation for immunizations • Accessible HPV vaccination services through schools, pharmacies, health departments, FQHCs, etc. • Community organizations that promote HPV vaccination • Community–clinical linkages • Supportive media environment • Community characteristics supportive of HPV vaccination promotion and service delivery
Policy	• Requirements for school and college attendance • Standing orders for nurses, pharmacists, and other clinical staff to provide HPV vaccination per protocol • Health insurance coverage for adolescent and young adult HPV vaccination

FQHC, Federally Qualified Health Center; HPV, human papillomavirus; VFC, Vaccines for Children program.

serves 30,000 patients annually. In January 2014, the FQHC team, led by the continuous quality improvement (CQI) nurse, decided to make improvements in HPV vaccination among adolescent patients, subsequently setting a goal of increasing HPV vaccination by 20% in a 1-year period. To achieve the goal, the FQHC employed multiple system interventions that aligned with its usual model of care delivery, including client-, provider-, and staff-based education; individual patient outreach and tracking; provider reminders; empowerment of support staff (e.g., front desk, checkout, and medical assistants) to deliver HPV vaccination messages; and standing immunization orders recommended by The Community Guide. A "plan–do–study–act" cycle and CQI approach guided clinical team interactions. As a result of these implementation strategies, the HPV vaccination rate increased from 11% in January 2014 to 57% by December 2014; the annual average was 64% (range, 11–86%). As of August 2015, the HPV vaccination rate was 72%, with a year-to-date average from January to August 2015 of 68% (range, 52–82%). Despite its success, the most common challenge was reluctance of parents/caregivers to vaccinate their children despite the multilevel approach. In light of this challenge, this example demonstrates the potential of implementation science to accelerate the adoption and integration of recommended strategies into existing organizational/clinical systems to increase HPV vaccination.

As advocated by the 2012–2013 President's Cancer Panel, provision of HPV vaccination in settings outside the medical home may be a viable approach to increasing population-level immunization rates.[30] Pharmacies are an ideal venue given their convenient locations; extended evening, weekend, and holiday hours; pharmacists' ability to provide vaccinations (e.g., flu and pneumonia); and prescription reminder/recall and tracking systems.[31,32] However, variation in state pharmacy immunization policies make it challenging for a coordinated, national approach.[33,34] In turn, local projects in states such as North Carolina, Iowa, Michigan, and Kentucky have been implemented to promote HPV vaccination in pharmacy settings with some success. These projects are not without challenges, however, including varied support from local health care providers, age-restricted prescription policies, limited pharmacy participation in the VFC program, low community demand, competing business and clinical priorities within pharmacies, and limited coverage of immunizations

in pharmacies by insurance payers.[31,35,36] In order to have a population-based impact, implementation science is needed to translate and scale-up traditional immunization services in pharmacy settings to the HPV vaccine context, paying special attention to patient/parent acceptability, feasibility, uptake, penetration, and cost.

With adaptation and ingenuity, these three highlighted initiatives have positively impacted HPV vaccination outcomes; however, most benefit was only realized locally. It is obvious that these and other initiatives could benefit from innovative implementation science conducted at multiple levels to improve HPV-related health outcomes across the population.[37,38] As such, we conclude with Table 7A.1, which outlines levels of influence that are known to collectively impact HPV vaccination and must be considered when promoting HPV vaccination education and immunization services. In addition, we suggest priority implementation science targets for HPV vaccination within each of these levels of influence.

REFERENCES

1. Human papillomavirus (HPV). Centers for Disease Control and Prevention website. https://www.cdc.gov/hpv. Updated November 15, 2016. Accessed November 28, 2016.
2. Chesson HW, Dunne FE, Hariri SE, Markowitz LE. The estimated lifetime probability of acquiring human papillomavirus in the United States. *Sex Transm Dis.* 2014;41(11):660–664.
3. How many cancers are linked with HPV each year? Centers for Disease Control and Prevention website. https://www.cdc.gov/cancer/hpv/statistics/cases.htm. Updated March 3, 2017. Accessed June 27, 2017.
4. Chesson HW, Ekwueme DU, Saraiya M, Watson M, Lowy DR, Markowitz LE. Estimates of the annual direct medical costs of the prevention and treatment of disease associated with human papillomavirus in the United States. *Vaccine.* 2012;30(42):6016–6019.
5. Markowitz LE, Dunne EF, Saraiya, M, Lawson HW, Chesson H, Unger ER. Quadrivalent human papillomavirus vaccine recommendations of the Advisory Committee on Immunization Practices (ACIP). *MMWR Morb Mortal Wkly Rep.* 2007;56(Early Release):1–24.
6. Meites E, Kempe A, Markowitz LE. Use of a 2-dose schedule for human papillomavirus

vaccination—Updated recommendations of the Advisory Committee on Immunization Practices. *MMWR Morb Mortal Wkly Rep.* 2016;65:1405–1408.

7. 2020 topics and objectives: immunization and infectious diseases. HealthyPeople.gov website. https://www.healthypeople.gov/2020/topics-objectives/topic/immunization-and-infectious-diseases/objectives. Accessed November 28, 2016.

8. Reagan-Steiner S, Yankey D, Jeyarajah J, et al. National, regional, state, and selected local area vaccination coverage among adolescents aged 13–17 years—United States, 2015. *MMWR Morbid Mortal Wkly Rep.* 2016;65:850–858.

9. Accelerating HPV vaccine uptake: Urgency for action to prevent cancer. A report to the President of the United States from the President's Cancer Panel. National Cancer Institute website. 2014. http://deainfo.nci.nih.gov/advisory/pcp/annualReports/HPV/PDF/PCP_Annual_Report_2012-2013.pdf.

10. Reducing the burden of HPV-associated cancer and disease through vaccination in the US. Centers for Disease Control and Prevention website. https://www.cdc.gov/grand-rounds/pp/2013/20130219-hpv-vaccine.html. Updated 2013. Accessed November 28, 2016.

11. The HPV vaccine: Access and use in the U.S. The Henry J. Kaiser Family Foundation website. https://www.kff.org/womens-health-policy/fact-sheet/the-hpv-vaccine-access-and-use-in. Accessed November 28, 2016.

12. Marlow LA, Zimet GD, McCaffery KJ, Ostini R, Waller J. Knowledge of human papillomavirus (HPV) and HPV vaccination: An international comparison. *Vaccine.* 2013;31(5):763–769.

13. Abiola SE, Colgrove J, Mello MM. The politics of HPV vaccination policy formation in the United States. *J Health Polit Policy Law.* 2013;38(4):645–681.

14. Casper MJ, Carpenter LM. Sex, drugs, and politics: The HPV vaccine for cervical cancer. *Sociol Health Illn.* 2008;30(6):886–899.

15. Gallagher KE, Kadokura E, Eckert LO, et al. Factors influencing completion of multi-dose vaccine schedules in adolescents: A systematic review. *BMC Public Health.* 2016;16:172.

16. Gilkey MB, McRee AL. Provider communication about HPV vaccination: A systematic review. *Hum Vaccin Immunother.* 2016;12(6):1454–1468.

17. What works: Increasing appropriate vaccination. The Community Guide website. https://www.thecommunityguide.org/sites/default/files/assets/What-Works-Vaccines-factsheet-and-insert.pdf. Updated May 2013. Accessed November 28, 2016.

18. Research-Tested Intervention Programs (RTIPs). National Cancer Institute website. https://rtips.cancer.gov/rtips/index.do. Accessed November 29, 2016.

19. Smulian EA, Mitchell KR, Stokley S. Interventions to increase HPV vaccination coverage: A systematic review. *Hum Vaccin Immunother.* 2016;12(6):1566–1588.

20. Niccolai LM, Hansen CE. Practice- and community-based interventions to increase human papillomavirus vaccine coverage: A systematic review. *JAMA Pediatr.* 2015;169(7):686–692.

21. Fu LY, Bonhomme LA, Cooper SC, Joseph JG, Zimet GD. Educational interventions to increase HPV vaccination acceptance: A systematic review. *Vaccine.* 2014;32(17):1901–1920.

22. Research-Tested Intervention Programs (RTIPs): Intervention programs: HPV vaccination. National Cancer Institute website. https://rtips.cancer.gov/rtips/searchResults.do. Accessed May 1, 2017.

23. The National HPV Vaccination Roundtable. American Cancer Society website. https://www.cancer.org/healthy/informationforhealthcareprofessionals/nationalhpvvaccinationroundtable. Accessed November 29, 2016.

24. NACCHO's Supporting Local Health Departments to Increase HPV Vaccination Rates Project. National Association of County and City Health Officials (NACCHO) website. http://archived.naccho.org/topics/HPDP/immunization/upload/HPV-Project-One-pager_final.pdf. Accessed April 24, 2018.

25. Lehmann CE, Brady RC, Battley RO, Huggins JL. Adolescent vaccination strategies: Interventions to increase coverage. *Pediatr Drugs.* 2016;18(4):273–285.

26. Human papillomavirus (HPV): For parents and public. Centers for Disease Control and Prevention website. https://www.cdc.gov/hpv/parents/index.html. Accessed November 28, 2016.

27. Human papillomavirus (HPV): For clinicians. Centers for Disease Control and Prevention website. https://www.cdc.gov/hpv/hcp/index.html. Accessed November 28, 2016.

28. Vanderpool RC, Cohen E, Crosby RA, Jones MG, Bates W, Casey BR, Collins T. "1-2-3 Pap" intervention improves HPV vaccine series completion among Appalachian women. *J Commun.* 2013;63(1):95–115.

29. Cohen EL, Head KJ, McGladrey MJ, et al. Designing for dissemination: Lessons in message design from "1-2-3 Pap." *Health Commun.* 2015;30(2):196–207.

30. Accelerating HPV vaccine uptake: Urgency for action to prevent cancer. A report to the President of the United States from the President's Cancer Panel. National Cancer Institute website. https://deainfo.nci.nih.gov/advisory/pcp/annualreports/HPV/index.htm. 2014.

31. Rothholz M, Tan LL. Promoting the immunization neighborhood: Benefits and challenges of pharmacies as additional locations for HPV vaccination. *Hum Vaccin Immunother.* 2016;12(6):1646–1648.

32. Goad JA, Taitel MS, Fensterheim LE, Cannon AE. Vaccinations administered during off-clinic hours at a national community pharmacy: Implications for increasing patient access and convenience. *Ann Fam Med.* 2013;11(5):429–436.

33. Brewer NT, Chung JK, Baker HM, Rothholz MC, Smith JS. Pharmacist authority to provide HPV vaccine: Novel partners in cervical cancer prevention. *Gynecol Oncol.* 2014;132(Suppl 1):S3–S8.

34. Skiles MP, Cai J, English A, Ford CA. Retail pharmacies and adolescent vaccination—An exploration of current issues. *J Adolesc Health.* 2011;48(6):630–632.

35. Trogdon JG, Shafer PR, Shah PD, Calo WA. Are state laws granting pharmacists authority to vaccinate associated with HPV vaccination rates among adolescents? *Vaccine.* 2016;34(38):4514–4519.

36. Vanderpool RC, Pilar M, Barker J, Freeman PR. Increasing HPV Vaccination through Community Pharmacy Partnerships: Lessons Learned from a Pilot Project. *The Kentucky Pharmacist.* 2017; July/August.

37. Paskett E, Thompson B, Ammerman AS, Ortega AN, Marsteller J, Richardson D. Multilevel interventions to address health disparities show promise in improving population health. *Health Aff (Millwood).* 2016;35(8):1429–1434.

38. Emmons KM, Colditz GA. Realizing the potential of cancer prevention—The role of implementation science. *N Engl J Med.* 2017;376:986–990.

Case Study 7B

CANCER PREVENTION THROUGH SCALING-UP THE PROCESS OF EVIDENCE-BASED DECISION-MAKING IN A STATE HEALTH DEPARTMENT

Peg M. Allen, Linda J. Ahrendt, Kiley A. Hump, and Ross C. Brownson

EVIDENCE-BASED DECISION-MAKING (EBDM) in public health settings involves applying program planning and quality improvement frameworks, engaging the community in assessment and decision-making, adapting and implementing evidence-based interventions for specific populations or settings, conducting sound evaluation, and using evaluation findings to improve programs and policies.[1,2] Efforts to build capacity for and use of EBDM among governmental public health organizations have increased in recent years in Canada, Australia, the United States, Europe, and elsewhere.[3–5]

A critical issue for implementation science is knowing how to more effectively and efficiently scale up evidence-based policies and programs. To scale up the process of EBDM,[6] a series of key skills and characteristics are needed in a public health organization: leadership support; workforce development; a supportive organizational climate and culture; relationships and partnerships; and financial practices, especially outcomes-based

contracting with funded partners.[3–5,7–11] Although no individuals are expected to have all the EBDM competencies, the following skill sets for EBDM need to be available within or to the public health organization: quantifying the issue, community assessment, prioritization, action planning, evaluation designs, use of economic evaluation data in decision-making, adapting interventions, qualitative evaluation, quantitative evaluation, and communicating evidence to policymakers.[1,12,13] Despite a narrowing of skill gaps in recent years in national studies, gaps persist, especially in the capacity to apply evaluation designs, use economic evaluation information, communicate evidence to policymakers, and adapt interventions for local populations and settings.[12]

In addition to initial education and training, workplace opportunities, expectations, and guidance for ongoing skill building and use of EBDM can be identified and supported through management practices. Such practices may include leaders allocating funding, informational resources, and staff time for EBDM; consistently communicating expectations for EBDM; seeking and incorporating input into participatory decision-making; providing face-to-face meetings to share lessons learned and compare experiences; identification of training opportunities in specific EBDM skills; and incorporating EBDM objectives in job descriptions, individual employee work plans and performance reviews, and program work plans.[7] EBDM skill sets are also needed in the many partnering organizations that public health organizations rely on and fund to locally plan, implement, and evaluate evidence-based interventions.[14–16]

THE SETTING

The South Dakota Department of Health (DOH) Office of Chronic Disease Prevention and Health Promotion (OCDPHP) has an in-house staff of approximately 20 people and relies heavily on contractors and funded partnering organizations to implement evidence-based interventions to prevent and detect cancers. OCDPHP is funded by the Centers for Disease Control and Prevention (CDC) to contract with partnering organizations to address risk factors for cancer and other chronic diseases, especially tobacco control and obesity prevention through promotion of physical activity and healthy eating. CDC funding is also provided to OCDPHP to support clinical partners to use Community Guide[17] recommended evidence-based interventions to increase breast, cervical, and colorectal cancer screening rates among low-income South Dakotans. South Dakota is a rural state with nine federally qualified tribes and a 2010 population of 816,463, including 154,473 in Sioux Falls, its largest city and home to the single city governmental health department. Additional partnering organizations include universities, regional health care systems and non-profits, and organizations serving tribes.

BUILDING CAPACITY FOR EBDM

In March 2014, 35 people attended a multi-day EBDM course in Pierre, South Dakota: 17 who worked in OCDPHP, 6 contractors, and 12 partners from eight different organizations. After the EBDM course, training participants brainstormed and prioritized ideas for how to keep building capacity for and use of EBDM processes with input from the study team.[18] The chronic disease director at

OCDPHP initiated several selected activities to further enhance EBDM capacity and application: (1) staff development of employee EBDM objectives included initially in individual employee work plans and later in performance reviews; (2) formation of an ad hoc group of staff and partners to develop common language for EBDM to apply across program areas; (3) incorporation of EBDM into the periodic conference calls with all staff and funded partners and the annual in-person partners meeting; (4) revision of statewide program area plans in cancer and other chronic diseases to incorporate EBDM processes and evidence-based policies and programs; (5) restructuring of programs to use data-driven planning; (6) program-specific supplemental training webinars in evidence-based approaches; (7) additional data collection to support data-driven decision-making and publicly posted data and reports for partners to use; (8) restructuring requests for proposals for performance-based contracting to fund menus of evidence-based policies and programs to address needs found in community health assessments or prioritized in the revised state plans; and (9) ongoing training and technical assistance with partners through workgroups, listserv sharing, phone calls, and visits.

Using materials from the initial training, the cancer program manager provided an EBDM overview training with the comprehensive cancer statewide coalition. Together, the coalition and program manager restructured both the coalition and the cancer program. The cancer coalition established a new subcommittee to ensure adoption of evidence-based policy, system, and environmental approaches and also a subcommittee that focuses on data and evaluation. The coalition then revised the statewide comprehensive cancer plan, ensuring inclusion of EBDM processes and evidence-based interventions. The tobacco program and coalition underwent a similar restructuring and state plan revision.

FINDINGS

Of the 91 staff working in prevention, detection, and management of cancer and other chronic conditions who completed both the 2014 baseline and the 2016 post survey, 27 were from the state health department. Response was high (87% at baseline and 79% at post survey). Most were female, 37% had graduate degrees, 24% had nursing backgrounds, 51% were program managers, and participants had worked in their agency an average of 7.8 years. Sixteen of the survey participants also completed 1-hour individual phone interviews during March through July 2016—5 from DOH and 11 contractors and partners from eight organizations. On average, interview participants had worked in their agencies 7.2 years. Participants described management practices to enhance EBDM capacity and use, discussed internal and external facilitators and challenges, and recommended ways to sustain EBDM capacity in the future.

Table 7B.1 shows survey measures and findings on management practices for EBDM skills and research evidence use for job tasks. Perceived gaps in importance and work unit availability of EBDM competencies were smaller in 2016 than in 2014 overall, with the largest remaining gaps in communicating research to policymakers, using economic evaluation information, and adapting interventions. Among partners ($n = 64$), the significant pre–post changes were lowered skill gaps in prioritization ($p = .003$), adapting interventions ($p = .04$), and evaluation designs ($p = .004$). It is noteworthy that some partners were trained and experienced in EBDM processes prior to the 2014 baseline survey, especially university partners.

Facilitators

Multiple interview participants emphasized three facilitators of EBDM: CDC funding requirements; leadership support, both formal and informal; and the initial in-state training. Participants discussed the strong influence of CDC's promotion and increasingly stringent requirements for use of evidence-based interventions to state health departments in affecting state health departments' requests for in-state proposals and contracts to carry out much of the work. Participants lauded the leadership support of DOH's chronic disease director, describing her support as a "key driver" and "big push":

DOH staff: I think [her] vision for it [EBDM] was a key driver, just to have a leader who was sold on it and was continuing to bring it up and lead by example, I think that was an important contributor to why it got incorporated more.

Partner: She was a big push. I think that helped catapult it [EBDM] statewide, especially working with so many partners and collaborators.

Several partners also discussed informal leadership roles that partners trained and experienced

in EBDM have taken in joint meetings to revise statewide plans. The in-state EBDM course was discussed as a key facilitator because it "grounded us with the common understanding and the common language moving forward" and "helped us to be more uniform across our programs in how we use evidence and incorporate it into our work."

Challenges

The main challenges discussed by the majority of those interviewed were the following: EBDM takes more time; buy-in—getting partners and colleagues onboard, especially volunteer partners not funded by DOH; limited data, especially tribal data; limited intervention evidence in some program areas and with tribes; and limited understanding among those not trained. Similar barriers have been found previously.[11,19,20]

Participants discussed several approaches to increase buy-in: ongoing EBDM conversation, making decisions together, building strong partnering relationships over time, and seeing successes. Buy-in was perceived after seeing improvement in implementation indicators that came after the time-consuming program and coalition restructuring and evaluation efforts. Examples included sharing success stories at meetings with partners; increased human papillomavirus vaccine completion rates; and measurable progress in reaching colorectal cancer program objectives, as seen in the South Dakota Comprehensive Cancer Control State Plan and reports.

Participant Recommendations

Two themes among DOH staff interview recommendations on ways to further EBDM in South Dakota were ongoing remotely delivered training and more full and systematic integration of EBDM into more programs. EBDM orientation of new DOH staff across the agency was recommended. Ongoing short remote trainings for staff and partners and refresher trainings were also recommended.

Among the partners interviewed, three themes emerged: future ongoing training, increased collaboration, and data-related recommendations. For training, several recommended remotely delivered and archived trainings on EBDM overall, including an advanced option; how to adapt evidence-based interventions for specific setting or populations;

Table 7B.1. EBDM Capacity Pre–Post Survey Findings in South Dakota, 2014–2016 (*N* = 91)

SURVEY ITEM	OVERALL (N = 91)			STATE HEALTH DEPARTMENT (N = 27)		
	BASELINE MEAN (SD)	POST MEAN (SD)	PAIRED *T*-TEST *P* VALUE	BASELINE MEAN (SD)	POST MEAN (SD)	PAIRED *T*-TEST *P* VALUE
Agreement: (7-point Likert, where 1 = strongly disagree and 7 = strongly agree)						
I use EBDM in my work.	5.68 (1.10)	5.91 (1.08)	.06	5.67 (1.30)	6.11 (1.16)	.05
My work unit has the resources (e.g., staff, facilities, partners) for EBDM.	5.08 (1.38)	5.43 (1.17)	.03	5.19 (1.44)	5.59 (0.89)	.18
My work unit has access to current research evidence for EBDM.	5.53 (1.25)	5.74 (1.12)	.12	5.63 (1.36)	5.74 (1.23)	.65
My direct supervisor expects EBDM, values supports for EBDM, and evaluates my performance on how well I use EBDM (mean of 3 items).	5.23 (1.23)	5.34 (1.10)	.47	5.32 (1.35)	5.85 (1.08)	.03
Skill gaps: (11-point Likert perceived importance minus perceived work unit availability of skill)						
EBDM skills gaps (10-item sum)	16.33 (16.34)	11.91 (16.86)	.02	12.67 (18.30)	11.15 (17.60)	.56
Prioritization skill gap	1.71 (1.79)	0.94 (1.83)	.002	1.12 (1.82)	0.65 (1.72)	.29
Adapting interventions skill gap	1.89 (2.26)	1.34 (1.96)	.07	1.23 (2.30)	1.19 (1.86)	.94
Evaluation designs skill gap	1.84 (2.70)	1.07 (2.40)	.009	1.35 (3.14)	1.00 (2.64)	.58
Community assessment skill gap	1.22 (1.72)	0.95 (2.04)	.28	1.04 (1.85)	0.44 (1.50)	.14
Communicating research to policy makers skill gap	2.22 (2.69)	1.66 (2.58)	.10	2.07 (3.40)	1.41 (2.52)	.29

(continued)

SURVEY ITEM	OVERALL (N = 91)			STATE HEALTH DEPARTMENT (N = 27)		
	BASELINE MEAN (SD)	POST MEAN (SD)	PAIRED *T*-TEST *P* VALUE	BASELINE MEAN (SD)	POST MEAN (SD)	PAIRED *T*-TEST *P* VALUE
How often use research evidence to: (1–4, where 1 = seldom/never and 4 = always)						
Write a grant application	1.62 (1.06)	1.67 (0.94)	.53	1.67 (1.06)	1.76 (0.83)	.56
Justify intervention selection to funders, agency leadership, partners	1.67 (0.94)	1.88 (0.91)	.36	1.65 (1.03)	2.17 (0.89)	.04
Evaluate interventions	1.70 (0.93)	1.93 (0.88)	.02	1.52 (1.05)	2.17 (0.76)	<.001

and how to evaluate implementation. Partners wanted to work together more and see more information and resources shared across programs and organizations: One stated, "I'd like to see us always thinking about how we can come together to leverage funding, to build that evidence-base together."

Data-related recommendations from partners included the following: (1) Collect additional tribal data representative of South Dakota (Sioux Nation) tribes, (2) build more evidence of what works in tribal communities, (3) customize data locally and provide local fact sheets to community partners, (4) identify data needs through a survey, (5) guide data interpretation and use, (6) provide state demographics summaries, and (7) continue to align and organize available data.

SUMMARY AND IMPLICATIONS

A key challenge for implementation science involves how to build organizational capacity for EBDM.[1-4,6,11,21] To illustrate one approach for capacity building, our case study highlights a collaboration between a university and a public health agency to address core public health functions and enhance the use of research evidence in EBDM.[15,21] Such collaborations are a growing phenomenon, with more than half of accredited US schools and

programs in public health responding to a recent survey reporting relationships with one or more public health practice partner organizations.[22] DOH also has strong ongoing partnering relationships with South Dakota State University faculty and staff, who provide evaluation expertise and informal leadership in statewide planning groups.

In addition to the previously mentioned recommendations from participants, we recommend the following: (1) Continue to document EBDM successes and share successes more broadly to enhance buy-in; (2) consider including skill-building trainings with DOH staff and partners on how to communicate evidence to decision-makers, create evaluation plans using both quantitative and qualitative methods, use economic evaluation information, and adapt evidence-based strategies for use and testing with tribes and other rural communities; (3) acknowledge and support the informal leadership and EBDM promotion provided by partners experienced in EBDM who serve on planning work groups and in coalitions; and (4) continue to institutionalize EBDM for sustainability through employee performance review EBDM incorporation, ensuring supervisors communicate expectations that staff and partners use EBDM, performance-based contracting, ensuring staff are well prepared for participatory decision-making with partners, asking about knowledge of EBDM processes in job interviews, and incorporating EBDM in partner meetings. The cancer program's strategic restructuring and systematic incorporation of EBDM internally and externally provide a transition process that others may find useful as well.

This case study has several limitations. Findings may not be generalizable to other states, both because of the purposive survey sampling and because of the uniqueness of South Dakota, with its rurality and small population that includes nine tribal nations. The 2-year lag time from the baseline survey to the post survey was intended to allow time for OCDPHP to institute the management practices planned after the initial training, but the lag time also resulted in survey loss to follow-up due to staff turnover. DOH staff had the highest knowledge dissemination exposure but were a small sample, whereas the larger sample of partners had diluted exposure.

Although this single-state sample was too small to assess potential moderators, in our study team's 12-state baseline survey with 1,237 participants, increased numbers of EBDM work unit supports were associated with higher odds of frequent research evidence use.[23] And similar to Zardo and Collie,[8] but different from Larsen et al.,[5] our 12-state baseline study found participants with a master's degree or higher or those in leadership or middle management were likely to use research evidence more frequently than others.[23] Dissemination of research evidence also needs to take into account the general training levels of agency staff; capacity readiness to apply the evidence; and variation in resources, political contexts, cultural considerations, and readiness.[4,5,16]

Although the settings, contexts, and targeted levels for public health interventions are diverse within and across states and countries, underlying EBDM skill sets and characteristics apply. Implementation science can continue to narrow the gap between discovery of intervention evidence and what it takes to apply EBDM processes in agencies and communities. Future research can further test scale-up of lessons learned in practice-based research on aspects of leadership support, workforce development, relationships and partnerships, organizational climate and culture, and financial practices associated with improved public health performance and population health. Community-based participatory research and network research can continue to inform partnership best practices.

Improvements in data systems nationally and within states, and development of online centralized data repositories in a number of state health departments, have increased availability and accessibility of both disease burden data and intervention evidence. Yet important gaps remain in availability of tribal data and local data needed for decision-making.

Due in large measure to research supported by the National Cancer Institute and CDC's funding requirements, the use of evidence-based interventions is increasingly the norm in prevention and early detection of cancers and other chronic conditions.[24,25] Yet much work remains to spread EBDM beyond chronic disease prevention and to learn how best to build, support, and sustain EBDM capacity in public health organizations and diverse partnering organizations to effectively apply the evidence, continually improve state and local application, and improve population health.

REFERENCES

1. Brownson RC, Baker EA, Deshpande AD, Gillespie KN. *Evidence-Based Public Health*. 3rd ed. New York: Oxford University Press; 2018.

2. Brownson RC, Fielding JE, Maylahn CM. Evidence-based decision making to improve public health practice. *Front Public Health Serv Syst Res*. 2013;2(2).

3. Yost J, Dobbins M, Traynor R, DeCorby K, Workentine S, Greco L. Tools to support evidence-informed public health decision making. *BMC Public Health*. 2014;14(1):1–13.

4. Pettman TL, Armstrong R, Pollard B, Evans R, Stirrat A, Scott I, Davies-Jackson G, Waters E. Using evidence in health promotion in local government: Contextual realities and opportunities. *Health Promot J Austr*. 2013;24(1):72–75.

5. Larsen M, Gulis G, Pedersen KM. Use of evidence in local public health work in Denmark. *Int J Public Health*. 2012;57(3):477–483.

6. Brownson RC, Colditz GA, Proctor EK, eds. *Dissemination and Implementation Research in Health: Translating Science to Practice*. 2nd ed. New York: Oxford University Press; 2018.

7. Brownson RC, Allen P, Duggan K, Stamatakis KA, Erwin PC. Fostering more effective public health by identifying administrative evidence-based practices: A review of the literature. *Am J Prev Med*. 2012;43(3):309–319.

8. Zardo P, Collie A. Predicting research use in a public health policy environment: Results

of a logistic regression analysis. *Implement Sci.* 2014;9(1):1–10.

9. Ward M, Mowat D. Creating an organizational culture for evidence-informed decision making. *Healthc Manage Forum.* 2012;25(3):146–150.

10. Yousefi-Nooraie R, Dobbins M, Marin A, Hanneman R, Lohfeld L. The evolution of social networks through the implementation of evidence-informed decision-making interventions: A longitudinal analysis of three public health units in Canada. *Implement Sci.* 2015;10(1).

11. Zardo P. Organisational factors affecting policy and programme decision making in a public health policy environment. *Health Policy.* 2015;11(4):509–527.

12. Jacob RR, Baker EA, Allen P, Dodson EA, Duggan K, Fields R, Sequeira S, Brownson RC. Training needs and supports for evidence-based decision making among the public health workforce in the United States. *BMC Health Serv Res.* 2014;14(1):564.

13. Jacobs JA, Duggan K, Erwin P, et al. Capacity building for evidence-based decision making in local health departments: Scaling up an effective training approach. *Implement Sci.* 2014;9(1):124.

14. Institute of Medicine. *The Future of the Public's Health in the 21st Century.* Washington, DC: National Academies Press; 2003.

15. Brownson RC. Practice–research partnerships and mentoring to foster evidence-based decision making. *Prev Chronic Dis.* 2014;11:E92.

16. Stamatakis KA, Vinson CA, Kerner JF. Dissemination and implementation research in community and public health settings. In: Brownson RC, Colditz GA, Proctor EK, eds. *Dissemination and Implementation Research in Health.* New York: Oxford University Press; 2012:359–383.

17. Centers for Disease Control and Prevention. Guide to community preventive services.

2016. Available from https://www.thecommunityguide.org/index.html.

18. Allen P, Sequeira S, Jacob RR, et al. Promoting state health department evidence-based cancer and chronic disease prevention: A multi-phase dissemination study with a cluster randomized trial component. *Implement Sci.* 2013;8(1):1–28.

19. Jacobs JA, Dodson EA, Baker EA, Deshpande AD, Brownson RC. Barriers to evidence-based decision making in public health: A national survey of chronic disease practitioners. *Public Health Rep.* 2010;125(5):736–742.

20. Dodson EA, Baker EA, Brownson RC. Use of evidence-based interventions in state health departments: A qualitative assessment of barriers and solutions. *J Public Health Manag Pract.* 2010;16(6):E9–E15.

21. Hardy AK, Nevin-Woods C, Proud S, Brownson RC. Promoting evidence-based decision making in a local health department, Pueblo City–County, Colorado. *Prev Chronic Dis.* 2015;12:E100.

22. Erwin PC, Harris J, Wong R, Plepys CM, Brownson RC. The academic health department: Academic–practice partnerships among accredited U.S. schools and programs of public health, 2015. *Public Health Rep.* 2016;131(4):630–636.

23. Jacob RR, Allen P, Ahrendt LJ, Brownson RC. Learning about and using research evidence among public health practitioners. *Am J Prev Med.* 2017;52(353):S304–S308.

24. Steele CB, Rose JM, Townsend JS, Fonseka J, Richardson LC, Chovnick G. Comprehensive cancer control partners' use of and attitudes about evidence-based practices. *Prev Chronic Dis.* 2015;12:E113.

25. National Cancer Institute. Cancer Control P.L.A.N.E.T. (Plan, Link, Act, Network with Evidence-Based Tools). 2016. http://cancercontrolplanet.cancer.gov.

Case Study 7C

IMPLEMENTING EVIDENCE-BASED MEDIA ENGAGEMENT PRACTICES TO ADDRESS CANCER DISPARITIES

Racquel E. Kohler, Shoba Ramanadhan, and K. Viswanath

THIS CASE study on disparities provides an example of efforts that focus on how disseminating evidence about the influence of social determinants of health (SDH) can be used to promote implementation of strategic communication activities among community-based organizations (CBOs). That is, instead of typical implementation study of a specific evidence-based program or intervention, the focus of this case study is on how communication activities of CBOs can be evidence-informed. Specifically, we drew on the literatures on SDH and occupational practices of journalists—their reliance on news sources and tendency to frame stories. We describe how this evidence-based approach was implemented among CBO members in order to change their media engagement practices to attend to disparities and frame them in the context of SDH.

CANCER DISPARITIES AND SOCIAL DETERMINANTS OF HEALTH

In the United States, socioeconomic and racial/ethnic disparities exist for health broadly and for specific cancer indicators.[1] The socioeconomic gradient is evident for multiple cancer risk factors (e.g., tobacco use, alcohol consumption obesity), receipt of screening and treatment services, and outcomes (e.g., incidence, stage at diagnosis, and survival). For example, tobacco consumption is high among low-income and vulnerable populations,[2,3] and smokers with low socioeconomic position (SEP) tend to have worse health outcomes.[4] Low educational attainment and low family income are linked to increased risk of some cancers, advanced stage diagnosis,[5] and higher mortality.[6] Place and geography are also important: poor counties have worse survival compared to more affluent communities.[7] Additional racial/ethnic disparities persist: overall, Blacks/African Americans have higher incidence and mortality rates than any other racial/ethnic group and have the highest national rates for all cancers.[8] Differential access to care, such as minority groups being less likely to receive appropriate treatment,[9] also contributes to worse outcomes.[10]

The social, economic, and cultural drivers of health disparities are well documented[11,12] and involve complex pathways, which can be difficult to understand and study because they cross multiple sectors (e.g., education, housing, labor, and health). Geography, income, education, occupation, social class, gender, and race/ethnicity are the most important stratifying indicators that contribute to extant health disparities within and between countries throughout the world.[13]

The multiple and dynamic interactions of SDH require systemic approaches to change them, such as public policies. However, the public arena, including the information environment, is often less hospitable or even hostile to such policy changes because they affect specific groups differently and involve public expenditures. Also, few Americans are aware of the connection between social determinants and unequal health outcomes.[14,15]

MEDIA INFLUENCE AND COMMUNICATION STRATEGIES

The media play a role in raising awareness about health and social problems, reasons for those problems, and potential solutions.[16] Media also influence the salience, or prominence, of topics, which in turn influences public opinion and public support.[17] How media cover (or do not cover) SDH and disparities may contribute to low public awareness and shape the public discussion on causes and solutions of health disparities.

Evidence from sociology of journalism shows that news media, specifically health journalists, rely largely on news sources such as spokespersons, news releases, and press conferences to develop ideas for stories on health and angles or frames they chose to use in those stories.[18-20] Thus, active engagement with journalists requires establishing a communications plan, building effective media relations, pitching and responding to media queries, and using exemplars and angles in communications. Key to this is framing. It is well documented that the

structure of the message is as powerful as the content of the message in influencing the public perception of a topic and support for health issues and policies.[21,22]

PROJECT IMPACT: INFLUENCING THE MEDIA AND PUBLIC AGENDA ON CANCER AND TOBACCO DISPARITIES

Project IMPACT was a multilevel, community-based participatory research (CBPR) project aimed at building capacity in CBOs to change the public agenda on health and tobacco-related disparities with the assumption that it may eventually lead to support for structural policy changes to address these disparities. Drawing on the large bodies of work on SDH and communication science, Project IMPACT sought to influence the information environment by implementing an evidence-based approach for SDH-informed strategic media engagement among CBOs. The approach focused on building skills to infuse evidence on SDH within the communication activities of CBO staff.

Specifically, the project focused on CBOs working with underserved and ethnic minority groups, and the intervention trained CBO staff on (1) evidence of SDH and (2) evidence-based communication strategies (e.g., framing news stories for journalists) to change media engagement practices. The project utilized a CBPR approach, which emphasizes equitable partnership between researchers and stakeholders, drawing on their diverse strengths in the effort to support research and action that address health disparities.[23] This research approach is well-suited for disparities-related policy work, and partnerships are increasingly focused on effecting policy changes to promote health and create healthy environments.[24,25] CBPR collaborations have been helpful in shifting how issues are framed among various groups to promote change,[26] and partners' knowledge and skills are key factors of successful policy change and implementation.[27]

Intervention Setting

Project IMPACT was led by a Community Project Advisory Committee that included academic researchers, CBOs, Departments of Public Health, and a health coalition.[28,29] Project IMPACT was conducted in Lawrence, Massachusetts, a former textile mill town of approximately 76,000 residents, more than 70% of whom identify as Hispanic/ Latino. Approximately 30% have incomes below the federal poverty level, and nearly two-thirds of adults have the equivalent of a high school diploma or less. Despite statewide health insurance coverage, disparities in obesity, cardiovascular disease, hypertension, diabetes, and cancer persist in Lawrence. At the same time, the city places tremendous emphasis on improving health and has rich, intersectoral collaborations to support these efforts, as well as support from city leadership.

Initial Work That Informed the Intervention

PUBLIC AND COMMUNITY LEADERS' OPINION OF HEALTH DISPARITIES

Prior to the intervention, we conducted a door-to-door public opinion survey and found that although some respondents acknowledged SDH, individual responsibility was the dominant causal frame to explain disparities.[28] For example, when asked to give reasons why some people experienced worse health compared to others, individual lifestyle behaviors (e.g., lack of willpower to quit smoking) dominated

Table 7C.1. Project IMPACT Intervention Package and Objectives

INTERVENTION COMPONENT	OBJECTIVE
• Workshops with didactic sessions and interactive in-class exercises • Training manual for media engagement • Wiki providing additional resources • Networking events and booster sessions	• Increase awareness of SDH, health disparities, and the media's role in setting public agenda • Equip CBOs with strategies to engage media • Change communication practices of CBOs to reframe disparities in light of SDH

CBOs, community-based organizations; SDH, social determinants of health.

over other reasons (e.g., limited access to cessation resources).

We also interviewed community leaders to assess their perspectives on health disparities.[30] Nearly all of the leaders acknowledged disparities were an issue in Lawrence, and most attributed them to both individual-level (e.g., biological and lifestyle factors) and structural-level causes (e.g., environmental, community, and social factors). In addition, most leaders thought there was no or poor media coverage of disparities and that more discussions among local leaders were needed. The disconnect between attributions made by the public and those by community leaders highlights the need to bring attention to structural drivers of disparities.

PUBLIC NEWS MEDIA COVERAGE OF HEALTH DISPARITIES

A content analysis of local mainstream (English) and ethnic (Spanish) media highlighted missed opportunities in media coverage. The analysis found that health disparities received little attention, and when covered, media framed causes and solutions to health disparities more as individual or behavioral factors compared to SDH.[31] The few stories that included discussions on disparities often compared different racial groups, whereas other SDHs received little attention.

Intervention Package

The training workshop for CBO staff members included a variety of components (Table 7C.1). Workshops included training on the ways in which unequal distribution of social resources can determine the risk individuals face in terms of getting sick, being able to prevent illnesses, and opportunities to access treatment.[32] The training also emphasized tobacco-related examples, including environmental factors that may influence disparities and multilevel determinants and solutions, such as smoking cessation policies, product availability, and pro- and anti-tobacco messaging. The strategic media engagement components focused on ways to foster media relations, use different media channels, write press releases and op-eds, and pitch stories to journalists. The goal was to provide high-level training as well as concrete examples and templates to promote utilization of the evidence-based approach to strategic media engagement.

We held four workshops that were attended by a total of 61 participants from 30 CBOs, including private non-profit, public/government, advocacy, foundation/charity, and other organizations. A variety of community interests were represented, such as public/mental health, social services, and education. Participants were mainly female (80%) and racial/ethnically diverse: 60% were Hispanic/Latino, 42% White, and 11% Black/African American. The initial day-long workshop was followed by optional booster sessions and ongoing technical assistance.

Training Outcomes

After the training, participants reported having a better understanding about how people's living and working environments can affect their health and that they intended to use the learned strategies for communicating health inequalities and for interacting with the media. We found significant increases in confidence across media-related activities (Figure 7C.1) from the pre- and post-survey responses. Immediately after the workshop, 72% of participants indicated it was very likely that they would use the communication practices with the media, and 82% said it was very likely that they would share SDH information with others.

At a 6-month follow-up assessment, participants reported using the communication and media practices (Table 7C.2). Nearly half of participants

(49%) reported using social media to promote their CBO, and one-third had written a press release.

As part of a process evaluation of the intervention, we discovered that participants wanted continued hands-on training to practice writing, to interact with local media representatives, and to have more networking opportunities. We held two optional booster events tailored to these requests. The first event included an exercise on writing press releases, a panel of local media, and dedicated time to network with media and other alumni. Participants reported increased social capital and communication skills. A separate social media training event demonstrated how to use social media to engage and interact with different audiences.

CONCLUSION

This case is an illustration of how CBO staff's communication practices can be changed through drawing on evidence from two areas—the influence of SDH on disparities and communication science. Disseminating and implementing a more abstract health innovation can make measuring adoption more challenging compared to a concrete tool or practice.[33] However, we successfully sensitized members of CBOs on structural drivers of disparities, and participants reported that new SDH and communication skills gained during training were shared with other staff members,

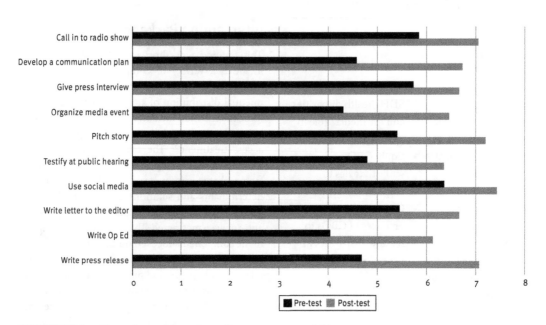

FIGURE 7C.1   Change in confidence in media-engagement activities.

Table 7C.2. Use of Strategic Media Engagement Practices 6 Months After Training

PRACTICE	%
Called in to a radio show	19
Developed a communication plan	21
Gave an interview to the press	17
Organized a media event	6
Pitched a story to a journalist	15
Testified at a public hearing	11
Used social media for promotion	49
Wrote a press release	32

CBOs, and media. This example also highlights the importance of building capacity and leveraging local community assets in order to reduce disparities and improve health.

Even though cancer disproportionately affects racial/ethnic and low SEP groups, implementation studies in diverse settings and with diverse populations is lacking.[34] More research on the implementation of disparities-focused interventions in contexts relevant to vulnerable populations is needed, especially as cancer interventions move upstream from narrow clinical practices to broader social policies affecting where people live and work. Understanding factors that affect implementation of disparities-focused interventions will provide critical insight into how, when, where, and for whom solutions are most likely to be successful. This type of work is critical to ensure that implementing evidence-based programs narrows disparities and does not widen them.

REFERENCES

1. Ryerson AB, Eheman CR, Altekruse SF, et al. Annual report to the nation on the status of cancer, 1975–2012, featuring the increasing incidence of liver cancer. *Cancer.* 2016;122(9):1312–1337.
2. Cook BL, Wayne GF, Kafali EN, Liu Z, Shu C, Flores M. Trends in smoking among adults with mental illness and association between mental health treatment and smoking cessation. *JAMA.* 2014;311(2):172–182.
3. Baggett TP, Tobey ML, Rigotti NA. Tobacco use among homeless people—Addressing the neglected addiction. *N Engl J Med.* 2013;369(3):201–204.
4. Campaign for Tobacco-Free Kids. *Tobacco and Socioeconomic Status.* Washington, DC: Campaign for Tobacco-Free Kids; 2016.
5. Clegg LX, Reichman ME, Miller BA, et al. Impact of socioeconomic status on cancer incidence and stage at diagnosis: Selected findings from the surveillance, epidemiology, and end results: National Longitudinal Mortality Study. *Cancer Causes Control.* 2009;20(4):417–435.
6. Albano JD, Ward E, Jemal A, et al. Cancer mortality in the United States by education level and race. *J Natl Cancer Inst.* 2007;99(18):1384–1394.
7. Ward E, Jemal A, Cokkinides V, et al. Cancer disparities by race/ethnicity and socioeconomic status. *CA Cancer J Clin.* 2004;54(2):78–93.
8. SEER cancer statistics review, 1975–2013. National Cancer Institute website. 2016. https://seer.cancer.gov/csr/1975_2013. Accessed December 2016.
9. Shavers VL, Brown ML. Racial and ethnic disparities in the receipt of cancer treatment. *J Natl Cancer Inst.* 2002;94(5):334–357.
10. DeLancey JOL, Thun MJ, Jemal A, Ward EM. Recent trends in Black–White disparities in cancer mortality. *Cancer Epidemiol Biomarkers Prev.* 2008;17(11):2908–2912.
11. Marmot M. Social determinants of health inequalities. *Lancet.* 365(9464):1099–1104.
12. Woodward A, Kawachi I. Why reduce health inequalities? *J Epidemiol Commun Health.* 2000;54(12):923–929.
13. Solar O, Irwin A. *A Conceptual Framework for Action on the Social Determinants of Health.* Geneva, Switzerland: World Health Organization; 2007.
14. Booske BC, Robert SA, Rohan AMK. Awareness of racial and socioeconomic health disparities in the United States: The National Opinion Survey on Health and Health Disparities, 2008–2009. *Prev Chronic Dis.* 2011;8(4):A73.
15. Robert SA, Booske BC. US opinions on health determinants and social policy as health policy. *Am J Public Health.* 2011;101(9):1655–1663.
16. Kim AE, Kumanyika S, Shive D, Igweatu U, Kim SH. Coverage and framing of racial and ethnic health disparities in US newspapers,

1996–2005. *Am J Public Health.* 2010;100(Suppl 1):S224–S231.

17. Iyengar S, Kinder DR. *News That Matters: Television and American Opinion.* Chicago: University of Chicago Press; 2010.

18. McCauley MP, Blake KD, Meissner HI, Viswanath K. The social group influences of US health journalists and their impact on the newsmaking process. *Health Educ Res.* 2013;28(2):339–351.

19. Viswanath K, Blake KD, Meissner HI, et al. Occupational practices and the making of health news: A national survey of US health and medical science journalists. *J Health Commun.* 2008;13(8):759–777.

20. Wallington SF, Blake K, Taylor-Clark K, Viswanath K. Antecedents to agenda setting and framing in health news: An examination of priority, angle, source, and resource usage from a national survey of U.S. health reporters and editors. *J Health Commun.* 2010;15(1):76–94.

21. Viswanath K, Emmons KM. Message effects and social determinants of health: Its application to cancer disparities. *J Commun.* 2006;56:S238–S264.

22. Chong D, Druckman JN. Framing theory. *Annu Rev Polit Sci.* 2007;10:103–126.

23. KHSP—Community track. Kellogg Health Scholars Program website. http:// cultureofhealthequity.org/our-work/khsp/khsp-community-track. Accessed June 2017.

24. Themba-Nixon M, Minkler M, Freudenberg N. The role of CBPR in policy advocacy. In: Minkler M, Wallerstein N, eds. *Community-Based Participatory Research for Health: From Process to Outcomes.* San Francisco, CA: Jossey-Bass; 2008:307–322.

25. Minkler M. Linking science and policy through community-based participatory research to study and address health disparities. *Am J Public Health.* 2010;100(S1):S81–S87.

26. Petersen D, Minkler M, Vásquez VB, Baden AC. Community-based participatory research as a tool for policy change: A case study of the Southern California Environmental Justice Collaborative. *Rev Policy Res.* 2006;23(2):339–354.

27. Israel BA, Coombe CM, Cheezum RR, et al. Community-based participatory research: A capacity-building approach for policy advocacy aimed at eliminating health disparities. *Am J Public Health.* 2010;100(11):2094–2102.

28. Ramanadhan S, Nagler RH, McCauley MP, et al. Much ventured, much gained: Community-engaged data collection by adolescents and young adults. *Prog Community Health Partnersh.* 2016;10(2):217–224.

29. Koh HH, Oppenheimer SC, Massin-Short SB, Emmons KM, Geller AC, Viswanath K. Translating research evidence into practice to reduce health disparities: A social determinants approach. *Am J Public health.* 2010;100(Suppl 1):S72–S80.

30. McCauley MP, Ramanadhan S, Viswanath K. Assessing opinions in community leadership networks to address health inequalities: A case study from Project IMPACT. *Health Educ Res.* 2015;30(6):866–881.

31. Nagler RH, Bigman CA, Ramanadhan S, Ramamurthi D, Viswanath K. Prevalence and framing of health disparities in local print news: Implications for multilevel interventions to address cancer inequalities. *Cancer Epidemiol Biomarkers Prev.* 2016;25(4):603–612.

32. Marmot M, Friel S, Bell R, Houweling TA, Taylor, S; Commission on Social Determinants of Health. Closing the gap in a generation: Health equity through action on the social determinants of health. *Lancet.* 2008;372(9650):1661–1669.

33. Elliott SJ, O'Loughlin J, Robinson K, et al. Conceptualizing dissemination research and activity: The case of the Canadian Heart Health Initiative. *Health Educ Behav.* 2003;30(3):267–282.

34. Rabin BA, Glasgow RE, Kerner JF, Klump MP, Brownson RC. Dissemination and implementation research on community-based cancer prevention: A systematic review. *American J Prev Med.* 2010;38(4):443–456.

Case Study 7D

IMPLEMENTATION SCIENCE IN RETAIL TOBACCO CONTROL POLICY

Todd B. Combs, Laura Brossart, Kurt M. Ribisl, and Douglas A. Luke

THE IMPLEMENTATION of tobacco control programs and policies during the past half century is largely responsible for the greater than 50% decline in smoking rates since the 1964 publication of the first Surgeon General's Report, "Smoking and Health."[1] However, tobacco use continues to be the leading preventable cause of death and disability in the United States, and more than 36 million Americans still smoke cigarettes.[1,2] Accelerated implementation of policies is needed to ensure protection for all citizens from tobacco-related cancers and other diseases and to eliminate tobacco-related disparities.[1]

While states and localities continue to implement traditional tobacco control strategies, such as strengthening smoke-free air policies and increasing excise taxes, a growing body of evidence now also points to the critical importance of policies that directly address the tobacco retail environment.[3,4] The 1998 Master Settlement Agreement that banned many types of tobacco marketing left retail promotion of tobacco largely unregulated.[5] As a result,

tobacco companies now spend the vast majority of their annual marketing budget ($9.5 billion in 2013)[6] in the retail environment. In-store advertising, promotions, and discounts increase impulse purchases, normalize the presence of tobacco products, encourage initiation, discourage cessation, and contribute to tobacco-related disparities.[7–9] The 2009 Family Smoking Prevention and Tobacco Control Act (FSPTCA) gave the US Food and Drug Administration greater control to regulate tobacco and reiterated the powers of states and localities to restrict aspects of tobacco advertising and promotion.[10]

The recent proliferation of retail tobacco control policies creates a significant opportunity for implementation science in public health. At a 2015 meeting funded by the National Cancer Institute's State and Community Tobacco Control (SCTC) initiative, tobacco control program managers, policymakers, legal experts, and researchers identified two main priorities for implementation in retail tobacco policy: (1) building an evidence base for policy and (2) developing strategies for translation and dissemination of policy-relevant data and information to the public and policymakers.[11] This case study considers how implementation science can enhance retail tobacco control policy efforts.

RETAIL TOBACCO CONTROL POLICY

Retail-focused tobacco control policies aim to reduce the availability and accessibility of tobacco products and can be categorized into four domains: place, price, promotion, and product availability.[12-15] Policies addressing *place* focus on reducing tobacco retailer density (e.g., the number of retailers per 1,000 residents or per square mile) and include limiting the number of tobacco retailer licenses available, restricting the proximity of retailers to each other or to youth-oriented locales such as schools and parks, and banning tobacco sales at pharmacies.[16,17]

Policies focused on increasing the *price* of tobacco products through non-tax approaches include enacting minimum price laws, banning price discounts and coupons, and establishing minimum packaging and prices for non-cigarette products such as cigarillos.[18-21] Strategies to curtail tobacco product *promotion* address the manner and quantity of advertisements or display of products in retailers. Tobacco advertising can be restricted by geographic location (e.g., near schools) or in conjunction with all types of window advertising (i.e., content-neutral advertisement space limits).[16,22] Policies focused on limiting *product availability* include raising the minimum legal sales age for tobacco products, banning

the sale of flavored products, and restricting sales to certain types of stores (e.g., adult-only specialty tobacco shops).[23]

Burgeoning tobacco control strategies focused on the retail environment create opportunities for D&I research to improve the impact of policies and practices. Figure 7D.1 illustrates the stages of retail tobacco policy implementation, from assessing retailers to disseminating process and policy evaluations. At each stage, early implementation has begun to enhance efforts and establish best practices.

ASSESSING THE RETAIL TOBACCO PROBLEM

Retail tobacco control policy efforts generally begin by assessing the nature and pervasiveness of tobacco in a community through assessments of tobacco sellers. Tobacco control programs and partners identify the locations of tobacco retailers through licensing lists, commercial business lists, and lists developed for enforcing laws banning tobacco sales to minors. Stakeholders can use maps and calculations of tobacco retailer density to demonstrate the pervasiveness of tobacco in communities. Implementation studies have described strategies at this stage.[24,25] For example, youth advocates in San Francisco used maps of retailers and comparative densities in the city's 11 districts to show that tobacco retailers were much more prevalent in low-income neighborhoods and those with higher proportions of people of color and young people.[25]

Tobacco prices, marketing, and promotion also differ across contexts.[13,26,27] Recognizing the

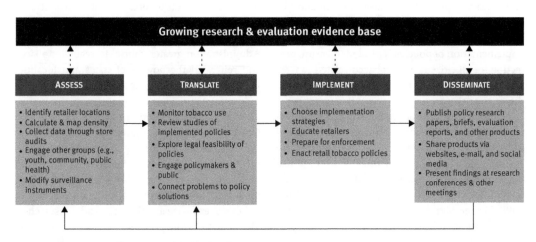

FIGURE 7D.1   Retail tobacco policy implementation.

need for a standardized instrument for retailer assessments, efforts from the National Cancer Institute's SCTC initiative resulted in the 2014 release of the Standardized Tobacco Assessment for Retail Settings (STARS).[28,29] Although other audit instruments already existed, STARS was developed by a group of tobacco control researchers explicitly to inform policy efforts and to facilitate comparisons across neighborhoods, cities, and states.[30]

By 2015, just 1 year after its release, programs in almost two-thirds of states (64%) had used or were actively planning to use STARS.[16] STARS was designed to be used by non-professional, self-trained assessors; a fidelity study found the majority of items on STARS exhibit high or moderate reliability between professional and self-trained assessors.[30] Case studies of STARS use in Indiana, Oregon, Texas, and Vermont detailed how results were disseminated to communities and policymakers.[24]

TRANSLATING PROBLEMS AND POLICY SOLUTIONS FOR COMMUNITIES

Communities also monitor tobacco use and investigate how prevalence rates and tobacco-related disparities are influenced by the accessibility and availability of tobacco products. Evidence linking higher tobacco retailer density with higher prevalence rates and increased disparities continues to grow.[25,26,31–35] As a way of enhancing and extending existing national and state health risk behavior surveillance systems,[36,37] states and localities are starting to add items to health surveys to help determine local policy priorities and feasibility. Minnesota added a question to its state survey about how smokers would react to a ban on menthol products in the state,[38] and New York City augmented its city survey with items asking about the use of coupons and discounts.[18] Once stakeholders have compiled evidence of tobacco problems from surveillance and store audits, policy solutions can be identified and compared to determine their potential for addressing problems in specific contexts. For example, states and communities have several mechanisms from which to choose when aiming to monitor and reduce tobacco retailer density, including licensing laws, zoning laws, conditional use permits, and direct regulation.[22,39] Tobacco control programs in at least 90% of states seek legal guidance to help choose specific policy solutions.[16] Since the 2009 FSPTCA, implementation researchers and public health legal experts

such as the Tobacco Control Legal Consortium[40] have produced several translational products that explain various retail tobacco policy options, their applicability to specific problems, and their legal defensibility.[12,22]

Engaging stakeholders is a crucial practical component of moving from problems to policy solutions and an important tenet of implementation science.[41] A case study of recent tobacco control efforts in New York City highlighted the practical ways many stakeholders took part in policy development. Several groups, including youth interns from the city's LGBT Center and representatives from Asian Americans for Equality, met with city councilors, spoke at community forums, and testified at public hearings. These groups helped not only in connecting tobacco-related problems to policy solutions but also in garnering public and policymaker support for implementation of the interventions. The case study, widely disseminated to tobacco control programs and partners, has become a tool for other communities.[16,18]

IMPLEMENTING RETAIL TOBACCO CONTROL POLICIES

Translational products such as legal tool kits and studies describing previous policy processes have also offered insights useful during policy adoption. For example, case studies of Providence, Rhode Island, and New York City showed that retailer education and engagement initiatives are important for setting feasible timelines for implementation. Whereas Providence's discount restrictions were scheduled to take effect 3 months after passage, similar laws in New York City were rolled out over 6 months. Practical and contextual factors (e.g., the number of retailers and tobacco control program and enforcement agency resources) influenced these and other decisions that stakeholders believe helped ensure timely compliance.[18,19] Other highlights for the implementation stage from translational products include how legal experts can help when choosing between and promoting different implementation strategies (e.g., grandfathering existing licensees when reducing the number of available tobacco retailer licenses)[22] and how early engagement of agencies that will take part after implementation (i.e., those charged with enforcement and evaluation) can help smooth policy roll-outs.[18,25]

BUILDING AND DISSEMINATING THE EVIDENCE BASE

Tobacco control programs and partners need confirmation that specific policies address specific problems (e.g., that raising the sales age to 21 years *decreases* youth prevalence rates or that retailer proximity buffers *reduce* disparities in prevalence). Given that most communities are just starting to develop retail interventions (e.g., the majority of jurisdictions implementing Tobacco 21 have done so in the past 2 years),[42] there is unsurprisingly a lack of evidence regarding long-term public health outcomes. However, in some cases, shorter term policy impacts are more readily observable; for example, San Francisco witnessed an 8% reduction in the number of tobacco retailers within 1 year of implementing its retailer reduction strategies.[25]

Studying policy effects in real communities takes time. Computational modeling of retail policy effects represents an alternative research strategy. Agent-based models have recently been used to estimate that tobacco retailer reduction policies may increase search and purchase costs for tobacco products, that different policies exhibit quite diverse impacts on cost, and that these impacts may differ significantly across context (e.g., urban vs. suburban neighborhoods).[43]

As evidence from scientific studies of retail tobacco policy continues to build, translation and dissemination of results remains a high priority. Dissemination through traditional and new media of case studies and other reports of communities' experiences[12,18,19,24,25,44,45] plays a critical role in information sharing and policy diffusion across locales. Although presentations at scientific conferences and peer-reviewed publications remain important strategies for building the evidence base, translational research products and tools designed for tobacco control programs can often be more quickly disseminated and adapted to local needs.

EMERGING OPPORTUNITIES FOR IMPLEMENTATION SCIENCE IN RETAIL TOBACCO CONTROL POLICY

Expanding implementation science in retail tobacco control can enhance policy activities through building the evidence base, establishing best practices, and targeting dissemination efforts. For example, studies guided by the theory of *diffusion of innovations*[46] can investigate how the lessons learned by early adopters of tobacco retail policies are shared with other communities and how policies are adapted in different environments, as well as how connections between researchers and tobacco control programs influence the dissemination of scientific findings and eventual policy adoption. With the help of Kingdon's Multiple Streams framework,[47] implementation science in retail tobacco policy might focus on the processes of *problem definition* (e.g., higher retailer density exacerbates tobacco-related disparities), *policy development* (e.g., connecting problems to specific policies), or the *politics* of retail tobacco policy (e.g., how evidence is best communicated to policymakers and how potential legal challenges or lobbying from the tobacco industry can be circumvented).

Evaluations of implemented policies are invaluable for demonstrating the effectiveness of retail-focused tobacco control strategies. As pioneering policies mature, evidence and lessons from evaluations will become even more central in designing, adopting, and implementing future policies. In the meantime and beyond, systems science approaches in implementation science can help build evidence. Applications of agent-based modeling to retail tobacco policy show promise for helping states and communities understand and predict the impact of retail tobacco policy. Other systems science methods, such as system dynamics modeling, could situate the tobacco retail problem in the context of the complex system of state and local policymaking bodies, public health departments, and communities.[48] Studies using network analysis that focus on the linkages between tobacco control programs can investigate the extent and quality of connections between programs as well as identify those that may be isolated from others.[49]

While most implementation science in cancer prevention is focused on translating established evidence bases into practice, retail tobacco policy is still in the early stages, and implementation of big "P" policies (e.g., government legislation and ordinances) in tobacco control comes with unique political and legal impediments. Both of these present unique challenges and opportunities for implementation science. Continuing to collect evidence is of paramount importance, as are strategies for rapid dissemination of this information. As retail tobacco policies proliferate, opportunities expand for building on successful strategies. Implementation science can help connect policy implementation with long-term public health outcomes, reduce political and legal obstacles, and advance the role of science in policy.

ACKNOWLEDGMENTS

This research was informed by the work of the Advancing Science in the Retail Environment (ASPiRE) project, funded by the National Cancer Institute's State and Community Tobacco Control Research initiative, grant No. CA154281. ASPiRE is a collaboration between researchers from the Center for Public Health Systems Science at Washington University, the Stanford Prevention Research Center, and the University of North Carolina Gillings School of Global Public Health.

REFERENCES

1. US Department of Health and Human Services. *The Health Consequences of Smoking—50 Years of Progress: A Report of the Surgeon General*. Atlanta, GA: US Department of Health and Human Services, Centers for Disease Control and Prevention, National Center for Chronic Disease Prevention and Health Promotion, Office on Smoking and Health; 2014.

2. Centers for Disease Control and Prevention. Current Cigarette Smoking Among Adults — United States, 2005–2015. *MMWR Morbid Mortal Wkly Rep*. 2016; 65(44):1205–1211.

3. National Cancer Institute. *The Role of the Media in Promoting and Reducing Tobacco Use*. Bethesda, MD: National Institutes of Health; 2008.

4. Moreland-Russell S, Combs T, Jones J, Sorg AA. State level point-of-sale policy priority as a result of the FSPTCA. *AIMS Public Health*. 2015;2(4):681–690.

5. Master settlement agreement. Public Health Law Center at Mitchell Hamline School of Law website. 2015. http://publichealthlawcenter. org/topics/tobacco-control/tobacco-control-litigation/master-settlement-agreement. Accessed November 18, 2016.

6. Federal Trade Commission. *Federal Trade Commission Cigarette Report for 2013*. Washington, DC: Federal Trade Commission; 2016.

7. Paynter J, Edwards R. The impact of tobacco promotion at the point of sale: A systematic review. *Nicotine Tob Res*. 2009;11(1):25–35.

8. Slater SJ, Chaloupka FJ, Wakefield M, Joynston LD, O'Malley PM. The impact of retail cigarette marketing practices on youth smoking uptake. *Arch Pediatr Adolesc Med*. 2007;161(5):440–445.

9. Wakefield M, Germain D, Henriksen L. The effect of retail cigarette pack displays on impulse purchase. *Addiction*. 2007;103(2):322–328.

10. About the FSPTCA. National Institutes of Health, Office of Disease Prevention website. 2009. https://prevention.nih.gov/tobacco-regulatory-science-program/about-the-FSPTCA. Accessed November 18, 2016.

11. Advancing science and policy in the retail environment: Closing plenary discussion. Paper presented at Using Science and Law to Advance Tobacco Retail Policy 2015, Chapel Hill, NC.

12. McLaughlin I, Schultzman M. *Point of Sale Playbook*. Oakland, CA: ChangeLab Solutions; 2016.

13. Lee JG, Henriksen L, Shyanika RW, Moreland-Russell S, Ribisl KM. A systematic review of neighborhood disparities in point-of-sale tobacco marketing. *Am J Public Health*. 2015;105(9):8–18.

14. Henriksen L. Comprehensive tobacco marketing restrictions: promotion, packaging, price and place. *Tob Control*. 2012;21(2):147–153.

15. Shiu E, Hassan LM, Walsh G. Demarketing tobacco through governmental policies—The 4Ps revisited. *J Bus Res*. 2009;62(2):269–278.

16. Center for Public Health Systems Science. *Point-of-Sale Report to the Nation: Realizing the Power of States and Communities to Change the Tobacco Retail and Policy Landscape*. St. Louis, MO: Center for Public Health Systems Science at the Brown School at Washington University, National Cancer Institute, State and Community Tobacco Control Research; 2016.

17. Tobacco-free pharmacies. Americans for Nonsmokers' Rights website. 2016. https://no-smoke.org/wp-content/uploads/pdf/pharmacies.pdf. Accessed November 29, 2016.

18. Center for Public Health Systems Science. *Reducing Cheap Tobacco & Youth Access: New York City. Innovative Point-of-Sale Policies: Case Study #3*. St. Louis, MO: Center for Public Health Systems Science at the Brown School at Washington University, National Cancer Institute, State and Community Tobacco Control Research; 2015.

19. Center for Public Health Systems Science. *Regulating Price Discounting in Providence, RI. Innovative Point-of-Sale Policies: Case Study #1*. St. Louis, MO: Center for Public Health Systems Science at the Brown School at Washington University, National Cancer Institute, State and Community Tobacco Control Research; 2015.

20. Feighery EC, Ribisl KM, Schleicher NC, Zellers L, Wellington N. How do minimum cigarette price laws affect cigarette prices at the retail level? *Tob Control.* 2005;14:80–85.

21. Ribisl KM., Patrick R, Eidson S, Francis J. State cigarette minimum price laws—United States, 2009. *MMWR Morbid Mortal Wkly Rep.* 2010;59(13):389–392.

22. Center for Public Health Systems Science. *Point-of-Sale Strategies: A Tobacco Control Guide.* St. Louis, MO: Center for Public Health Systems Science at the Brown School at Washington University, Tobacco Control Legal Consortium; 2014.

23. State by state. Preventing Tobacco Addiction Foundation website. 2014. http://tobacco21. org/state-by-state. Accessed December 22, 2014.

24. Center for Public Health Systems Science. *Assessing Retail Environments with STARS: Standardized Tobacco Assessment for Retail Settings.* St. Louis, MO: Center for Public Health Systems Science at the Brown School at Washington University, National Cancer Institute, State and Community Tobacco Control Research; 2015.

25. San Francisco Tobacco-Free Project Mission. *Reducing Tobacco Retail Density in San Francisco: A Case Study.* San Francisco, CA: San Francisco Department of Public Health, Bright Research Group; 2016.

26. Henriksen L, Schleicher NC, Dauphinee AL, Fortmann SP. Targeted advertising, promotion, and price for menthol cigarettes in California high school neighborhoods. *Nicotine Tob Res.* 2012;14(1):116–121.

27. Siahpush M, Jones PR, Singh GK, Timsina LR, Martin J. The association of tobacco marketing with median income and racial/ethnic characteristics of neighbourhoods in Omaha, Nebraska. *Tob Control.* 2010;19(3):256–258.

28. STARS. CounterTobacco.org website. 2017. http://countertobacco.wpengine.com/ resources-tools/store-assessment-tools/stars. Accessed January 8, 2017.

29. Addressing high-priority gaps in tobacco control research. State and Community Tobacco Control Research website. 2016. http://www.sctcresearch. org. Accessed November 6, 2016.

30. Henriksen L, Ribisl KM, Rogers T, et al. Standardized Tobacco Assessment for Retail Settings (STARS): Dissemination and implementation research. *Tob Control.* 2016;25(1):i67–i74.

31. Hyland A, Travers MJ, Cummings KM, Bauer J, Alford T, Wieczorek WF. Demographics and tobacco outlet density. *Am J Public Health.* 2003;93(11):1794.

32. Loomis BR, Kim AE, Goetz JL, Juster HR. Density of tobacco retailers and its association with sociodemographic characteristics of communities across New York. *Public Health.* 2013;127(4):333–338.

33. McCarthy WJ, Mistry R, Lu Y, Patel M, Zheng H, Dietsch B. Density of tobacco retailers near schools: Effects on tobacco use among students. *Am J Public Health.* 2009;99(11):2006–2013.

34. Peterson AN, Yu D, Morton CM, Reid RJ, Sheffer MA, Schneider JE. Tobacco outlet density and demographics at the tract level of analysis in New Jersey: A statewide analysis. *Drugs Educ Prev Policy.* 2011;18(1):47–52.

35. Rodriquez D, Carlos HA, Adachi-Mejia AM, Berke EM, Sargent JD. Predictors of tobacco outlet density nationwide: A geographic analysis. *Tob Control.* 2013;22(5):349–355.

36. Behavioral Risk Factor Surveillance System Survey (BRFSS). US Department of Health and Human Services, Centers for Disease Control and Prevention website. 2011–2015. http:// www.cdc.gov/brfss/annual_data/annual_data. htm. Accessed November 18, 2016.

37. Youth Risk Behavior Survey (YRBS). US Department of Health and Human Services, Centers for Disease Control and Prevention website. 2005–2015. http://www.cdc.gov/ healthyyouth/data/yrbs/data.htm. Accessed November 18, 2016.

38. MATS: The Minnesota Adult Tobacco Survey. ClearWay Minnesota and the Minnesota Department of Health website. 2014. http:// www.mnadulttobaccosurvey.org. Accessed September 12, 2016.

39. Ackerman A, Etow A, Bartel S, Ribisl KM. Reducing the density and number of tobacco retailers: Policy solutions and legal issues. *Nicotine Tob Res.* 2017;19(2):133–140.

40. Tobacco Control Legal Consortium. Public Health Law Center at Mitchell Hamline School of Law website. 2016. http:// publichealthlawcenter.org/programs/tobacco- control-legal-consortium. Accessed October 17, 2016.

41. Brownson RC, Jacobs JA, Tabak RG, Hoehner CM, Stamatakis KA. Designing for dissemination among public health researchers: Findings from a national survey in the United States. *Am J Public Health.* 2013;103(9):1693–1699.

42. Tobacco Twenty-One. Preventing Tobacco Addiction Foundation website. 2016. http:// tobacco21.org. Accessed October 17, 2016.

43. Luke DA, Hammond RA, Combs T, et al. Tobacco Town: Computational modeling of policy options to reduce tobacco retailer density. *Am J Public Health*. 2017;107(5):740–746.

44. Center for Public Health Systems Science. *Regulating Pharmacy Tobacco Sales: Massachusetts. Innovative Point-of-Sale Policies: Case Study #2*. St. Louis, MO: Center for Public Health Systems Science at the Brown School at Washington University, National Cancer Institute, State and Community Tobacco Control Research; 2014.

45. Tobacconomics: Economic research informing tobacco control policy. University of Illinois at Chicago, Institute for Health Research and Policy website. 2016. http://tobacconomics.org. Accessed November 29, 2016.

46. Rogers EM. *Diffusion of Innovations*. 5th ed. New York: Free Press; 2003.

47. Kingdon JW. *Agendas, Alternatives, and Public Policies*. 2nd ed. London: Longman; 2011.

48. Luke DA, McCay V, Morshed A, Combs TB. Systems science methods in dissemination and implementation research. In: Brownson RC, Colditz GA, Proctor EK, eds. *Dissemination and Implementation Research in Health: Translating Science to Practice*. 2ond ed. New York: Oxford University Press; 2018:157–174.

49. Schoen M, Moreland-Russell S, Prewitt K, Carothers B. Social network analysis of public health programs to measure partnership. *Soc Sci Med*. 2014;123:90–95.

8

CANCER DETECTION AND SCREENING

OVERVIEW OF CASE STUDIES

Gloria D. Coronado

LUNG AND colorectal cancer exact a staggering human and economic toll. Indeed, these cancers account for 34% of all cancer deaths in the United States, and medical expenditures to treat these cancers are projected to reach $26 billion by 2020.[1,2] Fortunately, screening programs have substantially reduced the incidence of and mortality from colorectal and lung cancers. To ensure their effectiveness, clinical guidance groups such as the US Preventive Services Task Force (USPSTF) continually review the evidence for screening for both these cancers to help guide their clinical implementation and ensure programs are based on the highest quality evidence available. For colorectal cancer, since 2002 the USPSTF has recommended screening for individuals aged 50–75 years, including colonoscopy, flexible sigmoidoscopy, and high-sensitivity fecal occult blood testing. Recently, the USPSTF updated its recommendations to include two additional screening modalities: fecal immunochemical (FIT) DNA testing and computed tomography (CT) colonography.[3] Similarly, the USPSTF

introduced new recommendations for lung cancer screening in 2013, calling for low-dose CT screening in adults aged 55–80 years who have a 30 pack-year smoking history and who currently smoke or have quit within the past 15 years.[4] The recommendations were based on evidence which showed that regular screening can reduce lung cancer deaths by 14%.[4] Taken together, screening programs for lung and colorectal cancer have saved countless lives. Despite these robust screening guidelines, however, a startling number of people still die from these cancers.

Lung and colorectal cancers account for high numbers of preventable deaths. Because of this, scaling-up effective interventions to increase routine screening and lower tobacco use is critically important. Screening programs for these diseases vary greatly in their anticipated outcomes. Colorectal cancer screening can both prevent colorectal cancer and identify it in early, treatable stages. Screening for lung cancer, on the other hand, cannot prevent most lung cancer-related deaths, and up to 80% of deaths could be averted from smoking cessation, making counseling for smoking cessation an important public health priority. An estimated 10 million US adults qualify for screening under USPSTF recommendations, of which 5 million are thought to be current smokers who may be highly motivated to quit or undergo tobacco dependence treatment.[5,6] As such, programs that include smoking cessation counseling are especially important for reducing mortality from lung cancer.

In this complicated environment for ongoing refinement of screening programs, the two case studies presented in this chapter showcase promising interventions for addressing the troubling high rates of mortality from lung and colorectal cancers. They underscore the value of designing experiments considering long-term implementation, aligning the intervention with existing clinic workflows and processes, and incorporating end user feedback.

The research conducted by Ostroff and Shelley, for example, highlights the importance of designing studies with scale-up and long-term dissemination in mind. Their research is based on the premise that lung cancer screening itself represents a "teachable moment" to counsel patients on smoking cessation and offer treatments to reduce smoking dependence. Although this counseling is widely considered critical, the scientific literature provides little guidance on how best to deliver it. To address this issue, Ostroff and Shelley designed an implementation–effectiveness study to report on clinical effectiveness outcomes as well as implementation outcomes needed to accelerate the program's adoption and scale-up. These dual outcomes will be reported using a multiphase optimization strategy that involves multiple, randomized experiments to test the individual and combined effects of promising cessation treatment interventions. The interventions are motivational interviewing, the nicotine replacement therapy patch, the nicotine replacement therapy lozenge, and message framing (gain vs. loss). These intervention components, tested individually and in combination, will comprise an intervention that is optimally effective and can be delivered with minimal burden on clinic staff. Scaling-up and disseminating a program relies on knowing which combination of intervention components works best.

Ostroff and Shelley selected implementation outcomes by applying two dissemination frameworks: Proctor's conceptual model for implementation science and the Consolidated Framework for Implementation Research (CFIR).

Proctor's model offers a taxonomy of implementation outcomes, including acceptability (satisfaction with content/delivery of the tobacco cessation interventions), adoption (uptake), appropriateness (relevance), cost, treatment fidelity/adaptation (the extent to which tobacco treatment interventions are delivered as planned as well as the type of treatment modifications made), penetration (reach), and sustainability. CFIR offers a taxonomy of constructs within five general domains (i.e., outer and inner setting, intervention characteristics, individual characteristics, and process) that were compiled from a comprehensive review of key theories and conceptual models informing implementation science and that offer an in-depth way to assess multilevel barriers at the patient, provider, intervention, and systems levels. By applying two distinct, yet complementary, frameworks to address tobacco treatment delivery, Ostroff and Shelley offer a deliberate and reasoned approach to long-term implementation planning.

Although designing for implementation is important, the case study by Potter and colleagues underscores the importance of additional efforts to support the broad implementation of evidence-based interventions. Potter and colleagues' case study describes the successful testing and scale-up of a program that distributes fecal tests to adults who attend routine flu shot clinics (FluFIT). Notably, Potter and colleagues attribute the success of the FluFIT program as much to its initial plans for implementation and scale-up as to efforts undertaken to align program elements with standard clinical processes, to encourage and learn from program adaptations, and to incorporate input from end users.

By combining FIT testing with a standard clinical process—a flu shot clinic—Potter and his team aligned clinical processes and promotional messages. Potter et al. designed clinic workflows that guided clinic staff to identify flu clinic patients who were due for colorectal cancer screening and offer them a FIT kit. In addition to embedding FIT distribution into a standard clinical process (i.e., the flu clinic), Potter and colleagues aligned promotional messages for the two prevention activities. Because both the flu shot and the FIT test are recommended annually, the flu clinic served to reinforce the message that "just like a flu shot, you need to get FIT every year." Promoting this message to screening advocates, practitioners, and patients contributed to local and national screening efforts.

Potter and colleagues offer a broad approach to implementation and scale-up that emphasized testing adaptations to the program. This included testing the program as integrated during primary care visits rather than in a dedicated FluFIT clinic, testing the program's effectiveness as a "FluFIT program" in a high-volume integrated care setting, and pilot testing the program's feasibility when deployed by pharmacy students during flu shot campaigns at local commercial pharmacies. The FluFIT program's efficacy was initially demonstrated in smaller controlled studies that were followed by a series of larger practice-based effectiveness studies that helped define the program's core elements while promoting local adaptation. Through these adaptations, the authors observed that the program could work with many variations.

Although Potter and his team disseminated their research through traditional scientific channels, publishing the program's scientific results in medical journals, they also actively promoted it to stakeholders and funders and received significant ongoing investments in technical support by the American Cancer Society, whose staff delivered technical assistance to health systems throughout the country. Ultimately, these end users will continue to weigh the benefits of FluFIT activities relative to other clinical interventions in an evolving context of possible changes in the evidence for effective interventions for FIT for screening in underserved populations and changing options for how influenza and colorectal cancer prevention are delivered.

Screening and prevention programs for lung and colorectal cancers have saved countless lives, yet a startling number of people still die from these cancers. Finding ways to promote broad adoption of evidence-based clinical guidelines and smoking cessation programs is a public health priority, especially because these cancers are highly preventable. Implementation Science can accelerate the adoption of evidence-based interventions into widespread use. These two case studies illustrate the importance of designing for implementation, learning from program adaptations, and incorporating input from end users. Applying these principles may support uptake of approaches that prevent cancers from occurring, identify early treatable cancer forms, and ultimately save lives from colorectal and lung cancers.

REFERENCES

1. Mariotto AB, Yabroff KR, Shao Y, Feuer EJ, Brown ML. Projections of the cost of cancer care in the United States: 2010–2020. *J Natl Cancer Inst.* 2011;103(2):117–128.
2. Siegel RL, Miller KD, Jemal A. Cancer statistics, 2017. *CA Cancer J Clin.* 2017;67(1):7–30.
3. Berger BM, Parton MA, Levin B. USPSTF colorectal cancer screening guidelines: An extended look at multi-year interval testing. *Am J Manag Care.* 2016;22(2):e77–81.
4. Moyer VA. Screening for lung cancer: U.S. Preventive Services Task Force recommendation statement. *Ann Intern Med.* 2014;160(5):330–338.
5. Doria-Rose VP, White MC, Klabunde CN, et al. Use of lung cancer screening tests in the United States: Results from the 2010 National Health Interview Survey. *Cancer Epidemiol Biomarkers Prev.* 2012;21(7):1049–1059.
6. Humphrey LL, Deffebach M, Pappas M, et al. Screening for lung cancer with low-dose computed tomography: A systematic review to update the US Preventive Services Task Force recommendation. *Ann Intern Med.* 2013;159(6):411–420.

Case Study 8A

THE FLUFIT PROGRAM

A COLORECTAL CANCER SCREENING INTERVENTION DESIGNED AND TESTED FOR SUCCESSFUL IMPLEMENTATION

Michael B. Potter, Debbie Kirkland, Judith M. E. Walsh, Carol P. Somkin,
Vicky Gomez, and Lawrence W. Green

INCREASED ACCESS to screening, along with more effective treatment, has contributed to significant reductions in colorectal cancer (CRC) incidence and mortality in the United States during the past three decades.[1] Yet, CRC remains the second leading cause of US cancer mortality among adults, with more than 50,000 deaths from CRC expected in 2017.[2] According to the most recent National Health Interview Survey data, 62.4% of eligible Americans were up-to-date with screening in 2015.[3] The public health impact of increasing the national screening rate to 80% by 2018 would be expected to lead to approximately 200,000 fewer cancer deaths by 2030.[4] The US Preventive Services Task Force has endorsed several evidence-based colorectal cancer screening (CRCS) tests for average-risk individuals between the ages of 50 and 75 years, including high-quality annual fecal occult blood tests (FOBT).[5] High-quality FOBT include fecal immunochemical tests (FIT) and high-sensitivity guaiac tests (HSgFOBT). They are endorsed because compared to colonoscopy, they cost less, are

widely available even in resource-limited settings, and can be as effective in reducing CRC mortality when used as part of a comprehensive screening program.[6,7]

CRCS rates have been increasing rapidly in clinical settings with resources to offer a full range of screening options and testing strategies, but less so in settings with more limited resources and a focus on care of the poor and uninsured.[3,8] For example, screening rates in the majority of federally qualified health centers remained under 50% as of 2015.[9] In these settings, access to colonoscopy for average-risk patients is often limited, and the primary initial screening modality is FOBT, given its low cost and relative ease of use. Yet, ensuring timely access to annual FOBT for every eligible patient can be a labor-intensive task. Interventions that facilitate higher rates of FOBT remain important to address CRCS disparities.

In 2005, when the idea to develop the "FluFOBT program" was developed, CRCS was receiving much less attention than it is today. Colonoscopy was less available, and when FOBT was offered, it was usually with lower sensitivity guaiac tests requiring multiple specimens collected after several days of dietary restriction. Seeking models to deliver timely annual FOBT, we (the original research team, including MP, JW, and Dr. Stephen McPhee) observed the success of annual clinic-based influenza vaccination campaigns and wondered whether such campaigns could be leveraged to offer CRCS to eligible patients. We hypothesized that FOBT might be a simple enough test to be provided independently by ancillary clinic staff as an additional service to patients seeking flu shots, presumably at a moment when they were thinking about prevention. In addition to our goal that more people would obtain screening, we wanted to test whether the FluFOBT campaign could provide an opportunity to educate patients and train staff about the importance of CRCS, using a new and potent normative behavioral message for clinical teams and patients alike that "just like a flu shot, adults over 50 should get colorectal cancer screening every year."

A first step to test our hypothesis was to explore the potential reach of a FluFOBT program if widely adopted and implemented successfully in community settings. We modeled the potential increase in CRCS rates that would occur if everyone in the target age group who received a flu shot during the previous year also had up-to-date CRCS. Using California Health Interview Survey data for 2004, we estimated, in this scenario, screening rates would increase by approximately 15 percentage points for all Californians and by 20 percentage points for Californians living in households earning below 200% of the federally defined poverty line. We also reviewed local data at San Francisco General Hospital (SFGH), where we hoped to test the intervention, learning that under this scenario the screening rate increase would be even greater. With these epidemiological and clinical justifications, the principal investigator secured a career development award from the American Cancer Society to develop and test the first FluFOBT program at SFGH's Family Health Center (FHC). The FHC, a residency-run clinic, serves a large, ethnically and linguistically diverse, socioeconomically disadvantaged patient population. The specifics of the intervention were developed with input from doctors, nurses, medical assistants, and clerical staff, as well as lay health workers and patients representative of the multiethnic population served by the clinic. Materials developed included multilingual patient messages about the importance of getting screened,

simplified multilingual FOBT instructions, and wordless FOBT instructions. Through role plays with the clinic team in advance of the intervention, we developed scripts for staff to use with patients. In addition, we designed algorithms to identify patients eligible for FOBT by accessing electronic laboratory data either before or during the course of the flu shot clinic. Scripts for telephone reminders from language-concordant staff during the weeks after the intervention were created.

By the fall of 2007, we were ready to test and evaluate the FluFOBT intervention in a randomized clinical trial using the previously discussed tools. Flu shot clinic dates were randomized to be either "FluFOBT" days, when we would provide the intervention with three-sample guaiac tests currently available, or "Flu-only" days, when we would provide usual care and provide flu shots without offering FOBT. Screening rates among 268 participants in the intervention arm increased by 29.8 percentage points versus 4.4 percentage points in the usual care arm.[10] These results were impressive, but as an efficacy study, the intervention was implemented with extensive supervision by the research team. Effectiveness research was needed to determine whether the program would be worthy of widespread dissemination and implementation.

The FluFOBT program was adapted and tested in additional settings and populations during the next several years, with expansion of the research team and additional research funding secured from the HMO Cancer Research Network, the American Cancer Society (ACS), the Centers for Disease Control and Prevention (CDC), and the Alexander and Margaret Stewart Trust. Variations in procedures and levels of support from the research team produced sometimes less potent but still clinically significant and beneficial results. Examples of adaptations included testing the program as integrated during primary care visits at public health clinics rather than in a dedicated FluFOBT clinic,[11] testing the program's effectiveness as a "FluFIT program" offering single-sample FIT kits during high-volume flu shot clinics serving thousands of patients at Kaiser Permanente Northern California,[12,13] and pilot testing the feasibility of the program when deployed by pharmacy students during annual flu shot campaigns at local commercial pharmacies.[14] We observed that the program could work with many variations. Clinic teams, in particular, preferred FIT to guaiac FOBT because of FIT's simpler patient instructions and superior test properties. In addition, the term "FIT" seemed to generate more positive connotations of good health prevention among both clinical teams and patients compared to the term "FOBT." The research results were presented locally, and most safety net clinics in San Francisco have switched to FIT, with many continuing to use the FluFIT program in various iterations.[15] Clinical teams at many Kaiser Permanente facilities continue to use the FluFIT program as well.[16] The FluFIT program was not maintained in local pharmacies, however, due to logistics and payment issues and also the challenges of providing patient follow-up for test results, although others have pursued adaptations in the hope of overcoming these barriers.

Our team disseminated the results through several channels, presenting the results at academic meetings and publishing them in journals targeting varied groups of clinicians, health care administrators, and public health practitioners. We also presented our findings at national stakeholder meetings such as those of the National Colorectal Cancer Roundtable and in webinars for CRC advocates throughout the United States. In addition, we used grant funding to develop a publicly available website, http://flufit.org, and step-by-step instructions and downloadable materials that serve as an enduring resource for health care teams to replicate and adapt the program for new clinical settings.

We kept in close contact with the funders of our research, who were supportive of our efforts to further disseminate the intervention. For example, the National Cancer Institute wrote a comprehensive digest of our research and featured it on their Research-Tested Interventions Programs website.[17] The program was also highlighted through its "Research to Reality" webinar series.[18] The CDC's Colorectal Cancer Control Program promoted the FluFIT program as one of a variety of practical interventions in meetings of state grantees and in its promotional materials for health practitioners. Many state and local health departments developed their own FluFIT promotional campaigns and materials with minimal consultation from our research team. The Agency for Healthcare Research and Quality featured our program on its Innovations Exchange website,[20] and the Prevent Cancer Foundation recognized the program with its annual Laurel for Innovative Programs.

Implementation activities intensified with substantial resources invested by the ACS. We granted ACS permission to disseminate the program nationally. The ACS's first step was a pilot (led by DK, Durado Brooks, and other ACS staff) in five Federally Qualified Health Centers (FQHCs), geographically distributed across rural and urban areas in several states. This helped determine the feasibility of providing national implementation support through ACS staff working with FQHCs. The ACS implementation team developed trainings for local ACS staff to engage with FQHC staff, including an ACS program implementation guide and a webpage on the ACS website to house project materials.[21] ACS chose to promote it as the "FluFOBT program," positing that the generic term FOBT might be more acceptable to clinical teams that had not yet switched to FIT—although it turned out that most sites choosing to participate were already using FIT. The ACS Statistics and Evaluation Center (SEC) developed an evaluation plan and data collection methods for the pilot, including both quantitative and qualitative data. In addition, the SEC staff conducted telephone interviews with FQHC staff and ACS staff after the pilot period ended to obtain more detailed process information about program implementation, perceptions of the training, staffing, resources utilized, and successes and challenges. The pilot was deemed successful, and several lessons learned were incorporated into ACS training materials. ACS staff began to promote the FluFOBT program more broadly to FQHCs and other partners. As of 2016, the ACS staff had documented support for 164 FluFOBT initiatives in 144 FQHCs and health systems throughout the United States. Partners have been motivated to implement a FluFOBT program for unique reasons, although they often cite preexisting active flu vaccination programs and a desire to leverage these programs as an opportunity to increase CRCS rates as important.

To sustain and scale-up success, the core program components and flow (Figure 8A.1) must be supported, while allowing local adaptations as needed. For example, ACS staff members have often found the need to remind clinics that the success of the program is jeopardized when test completion reminders or navigation to colonoscopy for individuals with abnormal tests are omitted. In one ACS-supported program, an FQHC made the program more accessible by offering it to migrant farmworkers in the fields where they worked. In another ACS-supported program, the emphasis on a FluFOBT program led to the recognition of deficiencies in offering FOBT as a year-round activity, in turn leading to additional clinic-based

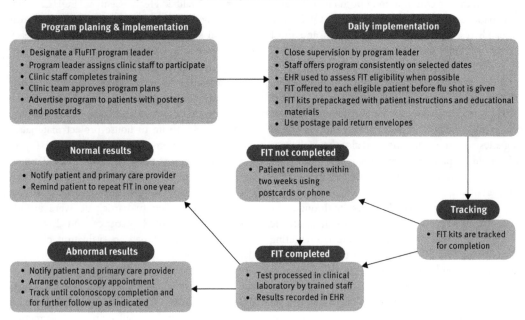

FIGURE 8A.1   FluFIT program flow diagram.

activities that supported more intensive efforts to increase screening. As ACS has introduced the FluFOBT programs to hospitals, it has learned that these programs must often be preceded by educational efforts to convince clinical teams that FOBT is a viable noninvasive alternative to colonoscopy for patients with average risk. In their work with these hospitals, ACS teams have helped tailor FluFOBT programs not only for hospital-based clinic patients but also for employees and outside the hospital as a service to the community.

In another innovative pilot, the ACS is collaborating with a statewide FQHC association and Medicaid managed care plans to promote wider use of the FluFOBT program. In this model, each collaborator will have a complementary role: The statewide association recruits FQHCs to participate in the pilot and provide technical and data support and analysis; health plans champion and promote the pilot to the FQHCs, serve as the conduit of information and resources between the collaborating organizations, and encourage member participation in the pilot; ACS staff provide implementation training and ongoing support to individual FQHCs and health plan staff, and they serve as a linkage point for all involved organizations. Results of this pilot partnership will be evaluated in the near future.

Beyond these ACS-supported activities, other programs modeled after the FluFIT program have emerged independently. An informal internet search for the term "FluFIT" in November 2016 as preparation for writing this chapter identified efforts to implement the FluFIT program in nearly all 50 states during the previous 5 years. Some of these programs have incorporated new innovations. For example, the Cancer Prevention Research Institute of Texas has funded "FluFIT on the Frontera," an ambitious program along the Texas–Mexico border that pairs the FluFIT program with patient navigation.[21]

One important question emerges as our program has been widely disseminated and implemented: To what extent will the FluFIT program ultimately contribute to increasing population screening rates and to the ultimate desired outcomes of reducing CRC mortality and disparities? Effectiveness on this level is difficult to measure because the FluFIT program is typically just one of many programs and activities used in clinical settings to increase screening rates. In San Francisco's public health clinics, sustained benefits of the program were documented during the year after our research program concluded, with increases in both the number of flu shots provided and the proportion of flu shot recipients who had up-to-date screening over time.[15] Yet, most of the success stories outside of our research program are anecdotal. For example, the National Colorectal Cancer Roundtable surveyed its stakeholders about their efforts to achieve an 80% screening rate and received reports from some, such as "Our local FluFIT campaign was instrumental in improving our overall CRCS rates" and "FluFIT increased the number of persons screened for CRC tremendously." ACS has collected success stories from FQHCs that it has supported, such as an Oklahoma clinic that increased its screening rate from 8% to 23% over 1 year, and another in North Carolina attributed FluFIT activities as an important contributor to increasing the screening rate from 13% to 56% over 2 years. These anecdotes do not substitute for rigorous evaluation, but clearly FluFIT programs can be effective when properly supported, and they likely have the greatest impact when introduced in settings in which robust screening activities have not yet taken hold or reached a sufficient proportion of the target population.

Of course, the mere existence of an evidence-based FluFIT program does not guarantee its use, nor should it. For adoption and implementation to occur, clinic leaders must prioritize CRCS; become aware of the program; and believe that it can be an affordable, feasible, and effective local strategy to increase screening rates. They must also believe that the benefits of the program are worth the investment of time and effort relative to other interventions. In addition, a series of decisions will determine its ultimate success, such as who is selected as the clinical champion and how the implementation process is tailored to overcome local barriers. We have seen seemingly small issues, such as an unexpected change in personnel or lack of access to electronic health records at the location where flu shots are being given, stop a FluFIT program in its tracks. We have also witnessed seemingly insurmountable barriers, including the unwillingness of patients in some settings to wait after their flu shot to pick up their FIT kit, overcome by simple changes such as providing the FIT kit first and the flu shot second. Also, we have seen FluFIT programs appropriately abandoned in cases in which timely colonoscopy referrals for abnormal FIT results are not available or when other programs, such as those focusing on colonoscopy and/or mailed FIT kits, are so successful that screening rates well over 80% have been achieved. Rather than being advocated as a program that everyone *should* adopt, the FluFIT program stands as an evidence-based tool that any health care organization *can use and adapt as needed* to achieve its goals.

In conclusion, we attribute the remarkable success of the FluFIT program to the fact that it was designed with the goal of dissemination and implementation. The program was built to complement activities that many clinical teams have already embraced (providing annual flu shots), justified by behavior change theory and epidemiologic evidence, and developed with input from providers and patients who would be end users and beneficiaries of the program. The efficacy of the program was demonstrated in smaller controlled studies and followed up with a series of larger practice-based effectiveness studies that helped define core elements of the program while also allowing and encouraging local adaptation. Where possible, the lasting effects of these interventions have been documented. The results were published in medical journals but also actively promoted to stakeholders by the investigators and the funders of the research, with significant ongoing investment in technical support by ACS. With the many types of FluFIT activities now in the field, program evaluation is best left to end users who must weigh the benefits of FluFIT activities relative to other clinical interventions. In fact, as activities that increase the FIT for screening in underserved populations continue to evolve, or as the options for influenza prevention or CRCS evolve, the FluFIT program could eventually and rightly be supplanted by new innovations. For now, the message that "just like a flu shot, you need to get FIT every year" has penetrated the consciousness of many cancer screening advocates, practitioners, and patients, contributing to local and national screening efforts.

REFERENCES

1. Potter MB. Strategies and resources to address colorectal cancer screening rates and disparities in the United States and globally. *Ann Rev Pub Health*. 2013;34:412–428.
2. Siegel RL, Miller KD, Jamal A. Cancer statistics, 2017. *CA Cancer J Clin*. 2017;67:7–30.
3. White A, Thompson TD, White MC, Sabatino SA, de Moor J, Doria-Rose PV, Geiger AM, Richardson LC. Cancer screening test use—United States, 2015. *MMWR Morb Mortal Wkly Rep*. 2017;66(8):201–206.
4. Meester RG, Doubeni CA, Zauber AG, Goede SL, Levin TR, Corley DA, Jemal A,

Lansdorp-Vogelaar I. Public health impact of achieving 80% colorectal cancer screening rates in the United States by 2018. *Cancer.* 2015;121(13):2281–2285.

5. Bibbins-Domingo K, Grossman DC, Curry SJ, et al. Screening for colorectal cancer: US Preventive Services Task Force recommendation statement. *JAMA.* 2016;315:2564–2575.

6. Tinmouth J, Lansdorp-Vogelaar I, Allison JE. Faecal immunochemical tests versus guaiac faecal occult blood tests: What clinicians and colorectal cancer screening programme organisers need to know. *Gut.* 2015;64(8):1327–1337.

7. Lieberman D, Ladabaum U, Cruz-Correa M, Ginsburg C, Inadomi JM, Kim LS, Giardiello FM, Wender RC. Screening for colorectal cancer and evolving issues for physicians and patients: A review. *JAMA.* 2016;316(2):2135–2145.

8. Klabunde CN, Cronin KA, Breen N, Waldron WR, Ambs AH, Nadel MR. Trends in colorectal cancer test use among vulnerable populations in the United States. *Cancer Epidemiol Biomarkers Prev.* 2011;20(8):1611–1621.

9. Steps for increasing colorectal cancer screening rates. American Cancer Society website. http://nccrt.org/wp-content/uploads/0305.60-Colorectal-Cancer-Manual_FULFILL.pdf.

10. Potter MB, Phengrasamy L, Hudes ES, McPhee SJ, Walsh JM. Offering annual fecal occult blood tests at annual flu shot clinics increases colorectal cancer screening rates. *Ann Fam Med.* 2009;7:17–23.

11. Potter MB, Walsh JM, Yu TM, Gildengorin G, Green LW, McPhee SJ. The effectiveness of the FLU-FOBT program in primary care: A randomized trial. *Am J Prev Med.* 2011;41:9–16.

12. Potter MB, Somkin CP, Ackerson LM, Gomez V, Dao T, Horberg MA, Walsh J ME. The FLU-FIT program: An effective colorectal cancer screening program for high volume flu shot clinics. *Am J Manag Care.* 2011;17(8):577–583.

13. Potter MB, Ackerson LM, Gomez V, Walsh JM, Green LW, Levin TR, Somkin CP. Effectiveness and reach of the FLU-FIT program in an integrated health care system: A multisite randomized trial. *Am J Public Health.* 2013 Jun;103(6):1128–1133.

14. Potter MB, Gildengorin G, Wang Y, Wu M, Kroon L. Comparative effectiveness of two pharmacy-based colorectal cancer screening interventions during an annual influenza vaccination campaign. *J Am Pharm Assoc.* 2010;50:181–187.

15. Walsh JM, Gildengorin G, Green LW, Jenkins J, Potter MB. The FLU-FOBT program in community clinics: Durable benefits of a randomized controlled trial. *Health Educ Res.* 2012;27(5):886–894.

16. Levin TR. Optimizing colorectal cancer screening by getting FIT right. *Gastroenterology.* 2011;141:1551–1555.

17. Research-Tested Intervention Programs (RTIPs). National Cancer Institute website. http://rtips.cancer.gov.

18. Research to Reality. National Cancer Institute website. http://researchtoreality.cancer.gov.

19. Meissner HI, Glasgow RE, Vinson CA, Chambers D, Brownson RC, Green LW, Ammerman AS, Weiner BJ, Mittman B. The U.S. Training Institute for Dissemination and Implementation Research in Health. *Implement Sci.* 2013;8(12).

20. Agency for Healthcare Research and Quality website. https://ahrq.innovations.gov.

21. ColonMD: Clinicians' information source. American Cancer Society website. https://www.cancer.org/health-care-professionals/colon-md.html.

22. Hurd TC, Lozano C, Sotelo S, Adame S, Rodriguez R, Guerra H, Sunil T. Colorectal cancer screening in rural and frontier communities: The FluFIt on the Frontera Project. *Cancer Epidemiol Biomarker Prev.* 2017;26(2).

Case Study 8B

IMPLEMENTATION OF AN EVIDENCE-BASED TOBACCO USE TREATMENT INTERVENTION IN THE CONTEXT OF LUNG CANCER SCREENING

Jamie S. Ostroff and Donna Shelley

LUNG CANCER is the second most commonly diagnosed cancer in both men and women, accounting for approximately 14% of all new cancer diagnoses.[1] Cigarette smoking is by far the leading risk factor, with approximately 85% of lung cancer cases caused by exposure to carcinogens in cigarettes and other combustible tobacco products. The overall 5-year survival rate for lung cancer is much lower than that of many other leading cancer sites, and more than half of patients with lung cancer die within 1 year of diagnosis. Historically, the poor prognosis has been attributable to lack of methods for early detection, such that most patients (>75%) present with relatively late stage III or IV disease, rarely curable with current therapies. However, for cases detected when the disease is still localized, the prognosis is much improved. Until recently, there was not an effective method to screen for lung cancer in high-risk individuals, and the majority of cases have been detected at an advanced stage.[2]

In 1999, the Early Lung Cancer Action Project reported that annual screening with low-dose computed tomography (LDCT) could detect lung cancer at an early stage such that approximately 80% of patients diagnosed with lung cancer had clinical stage I cancer.[3] Launched in 2002 and supported by the National Cancer Institute to test the efficacy of lung cancer screening, the National Lung Screening Trial (NLST) randomly assigned 53,454 asymptomatic, current or former heavy smokers aged 55–74 years to receive three annual screens with either LDCT or standard chest X-ray. The study findings demonstrated that screening with the use of LDCT reduced lung cancer mortality.[4] In 2013, in response to the encouraging NLST findings, the US Preventive Services Task Force (USPSTF) recommended that adults aged 55–80 years with a 30 pack-year smoking history (who currently smoke or have quit in the past 15 years) undergo annual LDCT lung cancer screening.[5]

Recognizing the substantial challenges to developing effective lung cancer screening programs in clinical practice, the National Cancer Policy Forum of the National Academies of Sciences, Engineering, and Medicine sponsored a June 2016 workshop, "Implementation of Lung Cancer Screening," and subsequently published proceedings that summarized the evidence base for lung cancer screening along with the current implementation challenges and opportunities to overcome them. As noted in the workshop proceedings, many factors need to be considered for broad implementation of lung cancer screening in clinical practice, including (1) understanding the balance of potential benefits and harms of lung cancer screening; (2) facilitating informed, shared decision-making; (3) defining and reaching eligible high-risk populations; (4) determining health system needs, infrastructure requirements, and capacity constraints; (5) monitoring individual and population health outcomes; (6) addressing health disparities; and (7) integrating screening efforts with smoking cessation interventions.[6]

Lung cancer screening with LDCT provides a crucial opportunity or "teachable moment" to deliver smoking cessation services to current cigarette smokers. There are several reasons to consider that delivering smoking cessation treatment in the context of lung cancer screening will further reduce smoking-related morbidity and mortality.[7] First, it is estimated that as many as 10 million adults are eligible for lung cancer screening in the United States.[8] Approximately 50% of all high-risk individuals who undergo lung cancer screening are likely to be current smokers.[9] Second, several studies have found that the majority of smokers seeking lung cancer screening are indeed motivated to quit and may be interested in tobacco dependence treatment options.[10,11] Third, lung cancer screening provides several touchpoint clinical encounters (pre-screening shared decision-making discussion, screening visit, subsequent disclosure of screening results, and annual repeat screening) when health care providers can assess for stage of readiness for smoking cessation and delivery of evidence-based cessation interventions.[12] Clinical practice guidelines for treatment of tobacco use and dependence in health care settings exist and provide clear guidelines for smoking cessation best practices, including asking about current smoking status, advising all current smokers to quit, and providing access to behavioral counseling and cessation medications.[12] Conversely, critics of lung cancer screening have cautioned that negative screening results may mitigate current smokers' concerns about the health consequences of smoking, thereby reducing motivation to quit.[13]

Recognizing this potential opportunity, the USPSTF and virtually all lung cancer screening guidelines highlight the importance of providing cessation advice and assistance to current smokers seeking lung cancer screening.[14,15] The Lung Cancer Alliance has also identified smoking cessation treatment delivery as one of the hallmarks of high-quality screening.[16] Two recent modeling and cost–utility analysis papers[17] support the additional public health benefit of incorporating smoking cessation interventions into lung cancer screening protocols. Moreover, the few randomized cessation clinical trials conducted in the context of lung cancer screening have shown promising overall quit rates results, particularly for those studies testing more intensive smoking cessation interventions.[18–22]

With this support and evidence, as part of its national coverage determinations, the Center for Medicare and Medicaid Services (CMS) required that current smokers seeking LDCT must receive counseling on the importance of smoking cessation and information about smoking cessation interventions. However, a recent systematic review concluded that simply undergoing cancer screening (without integration of evidence-based tobacco treatment) does not adequately promote smoking abstinence or utilization of evidence-based cessation strategies.[23] Unfortunately, CMS requirements for shared decision-making do not provide specific guidance regarding how to implement evidence-based smoking cessation treatment in the context of lung cancer screening programs, and there is a paucity of data on strategies for promoting the effectiveness, acceptability, and optimal implementation of evidence-based tobacco treatment in these settings.

In addition, the readiness and capacity of lung cancer screening sites to integrate smoking cessation treatment are largely unknown. Ostroff and colleagues[24] conducted a national survey of lung cancer screening site coordinators from 93 screening sites within the United States and assessed their organizational priority, current practice patterns, and barriers for delivery of evidence-based, tobacco use treatment in the context of a lung cancer screening setting. Most sites reported that at the initial visit, patients are routinely asked about their current smoking status (98.9%) and that current smokers are advised to quit (91.4%). However, fewer (57%) sites reported providing cessation counseling, referring smokers to a quitline (60.2%), and even fewer (36.6%) routinely recommend cessation medications. During follow-up screening visits, respondents reported less attention to delivery of smoking cessation advice and treatment. Lack of patient motivation and resistance to cessation advice and treatment, lack of staff training, and lack of reimbursement were the most frequently cited barriers to delivering smoking cessation treatment. Several site characteristics were examined to explain variation in tobacco treatment delivery. Organizational priority for promoting smoking cessation was viewed as a key driver for successful implementation of tobacco treatment services.

Currently, several tobacco treatment models are emerging for use in lung cancer screening settings. These range from a low resources model, whereby screening sites may provide self-help materials and rely heavily on primary care provider advice and referral to quitline, to a moderate resources model, whereby sites assess readiness to quit and refer interested smokers to either quitline or affiliated tobacco treatment program, and a more high resources embedded tobacco treatment model,[25] whereby trained tobacco treatment specialists provide on-site or telephonic counseling and cessation medication recommendations for all current smokers. Some promising tobacco treatment models place particular emphasis on the results of the lung scan in order to personalize the harms of persistent smoking.[26] However, there is no consensus on the optimal approach to intervening with tobacco users who are undergoing screening or the most effective strategies for integrating tobacco treatment delivery into lung cancer screening protocols.

Recognizing the importance of building an evidence base for this research priority, the National Cancer Institute (NCI) developed a targeted funding announcement (RFA-CA-15-011) and awarded six grants to support research on the design and implementation of smoking cessation interventions in lung cancer screening settings. With leadership from the NCI Tobacco Control Research Branch, these RFA-funded projects as well as an additional NCI-funded trial, and another project funded by the Veterans Health Administration, have formed the Smoking Cessation and Lung Cancer Screening (SCALE) collaboration to facilitate harmonization of measurement, data sharing, and peer feedback and to maximize the knowledge to be gained from the ongoing clinical trials.[27]

One of the SCALE projects, led by the co-authors of this case study, is using the Multiphase Optimization Strategy (MOST)[28] to design an optimized, scalable evidence-based tobacco treatment package that can be readily integrated within lung cancer screening sites. MOST involves highly efficient, randomized experimentation to precisely quantify the effects of individual treatment components and identify synergistic effects by combining them into an effective tobacco treatment package. This information then guides assembly of an optimized treatment package that achieves target outcomes with minimal resource consumption and staff burden. The rationale for using this MOST methodology is that once an optimized tobacco treatment package is established, future comparative effectiveness trials can examine strategies for wider implementation and dissemination in LDCT lung cancer screening settings. In partnership with the Lung Cancer Alliance, a leading lung cancer advocacy organization that has established the National Framework for Excellence in Lung Cancer Screening, we will identify 18 heterogeneous lung cancer screening sites throughout the United States that will serve as study sites. Sixty-four current smokers will be recruited from each of the participating screening sites (total $N = 1,152$). The specific aims of our project are (1) to use MOST to identify which of four evidence-based, tobacco treatment components—motivational interviewing (yes vs. no), nicotine replacement therapy (NRT) patch (yes vs. no), NRT lozenge (yes vs. no), and message framing (gain vs. loss)—contribute to superior cessation endpoints; (2) to estimate the cost and incremental cost-effectiveness of evidence-based tobacco treatment components, delivered alone and in combination; and (3) to assess factors that may influence implementation process and sustainability for delivering effective models of smoking cessation treatment in lung cancer screening settings.

This case describes the hybrid clinical trial design in which the effectiveness of the tobacco treatment interventions (AIM 1) and the implementation processes and outcomes (AIM 2 and AIM 3) are studied concurrently.[29] In blending clinical effectiveness and implementation science methods, the goal is to collect data concurrently on clinical outcomes (i.e., smoking abstinence) and the implementation outcomes needed to inform and facilitate more rapid adoption and scale-up of evidence-based clinical protocols for delivery of tobacco dependence treatment in LDCT clinical settings. To obtain data on the latter (AIM 2 and AIM 3), we are conducting a mixed methods evaluation guided by two conceptual frameworks: Proctor et al.'s model of implementation research and the Consolidated Framework for Implementation Research (CFIR).[30,31] Both models guide collection of key factors that are associated with effective implementation and provide insights into potential barriers and facilitators of implementation and future scale-up.

Proctor et al.'s model offers a taxonomy of implementation outcomes.[30] These include acceptability (satisfaction with content/delivery of the tobacco cessation interventions); adoption (uptake); appropriateness (relevance); cost; and treatment fidelity/adaptation (the extent to which tobacco treatment interventions are delivered as planned, as well as the type of treatment modifications made), penetration (reach), and sustainability.

CFIR includes a set of constructs within five domains (i.e., outer and inner setting, intervention characteristics, individual characteristics, and process) that were compiled from a comprehensive review of key theories and conceptual models informing implementation science.[31] CFIR complements Proctor et al.'s model by providing a blueprint for assessing, in more depth, multilevel barriers at the patient, provider, intervention, and systems levels that may impact tobacco treatment delivery. Identifying these barriers guides intervention design and redesign, with the goal to maximize implementation effectiveness and the benefit of integrating various models of smoking cessation into lung cancer screening protocols. In this case, CFIR informs an evaluation of contextual factors operationalized in lung cancer screening programs as (1) the intervention (e.g., the complexity of the specific tobacco treatment components and the delivery model), (2) the inner setting (e.g., leadership engagement, organizational priority for integrating tobacco dependence, compatibility with current workflow, and organizational structure), (3) the outer setting (e.g., CMS coverage requirements and clinical practice guidelines), (4) the individual characteristics of those involved (e.g., site coordinators' self-efficacy for tobacco treatment delivery), and (5) process (site and stakeholder engagement and implementation strategies such as clinical documentation and monitoring).

Findings from the investigators' national survey of lung cancer screening programs suggested several "intervention and inner setting" characteristics that may create barriers to implementation.[24] For example, most lung cancer screening programs are staffed by a single site coordinator or nurse navigator who guides participants throughout the screening process from pre-visit shared decision-making to the initial scan visit and any necessary follow-up. Fewer staff may amplify the most common barrier often cited by clinicians for not adopting tobacco use treatment—time constraints related to competing demands.[32] As such, the combination of tobacco treatment interventions selected for this study was designed specifically to limit the time required for training and the time needed to provide the intervention components. For example, site coordinators will be trained to offer brief motivational interviewing rather than more intensive counseling that may be more effective but would not be pragmatic given the staffing model in these sites. Early adaptations based on this formative work, however, may not adequately address site-specific multilevel constraints related to treating tobacco use in these settings. Therefore, guided by CFIR, at both the start of and after the study, we will obtain staff feedback on the perceived complexity of the intervention and site coordinators' ability to integrate and adapt the intervention to current workflow. These data will inform the design elements of effective strategies for implementing and disseminating treatment models in the wide range of screening programs in the United States.

Our survey also found that there is wide variation in lung cancer screening sites with regard to clinical volume, workflow and staffing patterns, access to trained tobacco treatment specialists, and infrastructure—all factors likely to influence organizational readiness and capacity to deliver evidence-based tobacco treatment services.[31] Again, CFIR will guide an assessment of these inner setting factors at each study site and therefore help us identify adaptations to the intervention that may be needed in the varying program contexts to enhance implementation while maintaining fidelity to core intervention components shown to be effective.[33] Finally, engagement of key staff and program leadership (i.e., process) to increase the relative priority of tobacco use treatment in these settings (i.e., inner setting) is likely a critical driver of successful implementation.

Based on a recent systematic review of the use of CFIR, most studies have applied the framework to assess barriers and facilitators to guideline implementation in the post-implementation phase.[34] However, the use of CFIR in the pre-implementation stage may help guide early adaptations that can address important aspects of effective implementation. In fact, assessing CFIR constructs as part of the initial site engagement is allowing us to formulate plans for local adaptation. For instance, we have discovered much variation in the current implementation of the required shared decision-making encounter and the workflow of smoking cessation treatment.

Finally, it not uncommon to apply more than one implementation framework in a single study to provide a more comprehensive evaluation of factors that drive effective implementation.[35,36] However, there is often overlap in measures. In this case, Proctor et al.'s measure of appropriateness overlaps with the CFIR inner setting construct of compatibility. The choice of which factors to evaluate and whether to do so using qualitative versus quantitative methods was driven by the research questions and hypothesized barriers in this study setting.

Qualitative and quantitative data will be collected from study participants, site coordinators, primary care providers, and electronic health record documentation. Table 8B.1 summarizes a

Table 8B.1. Required (Core) and Optional (Opt-In) Items[a]

OUTCOMES	VARIABLE	DEFINITION/ITEM	DATA SOURCE
Smoking cessation outcomes (effectiveness)	Point abstinence	Have you smoked a cigarette, even a puff, in the past 7 days?	Patient survey
	Continuous abstinence	During the past 3 months/6 months, have you smoked a cigarette, even a single puff?	Patient survey
	Quit attempt	Since you enrolled in the lung cancer screening program, have you made a 24 hour attempt to quit smoking?	Patient survey
	Smoking reduction	Have you cut down your daily smoking by more than 50% since you enrolled in the lung cancer screening program?	Patient survey
Implementation outcomes[30]	Feasibility	Perceived feasibility of implementing cessation interventions	Site coordinator survey
	Acceptability	Perceived acceptability of implementing cessation interventions	Site coordinator survey
		Satisfaction with smoking cessation intervention	Patient survey
	Appropriateness	Perceived appropriateness of implementing cessation interventions	Site coordinator survey
	Fidelity	Delivery of smoking cessation intervention components	Patient and site coordinator survey
	Sustainability	Sustained delivery of tobacco treatment, perceived barriers and facilitators of sustainability	Site coordinator survey and qualitative interviews
Outer setting	Payment policies	Current reimbursement mechanisms, state or federal incentive programs	Site coordinator survey and interviews

(*continued*)

Table 8B.1 Continued

OUTCOMES	VARIABLE	DEFINITION/ITEM	DATA SOURCE
Inner setting Organization structural characteristics	Volume	Volume of initial/baseline and follow-up/repeat scans past month	Site coordinator survey
	Geographic location	Urbanized areas of 50,000 or more people Urban clusters >2,500 and <50,000 people "Rural" (encompasses all population, housing, and territory not included within an urban area/cluster)	Site coordinator survey
	Payer mix	Classification of insurance coverage Medicare Medicaid Private commercial No insurance Other	Site coordinator survey
Organizational priority	Relative priority	Perceived priority for delivery of smoking cessation	Site coordinator survey

ªSCALE measures: https://www.gem-beta.org/Public/wsoverview.aspx?wid=33&cat=8.

relevant subset of required (core) and optional (opt-in) items being used to measure cessation outcomes, implementation processes, as well as the characteristics of the participating lung cancer screening sites.

Semi-structured focus group interviews, guided by both implementation frameworks, will be conducted in order to advance our understanding of factors that may impede or facilitate implementation within the lung cancer screening context. By doing so, we will be able to answer important implementation questions about not only which tobacco treatment intervention components work best in this setting but also for whom (participant characteristics) and under what (screening site) conditions.

CONCLUSION

Implementation science theories and methods can contribute to accelerating the translation of evidence-based interventions into routine practice. There is strong evidence for tobacco use treatment interventions, but given the nascent phase of implementation of smoking cessation in the context of lung cancer screening, it is essential that tobacco treatment effectiveness and implementation processes are studied concurrently so as to guide the development of effective, scalable clinical protocols for delivery of high-quality tobacco dependence treatment in LDCT settings. Ultimately, the findings from this study will guide assembly of an optimized and scalable cessation treatment package that achieves superior cessation outcomes with attention to minimizing burden in lung cancer screening sites.

ACKNOWLEDGMENT

This work was supported by NCI grant R01CA207442 (Optimizing Tobacco Treatment for Smokers Seeking Lung Cancer Screening).

REFERENCES

1. Cancer facts and figures. American Cancer Society website. 2016. https://www.cancer.org/research/cancer-facts-statistics/all-cancer-facts-figures/cancer-facts-figures-2016.html.

2. Ma J, Ward EM, Smith R, Jemal A. Annual number of lung cancer deaths potentially avertable by screening in the United States. *Cancer.* 2013;119(7):1381–1385.

3. Henschke CI, McCauley DI, Yankelevitz DF, et al. Early Lung Cancer Action Project: Overall design and findings from baseline screening. *Lancet.* 1999;354(9173):99–105.

4. Aberle DR, Adams AM, Berg CD, et al. Reduced lung-cancer mortality with low-dose computed tomographic screening. *N Engl J Med.* 2011;365(5):395–409.

5. Moyer VA, LeFevre ML, Siu AL, et al. Screening for lung cancer: U.S. Preventive Services Task Force recommendation statement. *Ann Intern Med.* 2014;160(5):330–338.

6. The National Academies of Sciences, Engineering, and Medicine. *Implementation of Lung Cancer Screening: Proceedings of a Workshop.* Washington, DC: National Academies Press; 2017.

7. Pastorino U, Boffi R, Marchiano A, et al. Stopping smoking reduces mortality in low-dose computed tomography screening participants. *Thorac Oncol.* 2016;11(5):693–699.

8. Doria-Rose VP, White MC, Klabunde CN, et al. Use of lung cancer screening tests in the United States: Results from the 2010 National Health Interview Survey. *Cancer Epidemiol Biomarkers Prev.* 2012;21(7):1049–1059.

9. Humphrey LL, Deffebach M, Pappas M, et al. Screening for lung cancer with low-dose computed tomography: A systematic review to update the US Preventive Services Task Force recommendation. *Ann Intern Med.* 2013;159(6):411–420.

10. Park ER, Streck JM, Gareen IF, et al. A qualitative study of lung cancer risk perceptions and smoking beliefs among national lung screening trial participants. *Nicotine Tob Res.* 2014;16(2):166–173.

11. Hahn EJ, Rayens MK, Hopenhayn C, Christian WJ. Perceived risk and interest in screening for lung cancer among current and former smokers. *Res Nurs Health.* 2006;29(4):359–370.

12. Fiore MC, Jaen CR, Baker TB, et al. Treating tobacco use and dependence: 2008 update. Clinical practice guideline. US Department of Health and Human Services- Public Health Service. 2008. https://bphc.hrsa.gov/buckets/treatingtobacco.pdf.

13. Bach PB, Mirkin JN, Oliver TK, et al. Benefits and harms of CT screening for lung cancer: A systematic review. *JAMA.* 2012;307(22):2418–2429.

14. Fucito LM, Czabafy S, Hendricks PS, Kotsen C, Richardson D, Toll BA. Pairing smoking-cessation services with lung cancer screening: A clinical guideline from the Association for the Treatment of Tobacco Use and Dependence and the Society for Research on Nicotine and Tobacco. *Cancer.* 2016;122(8):1150–1159.

15. Watson KS, Blok AC, Buscemi J, et al. Society of Behavioral Medicine supports implementation of high quality lung cancer screening in high-risk populations. *Transl Behav Med.* 2016;6(4):669–671.

16. Screening Centers of Excellence designation. Lung Cancer Alliance website. 2017. https://lungcanceralliance.org/for-professionals/screening-centers-of-excellence-designation.

17. Villanti AC, Jiang Y, Abrams DB, Pyenson BS. A cost–utility analysis of lung cancer screening and the additional benefits of incorporating smoking cessation interventions. *PLoS One.* 2013;8(8):e71379.

18. Clark MM, Cox LS, Jett JR, et al. Effectiveness of smoking cessation self-help materials in a lung cancer screening population. *Lung Cancer.* 2004;44(1):13–21.

19. Ferketich AK, Otterson GA, King M, Hall N, Browning KK, Wewers ME. A pilot test of a combined tobacco dependence treatment and lung cancer screening program. *Lung Cancer.* 2012;76(2):211–215.

20. Marshall HM, Courtney DA, Passmore LH, et al. Brief tailored smoking cessation counseling in a lung cancer screening population is feasible: A pilot randomized controlled trial. *Nicotine Tob Res.* 2016;18(7):1665–1669.

21. Pozzi P, Munarini E, Bravi F, et al. A combined smoking cessation intervention within a lung cancer screening trial: A pilot observational study. *Tumori.* 2015;101(3):306–311.

22. van der Aalst CM, de Koning HJ, van den Bergh KA, Willemsen MC, van Klaveren RJ. The effectiveness of a computer-tailored smoking cessation intervention for participants in lung cancer screening: A randomised controlled trial. *Lung Cancer.* 2012;76(2):204–210.

23. Slatore CG, Baumann C, Pappas M, Humphrey LL. Smoking behaviors among patients receiving computed tomography for lung cancer screening: Systematic review in support of the U.S. Preventive Services Task Force. *Ann Am Thorac Soc.* 2014;11(4):619–627.

24. Ostroff JS, Copeland A, Borderud SP, Li Y, Shelley DR, Henschke CI. Readiness of lung cancer screening sites to deliver smoking cessation treatment: Current practices, organizational priority, and perceived barriers. *Nicotine Tob Res.* 2016;18(5):1067–1075.

25. Taylor KL, Hagerman CJ, Luta G, et al. Preliminary evaluation of a telephone-based smoking cessation intervention in the lung cancer screening setting: A randomized clinical trial. *Lung Cancer.* 2017;108:242–246.

26. Pua BB, Dou E, O'Connor K, Crawford CB. Integrating smoking cessation into lung cancer screening programs. *Clin Imaging.* 2016;40(2):302–306.

27. Joseph AM, Rothman AJ, Almirall D, et al. Lung cancer screening and smoking cessation clinical trials: SCALE (Smoking Cessation within the Context of Lung Cancer Screening) Collaboration. *Am J Respir Crit Care Med.* 2018;197(2):172-182.

28. Collins LM, Baker TB, Mermelstein RJ, et al. The multiphase optimization strategy for engineering effective tobacco use interventions. *Ann Behav Med.* 2011;41(2):208–226.

29. Curran GM, Bauer M, Mittman B, Pyne JM, Stetler C. Effectiveness–implementation hybrid designs: Combining elements of clinical effectiveness and implementation research to enhance public health impact. *Med Care.* 2012;50(3):217–226.

30. Proctor E, Silmere H, Raghavan R, et al. Outcomes for implementation research: Conceptual distinctions, measurement challenges, and research agenda. *Admin Policy Ment Health.* 2011;38(2):65–76.

31. Damschroder LJ, Aron DC, Keith RE, Kirsh SR, Alexander JA, Lowery JC. Fostering implementation of health services research findings into practice: A consolidated framework for advancing implementation science. *Implement Sci.* 2009;4:50.

32. Schroeder SA. What to do with a patient who smokes. *JAMA.* 2005;294(4):482–7.

33. Stirman SW, Miller CJ, Toder K, Calloway A. Development of a framework and coding system for modifications and adaptations of evidence-based interventions. *Implement Sci.* 2013;8:65.

34. Kirk MA, Kelley C, Yankey N, Birken SA, Abadie B. A systematic review of the use of the Consolidated Framework for Implementation Research. *Implement Sci.* 2016;11:72.

35. Nilsen P. Making sense of implementation theories, models and frameworks. *Implement Sci.* 2015;10:53.

36. Birken SA, Powell BJ, Presseau J, et al. Combined use of the Consolidated Framework for Implementation Research (CFIR) and the Theoretical Domains Framework (TDF): A systematic review. *Implement Sci.* 2017;12(1):2.

9

PROVIDER-LEVEL FACTORS INFLUENCING IMPLEMENTATION

OVERVIEW OF CASE STUDIES

Alex H. Krist and Vivian Jiang

CANCER TREATMENT is increasingly complex. The tools for diagnosis, staging, and predicting prognosis are rapidly evolving, as are the therapies, treatment modalities, and treatment protocols. Fortunately, there are robust evidence-based and evidence-guided cancer treatment guidelines from the National Cancer Control Network, American Society of Clinical Oncology, and others to help direct cancer care. Yet, ensuring patients get the right care in a timely manner is dependent on more than just providers knowing the guidelines; systems and supports for providers and patients are critically needed. These systems and supports are particularly important for cancer care because treatment involves a multidisciplinary team from multiple specialties, such as oncology (e.g., radiation, surgical, and medical), palliative care, primary care, and mental health. Care also occurs across multiple settings, including hospitals, surgical and radiation centers, outpatient offices, and the home. In addition, patient factors, especially the social

determinants of health, strongly correlate with disparities in quality of care, timeliness of treatment, adherence to medical recommendations, and overall health outcomes.[1] Patients with lower health literacy levels ask fewer questions during office visits and have more difficulty understanding complex information.[2] Individuals of lower socioeconomic status are less frequently educated about and enrolled in clinical trials.[3] Clinicians are more verbally dominant and engage less in patient-centered communication during encounters with ethnic minority patients and older patients.[4,5] Collectively, the complexity of care, the need for a multidisciplinary team across settings, and patient-level factors all present providers with a unique set of challenges.

Adding to these issues, medicine has shifted from previously paternalistic models of care delivery to more patient-centered approaches involving partnerships between patients and providers. Accordingly, patients, caregivers, and their families must also be considered and included as part of the care team. Numerous studies have demonstrated that effective patient engagement significantly improves the quality of care delivered and clinical outcomes.[6,7] This is particularly true for cancer care. A new suspicion or diagnosis of cancer comes with a tremendous emotional burden. Patients and their loved ones rely on their cancer care team for emotional guidance, reassurance, and hope. Often, there are multiple treatment options, with different potential benefits and risks, that require shared decisions between patients and their providers. Once treatment is underway, adherence to complex regimens, management of side effects, attention to caregiver needs, and monitoring response to treatment all require active involvement of patients and caregivers. Research clearly shows that increased patient engagement leads to increased perceptions of personal control, increased trust, and decreased feelings of uncertainty or later regret for decisions.[8,9] Indeed, cancer patients surveyed in several studies report a strong desire to actively participate in medical decision-making with their providers.[10] Although a patient's preference for degree of involvement may vary throughout his or her cancer treatment course, studies have shown that patients consistently play a less active role in decision-making than they would like.[11] Barriers to shared decision-making at the provider level are numerous and include limited time during visits, limited training in shared decision-making techniques, few patient or provider tools to support shared decision-making, fee-for-service rather than value-based payment structures, and lack of institutional support.[12]

Caring for patients with more aggressive or advanced cancer is particularly challenging. Making a quick and accurate diagnosis and initiating care can prove life-saving. Nonetheless, the prognosis, treatment needs, and goals of care can rapidly change. As the likelihood of cure decreases, refocusing on quality of life, aiming for attainable goals, and addressing psychological and spiritual needs become the new focus of cancer treatment. Although this can be a difficult transition for both patients and providers, refocusing care has been shown to improve patients' satisfaction with care, quality of life, and even length of life.[13-16] Accordingly, national guidelines and professional societies have endorsed the early integration of palliative care into cancer care for all patients diagnosed with advanced cancer; this is referred to as concurrent palliative care (CPC).[17,18] Despite these recommendations, CPC is put into practice less often and later in the course of treatment than desired.

The three case studies presented in this chapter explore strategies that help providers by (1) promoting and incorporating the routine use of shared decision-making in determining prostate cancer treatment, (2) supporting the adoption of CPC for patients with advanced cancer, and (3) ensuring low-income patients with breast cancer receive care consistent with guidelines through patient engagement and navigation. The specific challenges and needs for future implementation science are highlighted throughout each case.

The first case study by Kobrin and Conway reviews the need to implement shared decision-making (SDM) for early stage prostate cancer treatment decisions. Men diagnosed with early stage prostate cancer have three potential treatment options: radical prostatectomy, radiation therapy, or active surveillance (or variations of active surveillance).[19] Each treatment option has a different set of potential benefits and risks. This creates a need for men to be engaged in making treatment decisions so that their preferences and values can be accurately incorporated into care. For other decisions, SDM has been demonstrated to reduce decisional conflict, improve knowledge, and align decisions with patient values.[20] However, there is a lack of evidence to demonstrate that SDM improves health outcomes (i.e., increased quality or quantity of life) for any health decision. For early prostate cancer treatment, there is a paucity of studies to inform providers about how to implement SDM. Few tools are available for providers and patients to use, and most studied interventions are not feasible for routine implementation into practice. The authors identify many implementation questions that need to be answered about SDM and early prostate cancer treatment: Why isn't it done? Who should do it? How can it best be integrated into care? How can interventions be tailored to the individual patient's desired locus of decision control? How do we make time to incorporate SDM? Is it a worthwhile use of time?

In the second case study, Whisenant and Mooney present the need and barriers to CPC during the treatment of advanced cancers. They detail the implementation factors to consider for ensuring uptake of CPC, including acceptability, appropriateness, cost, feasibility, fidelity, penetration, and sustainability of interventions. Given the low use of CPC and limited evidence demonstrating its effectiveness, the authors pay particular attention to CPC acceptability and feasibility by providers.

The authors highlight the need for providers to have strategies to present CPC to patients and families and to change the treatment paradigm from being disease-centered to being patient-centered. They also discuss a need to expand the workforce and to develop new workflow models that support routine use of CPC. In considering workforce limitations and improving workflow, they identify health information technology (HIT) as a tool that may function as an extension of the providers, allowing the providers to interact with patients and caregivers between clinic visits. Using HIT, providers can monitor and manage patients' symptoms and side effects and reduce caregiver burden through virtual palliative care and automated coaching. Whisenant and Mooney conclude by summarizing the findings from the ENABLE, CHESS, and SCH studies that used technology to support palliative care in advance cancer patients.

In the final case study, Helzlsouer and Varanasi describe the need and challenges with helping providers and patients ensure adherence to guideline-based care. They highlight a pilot study that used technology-enhanced virtual navigation to help low-income women newly diagnosed with breast cancer. Through the intervention, women were provided with an online knowledge and communication resource that served as a gateway to their treatment plans. The patients were given computers, shown how to use the system, and connected with a navigator—a new care team member role—to provide a personal touch. The navigator coordinated care and support between providers, nurses, social workers, and other cancer care team members to ensure timely care delivery. Like the patient, the navigator had an interface with the online resource to document care and communicate with the patient. Prior to fielding, the program was iteratively created with representative patients to ensure that the informatics-based intervention did not further enhance the digital divide—a common experience for lower income, minority, low health literacy, and older patients.[21] During the study, several participants were found to have inadequate care and treatment plans that improved through informatics and navigator support. Participants generally liked the intervention, and the intervention was feasible for patients, providers, and health systems. Critical future research would include further demonstrating efficacy, generalizability to a range of settings, and dissemination of this model of patient and provider support to enhance guideline-based care.

In the dynamic world of cancer research, diagnostics, and treatment, innovative mechanisms to coordinate teams, new personnel roles, increased focus on patient-centered care, and HIT solutions can all help providers better deliver care across the cancer control and treatment continuum. Yet, more is needed to better understand the best ways to put these strategies and tools into routine practice, and implementation science can help us learn what works and how to put it into practice.

REFERENCES

1. Albain KS, Unger JM, Crowley JJ, Coltman CA, Jr., Hershman DL. Racial disparities in cancer survival among randomized clinical trials patients of the Southwest Oncology Group. *J Natl Cancer Inst.* 2009;101(14):984–992.

2. Katz MG, Jacobson TA, Veledar E, Kripalani S. Patient literacy and question-asking behavior during the medical encounter: A mixed-methods analysis. *J Gen Intern Med.* 2007;22(6):782–786.

3. Kim SP, Knight SJ, Tomori C, et al. Health literacy and shared decision making for prostate cancer patients with low socioeconomic status. *Cancer Investig.* 2001;19(7):684–691.

4. Cooper LA, Roter DL, Carson KA, et al. The associations of clinicians' implicit attitudes about race with medical visit communication and patient ratings of interpersonal care. *Am J Public Health.* 2012;102(5):979–987.

5. Amalraj S, Starkweather C, Nguyen C, Naeim A. Health literacy, communication, and treatment decision-making in older cancer patients. *Oncology (Williston Park).* 2009;23(4):369–375.

6. Laurance J, Henderson S, Howitt PJ, et al. Patient engagement: Four case studies that highlight the potential for improved health outcomes and reduced costs. *Health Aff (Millwood).* 2014;33(9):1627–1634.

7. Osborn R, Squires D. International perspectives on patient engagement: Results from the 2011 Commonwealth Fund Survey. *J Ambul Care Manage.* 2012;35(2):118–128.

8. Arora NK, Weaver KE, Clayman ML, Oakley-Girvan I, Potosky AL. Physicians' decision-making style and psychosocial outcomes among cancer survivors. *Patient Educ Couns.* 2009;77(3):404–412.

9. Nicolai J, Buchholz A, Seefried N, et al. When do cancer patients regret their treatment decision? A path analysis of the influence of clinicians' communication styles and the match of

decision-making styles on decision regret. *Patient Educ Couns*. 2016;99(5):739–746.

10. Chewning B, Bylund CL, Shah B, Arora NK, Gueguen JA, Makoul G. Patient preferences for shared decisions: A systematic review. *Patient Educ Couns*. 2012;86(1):9–18.

11. Tariman JD, Berry DL, Cochrane B, Doorenbos A, Schepp K. Preferred and actual participation roles during health care decision making in persons with cancer: A systematic review. *Ann Oncol*. 2010;21(6):1145–1151.

12. Woolf SH, Chan EC, Harris R, et al. Promoting informed choice: Transforming health care to dispense knowledge for decision making. *Ann Intern Med*. 2005;143(4):293–300.

13. Hearn J, Higginson IJ. Do specialist palliative care teams improve outcomes for cancer patients? A systematic literature review. *Palliat Med*. 1998;12(5):317–332.

14. Temel JS, Greer JA, Muzikansky A, et al. Early palliative care for patients with metastatic non-small-cell lung cancer. *N Engl J Med*. 2010;363(8):733–742.

15. McDonald J, Swami N, Hannon B, et al. Impact of early palliative care on caregivers of patients with advanced cancer: Cluster randomised trial. *Ann Oncol*. 2017;28(1):163–168.

16. Zimmerman EB, Woolf SH, Haley A. Understanding the relationship between education and health: A review of the evidence and an examination of community perspectives. In: Kaplan RM, Spittel ML, David DH, eds. *Population Health: Behavioral and Social Science Insights*. AHRQ Publication No. 15-0002. Rockville, MD: Agency for Healthcare Research and Quality and Office of Behavioral and Social Sciences Research, National Institutes of Health; 2015:347–384.

17. Ferrell BR, Temel JS, Temin S, Smith TJ. Integration of palliative care into standard oncology care: ASCO clinical practice guideline update summary. *J Oncol Pract*. 2017;13(2):119–121.

18. Levy MH, Smith T, Alvarez-Perez A, et al. Palliative care, Version 1.2014. Featured updates to the NCCN guidelines. *J Natl Compre Canc Netw*. 2014;12(10):1379–1388.

19. Wilt TJ, Ahmed HU. Prostate cancer screening and the management of clinically localized disease. *BMJ*. 2013;346:f325.

20. Stacey D, Legare F, Lewis K, et al. Decision aids for people facing health treatment or screenings. *Cochrane Database Syst Rev*. 2017;2017(10):CD001431.

21. Irizarry T, DeVito Dabbs A, Curran CR. Patient portals and patient engagement: A state of the science review. *J Med Internet Res*. 2015;17(6):e148.

Case Study 9A

TREATMENT FOR EARLY STAGE PROSTATE CANCER

THE NEED TO IMPLEMENT SHARED DECISION-MAKING

Sarah C. Kobrin and Alex Conway

MEN DIAGNOSED with early stage prostate cancer will very likely survive many years after their prostate cancer treatment, regardless of which standard treatment is used.[1] For younger men in particular, those diagnosed in their 50s or 60s with few other health issues, all standard treatments are supported by evidence. The choice of treatment is made by comparing the inconveniences and likely side effects of one treatment versus another. A man who is still working may prefer an option that minimizes work time lost during recovery; a man with an active sex life may prefer an option that minimizes the risk of persistent erectile dysfunction.

Making this treatment decision requires a partnership between the patient, who knows his preferences on these and other issues, and the doctor, who has expertise on the treatments and their risks and benefits. A process to help the patient and doctor deliberate together, each having expertise and relying on the other's expertise, is called *shared decision-making* (SDM).[2] Successful approaches to SDM have been developed for many other decisions that similarly require input about patient preferences as well as medical evidence.[3] However, few interventions have been developed for SDM concerning early stage prostate cancer, and those few have not been found to be effective.[4] Therefore, implementation of this generally effective intervention, SDM, remains a gap in early stage prostate cancer treatment decisions.

TREATMENT FOR EARLY STAGE PROSTATE CANCER

Standard treatment options for early stage prostate cancer include surgery or one of two types of radiation therapy.[5] The surgical option, prostatectomy, removes the prostate and therefore removes the cancer in the prostate. Surgery requires two or more nights in the hospital. In some cases, surgery is followed by radiation. Radiation therapy is often done as an outpatient procedure and does not carry the risks associated with surgery; however, radiation takes place daily for as many as 9 weeks. These treatment characteristics have different implications for men who are working or not, could work from home or not, and who can tolerate surgery or not. Each of these treatments has side effects; all carry a significant probability of affecting how easily a man passes urine and his ability to have an erection. However, the timing of these effects (i.e., immediately following treatments or years later), their duration, and their severity vary by treatment type. These side effect characteristics also have implications for men who want to have children or not, who can manage urinary problems or not, and who have active sex lives or not.

Prostate cancer is often very slow growing; many men live for many years with a diagnosis of prostate cancer with no symptoms and no effect on quality of life. Unfortunately, currently there is no way to distinguish a slow-growing, relatively harmless prostate cancer from an aggressive prostate cancer that threatens a man's life. An additional "treatment" option exists for men who are comfortable with choosing not to start any of the standard treatments. The approach is called "active surveillance," and it is characterized by routine observation with the plan to avoid active treatment as long as possible. The choice of active surveillance is appropriate for patients and families who can tolerate the uncertainty inherent in living with a diagnosis and choosing to watch for disease progression without starting treatment. Although the frequent testing can be uncomfortable and inconvenient, active surveillance has no effect on urine and sexual function. If the disease shows signs of progressing, men who chose this option then face the same decision among the standard surgical and radiation treatments.

SHARED DECISION-MAKING

Shared decision-making is broadly defined as a collaborative process through which health care professionals share information about the benefits and harms of proposed interventions, and patients (and their family and friends) share information about their relevant preferences and values.[2] Both types of information are essential and distinguish this process from other types of communication about health care interventions.

The importance of patient preferences and values for choosing among early stage prostate cancer treatments creates what is called a "preference-sensitive decision," for which SDM is ideally suited. Interventions have been created to promote SDM

for many other preference-sensitive decisions, including angina, joint arthritis, and back pain.[6] These take the form of print materials that guide doctors or patients through a collaborative process, web-based tools that share information back and forth between doctors and patients, and other approaches. Many have been successful in improving patient knowledge about risks and benefits, increasing the likelihood that patients make decisions that accord with their preferences and values[3] and that "high-quality" decisions are made.[7]

However, as discussed later, very few such approaches have been developed to support men who are making decisions about early stage prostate cancer treatment, and the few that have been developed have had limited success. In the following sections, we discuss possible barriers to development of these particular interventions and call for consideration of implementation challenges as part of the intervention development process.

DESCRIBING CURRENT GUIDELINES

Treatment guidelines for early stage localized prostate cancer are provided by professional organizations and national health programs. However, their recommendations vary.[8] This variability is most obvious in criteria for pursuing active surveillance or watchful waiting versus more aggressive treatment. Generally, guidelines are in agreement regarding clinical indicators that should be used to weigh treatment options: clinical stage of the tumor, serum prostate-specific antigen (PSA) level, Gleason score, and tumor volume or load. However, consensus does not extend to the *values* of each indicator that constitutes eligibility to pursue active surveillance. For instance, the European Association of Urology (EAU) guideline provides strict cut-offs for consideration of active surveillance (clinical stage of T1c–T2, serum PSA ≤ 10, and a Gleason score ≤ 6), whereas the American Urological Association's (AUA) recommendations are broader (clinical stage T1c–T2c, serum PSA from ≤ 10 to 20, and Gleason score from ≤ 6 to 10).

This lack of consensus on clinical cut-offs, combined with well-established evidence showing no significant differences in long-term efficacy among treatment options,[1] produces a need for consideration of patients' preferences and values when choosing a prostate cancer treatment. Reflecting this need for patient input, many prostate cancer treatment guidelines are cursory. Of 13 national, international, and provincial guidelines, only 7 make any mention of the need to consider potential side effects related to bowel, genitourinary, and sexual function; 9 mention the need to consider patient preference when choosing between active surveillance and active treatment.[8] In addition, the guidelines that do mention these factors do so briefly, mentioning the importance of these processes but providing no detail regarding how to incorporate preferences and side effects in decision-making. Only one national guideline, the UK's National Health Service's National Institute for Health and Clinical Excellence (NICE), mentions the use of a decision aid in the development of a treatment plan.[8]

Lack of attention to patient preferences and side effects is also seen in guidelines' recommendations regarding the transition from active surveillance to active treatment. Although there is slightly more agreement on clinical criteria for this transition—described as "clinical progression," usually in the form of increase in serum PSA levels and/or increase in Gleason score—patient preference is mentioned only briefly. Again, preferences are recommended for consideration with no discussion of how they should be considered. Only the NICE guideline takes the next step, recommending use of a provided decision aid.

In summary, many urological and cancer professional organizations accept active surveillance as a way to delay potentially unnecessary treatment and preserve a patient's current quality of life, but rarely are recommendations made for how the patient should be involved in this important decision.

DISCUSSING CURRENT INTERVENTIONS

The current state of prostate cancer treatment guidelines provides ample opportunity for the study and implementation of shared decision-making interventions. Several randomized controlled trials have been carried out in recent years, comparing the use of a decision aid either to usual treatment or to treatment with a different decision aid.[4] Results have been mixed, partially due to wide variety in both the measurement and outcomes of the decision aids used and the variety of study designs and types of decision aids.

In studies that report successful results, the most consistent findings are reductions in decisional

conflict and decisional regret and increases in cancer knowledge and decisional self-efficacy. For example, Hacking et al.[9] implemented a "decision navigation" intervention that provided a personal guide, or "navigator," to help patients through the treatment decision process. Intervention group participants met with the navigator to set expectations and prepare questions prior to talking with the physician specialist. Results were in the expected directions, with decisional self-efficacy improved more in the intervention group; decisional conflict lower in the intervention group; and, 6 months after the intervention, decisional regret also lower. In a subsequent qualitative study, interviews with six prostate cancer patients and all four participating doctors suggested the intervention enabled doctors to tailor consultations to each patient's prioritized concerns, helped patients organize and clarify their medical questions, and ensured those concerns were being attended to by doctors.[10]

In contrast, multiple studies have failed to show that decision aids increase choice of treatments that match patients' preferences and values. For instance, Bosco et al.[11] studied the effects of a computer-based decision aid on concordance between treatment decisions and reported side effects. Treatment choice was considered "concordant" if (1) men concerned with sexual function chose external beam radiotherapy or brachytherapy; (2) men concerned with bowel function chose prostatectomy; (3) men concerned with sex, bowel, and/or bladder function chose active surveillance; or (4) men not concerned with any side effect chose any treatment. However, there were no significant differences between the intervention and control group; radical prostatectomy was the most common treatment choice. Despite educating men about common symptoms and helping them rank their own anticipated reactions to those symptoms, the decision aid did not increase concordance between the men's own values and their treatment choices.

ROLE OF IMPLEMENTATION SCIENCE

The lack of data distinguishing the mortality benefit of one prostate cancer treatment from another and the likelihood of significant side effects following any active treatment combine to create a need for SDM when early stage prostate cancer is diagnosed. Decision aids to guide patients choosing among prostate cancer treatments are effective at increasing knowledge and reducing decisional conflict. This finding is similar to the the performance of SDM interventions to support other preference-sensitive decisions.[12] As such, they are ready for implementation. However, more complex interventions, reaching for the more important goal of helping each man choose the treatment best for *him*, have not been consistently found to match decisions to patients' preferences and values.[12] These trials have generally focused on efficacy of the SDM intervention at the individual level and given little consideration of feasibility in routine clinical practice.

Hybrid implementation science designs[13] may be the ideal next step for this area of research. Hybrid designs can test explanations for prior intervention failure (e.g., lack of adherence to the protocol and contamination between groups) and can measure interactions across levels affected by the intervention (e.g., patient, clinician, office staff, and organizational reimbursement practices). At the same time, a hybrid design can link effectiveness data to a specific implementation approach. Results from a hybrid study should move SDM more quickly into practice compared to the current approach of conducting numerous, unrelated efficacy tests of new decision aids or overly simple effectiveness tests of existing decision aids.

Implementing SDM interventions has proven challenging at every level of clinical practice. For practice change to outlast a funded intervention, *individuals* must be willing to take a role in their own medical decision-making and be given sufficient time to understand and ask questions. At the *clinician* level, similarly, doctors must be willing to share the decision-making, feel comfortable eliciting the relevant information, have support from their peers, and—trivially but importantly—have the time to enter into a real discussion. Lack of time is a challenge at the *clinic* level. Policies regarding time spent with patients, quality measures for talking about decisions rather than ordering a test, leadership supportive of SDM, and peer support of SDM are all clinic-level characteristics without which an intervention will either not succeed or not be maintained after the study. At a *public health* level, credible evidence and evidence synthesis about the treatment options and their consequences must be available and accessible in a wide range of reading levels, for people with different values and preferences, and for people who view the choices differently. Creating these materials is time-consuming, expensive, and currently funded through research. To address

these challenges together rather than piecemeal—and therefore promote adoption, implementation, and sustainability—a multilevel, implementation science-oriented approach is needed.

CONCLUSION

The recommendation for SDM research to move forward to implementation science is not limited to early stage prostate cancer treatment decisions. The growing number of cancer-related decisions for which current evidence cannot define a best choice creates a clear and broad public health need. Many of these decisions have significant and potentially long-term implications, making patients' preferences and values key factors in making a choice. Many decision aids have been developed for cancer treatments and screening, but few have been widely implemented.[14] We call for all tests of new and evidence-based SDM interventions to include plans for implementation and use of implementation science methods. These two steps are essential for the promise of SDM to be realized in everyday cancer care.

REFERENCES

1. NIH consensus and state-of-the-science statements: Role of active surveillance in the management of men with localized prostate cancer. 2011;28(1). https://consensus.nih.gov/2011/prostate.htm
2. Elwyn G, Lloyd A, May C, et al. Collaborative deliberation: A model for patient care. *Patient Educ Counc.* 2014;97(2):158–164.
3. Stacey D, Légaré F, Col NF, et al. Decision aids for people facing health treatment or screening decisions. *Cochrane Database Syst Rev.* 2014;2014(1):CD001431.
4. Violette PD, Agoritsas T, Alexander P, et al. Decision aids for localized prostate cancer treatment choice: Systematic review and meta-analysis. *CA Cancer J Clin.* 2015;65(3):239.
5. PDQ Adult Treatment Editorial Board. Prostate cancer treatment (PDQ): Health professional version. PDQ cancer information summaries. 2002. National Cancer Institute website. https://www.ncbi.nlm.nih.gov/pubmed/26389471.
6. Veroff D, Marr A, Wennberg DE. Enhanced support for shared decision making reduced costs of care for patients with preference-sensitive conditions. *Health Aff (Project Hope)* 2013;32(2):285–93. https://doi.org/10.1377/hlthaff.2011.0941.

7. Sepucha KR, Fowler FJ Jr, Mulley AG Jr. Policy support for patient-centered care: The need for measureable improvements in decision quality. *Health Aff.* 2004;VAR54-62.

8. Bruinsma SM, Bangma CH, Carroll PR, et al. Active surveillance for prostate cancer: A narrative review of clinical guidelines. *Nature Rev Urol.* 2016;13(3):151–167. https://doi.org/10.1038/nrurol.2015.313.

9. Hacking B, Wallace L, Scott S, Kosmala-Anderson J, Belkora J, McNeill A. Testing feasibility, acceptability and effectiveness of a "decision navigation" intervention for early stage prostate cancer patients in Scotland—A randomised controlled trial. *Psycho-Oncology.* 2013;22:1017–1024.

10. Hacking B, Scott SE, Wallace LM, Shepherd SC, Belkora J. Navigating healthcare: A qualitative study exploring prostate cancer patients' and doctors' experience of consultations using a decision-support intervention. *Psycho-Oncology.* 2014;23(6):665–671.

11. Bosco JL, Halpenny B, Berry DL. Personal preferences and discordant prostate cancer treatment choice in an intervention trial of men newly diagnosed with localized prostate cancer. *Health Qual Life Outcomes.* 2012;10:123. https://doi.org/10.1186/1477-7525-10-123.

12. Munro S, Stacey D, Lewis KB, Bansback N. Choosing treatment and screening options congruent with values: Do decision aids help? Sub-analysis of a systematic review. *Patient Educ Couns.* 2016;99(4):491–500.

13. Curran GM, Bauer M, Mittman B, Pyne JM, Stetler C. Effectiveness–implementation hybrid designs: Combining elements of clinical effectiveness and implementation research to enhance public health impact. *Med Care.* 2012;50(3):217–226.

14. Elwyn G, Scholl I, Tietbohl C, et al. "Many miles to go . . .": A systematic review of the implementation of patient decision support interventions into routine clinical practice. *BMC Med Inform Decis Mak.* 2013;13(Suppl 2):S14.

Case Study 9B

INTEGRATING CONCURRENT PALLIATIVE CARE INTO CANCER CARE DELIVERY SETTINGS

Meagan Whisenant and Kathi Mooney

ADVANCED CANCER brings a cascade of difficult decisions and challenges for patients and their family caregivers. Among the challenges are unpleasant symptoms related to the disease and treatment, psychological and spiritual challenges in coping with life-limiting cancer, and disruption in social and family roles.[1-3] When these needs are not adequately addressed, they result in poor coping, inadequate decision-making, and diminished quality of life.[4] Family caregivers also report significant burden related to caregiving tasks, deterioration in their own health, and disruptions in their normal activities and roles.[3]

Palliative medicine is a relatively new subspecialty developed in 2006 to address these care needs in conjunction with disease specialists who continue to provide the therapies directed at controlling the disease. Palliative care is defined as "the interdisciplinary prevention and relief of suffering of any kind—physical, psychological, social, or spiritual—experienced by adults and children living with life-limiting health problems. It promotes

dignity, quality of life and adjustment to progressive illnesses, using best available evidence" (p. 5).[5] Palliative care, concurrent with active disease treatment, has been recommended as part of standard cancer care for all patients with advanced cancer and any cancer patient with significant symptom burden.[6] Concurrent palliative care (CPC) may include symptom management, discussion of goals of care, psychosocial and spiritual distress management, and provision of support during transitions of care. CPC may result in improved symptom management, quality of life, survival, family caregiver well-being, health care resource utilization, and end-of-life outcomes.[7-9]

There is strong research evidence to support the usefulness of CPC in improving patient and family caregiver outcomes. Multiple randomized controlled trial (RCT) studies have demonstrated that advanced cancer patients who receive CPC have improved quality of life, less depression, and greater satisfaction with care.[9-14] At least 13 CPC intervention studies have demonstrated some aspect of benefit for advanced cancer patients and/or their family caregivers.[14–27] Patients who receive CPC are more likely to accurately understand their prognosis and optimize the timing of last chemotherapy and transition to hospice care compared to patients who receive standard care.[28,29] Importantly, there is evidence of longer survival with early CPC.[9,16,30]

Given the strong evidence in support of improved outcomes for patients receiving CPC, practice guidelines have been generated for adoption in the oncology setting. The most recent 2016 clinical practice guideline for palliative care from the American Society of Clinical Oncology (ASCO) includes evidence-based recommendations to oncology clinicians, patients, caregivers, and palliative care specialists that update the 2012 ASCO provisional clinical opinion and recommends for the integration of palliative care into standard oncology care for all patients diagnosed with advanced cancer.[31] In addition, the National Comprehensive Cancer Network (NCCN) provides interdisciplinary recommendations on CPC for cancer patients, including screening, assessment, and clinical management protocols; discussions about the benefits and risks of cancer treatment; and approaches to advance care planning.[32] Both ASCO and NCCN guidelines emphasize patient-centered care enhancement and early integration of palliative care.

ROLE FOR IMPLEMENTATION SCIENCE

Even with strong evidence in support of and professional organization advocacy for CPC, there is variable uptake of these guidelines and adoption in cancer care. Barriers to implementation include the need to increase awareness of existing evidence and guidelines and overcome stigma, adequacy of a workforce for scale-up, lack of effective models for integration and delivery, and restrictive reimbursement mechanisms.[31] Nearly 85% of large hospitals report having palliative care services, but most are limited to inpatient care, with less reporting outpatient services and very few with reach into the community through home care.[33] With advanced cancer, symptoms and caregiving burden can rapidly change, necessitating effective monitoring and care beyond inpatient settings. One of the goals of palliative care is to maximize time at home; thus, delivery models must consider delivery of services across settings. In addition, only a small percentage of patients with advanced cancer are referred for palliative care or referred early in the course of care.[34,35] Implementation science can serve as a framework to address barriers and improve adoption of CPC. Key implementation factors should be considered in designing studies and strategies to improve the uptake. These include acceptability, adoption, appropriateness, costs, feasibility, fidelity, penetration, and sustainability.[36]

Acceptability, or the perception among stakeholders that a given service is agreeable, involves convincing stakeholders that CPC is attractive and useful.[37–40] Palliative care and its association with end-of-life hospice care make integration early in the course of limiting disease difficult. This presents a problem for acceptability to patients and their families but also for oncology care providers, who are reluctant to refer to the palliative care team until patients are near death, if at all.[34,35] Achieving acceptability of CPC will require improved strategies to present palliative care services to patients, families, and oncologists knowing the stigma attached, even though there is increasing evidence that early palliative care may actually extend survival. It also requires adopting a broader treatment paradigm in cancer care, especially in cancer centers, from a disease-oriented treatment approach to a more patient-centered approach that emphasizes eliciting and concordance with patients' goals.[41] Research should continue to evaluate outcomes and determine the value and cost of palliative care services paired with strong dissemination efforts to oncology care providers, patients, and families, as well as the public.[41–43]

Appropriateness, or the perceived fit of an innovation for the practice, is difficult when the primary focus of cancer care is on treatment and cure to the exclusion of quality of life and coping management. Barriers related to achieving appropriateness of CPC may be particularly difficult where the trajectories of cancer and dying are variable and unpredictable.[43–45]

The *costs* associated with an intervention and its implementation must be considered as well. Extrinsic financial incentives are crucial for effectiveness of strategies to promote service adoption, and financial constraints can result in the truncation of CPC implementation.[37,39,40,42,44] Palliative care includes aspects of care and services that are not routinely reimbursed, such as chaplain care or support services to family caregivers. In addition, palliative care has been shown to reduce medical resource use, including hospitalizations and emergency department use. CPC provides better care at a cost that is more affordable.[31] Reimbursement models are key to adoption. Health care systems largely based on fee-for-service and with bed capacity may find reduced health care utilization a disincentive to palliative care adoption; conversely, reimbursement models based on value and population health would find it an incentive.

Adoption involves the motivation, interest, and intention to employ the innovation or evidence-based intervention.[39] Professional skill development for clinicians and palliative care specialists, as well as administrative leadership, professional organization advocacy, and policymaker endorsement are needed to facilitate adoption.[39–42,46] Stakeholder motivation to adopt CPC models will be enhanced by external pressure and appropriate incentives, such as performance measures, accreditation standards, and ensuring adequate reimbursement of time and effort.[38,39]

For palliative care, the overriding concerns with *feasibility*, or the extent to which the innovation can be successfully used within a setting, are related to workforce availability and the lack of demonstrated models to integrate palliative and cancer care seamlessly for the patient and family. As a new subspecialty, there is an inadequate workforce prepared to provide needed services. There is a need to evaluate different models of delivery to determine how care can be provided effectively, utilizing a variety of disciplines and adjuncts such as technology. Innovative approaches to training of both existing oncology care providers and students so that palliative care can be provided during oncology visits will be important to address feasibility.[45,47,48] Investigations of specific triggers for CPC referrals are limited, and further examination is needed to make referral seamless and efficient. Both the Center to Advance Palliative Care and the most recent ASCO guidelines endorse the use of triggers for oncologists to refer and will require training in basic palliative care assessment and treatment skills.[31]

An important feasibility consideration in upstreaming CPC into cancer care is how to efficiently monitor patient outcomes when patients are not hospitalized but are very ill. Mechanisms for reaching patients and family caregivers in between clinic visits are important for effective CPC. Technology, including the internet, interactive voice response (IVR) telephone systems, and mobile application interventions, has potential benefits as a mechanism for extending care, implementing palliative care into the existing workflow, and

overcoming issues of scalability and workforce limitations.[44,49] Technology may be useful for increasing feasibility of outpatient monitoring in palliative care (Table 9B.1). For example, a multicomponent, psycho-educational, telephone-delivered palliative care intervention (ENABLE) delivered weekly by an advanced practice nurse improved patient quality of life compared to usual care.[15,21] The ENABLE study, along with other studies, has also reported family caregiver benefit when using technology. Using a web-based lung cancer information, communication, and coaching system (CHESS), family caregivers of patients with advanced lung cancer reported less burden and less negative mood compared those who received usual care.[19] When CHESS added a patient symptom reporting component that family caregivers used to provide their perception of patient symptoms, caregivers reported less negative mood compared to caregivers who received only CHESS and no symptom reporting.[17] An automated system offers the opportunity to monitor the changing symptom experience, provide automated coaching based on the actual symptom presentation, and alert the care team of poorly controlled symptoms, while also addressing the caregiver's physical and psychological well-being.[50] When family caregivers of patients in home hospice daily reported both patient and caregiver symptoms using an automated IVR system, Symptom Care at Home (SCH), and received automated self-care coaching and clinician triage based on the reported patterns, patient symptom severity was significantly decreased and caregiver vitality and mood were significantly improved in comparison to usual hospice care.[51,52] Using the same SCH system adapted for patients receiving chemotherapy, symptom severity was once again significantly reduced overall and for 10 of the 11 symptoms monitored.[53] Use of technology as an adjunct to standard care aids implementation of CPC and overcomes barriers to uptake, including workforce and cost constraints.

Fidelity refers to the degree to which an intervention is implemented as designed. For CPC, recent national guidelines (ASCO and NCCN) can guide clinicians in integrating CPC into standard practice. However, these guidelines are often detailed and lengthy and not conducive to point-of-care use. New approaches to guideline support for clinicians are needed and may be facilitated by decisions support systems at the point of care, especially if they can be linked to the electronic health record. In addition,

Table 9B.1. Key Palliative Care in Advanced Cancer Intervention Studies Using Technology

INTERVENTION	REFERENCE	DESIGN	FINDINGS
ENABLE: Consisting of a multicomponent, psycho-educational, palliative care intervention with structured advanced practice nurse-delivered sessions and monthly follow-up	Bakitas et al. (2009)[15]	ENABLE vs. UC	Patients with intervention exposure: less depression (p =.02), better QOL (p = .02), symptoms (NS)[a]
	O'Hara et al. (2010)[21]	ENABLE vs. UC	Caregivers with intervention exposure: burden (NS)[a]
	Dionne-Odom et al. (2015)[18]	Early vs. delayed ENABLE	Caregivers with early intervention: less depression (p = .02, d = −.32), QOL (NS),[a] burden (NS)[a]
	Bakitas et al. (2015)[16]	Early vs. delayed ENABLE	Patients with intervention exposure: symptoms (NS),[a] resource use (NS)[a]
CHESS: Consisting of a web-based lung cancer information, communication, and coaching system for caregivers	DuBenske et al. (2014)[19]	CHESS vs. control	Caregivers with intervention exposure: less burden (p = .02, d = .39), less negative mood (p < .01, d = .44)
	Gustafson et al. (2013)[20]	CHESS vs. control	Patients with intervention exposure: less symptom distress (p = .03, d = .42 at 4 months; p < .01, d = .61 at 6 months; NS at 2 and 8 months)[a]
	Chih et al. (2013)[17]	CHESS vs. CHESS + symptom reporting	Caregivers with intervention plus: less negative mood (p < .01 at 6 months, p < .01 at 12 months), burden (NS at 6 and 12 months),[a] preparedness (NS at 6 and 12 months)[a]
Symptom Care at Home (SCH): Consisting of an automated system for reporting patient and caregiver symptoms, with automated coaching and provider triage when needed	Mooney et al. (2014, 2015)[51,52]	SCH vs. UC	Patients with intervention exposure: less total symptoms (p < .001, d = .55) Caregivers with intervention exposure: better vitality (p < .001, d = .47), better mood (p = .003, d = .36)

[a] NS, not significant; QOL, quality of life; UC, usual care.

there is limited study of the level of adoption and care concordance with palliative care guidelines.[31]

Penetration is defined as the integration of an innovation within subsystems of a practice setting, and *sustainability* is the extent to which a newly implemented treatment is maintained within a setting. Identifying ways to improve penetration of CPC is the current priority. Sustainability will become the focus once implementation science provides an understanding of the appropriate models for effective integration.[37-40]

CONCLUSION

Implementation science, with the purpose of integrating scientific methodologies into the point of care, is needed to develop and evaluate different delivery models that address barriers to CPC. There is significant evidence of the usefulness of CPC for improving cancer patient and family caregiver outcomes across the illness trajectory of advanced cancer. This evidence is substantial and undergirds national clinical practice guidelines and professional organization policy advocacy. Implementation science is poised to address the barriers currently inherit in CPC so that quality of life can be improved for those with life-limiting cancer and their families.

REFERENCES

1. Given B, Given C, Azzouz F, Stommel M. Physical functioning of elderly cancer patients prior to diagnosis and following initial treatment. *Nurs Res.* 2001;50(4):222–232.
2. Mazanec SR, Daly BJ, Douglas SL, Lipson AR. Work productivity and health of informal caregivers of persons with advanced cancer. *Res Nurs Health.* 2011;34(6):483–495.
3. Bevans M, Sternberg EM. Caregiving burden, stress, and health effects among family caregivers of adult cancer patients. *JAMA.* 2012;307(4):398–403.
4. Delgado-Guay MO, Hui D, Parsons HA, et al. Spirituality, religiosity, and spiritual pain in advanced cancer patients. *J Pain Symptom Manage.* 2011;41(6):986–994.
5. World Health Organization. *Planning and Implementing Palliative Care Services: A Guidebook for Programme Managers.* Geneva, Switzerland: World Health Organization; 2016.
6. Smith TJ, Temin S, Alesi ER, et al. American Society of Clinical Oncology provisional clinical opinion: The integration of palliative care into standard oncology care. *J Clin Oncol.* 2012;30(8):880–887.
7. Institute of Medicine, Committee on Approaching Death: Addressing Key End-of-Life Issues. *Dying in America: Improving Quality and Honoring Individual Preferences Near the End of Life.* Washington, DC: National Academies Press; 2015.
8. Basch E, Deal AM, Dueck AC, et al. Overall survival results of a trial assessing patient-reported outcomes for symptom monitoring during routine cancer treatment. *JAMA.* 2017;318(2):197–198.
9. Temel JS, Greer JA, Muzikansky A, et al. Early palliative care for patients with metastatic non-small-cell lung cancer. *N Engl J Med.* 2010;363(8):733–742.
10. McDonald J, Swami N, Hannon B, et al. Impact of early palliative care on caregivers of patients with advanced cancer: Cluster randomised trial. *Ann Oncol.* 2017;28(1):163–168.
11. Zimmermann C, Swami N, Krzyzanowska M, et al. Early palliative care for patients with advanced cancer: A cluster-randomised controlled trial. *Lancet.* 2014;383(9930):1721–1730.
12. Pirl WF, Greer JA, Traeger L, et al. Depression and survival in metastatic non-small-cell lung cancer: Effects of early palliative care. *J Clin Oncol.* 2012;30(12):1310–1315.
13. Grudzen CR, Richardson LD, Johnson PN, et al. Emergency department-initiated palliative care in advanced cancer: A randomized clinical trial. *JAMA Oncol.* 2016;2(5):591–598.
14. Dyar S, Lesperance M, Shannon R, Sloan J, Colon-Otero G. A nurse practitioner directed intervention improves the quality of life of patients with metastatic cancer: Results of a randomized pilot study. *J Palliat Med.* 2012;15(8):890–895.
15. Bakitas M, Lyons KD, Hegel MT, et al. The project ENABLE II randomized controlled trial to improve palliative care for rural patients with advanced cancer: Baseline findings, methodological challenges, and solutions. *Palliat Support Care.* 2009;7(1):75–86.
16. Bakitas MA, Tosteson TD, Li Z, et al. Early versus delayed initiation of concurrent palliative oncology care: Patient outcomes in the ENABLE III randomized controlled trial. *J Clin Oncol.* 2015;33(13):1438–1445.
17. Chih MY, DuBenske LL, Hawkins RP, et al. Communicating advanced cancer patients' symptoms via the internet: A pooled analysis of two randomized trials examining caregiver

preparedness, physical burden, and negative mood. *Palliat Med.* 2013;27(6):533–543.

18. Dionne-Odom JN, Azuero A, Lyons KD, et al. Benefits of early versus delayed palliative care to informal family caregivers of patients with advanced cancer: Outcomes from the ENABLE III randomized controlled trial. *J Clin Oncol.* 2015;33(13):1446–1452.

19. DuBenske LL, Gustafson DH, Namkoong K, et al. CHESS improves cancer caregivers' burden and mood: Results of an eHealth RCT. *Health Psychol.* 2014;33(10):1261–1272.

20. Gustafson DH, DuBenske LL, Namkoong K, et al. An eHealth system supporting palliative care for patients with non-small cell lung cancer: A randomized trial. *Cancer.* 2013;119(9):1744–1751.

21. O'Hara RE, Hull JG, Lyons KD, et al. Impact on caregiver burden of a patient-focused palliative care intervention for patients with advanced cancer. *Palliat Support Care.* 2010;8(4):395–404.

22. Sun V, Grant M, Koczywas M, et al. Effectiveness of an interdisciplinary palliative care intervention for family caregivers in lung cancer. *Cancer.* 2015;121(20):3737–3745.

23. Chochinov HM, Kristjanson LJ, Breitbart W, et al. Effect of dignity therapy on distress and end-of-life experience in terminally ill patients: A randomised controlled trial. *Lancet Oncol.* 2011;12(8):753–762.

24. Ferrell B, Sun V, Hurria A, et al. Interdisciplinary palliative care for patients with lung cancer. *J Pain Symptom Manage.* 2015;50(6):758–767.

25. Higginson IJ, Bausewein C, Reilly CC, et al. An integrated palliative and respiratory care service for patients with advanced disease and refractory breathlessness: A randomised controlled trial. *Lancet Respir Med.* 2014;2(12):979–987.

26. Hudson P, Trauer T, Kelly B, et al. Reducing the psychological distress of family caregivers of home-based palliative care patients: Short-term effects from a randomised controlled trial. *Psycho-Oncology.* 2013;22(9):1987–1993.

27. Hudson P, Trauer T, Kelly B, et al. Reducing the psychological distress of family caregivers of home-based palliative care patients: Longer term effects from a randomised controlled trial. *Psycho-Oncology.* 2015;24(1):19–24.

28. Greer JA, Pirl WF, Jackson VA, et al. Effect of early palliative care on chemotherapy use and end-of-life care in patients with metastatic non-small-cell lung cancer. *J Clin Oncol.* 2012;30(4):394–400.

29. Temel JS, Greer JA, Admane S, et al. Longitudinal perceptions of prognosis and goals of therapy in patients with metastatic non-small-cell lung cancer: Results of a randomized study of early palliative care. *J Clin Oncol.* 2011;29(17):2319–2326.

30. Basch E. Patient-reported outcomes—Harnessing patients' voices to improve clinical care. *N Engl J Med.* 2017;376(2):105–108.

31. Ferrell BR, Temel J, Temin S, et al. Integration of palliative care into standard oncology care: American Society of Clinical Oncology clinical practice guideline update. *J Oncol Pract.* 2017;13(2):119–121.

32. Levy MH, Smith T, Alvarez-Perez A, et al. Palliative care, Version 1.2014. Featured updates to the NCCN guidelines. *J Natl Comprehens Canc Netw.* 2014;12(10):1379–1388.

33. Rabow M, Kvale E, Barbour L, et al. Moving upstream: A review of the evidence of the impact of outpatient palliative care. *J Palliat Med.* 2013;16(12):1540–1549.

34. Fadul N, Elsayem A, Palmer JL, et al. Supportive versus palliative care: What's in a name? A survey of medical oncologists and midlevel providers at a comprehensive cancer center. *Cancer.* 2009;115(9):2013–2021.

35. Zimmermann C, Swami N, Krzyzanowska M, et al. Perceptions of palliative care among patients with advanced cancer and their caregivers. *CMAJ.* 2016;188(10):E217–227.

36. Proctor E, Silmere H, Raghavan R, et al. Outcomes for implementation research: Conceptual distinctions, measurement challenges, and research agenda. *Adm Policy Ment Health.* 2011;38(2):65–76.

37. Antunes B, Harding R, Higginson IJ. Implementing patient-reported outcome measures in palliative care clinical practice: A systematic review of facilitators and barriers. *Palliat Med.* 2014;28(2):158–175.

38. Bekelman DB, Rabin BA, Nowels CT, et al. Barriers and facilitators to scaling up outpatient palliative care. *J Palliat Med.* 2016;19(4):456–459.

39. van Riet Paap J, Vernooij-Dassen M, Brouwer F, et al. Improving the organization of palliative care: Identification of barriers and facilitators in five European countries. *Implement Sci.* 2014;9:130.

40. van Riet Paap J, Vissers K, Iliffe S, et al. Strategies to implement evidence into practice to improve palliative care: Recommendations of a nominal group approach with expert opinion leaders. *BMC Palliat Care.* 2015;14:47.

41. Grant M, Elk R, Ferrell B, Morrison RS, von Gunten CF. Current status of palliative

care—Clinical implementation, education, and research. *CA Cancer J Clin*. 2009;59(5):327–335.

42. Demiris G, Parker Oliver D, Capurro D, Wittenberg-Lyles E. Implementation science: Implications for intervention research in hospice and palliative care. *The Gerontologist*. 2014;54(2):163–171.

43. Vijeratnam SS, Bush H, Esan A, Davis C. Assessing the uptake of the Liverpool Care Pathway for dying patients: A systematic review. *BMJ Support Palliat Care*. 2014;4(3):227.

44. Andre B, Ringdal GI, Loge JH, Rannestad T, Kaasa S. Implementation of computerized technology in a palliative care unit. *Palliat Support Care*. 2009;7(1):57–63.

45. Hui D, Bruera E. Integrating palliative care into the trajectory of cancer care. *Nat Rev Clin Oncol*. 2016;13(3):159–171.

46. Back AL, Park ER, Greer JA, et al. Clinician roles in early integrated palliative care for patients with advanced cancer: A qualitative study. *J Palliat Med*. 2014;17(11):1244–1248.

47. Dalal S, Bruera S, Hui D, et al. Use of palliative care services in a tertiary cancer center. *The Oncologist*. 2016;21(1):110–118.

48. Kamal AH, Bull J, Wolf S, et al. Characterizing the hospice and palliative care workforce in the U.S.: Clinician demographics and professional responsibilities. *J Pain Symptom Manage*. 2016;51(3):597–603.

49. Glasgow RE, Kaplan RM, Ockene JK, Fisher EB, Emmons KM. Patient-reported measures of psychosocial issues and health behavior should be added to electronic health records. *Health Aff (Project Hope)*. 2012;31(3):497–504.

50. Kent EE, Rowland JH, Northouse L, et al. Caring for caregivers and patients: Research and clinical priorities for informal cancer caregiving. *Cancer*. 2016;122(13):1987–1995.

51. Mooney K, Berry P, Wong B, Donaldson G. The last 8 weeks of life: Family caregiver distress and patient symptoms. *J Pain Symptom Manage*. 2015;49(2):443–444.

52. Mooney K, Berry P, Wong B, Donaldson G. Helping cancer-family caregivers with end-of-life home symptom management: Initial evaluation of an automated symptom monitoring and coaching system. *J Clin Oncol*. 2014;32(31):85.

53. Mooney KH, Beck SL, Wong B, et al. Automated home monitoring and management of patient-reported symptoms during chemotherapy: Results of the symptom care at home RCT. *Cancer Med*. 2017;6(3):537–546.

Case Study 9C

ENHANCING FIDELITY TO CANCER TREATMENT GUIDELINES

Kathy J. Helzlsouer and Arti Patel Varanasi

Knowing is not enough; we must apply.
Willing is not enough; we must do.

—Johann Wolfgang von Goethe

BACKGROUND

Delivery of optimum care requires a balance between provider knowledge and expertise in prescribing the appropriate treatment and patient perspective and resources in overcoming barriers in adherence to the prescribed treatment plan. Clinical guidelines, based on evidence obtained from observational and clinical trials, provide the knowledge base but are underutilized.[1] Implementation of these guidelines requires further research to determine best practices for optimizing use of guidelines and delivering optimum care. This case study considers an approach to enhance the likelihood that patients receive treatment consistent with recognized cancer clinical guidelines. A virtual navigation program holds promise for educating the patient regarding best treatment practices, supporting self-care, and interfacing with the provider to facilitate the delivery of guideline-based care. The following case report describes the plight of a 45-year-old, low-income woman diagnosed with breast cancer and one approach to enhancing care delivery. This approach, combines health technology with a personal touch to create a virtual navigation program, and is discussed in detail.

SCENARIO

Ms. R.S. is a 45-year-old woman who was diagnosed with an advanced stage breast cancer. She presented for genetic counseling at the recommendation of a surgeon due to her age at presentation. During the course of her visit, it was noted that despite prompt referrals to the breast surgeon at the time of her diagnosis, her treatment had been delayed for nearly 6 months due to her struggles with the treatment decision-making process and the ability to have productive discussions with providers. Consistent with treatment guidelines, the initial recommendation for primary surgical treatment changed to neoadjuvant therapy followed by surgery and radiation therapy due to the noted growth of her breast cancer during this period of delay. Prior to her diagnosis, she had been under the care of a counselor and psychiatrist, but she had not been in contact with them since her diagnosis. Her ex-husband had died suddenly, and she was very distressed because she depended on him for both financial and emotional support despite being divorced. She was unemployed and lived with two teenage sons in a small single-family home. With multiple demands on her physically and emotionally, R.S. was unable to make a decision about where to receive treatment and to initiate therapy. She was offered enrollment in a clinical trial evaluating a centralized, virtual navigation program to improve adherence to recommended cancer treatment. She agreed to enroll in the clinical trial and was randomized to the intervention arm. R.S. was provided a netbook computer, brief computer training, internet access, and access to navigational support for a 10-year period with a nurse/social worker team, overseen by a medical oncologist, and the online breast cancer knowledge and communication resource, which included the recommended treatment plan.

INTRODUCTION TO THE TECHNOLOGY-ENHANCED NAVIGATION PROGRAM

Cancer treatment guidelines are complex and are based on equally complex staging guidelines. Multimodality treatments are commonly employed and include surgery, radiation, and systemic chemotherapy. Chemotherapy regimens are also increasingly complex, with combinations of intravenous and oral regimens given at varying intervals and accompanied by other medications to minimize side effects. Receiving optimum treatment depends on multiple provider and patient factors: timely diagnosis, appropriate staging, knowledgeable health care providers recommending state-of-the-art treatment, patients' access to providers, adequate health care insurance, ability to make complex decisions, attend treatment sessions, timely delivery of treatment, optimum dosing, and management of comorbidities and side effects. Breaks or gaps in any of these aspects along the continuum of care lead to less than optimum treatment and poorer cancer outcomes. Resources for providers exist, such as evidence-based treatment guidelines, However, these guidelines are underutilized,[1] and patterns of care studies demonstrate that disparities persist in the receipt of optimum treatment as defined by guidelines.[2-5] One approach is to improve patient knowledge of guidelines and the importance of treatment adherence while providing supportive care through the treatment period. This case study focuses on a patient-centered approach that may

be useful to implement treatment guidelines and minimize the observed disparities in receipt of appropriate treatment, particularly among socioeconomically disadvantaged patients.

DEFINING OPTIMUM CANCER TREATMENT

Defining optimum treatment can be challenging, and methods to develop clinical guidelines vary in rigor by the professional organizations producing them. Here, we briefly highlight several sources that cover the range of adult and pediatric cancer sites and are readily accessible online.

Although not providing guidelines per se, the PDQ™ (Physician Data Query) of the National Cancer Institute provides regularly updated evidence-based summaries of cancer treatment.[6] The editorial boards provide cancer treatment summaries for adult and pediatric cancers that are accompanied by level of evidence notations that indicate the strength of the available level of evidence supporting the treatment interventions. The PDQ™ clearly states the methods for reviewing the evidence and defining the strength of the evidence. The summaries are provided in different formats for health professionals and for patients.

A recognized source for cancer treatment guidelines is the National Comprehensive Cancer Network™ (NCCN).[7] The NCCN guidelines are updated annually through a consensus process. The process begins with a focused literature search for the specific cancer site and treatment-related studies using the PubMed database. The results are reviewed by a panel of experts from 27 member institutions who compose 48 individual panels that produce updated and new clinical guidelines addressing care in cancer prevention, treatment, and supportive care. The panels consider the extent of the literature, consistency, and quality (e.g., trial design) in their deliberations. The updated guidelines are published annotated with the category of the evidence base and level of consensus among the review panel.

The American Society of Clinical Oncology (ASCO) also has a consensus-based process for cancer treatment guideline development through its Clinical Practice Guidelines Committee.[8] The process includes a systematic review conducted by ASCO staff using multiple databases, including the Cochrane Library, Medline (via PubMed), and EMBASE. In the absence of an existing evidence base determined from the systematic review, the committee may formulate a recommendation based on expert opinion following a formally defined consensus process. Summary recommendations include statements with defined categories regarding the type of recommendations and evidence base (sufficient evidence exists to inform a recommendation), formal consensus, informal consensus, no recommendation (insufficient evidence or consensus agreement), as well as strength of the recommendation (strong, moderate, or weak).[9]

It is important to keep in mind that guideline development may vary greatly by organization, and the process may be more or less formalized and rigorous. In addition to guidelines produced by professional societies, health insurers may rely on their own evaluation process for determining appropriate treatment and thus payments, which in turn influence recommendations and access of patients to treatments.

Reliable sources, following evidence-based methodologies, exist to guide cancer treatment and are accessible online. This is only the first step in the process of ensuring receipt of the treatment by the patient. Disseminating and implementing these guidelines, knowledge transfer to the patients, and overcoming barriers to treatment, especially in vulnerable populations, remain particularly challenging.[1]

IMPLEMENTING CANCER TREATMENT GUIDELINES: PATIENT PERSPECTIVE

The National Academy of Sciences (formerly the Institute of Medicine) issued a report from a workshop calling for the provision of treatment plans to cancer patients.[10] With awareness of the plan, patients become partners in their care, which should translate into improved receipt of care. The plan should be consistent with treatment guidelines, and if it deviates from those guidelines, it should state the reasons for the deviation. However, a written plan is only one step in what should be an ongoing process to improve delivery of care in line with clinical treatment guidelines. In addition, treatment plans are dynamic and may change over time. The plan should be given, explained, and reviewed for appropriateness, and then steps should be taken to ensure that it is received and understood. During cancer treatment, plans may be revised due to lack of response or adverse effects of treatment. Revised

treatment plans should then go through the process again: They should be provided, explained, and reviewed and, most important, receipt and comprehension by the patient must be ensured. Providing this process to transfer knowledge of the plan to patients is challenging, especially for resource-poor patients and health care communities.

In addition to the understanding the plan, there are other barriers to overcome in receiving optimum care. Considering our case study, low socioeconomic status is one factor that has been associated with receipt of less than optimum cancer treatment. Compared to wealthier patients, the poor are more likely to not complete treatment or to experience treatment delays due to multiple factors, such as missed appointments, poor symptom management, psychological co-morbidities, and limited social and psychological support.[4, 11-14] Patient navigation may help overcome barriers and improve adherence.

FACILITATING ADHERENCE TO CLINICAL GUIDELINES: AN INTEGRATED APPROACH

The case study described here presents a scenario in which a centralized program of technology-enhanced virtual navigation facilitated patient adherence to cancer treatment guidelines.[14,15] Key to the acceptability and feasibility of the web-based application was the iterative development process involving low-income breast cancer survivors. A series of focus groups were held to assess the needs of the patients undergoing adjuvant therapy. Common themes and issues raised by the group included the sense of isolation they experienced during treatment, the need for information that was filtered and tailored to them, and the importance of being able to talk to someone who is knowledgeable about breast cancer and its treatment. Among those who had some computer experience, a common complaint was that internet searches on "breast cancer" produced an overwhelming number of sites; moreover, they lacked confidence in the information because it sometimes contradicted the advice of their doctors. The patients wanted access to websites and information that were specific and known to provide reliable information. They also desired personal interaction with someone knowledgeable with whom they could talk between appointments or who could teach them how to communicate with their health care team. Because computer experience

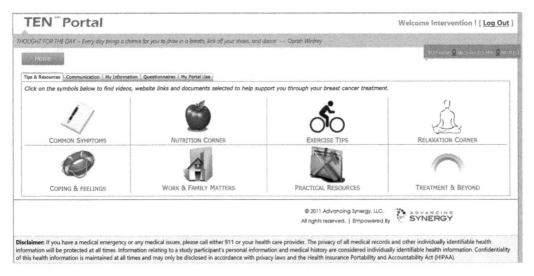

FIGURE 9C.1   Patient view.

was limited, the patients wanted an easy-to-use and simple interface that did not require much typing. The final web-based application included a dual interface: one for the patient (Figure 9C.1) and one for the navigator. The patient interface served as the gateway to the treatment plan and a vetted knowledge base, including websites, documents, and videos; it also provided access to communication channels (Table 9C.1). Through the navigator interface, the provider team, including the nurse, social worker, and coordinator, could document patient interactions and updates, complete administrative tasks, view the patient interface, and securely send and respond to messages within the application (Table 9C.2).

The virtual navigation program was evaluated in a pilot study that randomized low-income newly diagnosed breast cancer patients either to have access to the web-based application alone or to have the application plus navigational support with a nurse and/or social worker. Of a total of 101 patients who were randomized, 98 patients (49 on each arm of the study) completed the 1-year intervention.[14,15] All participants, like the woman in this case study, met the low-income definition according to published income criteria by the Department of Housing and Urban Development at the time of the study.[16] Sixty-four percent of participants were Black, approximately 50% had a high school education or less, 43% resided in rural locations, and all were treated in a variety of clinical practice settings throughout one state. Review of treatment plans

revealed 2 patients not being treated per guidelines. The navigators were able to detect the departure from guidelines and to intervene as appropriate. One patient, an 83-year-old woman, did not receive recommended chemotherapy treatment due to a co-morbid condition of clinically significant heart failure. One other patient was encouraged to seek a second opinion when review of medical records noted failure to follow recommended guidelines. The pilot study showed improved adherence with the addition of navigational support. Two patients randomized to receive navigational support and 6 randomized to the web-based application alone refused all or some of the recommended adjuvant treatment. With navigational support, only 2 of 146 recommended treatments were refused; among those without navigational support, 10 of 146 recommended treatments were refused (p value $_{\text{Fisher's Exact}}$ = 0.04). With respect to our case example, R.S. had interactions with the navigators approximately every 2 weeks. On multiple occasions, intense interactions were required by the navigation team to encourage her to complete therapy and smooth over conflicts between the patient and providers. With the help of the navigator, she reestablished her regular counseling visits. Ultimately, she completed all of her adjuvant chemotherapy and primary surgery, two-thirds of radiation treatment, and initiated hormone therapy. She expressed high satisfaction with the navigation program.

The pilot study demonstrated the feasibility of implementing a centralized technology-enhanced

Table 9C.1. Patient Modules

MODULE	CATEGORIES	ROLE
Tips & Resources	• Common Symptoms: Common symptoms and side effects that individuals going through breast cancer treatment may experience • Nutrition: Nutrition tips during and after chemotherapy • Exercise: Exercise guidance, including gentle exercise videos for individuals going through cancer treatment • Relaxation: Relaxation techniques, including guided imagery and music therapy videos • Coping & Feelings: Coping techniques for dealing with cancer diagnosis and treatment • Work & Family Matters: Issues that may arise both at work and within the family • Practical Resources: Practical needs, such as financial assistance and related matters • Treatment & Beyond: Cancer staging, chemotherapy treatment, and survivorship care plan	Provide patients with resources and information to support them during treatment and beyond.
Communication	• Videoconferencing: Communicate visually with the navigation team • My Messages: Send messages to navigator team • My Notes: Receive messages from the navigation team • My Schedule: Maintain appointment schedules	Enables patients to communicate through different channels with the navigator team.
My Information	• My Information: Patient-specific treatment plan • My Doctor: Information about patient's health care providers • My Team: Information about the navigator team • My Corner: A place for navigator team to provide patients with specific information and resources based on their individual treatment plan and needs	Patients can view and maintain information about their cancer treatment.
Questionnaires	• Quality of life • Functional assessment • Usability	Monitor the progress of patients and their use of the technology.

navigational support program that can operate independent of a given practice, thus enabling the use of a shared resource among multiple health care communities. The navigators tracked frequency, duration, and attempted personal interactions during the 12-month intervention period. Patients on the intervention arm were contacted an average of 29 times, with a median call duration of

Table 9C.2. Navigator Modules

MODULE	ROLE
Enrollment	Register new patients and track patient status.
Find Patient	Find specific patients and view the application from their perspective, including the treatment plan.
Patient Log	Enables the navigators to enter information on each contact with the patient and record results of interactions, including adherence to the treatment plan.
Send Message	Enables the navigators to send messages to specific patients or patient groups from within the web-based application.
Message Board	Enables the navigators to view all message correspondence.
Questionnaire Status	Enables the navigators to review and finalize all questionnaires.
Videoconferencing	Enables the navigators to communicate visually with patients.
Administration	Enables the administrator to create user accounts for eligible non-participant/patient users (staff, care providers, etc.).

30 minutes. The vast majority of contacts were by phone (90%). Considering the number of contacts and contact and documentation time, one full-time equivalent of a nurse and/or social worker could carry a patient load of 100 patients who have similar needs as those of the patients enrolled in the study. Not all patients require the level of interactions provided in the pilot study of low-income patients. With a different case distribution, requirements for caseloads may vary.

THE FUTURE

Disparities in the receipt of optimum cancer treatment exist, and reducing the disparities requires facilitating the process of treatment care and delivery from both the provider and the patient perspective. Advances in digital applications can enhance the delivery of care from both perspectives in accordance with evidence-based guidelines. Implementing guidelines requires outreach to both providers and patients. Electronic health records and increasing accessibility to the internet across age, geographic, and socioeconomic groups have helped overcome digital divides among subgroups. The resulting explosion of digital applications in health care has great potential to cost-effectively create awareness of treatment and supportive care guidelines for optimum care for both cancer patients and health care providers, enhance care delivery, and facilitate delivery and receipt of optimum treatment, but we should not lose sight of the importance of the personal touch. In developing the technology-enhanced program, our patient partners noted that internet sites produced an overwhelming amount of information, some of which contradicted information that they received from their health care provider. In addition to targeted, reliable information sources, the patients wanted access to a knowledgeable person who could help them navigate the information highway and help them communicate with their doctors. The results of the pilot study described here suggest that adherence to recommended treatment was enhanced with the addition of the personal navigator to the web-based application.[15] Research on implementation of best practices to enhance delivery of quality care is needed to ensure all patients receive optimum cancer treatment.

This case study focused on how a combined personal and web-based approach directly to the patient may help improve the delivery of care, especially among low-socioeconomic status groups, and thereby improve implementation of cancer treatment guidelines. Knowledge of what is the appropriate treatment as well as how to cope with that treatment can help patients to be partners in their care and improve completion of all aspects of their treatment.

REFERENCES

1. Gagliardi AR, Brouwers MC, Palda VA, Lemieux-Charles L, Grimshaw JM. How can we improve guideline use? A conceptual framework of implementability. *Implement Sci*. 2011;6:26.

2. Latosinsky S, Fradette K, Lix L, Hildebrand K, Turner D. Canadian breast cancer guidelines: Have they made a difference? *CMAJ*. 2007;176(6):771–776.

3. Bristow RE, Chang J, Ziogas A, Campos B, Chavez LR, Anton-Culver H. Sociodemographic disparities in advanced ovarian cancer survival and adherence to treatment guidelines. *Obstet Gynecol*. 2015;125(4):833–842.

4. Neugut AI, Hillyer GC, Kushi LH, et al. A prospective cohort study of early discontinuation of adjuvant chemotherapy in women with breast cancer: The Breast Cancer Quality of Care Study (BQUAL). *Breast Cancer Res Treat* 2016;158(1):127–138.

5. Losk K, Vaz-Luis I, Camuso K, Batista R, Lloyd M, Tukenmez M, Golshan M, Lin NU, Bunnell CA. Factors associated with delays in chemotherapy initiation among patients with breast cancer at a comprehensive cancer center. *J Natl Compr Canc Netw*. 2016;14(12):1519–1526.

6. PDQ—NCI's Comprehensive Database. National Cancer Institute website. https://www.cancer.gov/publications/pdq.

7. Development and update of the NCCN guidelines. National Comprehensive Cancer Network website. https://www.nccn.org/professionals/development.aspx.

8. Quality & guidelines: Guidelines, tools, & resources. American Society of Oncology website. http://www.asco.org/practice-guidelines/quality-guidelines/guidelines.

9. ASCO guidelines methodology manual: Secondary ASCO guidelines methodology manual. American Society of Oncology website. https://pilotguidelines.atlassian.net/wiki/display/GW/Guideline+Development+Process.

10. Institute of Medicine. *Patient-Centered Cancer Treatment Planning: Improving the Quality of Oncology Care: Workshop Summary*. Washington, DC: Institute of Medicine; 2011.

11. Murphy CC, Bartholomew LK, Carpentier MY, Bluethmann SM, Vernon SW. Adherence to adjuvant hormonal therapy among breast cancer survivors in clinical practice: A systematic review. *Breast Cancer Res Treat* 2012;134(2):459–478.

12. Bettencourt BA, Schlegel RJ, Talley AE, Molix LA. The breast cancer experience of rural women: A literature review. *Psycho-Oncology*. 2007;16(10):875–887.

13. Albain KS, Unger JM, Crowley JJ, Coltman CA Jr, Hershman DL. Racial disparities in cancer survival among randomized clinical trials patients of the Southwest Oncology Group. *J Natl Cancer Inst*. 2009;101(14):984–992.

14. Helzlsouer KJ, Appling, SE. Scarvalone S, Gallicchio L., Henninger D, Manocheh S, MacDonald R., Varanasi AP. Development and evaluation of a technology-enhanced interdisciplinary navigation program for low-income breast cancer patients. *J Oncol Navig Survivorship*.2016;7(4):10–18.

15. Helzlsouer KJ, Appling, SE, Scarvalone S, Gallicchio L, Henninger D, Manocheh S, MacDonald R, Varanasi AP. A pilot study of a virtual navigation program to improve treatment adherence among low-income breast cancer patients. *J Oncol Navig Survivorship*. 2016;7(7):20–29.

10

ORGANIZATION- AND SYSTEM-LEVEL FACTORS INFLUENCING IMPLEMENTATION

OVERVIEW OF CASE STUDIES

Stephanie B. Wheeler

ORGANIZATION- AND health system-level determinants of cancer outcomes are critical to understand. Studies focusing only on individual- or provider-level factors contributing to differential outcomes may mask the important, and often far-reaching, influence of organization- and system-wide structures, policies, norms, and behaviors that drive outcomes.[1] The National Cancer Institute (NCI) has defined health care organizations as those settings "in which individuals receive health-focused services across the cancer care continuum [including] clinics, hospitals, cancer centers, federally qualified health centers, integrated delivery systems, health departments, and community-based organizations."[2] This chapter summarizes implementation lessons learned from four case studies that describe how diverse health care organizations can influence cancer outcomes through implementing system-wide evidence-based interventions (EBIs) ranging from symptom and distress screening to universal Lynch syndrome testing and patient navigation.

The Chronic Care Model[3,4] elucidated the multilayered determinants of patients' functional and clinical outcomes, including the critical roles that health care organizations and health systems play in setting up delivery system design, decision support, clinical informatics, and self-management support. Wagner and colleagues noted that health care organizations and systems are embedded within a larger community and policy context and that these together lead to (ideally) productive, multiway interactions between informed, activated patients and prepared, proactive providers. They posited that sufficient management of complex illnesses requires appropriately organized and coordinated health care systems existing within, and cognizant of, community resources, constraints, policies, and norms. Cancer fits well within this model, due to the need to harmonize multiple moving clinical parts within a multispecialty care environment, the focus on patient self-management support, and the importance of routine monitoring and follow-up of patients across the cancer continuum, aided (or challenged) by ever-evolving clinical informatics systems.

Studies assuming that outcomes result only from patient- or provider-level factors through direct pathways fail to consider the complex nature of health care provided within multiple types of health care organizations, ranging from fully integrated to terribly fragmented systems. Fortunately, statistical advances have allowed us greater flexibility to define more precisely the contributions of organization- and systems-level determinants of differential outcomes, relative to individual- or provider-level determinants. In addition, implementation science approaches have further underscored the importance of understanding local organizational and system context as an essential element of implementation strategy selection, adaptation, and outcomes assessment. New instruments and measures to assess organizational climate and readiness for change,[5] as well as pragmatic implementation measures,[6] are essential tools to assess readiness and capacity and to implement and test EBIs within diverse organizations.

In this chapter, Dr. Angela Stover first presents a case study of implementation of patient-reported outcomes (PRO) symptom monitoring within a large academic medical center. PRO monitoring is essential to clinical care because burdensome symptoms are frequently undetected by care teams, resulting in unnecessary distress, poor functional status, and excess health care utilization and cost. When PRO integration is effective, patients and providers report better outcomes;[7] despite this evidence, routine PRO monitoring is rare in clinical practice. Stover describes a two-phase systematic process guided by the Organizational Model of Innovation Implementation[8] and the Theoretical Domains Framework,[9] consisting of developing and piloting a prototype PRO system informed by patients, multidisciplinary clinician teams, health system administrators, health services researchers, and PRO and informatics experts. Notable features of the PRO system design process include (1) leveraging existing, validated PRO measures of adverse events and quality of life (e.g., PRO-CTCAE and PROMIS); (2) providing graphical displays and hard-copy symptom summaries to both patients and clinicians; (3) mapping clinical workflows and assessing organizational readiness and capacity for change; and (4) attending to sustainability by assessing fit between organizational values and the PRO innovation, in addition to ensuring sufficient implementation support necessary to fully integrate and sustain the PRO innovation in the long term. Critical implementation questions still being assessed pertain to the timing and frequency of PRO monitoring and reporting, reimbursement, questionnaire standardization across cancer sites/clinics, visualization and accessibility of PRO data, and ensuring appropriate clinical response and follow-up after burdensome systems are reported.

Drs. Harold Freeman and Melissa Simon report on the example of cancer patient navigation programs to reduce social, economic, cultural, and system barriers to timely cancer care. Navigation across the cancer care continuum is intended to target organizational and health system barriers pertaining to lack of communication and information, medical system fragmentation and complexity, fear and distrust, and financial accessibility of care. As such, navigation has been particularly beneficial in reducing delays and ensuring receipt of evidence-based care for those patients most likely to encounter barriers, including poor, uninsured/underinsured, minority, and rural Americans. Since its inception in 1990,[10] patient navigation has expanded considerably and is now mandated by the American College of Surgeons' Commission on Cancer requirements of cancer centers seeking approval.[11] Freeman and Simon describe patient navigation as a health system support strategy designed to close the gap between scientific discovery and health care delivery. One of the clear conclusions of this work is that in order to be effective and sustainable, cancer navigation programs must (1) be truly patient-centered and culturally appropriate; (2) cross the cancer continuum; (3) define a clear scope of practice and roles/responsibilities that distinguish the navigator from other care providers; (4) be cost-effective and well resourced; (5) be cognizant of, and integrative across, disconnected systems of care; and (6) be coordinated within the organization itself, ideally through a system-wide navigation delivery team with clear leadership and institutional direction. Freeman and Simon describe several practical implementation challenges, however, that impede scale-up and sustainability of navigation programs that meet these criteria. Specifically, contextual or structural impediments, including lack of reimbursement for navigation, limit its expansion. Proponents of navigation have responded by producing cost-effectiveness research and research on targeting high-risk populations most in need of navigation to make a stronger case to motivate payer reimbursement and institutional commitment to funding navigators. Other barriers to implementation include poor fit between the navigation program and implementation setting, variation in navigator training and function, and lack of standardization or transparency about navigation program content. Opportunities include the national emphasis on navigation, increased availability of funding models to support it, and a growing appreciation that context-appropriate implementation of navigation models is essential to long-term sustainability.

Dr. Paul Montgomery and colleagues share how psychosocial support has been integrated into community-based and Veterans Administration (VA) oncology programs. Psychosocial distress screening is vital to understand which cancer patients are most in need to referrals to psychosocial support and is expected of Commission on Cancer-accredited centers.[11,12] However, appropriate use of distress screeners, such as the National Comprehensive Cancer Network's Distress Management Tool and the Personal Health Questionnaire-4, has been uneven in practice, with notable lapses in follow-up after screening and lack of consistency in application. Experience with a variety of distress screeners has yielded the following recommendations from Montgomery and colleagues: (1) Distress screening tools must be fully integrated into clinical practice, routinely captured, and readily available to all care providers via the medical record; (2) clear follow-up protocols must be established, with social workers and other psychosocial support staff co-located in close proximity to oncology care teams to ensure immediate assessment and follow-up of distressed patients; (3) use of distress screening tools must be accompanied by rigorous staff training to optimize and standardize collection of data; (4) organization of psychosocial support services should anticipate differential utilization of services by oncology service line; and (5) implementation of distress screening must attend to, and be tailored in light of, key organizational differences in the health care services environment in which it is being introduced. Care providers who have been sensitized to detect unmet psychosocial needs and who have been given clear guidelines for follow-up and referral are most likely to be successful in linking distressed cancer patients to needed psychosocial support; thoughtful vetting of staff

through awareness-raising training and coherent protocols for action are therefore essential.

Dr. Maren Scheuner and colleagues reflect on their experience implementing Lynch syndrome testing within a VA integrated health care system, noting several strategies that made implementation successful, including integrated health care system data warehousing, case management, and centralized technical assistance. They also note several challenges to sustainability, including low prevalence of Lynch syndrome among veterans, limited expertise with Lynch syndrome among clinic staff, organizational changes, and the rapidly changing field of precision oncology. Lynch syndrome testing is critical to informing treatment and surveillance options among colorectal cancer cases and other patients at high risk for colorectal cancer, including family members of positives (via cascade testing).[13,14] Preparation for Lynch syndrome testing in the VA population began with pre-implementation activities led by a multidisciplinary team with expertise in medical genetics, genetic counseling, colorectal cancer care, medical anthropology, organizational theory, and implementation science. Pre-implementation activities included semi-structured patient interviews, identification of a clinical program and champion to lead the effort, selection and setup of key implementation strategies such as a tracking registry, case management, and centralized technical assistance. Active implementation activities included monitoring implementation progress and data collection, as well as assessing fidelity, intensity, exposure, and local adaptation. During this process, the investigators noted a variety of emergent challenges pertaining to procedural and protocol issues, personnel and staffing issues, and organizational disruptions (e.g., consolidation). Post-implementation efforts focused on ensuring maintenance and sustainability and included progress reporting, consideration of protocol modifications and adaptation, and cost and value assessment. Although the Lynch syndrome testing program was widely considered to be successful, the authors acknowledged that the rapidly evolving field of precision oncology may eventually replace current procedures and warrant a different implementation approach.

One of the most interesting and impactful conclusions emerging from the four case studies is that "bottom-up" stakeholder-engaged implementation planning may conflict with traditional "top-down" quality improvement processes. That is, national priorities focused on implementing certain EBPs may be out of step with local realities and constraints that impose limits on real-world implementation. Importantly, given health system organizational complexity and the breadth of personnel expertise required to successfully implement complex innovations such as PRO monitoring, patient navigation, distress screening, and genetic testing, it is clear that in the absence of transformational, whole health care system reforms, more bottom-up implementation approaches that take into consideration local implementation context, resource and personnel constraints, and organizational culture will be needed in today's increasingly scattered, rapidly evolving health care systems.[15]

REFERENCES

1. Birken SA, Bunger AC, Powell BJ, et al. Organizational theory for dissemination and implementation research. *Implement Sci.* 2017;12(1):62.
2. Accelerating colorectal cancer screening and follow-up through implementation science. National Cancer Institute website. 2017. https://grants.nih.gov/grants/guide/rfa-files/RFA-CA-17-038.html.
3. Wagner EH, Austin BT, Von Korff M. Improving outcomes in chronic illness. *Manag Care Q.* 1996;4(2):12–25.
4. Bodenheimer T, Wanger EH, Grumbach K. Improving primary care for patients with chronic illness: The Chronic Care Model, Part 2. *JAMA.* 2002;288(15):1909–1914.
5. Shea CM, Jacobs SR, Esserman DA, Bruce K, Weiner BJ. Organizational readiness for implementing change: A psychometric assessment of a new measure. *Implement Sci.* 2014;9:7.
6. Powell BJ, Stanick CF, Halko HM, et al. Toward criteria for pragmatic measurement in implementation research and practice: A stakeholder-driven approach using concept mapping. *Implement Sci.* 2017;12(1):118.
7. Basch E, Deal A, Kris M, et al. Symptom monitoring with patient-reported outcomes during routine cancer treatment: A randomized controlled trial. *J Clin Oncol.* 2016;34:557–565.
8. Weiner BJ, Lewis MA, Linnan LA. Using organization theory to understand the determinants of effective implementation of worksite health promotion programs. *Health Educ Res.* 2008;24(2):292–305.
9. French SD, Green S, O'Connor D, et al. Developing theory-informed behavior change interventions to implement evidence into practice: A systematic approach using the Theoretical Domains Framework. *Implement Science.* 2012;7:38.
10. Freeman HP. Patient navigation: A community-centered approach to reducing cancer mortality. *J Cancer Educ.* 2006; 21(1 Suppl):S11–S14.
11. Greene F. *Cancer Program Standards 2012: Version 1.2.1.* Chicago: American College of Surgeons Commission on Cancer; 2012. https://www.facs.org/~/media/files/quality%20programs/cancer/coc/programstandards2012.ashx.
12. Lazenby M, Ercolano E, Grant M, Holland JC, Jacobsen PB, McCorkle R. Supporting commission on cancer-mandated psychosocial distress screening with implementation strategies. *J Oncol Pract.* 2015;11(3):e413–e420. https://www.ncbi.nlm.nih.gov/pubmed/25758447.
13. Hampel H, Frankel WL, Martin E, et al. Feasibility of screening for Lynch syndrome among patients with colorectal cancer. *J Clin Oncol.* 2008;26(35):5783–5788.
14. Hampel H. Genetic counseling and cascade genetic testing in Lynch syndrome. *Fam Cancer.* 2016;15(3):423–427.
15. Institute of Medicine. *Best Care at Lower Cost: The Path to Continuously Learning Healthcare in America.* Washington, DC: National Academies Press; 2012.

Case Study 10A

INTEGRATING PATIENT-REPORTED OUTCOMES INTO ROUTINE CANCER CARE DELIVERY

Angela M. Stover

PATIENT-REPORTED OUTCOME (PRO) measures are standardized questionnaires assessing symptoms, physical function, or care experiences (e.g., satisfaction with treatment). In 2009, the US Food and Drug Administration defined PROs as "measurement based on a report that comes directly from the patient . . . about the status of a patient's health condition without amendment or interpretation of the patient's response."[1,p32]

PROs are needed in cancer care delivery because burdensome symptoms are frequently undetected by care teams (up to half the time[2]), which may result in distress, decrements in physical function, and hospitalizations.[3] Systematic reviews have shown that integrating PRO measures into cancer care delivery improves communication between patients and clinicians, increases satisfaction with care, and reduces symptom burden.[3] Chemotherapy patients randomized to complete weekly symptom questionnaires (with results automatically fed back to nurses) are more likely to be alive at 1 year and have fewer emergency room visits.[4] The probable mechanism at work is that clinicians become aware of symptoms sooner and change treatment plans to avoid adverse outcomes. PRO integration also has benefits for clinicians. An implementation study at 17 cancer practices in Canada showed that identifying patients' distress with PRO measures increased clinicians' confidence in addressing symptoms.[5] Despite this evidence, PRO measures have not been widely integrated into cancer care delivery—an implementation problem.

Similar to other health care systems, UNC Healthcare has been working for several years to integrate PROs into routine care delivery across all outpatient units. The focus of this chapter is implementation planning at the North Carolina Cancer Hospital (NCCH). Cancer care delivery is a useful example for illustrating the principles of implementation science because multilevel barriers exist at the patient, clinician, clinic, and even national levels. Implementing PROs into cancer care delivery is also a good example because there is ample evidence for effectiveness but stalled implementation. The Organizational Model of Innovation Implementation[6] and the Theoretical Domains Framework[7,8] are used in this case study to illustrate the implementation planning process and the barriers encountered.

IMPLEMENTATION PLANNING

Phase I

Implementing PROs into cancer care delivery is challenging due to necessary changes in clinic operations and workflow, barriers to electronic health record (EHR) integration, and lack of clinician training.[9] No "turnkey" PRO implementation strategies exist; thus, each clinic or health care system has to make many complex implementation decisions on its own.

At NCCH, we have been using an iterative strategy for the past several years to make initial implementation planning decisions and to plan for live implementation (Figure 10A.1). We started with internal pilot funding to develop a prototype "Patient-Reported Symptom Monitoring" system and to pilot test it in real time during clinical visits.[10] The research team included five stakeholder groups: clinicians, patients, health care administrators, health services researchers, and

experts in PRO measurement. A two-part study was conducted. In Part 1, we identified important symptom areas to assess and PRO measures with high-quality psychometric properties.[10] In Part 2, we pilot tested PRO measures in real time[10] to examine common implementation science outcomes, such as feasibility and perceptions of acceptability.[11]

The research team conducted cognitive interviews with cancer patients to assess whether symptom questions were meaningful and comprehensible,[10] which are critical to providing better person-centered care.[12] The research team selected 16 symptoms based on a literature review,[13–15] clinical expertise, and consensus of stakeholder groups.

We followed recommendations from the International Society of Quality of Life[16] to develop our objectives for PRO implementation: (1) screener for common symptoms across cancer types experienced by patients during cancer care delivery, (2) enhancing care delivery by increasing detection of common burdensome symptoms, (3) meeting meaningful use[17] and distress screening[18] requirements, and (4) potentially using the PROs as a quality of care indicator in the future.[19] Common symptoms selected included the National Cancer Institute's list of recommended symptoms to assess in clinical trials (pain, nausea, etc.).[13]

PRO measures selected included the US National Cancer Institute's Patient-Reported

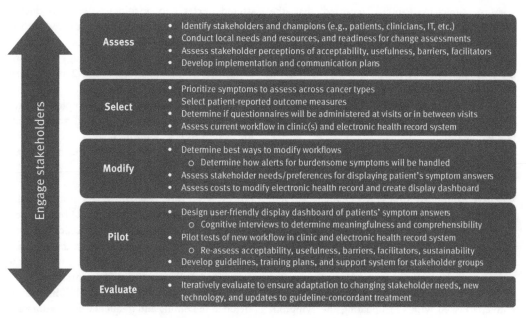

FIGURE 10A.1   Implementation process for integrating PROs into care delivery.

Outcomes version of the Common Terminology Criteria for Adverse Events (PRO-CTCAE).[20] Questions assessing quality of life were taken from the US National Institutes of Health's Patient-Reported Outcomes Measurement Information System (PROMIS) Global Health short form.[21] It was also important to stakeholders to include a question that gave the patient an opportunity to set an agenda for what he or she would like to talk about with clinicians to better personalize care. A hard-copy summary of patient responses was automatically generated that listed symptoms ordered from most to least severe with color coding. Summaries were provided to both patients and clinicians.

In Part 2 of the study, we examined feasibility and perceived acceptability of using PROs during active treatment with 39 cancer patients and 14 clinicians.[10] Three clinics at NCCH participated (Bone Marrow and Stem Cell Transplant, Breast Medical Oncology, and Radiation Oncology).

More than 80% of cancer patients reported that the PRO questionnaire was helpful in discussing symptoms with their clinicians, wanted to use the PRO system during future visits, and would recommend it to other patients.[10] An initial barrier identified by stakeholders was how many questions to administer to patients in the waiting room. We used a brief screener with 22 questions. More than 90% of cancer patients were willing to answer 10 additional questions,[10] although the feasibility of this number of questions was not tested.

Most clinicians (>60%) reported that the PRO summary was easy to interpret, helpful for communicating with patients, and that they would recommend it to future patients.[10] The PRO summary was perceived by clinicians to be most useful for documenting the Review of Systems. More than 75% of clinicians reported that incorporating the PRO summary into the visit did not change consultation time.[10]

Phase II

We have continued to use stakeholder engagement as we move toward PRO integration into the EHR at NCCH. A multidisciplinary committee was formed with six stakeholder groups: clinicians, patients, health care administrators, quality improvement experts, health services researchers and PRO experts, and informatics leadership. The committee is tasked with (1) updating the symptom areas and PROs to be assessed based on state and national initiatives and ongoing research initiatives, (2) integrating PROs into our EHR system (Epic), and (3) developing intuitive graphical displays of symptom scores for use during clinic visits. This broad mandate involves many implementation decisions and multidisciplinary solutions.

In Phase II, we are also examining broader implementation outcomes, such as (1) types of implementation support that will be needed, (2) mapping clinical workflow in each unit, (3) costs and capacity for changing the EHR system to include PROs and graphic visualization of scores, and (4) sustainability. The Organizational Model of Innovation Implementation[6] and the Theoretical Domains Framework[7,8] have informed our thinking about system-level factors that are important for implementation planning. For example, the Organizational Model of Innovation Implementation includes constructs for organizational readiness and capacity for change, fit between the values of the organization and the innovation, and implementation support necessary for integration and sustainability.[6] The Theoretical Domains Framework synthesizes 33 theories and more than 120 constructs into 14 domains to help apply theoretical approaches to care delivery change.[7,8]

We have been conducting in-depth interviews with stakeholder groups and reviewing state and national PRO initiatives to complete committee mandates and to make decisions regarding broader implementation issues. Focus groups with registered nurses and oncologists were conducted. Key informant interviews were conducted with 16 stakeholders at NCCN (10 patients with various types of cancer, 2 medical oncology clinicians, 2 health care administrators, and 2 health services researchers). Interview guides were used to elicit local barriers, types of implementation supports that will be needed, and acceptability for using PROs as a future quality of care metric. Transcripts were content analyzed using standard methodology.

Cancer patients reported barriers related to processes of care (e.g., providers not reviewing responses on PROs with the patient) but were enthusiastic about increasing communication with providers. Clinicians reported barriers that were also process oriented (e.g., changing clinic workflow to accommodate PRO review and potential issues with patient flow). Decisions related to EHR integration included the timing and frequency of questionnaire administration and also workflow changes to alert clinicians of burdensome symptoms. A structural barrier reported was that PRO data must be mined in real time for patient care and decision-making. Currently, there are no templates in most EHR systems for mining and visualizing PRO reports, although work is underway.

Clinicians and administrators reported structural barriers such as staff training and lack of reimbursement from insurance billing. Health services researchers participating in the in-depth interviews focused on standardization of questionnaires across NCCH clinics and selecting thresholds for burdensome symptom alerts. Perceived facilitators included dashboards to visually display symptom levels that are intuitive and easily accessible in the EHR. Displays for NCCH are being designed with our stakeholders to ensure graphics are meaningful, comprehensible, and meet stakeholder needs.[22]

The NCCH is approximately halfway toward our goal of PRO implementation into routine care delivery (for all patients). We are assessing workflow modifications in each clinic and how to handle burdensome symptom alerts in workflow. We are also obtaining cost estimates to modify our EHR and to create a display dashboard that is easy to use for clinicians and patients. Pilot testing in occurring in a small number of clinics to determine real-time barriers. We anticipate that the implementation planning process is going to take approximately 2 or 3 more years for a rollout to all patients.

Several health care systems can provide guidance for moving forward. For example, the Cleveland Clinic and Dartmouth–Hitchcock Medical Center have systematically integrated PRO measures into care delivery for a portion of their clinics.[23,24] Both health care systems use PRO data during care visits, for quality improvement, and for comparative effectiveness research.[23,24] The Cleveland Clinic has collected longitudinal PRO measures from more than 200,000 patients since 2007. More than 70% of its 17 disease-based clinics systematically collect PROs.[23] Approximately 30% of PRO data are collected through their Epic MyChart patient portal prior to visits. The PRO data collection system and EHR are linked through a web-based interface. The remaining 70% are collected in waiting rooms with tablet computers and kiosks.

Dartmouth–Hitchcock Medical Center has collected PRO data on pain, physical functioning, and emotional health from outpatients since 2011.[24]

PRO data are graphically displayed alongside vital signs in its EHR for clinicians to review with patients during visits. At the Dartmouth Spine Center, patients complete a PRO questionnaire prior to all visits, via either patient portal or tablet computer. A summary report is generated and automatically inserted into workflow for individual patient management. After the visit, PRO data are automatically combined with clinical data, claims, and diagnostic tests and sent to a data warehouse. Feedback reports stratified by diagnosis are generated for quality improvement.[24]

LESSONS LEARNED

We have found that multidisciplinary teams and stakeholder engagement are critical at every step of implementation planning for PROs. We used an iterative, bottom-up process in which stakeholders were engaged in implementation planning and decision-making beginning at the initial step. This level of stakeholder engagement may run counter to conventional quality improvement (QI), in which practice changes are generally made in a top-down approach over a short span of time.[25]

Our experience suggests that QI methodology alone may not be sufficient to overcome barriers to integrating PROs into routine care delivery. Instead, a blend of QI and implementation science is needed.[26-27] QI provides on-the-ground expert input and rapid cycles for testing parts of implementation planning. Theories and frameworks from implementation science may be better suited to increase adoption of PRO measures for care delivery.[26] We used implementation science theories to develop our interview guides for stakeholders, inform barriers and facilitators, and guide selection of strategies to overcome barriers. In the future, we also plan to use theory to measure the effectiveness of implementation.[28]

Implementation science theories focusing on practice integration[29] also suggest that ongoing evaluations will be needed for sustainability and to ensure that the PRO systems and EHR adapt to changing stakeholder needs, new technology, and updates to guideline-concordant treatment. This idea corresponds to the Institute of Medicine's idea of a "rapid learning healthcare system" in which science, informatics, healthcare delivery, and PRO methodology are seamlessly embedded in workflow, and new knowledge is a key derivative of care delivery.[30]

CONCLUSION

PRO measures reflect the patient experience and what is meaningful and important to patients during care delivery. PRO measures are effective in improving communication between patients and clinicians and reducing symptom burden, and they are correlated with survival and fewer hospital admissions. At NCCH, we have been using an iterative planning approach and a blend of QI and implementation science methodology to make initial decisions and plan for live integration of PROs into routine care delivery. Our experience is a useful case study for implementation science because effectiveness has been established but implementation is stalled across most US health care systems. No ready-made PRO implementation strategies exist; thus, health care systems have to make many complex implementation decisions on their own. Health care systems making these decisions in the future would benefit from a menu of adaptable implementation strategies (based on theory and accumulating evidence) that includes practical recommendations for making decisions during implementation steps, ways to increase stakeholder engagement in implementation planning, and recommendations on how to evaluate whether implementation is working.

REFERENCES

1. US Food and Drug Administration. *Guidance for Industry: Patient-Reported Outcome Measures: Use in Medical Product Development to Support Labeling Claims.* Washington, DC: US Food and Drug Administration; 2009.

2. Atkinson TM, Li Y, Coffey CW, et al. Reliability of adverse symptom event reporting by clinicians. *Qual Life Res.* 2012;21:1159–1164.

3. Kotronoulas G, Kearney N, Maguire R, et al. What is the value of the routine use of patient-reported outcome measures toward improvement of patient outcomes, processes of care, and health service outcomes in cancer care? A systematic review of controlled trials. *J Clin Oncol.* 2014; 32(14):1480–1501.

4. Basch E, Deal A, Kris M, et al. Symptom monitoring with patient-reported outcomes during routine cancer treatment: A randomized controlled trial. *J Clin Oncol.* 2016;34:557–565.

5. Tamagawa R, Groff S, Anderson J, et al. Effects of a provincial-wide implementation of screening for distress on healthcare professionals' confidence and understanding of person-centered care in oncology. *J Natl Compr Canc Netw.* 2016;14(10):1259–1266.

6. Weiner BJ, Lewis MA, Linnan LA. Using organization theory to understand the determinants of effective implementation of worksite health promotion programs. *Health Educ Res.* 2008;24(2):292–305.

7. French SD, Green SE, O'Connor D, et al. Developing theory-informed behavior change interventions to implement evidence into practice: A systematic approach using the Theoretical Domains Framework. *Implement Sci.* 2012;7:38.

8. Cane J, O'Connor D, Michie S. Validation of the theoretical domains framework for use in behavior change and implementation research. *Implement Science.* 2012;7:37.

9. Antunes B, Harding R, Higginson IJ. Implementing patient-reported outcome measures in palliative care clinical practice: A systematic review of facilitators and barriers. *Palliat Med.* 2014;28(2):158–175.

10. Stover AM, Irwin D, Chen RC, et al. Integrating patient-reported measures into routine cancer care: Cancer patients' and clinicians' perceptions of acceptability and value. *eGEMs.* 2015;2(1): Article 23. DOI:http://dx.doi.org/10.13063/2327-9214.1169.

11. Proctor E, Silmere H, Raghavan R, et al. Outcomes for implementation research: Conceptual distinctions, measurement challenges, and research agenda. *Adm Policy Ment Health.* 2011;38(2):65–76.

12. Institute of Medicine. *Crossing the Quality Chasm: A New Health System for the 21st Century.* Washington, DC: National Academies Press; 2001.

13. Reeve BB, Mitchell SA, Dueck AC, et al. Recommended patient-reported core set of symptoms to measure in adult cancer treatment trials. *J Natl Cancer Inst.* 2014;106(7):dju129. DOI:10.1093/jnci/dju129.

14. Cleeland CS, Zhao F, Chang VT, et al. The symptom burden of cancer: Evidence for a core set of cancer-related and treatment-related symptoms from the Eastern Cooperative Oncology Group Symptom Outcomes and Practice Patterns study. *Cancer.* 2013;119(24):4333–4340.

15. Kirkova J, Davis MP, Walsh D, et al. Cancer symptom assessment instruments: A systematic review. *J Clin Oncol.* 2006;24:1459–1473.

16. Aaronson N, Elliott T, Greenhalgh J, et al. *User's Guide to Implementing Patient-Reported Outcomes Assessment in Clinical Practice.* 2015.

International Society for Quality of Life Research website. http://www.isoqol.org/UserFiles/2015UsersGuide-Version2.pdf.

17. Meaningful use definition and objectives. HealthIT.gov. website. https://www.healthit.gov/providers-professionals/meaningful-use-definition-objectives.

18. National Comprehensive Cancer Network. Distress management clinical practice guidelines in oncology. *J Natl Compr Canc Netw.* 2003;1(3):344–374.

19. Stover AM, Basch EM. Using patient-reported outcomes as a quality indicator in routine cancer care. *Cancer.* 2016;122:355–357.

20. Basch EM, Reeve BB, Mitchell S, et al. Development of the National Cancer Institute's Patient-Reported Outcomes Version of the Common Terminology Criteria for Adverse Events (PRO-CTCAE). *J Natl Cancer Inst.* 2014;106(9):dju244.

21. Hays RD, Bjorner J, Revicki RA, et al. Development of physical and mental health summary scores from the Patient Reported Outcomes Measurement Information System (PROMIS) global items. *Qual Life Res.* 2009;18(7):873–880.

22. Smith KC, Brundage MD, Tolbert E, et al. Engaging stakeholders to improve presentation of patient-reported outcomes data in clinical practice. *Support Care Cancer.* 2016;24:4149–4157.

23. Versel N. Healthcare experts balance patient-reported data promise, problems. 2012. Information Week website. https://www.informationweek.com/healthcare/patient-tools/healthcare-experts-balance-patient-reported-data-promise-problems/d/d-id/1107205.

24. Nelson EC, Hivtfeldt H, Reid R, et al. Using patient-reported information to improve health outcomes and health care value: Case studies from Dartmouth, Karolinska, and Group Health. Lebanon, NH: Dartmouth Institute for Health Policy and Clinical Practice; 2012. https://ki.se/sites/default/files/using_patientreported_information_to_improve_health_outcomes_and_health_care_value.pdf.

25. Moranos J, Lemstra M, Nwanko C. Lean interventions in healthcare: Do they actually work? *Int J Qual Health Care.* 2016;28(2):150–165.

26. Mitchell SA, Chambers D. Leveraging implementation science to improve cancer care delivery and patient outcomes. *J Oncol Pract.* 2017;13(8):523–529.

27. Koczwara B, Stover AM, Davies L, et al. Harnessing the synergy between improvement science and implementation science in cancer: A call to action. *J Oncol Pract.* 2018;in press.

28. Glasgow RE, Vogt TM, Boles SM. Evaluating the public health impact of health promotion interventions: The RE-AIM framework. *Am J Public Health.* 1999;89(9):1322–1327.

29. Chaudoir SR, Dugan AG, Barr CH. Measuring factors affecting implementation of health innovations: A systematic review of structural, organizational, provider, patient, and innovation level measures. *Implement Sci.* 2013;8:22.

30. Institute of Medicine. *Best Care at Lower Cost: The Path to Continuously Learning Healthcare in America.* Washington, DC: National Academies Press; 2012.

Case Study 10B

PATIENT NAVIGATION AND CANCER CARE DELIVERY

Harold P. Freeman and Melissa A. Simon

PATIENT NAVIGATION may be seen, in some ways, as being similar to a mile relay race. In the relay, runners each carry a baton during their segment of the race, at the end of which they pass it on to the next runner on their team. In such a race, let us imagine that the runners are navigators and the baton is the patient. The object, of course, is to win the race, which is not over until the final runner crosses the finish line with the baton (patient) in hand. It is essential that the baton (patient) not be dropped when passed to the next runner. Similar to the mile relay, patient navigation, in its highly developed form, is a team effort in which navigators guide patients through various phases of health care to a defined point of resolution.

Often for many Americans, the mile relay race resembles relay race with hurdles added. Although the American health care system offers the very best care to many, the poor and uninsured typically face challenges in accessing timely health care even when faced with a life-threatening disease such as cancer.

Spurred by unmet patient needs and the growing complexity of health care delivery systems, patient navigation seeks to diminish social, economic, cultural, and medical system barriers to timely quality care. Implementation science, with its focused pursuit of knowledge and methods to enhance uptake of evidence-based practices into community, health care, and other real-world settings, has an instrumental role in the extent to which patient navigation programs can deliver on its promise. This is particularly true in the context of changing health care landscapes and challenging funding climates that threaten to diminish important patient support services and resources.

In this case study, we discuss patient navigation's emergence as a strategy for improving cancer outcomes, especially among vulnerable populations. We explore challenges and opportunities related to advancing successful implementation of patient navigation across the cancer care continuum. We seek to harness and apply the power and energy of patient navigators with the goal of guiding individuals across the health care continuum—from the communities in which they live all the way through screening, diagnosis, and treatment at clinical care sites.

PATIENT NAVIGATION FROM CONCEPT TO EVIDENCE-BASED INTERVENTION AND STANDARD OF CANCER CARE

Patient navigation has evolved as a strategy to improve outcomes in vulnerable populations by eliminating barriers to screening, timely diagnosis, and treatment of cancer and other chronic diseases. The seeds were planted in the "National Hearings on Cancer in the Poor" held by the American Cancer Society (ACS) in 1989, with testimony by Americans of diverse ethnic and racial groups who had been diagnosed with cancer. Based on the hearings, the ACS issued its "Report to the Nation on Cancer in the Poor."[1] Findings highlighted critical issues confronting poor people with cancer, including substantial barriers to obtaining timely cancer care, culturally insensitive cancer education programs, fatalism about cancer, and the greater pain and suffering poor people endure compared to other Americans. These findings led to the concept of patient navigation.

The nation's first patient navigation program was initiated by Freeman in 1990 at Harlem Hospital, a public hospital in New York City.[2] The original program focused on the critical window of opportunity to save lives by eliminating barriers to timely cancer care between the point of suspicious finding and the resolution of the finding by diagnosis and treatment. These barriers included financial, communication, and information barriers; medical system barriers; and fear, distrust, and emotional barriers. The aim was to diminish the high breast cancer death rate in a population of poor Black women, half of whom had presented with late-stage breast cancer. The combined interventions of free breast cancer screening and patient navigation applied at the point of abnormal finding through the time of diagnosis and treatment increased the 5-year breast cancer survival in this population from 39% to 70% in two separate time periods of study.[3,4]

The patient navigation model in Harlem paved the way for passage of the Patient Navigator Outreach

and Chronic Disease Prevention Act by Congress in 2005.[5] This legislation provided funds to the Health Resources and Services Administration to support patient navigation demonstration research. The Centers for Medicare and Medicaid Services, the Centers for Disease Control and Prevention, and the National Cancer Institute (NCI) subsequently invested significant resources to support patient navigation research and programs. Among the first set of research trials to solder an evidence-based platform for patient navigation was the national Patient Navigation Research Program (PNRP), a multicenter study that tested interventions aimed at reducing time to delivery of quality cancer care after a screening abnormality in underserved individuals at risk for cancer.

The weight of evidence from the PNRP studies indicates that patient navigation can reduce the time from abnormal finding to diagnosis in breast, cervical, and colorectal cancer.[6] Subsequent meta-analyses and systematic reviews with PNRP and other research studies have found patient navigation effective in increasing breast, cervical, and colorectal cancer screening rates, as well as completion of cancer care events such as follow-up of abnormal findings, diagnostic resolution, and treatment initiation.[7–10] Scaling of a patient navigation model to the county level also demonstrated efficacy with respect to timeliness outcomes.[11] Importantly, although patient navigation may possibly be beneficial to all patients, the body of literature suggests that navigation may be most effective in promoting early diagnosis and timely treatment when targeted to patients who are more likely to encounter significant barriers and delays to timely quality care. An analysis of 3,777 patients within the NCI-funded Patient Navigation Research Program concluded that patient navigation eliminated delays in diagnostic resolution that were known to exist by employment, housing type, and marital status.[12]

In 2012, the American College of Surgeons Commission on Cancer designated patient navigation as a standard of care to be met by cancer centers seeking accreditation. The Commission on Cancer's "Cancer Program Standards 2012" directive furthers the national expansion of patient navigation. It requires cancer centers to develop a patient navigation process driven by a community needs assessment to address health care disparities and barriers to patient care.[13] From origins in Harlem to designation as a standard of cancer care, patient navigation has evolved as a patient care support intervention with wide application potential throughout the nation.

PRINCIPLES OF PATIENT NAVIGATION

The core principle of patient navigation is the elimination of barriers to timely care across all phases of the health care continuum, including detection, diagnosis, treatment, and post-treatment quality of life. Patient navigation provides guidance and coordination of the journey of the individual across the care continuum.

The following are the principles of patient navigation developed and vetted based on 25 years of successful patient navigation programs:[14]

1. Patient navigation is a patient-centered health care delivery intervention.

2. The core function of patient navigation is to eliminate barriers to timely care across all phases of the health care continuum.

3. Patient navigation may serve to integrate a fragmented health care system for the individual patient.

4. In a given setting, patient navigation should be defined with a clear scope of practice that distinguishes the roles and responsibilities of the navigator from those of all other health care providers.

5. The determination of who should navigate should be based on the level of skills required in a given phase of navigation and within the context of a given health care setting (e.g., availability of resources and complement of supporting or "wraparound" services).

6. The delivery of patient navigation services should be cost-effective and commensurate with the level of skills to navigate an individual through a particular phase of the health care continuum.

7. In a given system of care, there is a need to define the point at which navigation begins and where it ends.

8. There is often a need to navigate patients across disconnected systems of care, such as primary care sites and tertiary care sites. Patient navigation can serve as the process that connects disconnected health care systems.

9. Patient navigation systems require coordination.

ADVANCING IMPLEMENTATION OF PATIENT NAVIGATION INTERVENTIONS

Declines in cancer mortality have been attributed to improved cancer prevention, screening, and detection measures, as well as the application of more effective treatments. However, some Americans have not fully benefited from this progress and are still more likely to die from cancer—particularly the poor, uninsured, and underinsured. According to the US Census Bureau, there were 40.6 million people in poverty in 2016.[15] Poverty is associated with low educational level, substandard living conditions, unemployment, risk-promoting lifestyle, and diminished access to timely health care. A disproportionate percentage of Blacks and Hispanics are poor, uninsured, and underinsured. Higher cancer mortality and lower cancer survival among some population groups suggest the existence of a disconnect between the nation's discovery and delivery enterprises—a disconnect between what we know and what we do.

Implementation science is vital to the scale-up and sustainment of patient navigation, to bridge the disconnect between discovery and delivery. Advancing uptake of patient navigation into routine practice, like that of any number of evidence-based health innovations, is a complex process. The success or failure of implementation efforts likely involves a constellation of variables related to the intervention components themselves; the local implementation context; program implementers; and structural, macro-level factors involving care delivery systems and public policy.[16] As it is, patient navigation interventions are particularly well suited, and relevant, for benefiting from—and advancing—implementation science.

Key findings from existing bodies of research suggest that patient navigation is an intervention strategy with opportunities for implementation in a variety of real-world settings. Multi-site efficacy trials alone have involved large variability in patient navigator roles, qualifications, responsibilities, and the settings in which they worked (e.g., community health centers, hospitals, primary care, and specialty practices).[17] Combined with the unique needs of each patient, the multitude of screening modalities and treatments, as well as continuous change within local delivery contexts, patient navigation is not a "one-size-fits-all" but, rather, an intervention in which adaptation is encouraged—and necessary—for successful implementation.

In advancing patient navigation through implementation science, we may be able to tackle numerous unanswered questions and challenges faced by researchers, practitioners, and systems and policy designers. Guided by multilevel frameworks in implementation science,[16,18] the following sections highlight several implementation challenges and areas of opportunity for patient navigation research and programs.

CONTEXTUAL CATALYSTS

Contextual or structural factors, such as those representing the political and financial environments in which organizations are nested, have played pivotal roles in furthering the expansion of patient navigation into health care settings. However, some of these same catalysts—such as mandates of patient navigation as standard of cancer care and funding availability for patient navigation research and programs—represent significant implementation challenges and raise questions of intervention sustainability. It may be difficult, for example, to maintain sustained employment for patient navigators funded by grants and philanthropic sources. A key impediment is that existing payment models do not cover patient navigation services; there is little incentive for organizations to create sustainable roles for patient navigation without recognition of navigation as a reimbursable, covered service for both public and private payers.[19]

In response, a growing vein of patient navigation research has been centered on cost-effectiveness to inform policy and practice. Studies have put forth evidence of cost savings and practice efficiency (e.g., fewer missed appointments).[20,21] Also in tune with shaping policy environments and payment models for successful implementation of navigation programs, another important thrust of patient navigation research is implementing navigation interventions for only those patients who would benefit from them the most. This is an outgrowth of research findings suggesting that not all high-risk patients need navigation and that some patients may only need elements of patient navigation during discrete points of time along the cancer care continuum. One example of how targeting might be achieved within health care systems involves leveraging population-based information technology systems to identify patients at high risk for non-adherence with completing screening.[22]

LOCAL IMPLEMENTATION SETTINGS

The successful implementation and sustainment of interventions may be related to the fit between the program and the implementation setting.[16,23] Site-specific differences, possibly with respect to resources, have been suggested as explanations for the observed differences in navigation benefits experienced at some sites participating in multisite efficacy trials relative to pooled analyses.[24] However, research focusing on understanding aspects of organizations in which patient navigation interventions are being implemented is in its nascent stages. Recommendations for needs assessments to guide patient navigation programs include assessment of organizational characteristics, such as resource capacity, organizational staffing structure, patient flow, space, organizational readiness for change, climate, and culture.[19] However, the standard measurement of these characteristics and the organizational factors most pertinent to the success of navigation interventions have not been systematically identified. In light of calls for needs assessments, the application and validation of organizational-level measures for patient navigation will be important steps in scaling implementation of patient navigation to a variety of settings. An example line of research toward measurement of characteristics is the development of tools to assess formal linkages, interorganizational relationships, and existing clinical service offerings of county organizations as a snapshot of capacity to conduct patient navigation.[25]

PROGRAM IMPLEMENTERS

Although there is general agreement regarding the core principles of patient navigation, there is substantial variability in the characteristics, qualifications, and responsibilities of patient navigators—the intervention implementers. Proposed models of patient navigators have included lay navigators, professional navigators such as nurses or social workers, and teams that include both lay and professional navigators.[6,26,27] Needs assessments are recommended to identify appropriate navigator skill sets and responsibilities for a particular implementation setting. But to complicate matters, strong correlations have been uncovered between provision of support services not directly related to navigating the diagnostic abnormality and timely diagnostic outcomes.[28] Moreover, implementation science findings also suggest that improvisation and relationship building are substantial components of navigator roles.[29]

Although various patient navigation models have demonstrated efficacy, furthering integration of patient navigation into health care settings may warrant task clarification and coordination, including of clinical and nonclinical support tasks.[30] It follows that navigators of different levels of knowledge and training are required to guide the individual across the health care continuum. However, a major challenge in training navigators is the lack of nationally established standards for patient navigation training or certification, in part stemming from lack of consensus regarding core competencies that navigators should possess.[31]

A few established training programs exist in the United States, including the Harold P. Freeman Patient Navigation Training Institute, the Colorado Patient Navigator Training Program, and the training curricula established by the PNRP. However, a systematic review of training of patient navigators nevertheless found wide variation across studies with respect to training content, format, duration, location, and trainer background.[27] With the movement toward credentialing of patient navigators to align with payment models that emphasize credentialing, implementation science that can inform task clarification may be instrumental toward development of national standards for training and patient navigation competencies.

ONGOING RESEARCH DIRECTIONS

From the first patient navigation program in Harlem to continuing expansion of patient navigation to community and clinical systems, research has played an important role in shaping patient navigation as an evolving implementation strategy for eliminating barriers to screening, timely diagnosis, and treatment of cancer. To enable more effective dissemination and implementation of patient navigation, ongoing comparative effectiveness research is necessary to answer research questions at the heart of what constitutes patient navigation services. These include untangling multicomponent navigation programs to identify the most beneficial

components for improving outcomes and also comparing the effectiveness of different patient navigation models with respect to intervention dose (e.g., delivery time, caseload, and contacts), delivery methods (e.g., in-person interactions, phone, and mail based), and staffing characteristics (e.g., lay navigators, professional navigators, or a combination of lay and professional navigators).[28,32,33]

Additional opportunities to shape patient navigation's role in cancer care delivery involve investigation into its long-term impact and efficacy in other areas within the cancer care continuum. Furthering the depth of patient navigation research may warrant assessment of the long-term impact of patient navigation on outcomes through development of methodologies to integrate increasing amounts of data from electronic health records as well as collection of patient-reported outcomes. Expanding the breadth of applications has already seen the emergence of patient navigation implementation for cancer clinical trials,[34] cancer survivorship,[8] and end-of-life care.[35]

CONCLUSION

Patient navigation had its origin as an intervention designed to reduce the exceedingly high breast cancer mortality in a poor Black community. When first applied, patient navigation was not an evidence-based intervention but, rather, a strategy initiated in response to the needs of patients in an underserved community. The effectiveness of patient navigation was later validated by extensive scientific studies. Patient navigation is now applied throughout the nation and has been designated as a standard of cancer care.[13] Patient navigation programs are a proven strategy for diminishing social, economic, cultural, and medical system barriers to timely quality care, especially among patients who would otherwise not make it to the finish line in their mile relay. Key to not dropping the baton are efforts that advance the context-appropriate implementation of patient navigation into routine practice and that enhance the long-term sustainment of patient navigation programs.

REFERENCES

1. A summary of the American Cancer Society Report to the Nation: Cancer in the poor. *CA Cancer J Clin.* 1989;39(5):263–265.
2. Freeman HP, Muth BJ, Kerner JF. Expanding access to cancer screening and clinical follow-up

among the medically underserved. *Cancer Pract.* 1995;3(1):19–30.

3. Freeman HP, Wasfie TJ. Cancer of the breast in poor Black women. *Cancer.* 1989;63(12):2562–2569.

4. Oluwole SF, Ali AO, Adu A, et al. Impact of a cancer screening program on breast cancer stage at diagnosis in a medically underserved urban community. *J Am Coll Surg.* 2003;196(2):180–188.

5. Patient Navigator Outreach and Chronic Disease Prevention Act of 2005, Public Law 109-18, Stat. 340 HR 1812.

6. Freeman HP. The origin, evolution, and principles of patient navigation. *Cancer Epidemiol Biomarkers Prev.* 2012;21(10):1614–1617.

7. Ali-Faisal SF, Colella TJ, Medina-Jaudes N, Benz Scott L. The effectiveness of patient navigation to improve healthcare utilization outcomes: A meta-analysis of randomized controlled trials. *Patient Educ Couns.* 2017;100(3):436–448.

8. Krok-Schoen JL, Oliveri JM, Paskett ED. Cancer care delivery and women's health: The role of patient navigation. *Front Oncol.* 2016;6(2).

9. Jojola CE, Cheng H, Wong LJ, Paskett ED, Freund KM, Johnston FM. Efficacy of patient navigation in cancer treatment: A systematic review. *J Oncol Navig Survivorship.* 2017;8(3).

10. Paskett ED, Harrop JP, Wells KJ. Patient navigation: An update on the state of the science. *CA Cancer J Clin.* 2011;61(4):237–249.

11. Simon MA, Tom LS, Nonzee NJ, et al. Evaluating a bilingual patient navigation program for uninsured women with abnormal screening tests for breast and cervical cancer: Implications for future navigator research. *Am J Public Health.* 2015;105(5):e87–e94.

12. Rodday AM, Parsons SK, Snyder F, et al. Impact of patient navigation in eliminating economic disparities in cancer care. *Cancer.* 2015;121(22):4025–4034.

13. American College of Surgeons, Commission on Cancer. *Cancer Program Standards 2012: Continuum of Care Services Standard 3.1.* Chicago: American College of Surgeons.

14. Freeman HP, Rodriguez RL. History and principles of patient navigation. *Cancer.* 2011;117(15 Suppl):3539–3542.

15. Semega JL, Fontenot KR, Kollar MA. Current population reports: Income and poverty in the United States: 2016. 2017. US Census Bureau website. https://census.gov/content/dam/Census/library/publications/2017/demo/P60-259.pdf.

16. Chaudoir SR, Dugan AG, Barr CH. Measuring factors affecting implementation of health innovations: A systematic review of structural, organizational, provider, patient, and innovation level measures. *Implement Sci.* 2013;8:22.

17. Gunn CM, Clark JA, Battaglia TA, Freund KM, Parker VA. An assessment of patient navigator activities in breast cancer patient navigation programs using a nine-principle framework. *Health Serv Res.* 2014;49(5):1555–1577.

18. Tabak RG, Khoong EC, Chambers DA, Brownson RC. Bridging research and practice: Models for dissemination and implementation research. *Am J Prev Med.* 2012;43(3):337–350.

19. Calhoun E, Esparza A, eds. *Patient Navigation: Overcoming Barriers to Care.* New York: Springer; 2017.

20. Rocque GB, Pisu M, Jackson BE, et al. Resource use and Medicare costs during lay navigation for geriatric patients with cancer. *JAMA Oncol.* 2017;3(6):817–825.

21. Ladabaum U, Mannalithara A, Jandorf L, Itzkowitz SH. Cost-effectiveness of patient navigation to increase adherence with screening colonoscopy among minority individuals. *Cancer.* 2015;121(7):1088–1097.

22. Percac-Lima S, Ashburner JM, Zai AH, et al. Patient navigation for comprehensive cancer screening in high-risk patients using a population-based health information technology system: A randomized clinical trial. *JAMA Intern Med.* 2016;176(7):930–937.

23. Chambers DA, Glasgow RE, Stange KC. The dynamic sustainability framework: Addressing the paradox of sustainment amid ongoing change. *Implement Sci.* 2013;8:117.

24. Battaglia TA, Darnell JS, Ko N, et al. The impact of patient navigation on the delivery of diagnostic breast cancer care in the National Patient Navigation Research Program: A prospective meta-analysis. *Breast Cancer Res Treat.* 2016;158(3):523–534.

25. Inrig SJ, Higashi RT, Tiro JA, Argenbright KE, Lee SJ. Assessing local capacity to expand rural breast cancer screening and patient navigation: An iterative mixed-method tool. *Eval Program Plann.* 2017;61:113–124.

26. Oncology Nursing Society, the Association of Oncology Social Work, and the National Association of Social Workers. Oncology Nursing Society, the Association of Oncology Social Work, and the National Association of Social Workers joint position on the role of

oncology nursing and oncology social work in patient navigation. *Oncol Nurs Forum.* 2010;37(3):251–252.

27. Ustjanauskas AE, Bredice M, Nuhaily S, Kath L, Wells KJ. Training in patient navigation: A review of the research literature. *Health Promot Pract.* 2016;17(3):373–381.

28. Gunn C, Battaglia TA, Parker VA, et al. What makes patient navigation most effective: Defining useful tasks and networks. *J Health Care Poor Underserved.* 2017;28(2):663–676.

29. Simon MA, Samaras AT, Nonzee NJ, et al. Patient navigators: Agents of creating community-nested patient-centered medical homes for cancer care. *Clin Med Insights Womens Health.* 2016;9:27–33.

30. Freund KM. Implementation of evidence-based patient navigation programs. *Acta Oncol.* 2017;56(2):123–127.

31. Byers T. Assessing the value of patient navigation for completing cancer screening. *Cancer Epidemiol Biomarkers Prev.* 2012;21(10):1618–1619.

32. DeGroff A, Schroy PC 3rd, Morrissey KG, et al. Patient navigation for colonoscopy completion: Results of an RCT. *Am J Prev Med.* 2017;53(3):363–372.

33. Molina Y, Kim SJ, Berrios N, et al. Patient navigation improves subsequent breast cancer screening after a noncancerous result: Evidence from the Patient Navigation in Medically Underserved Areas Study. *J Womens Health (Larchmt).* 2017. [Epub ahead of print]

34. Fouad MN, Acemgil A, Bae S, et al. Patient navigation as a model to increase participation of African Americans in cancer clinical trials. *J Oncol Pract.* 2016;12(6):556–563.

35. Colligan EM, Ewald E, Ruiz S, Spafford M, Cross-Barnet C, Parashuram S. Innovative oncology care models improve end-of-life quality, reduce utilization and spending. *Health Aff (Millwood).* 2017;36(3):433–440.

Case Study 10C

IMPLEMENTING DISTRESS SCREENING IN A COMMUNITY AND VETERAN'S ADMINISTRATION ONCOLOGY CLINIC

Paul Montgomery, Nicole Thurston, Michelle Betts, and C. Scott Smith

CASE STUDY OF DISTRESS TOOL ADOPTION

Keith (names and details of cases have been changed to ensure anonymity) is a 65-year-old man who was discovered to have metastatic non-small cell lung cancer after evaluation for a chronic cough unresponsive to antibiotics. He was the primary caregiver for his disabled wife, who could not drive, keep house, nor cook. He had three grown daughters, but none lived nearby. Keith drove himself to his first two rounds of platinum-based chemotherapy, which were complicated by diarrhea. Managing the diarrhea while caring for his wife had become progressively difficult. Keith had lost 25 pounds; his Karnofsky performance index dropped from 90 to 60; and he looked tired, pale, and careworn. He stated that he could just barely get up and cook breakfast for he and his wife and was frequently short of breath. His radiographic imaging showed progression of his disease.

Dealing with Keith's cancer when his condition was deteriorating required a different approach than a new drug. Many of Keith's challenges were medical issues, but there were other stressors, including existential/mortality threat, functional status decline, role and identity changes, relationship tensions, financial burdens, pain, transportation, coordination of care, and, simply, clinic parking. A brief internet blog search easily reveals that cancer patients in the community have little or no familiarity with tools that deal with the anxiety, depression, and stress brought on by the challenges of cancer. Both the Institute of Medicine and the American College of Surgeons Commission on Cancer accreditation program emphasize detecting distress and providing psychological support.[1,2] Despite this encouragement from major institutions, incorporating the evolving science of psychosocial support into community oncology clinics has followed an uneven course.[3] Although the US Department of Veterans Affairs (VA) system has integrated psychosocial support for primary care of veterans, there remain significant challenges for those with cancer.[4] To find acceptable and efficacious ways to support patients such as Keith, a cancer care system needs to determine the depth, breadth, and remediable causes of distress and build a comprehensive and sustainable program to address patient needs. In this case study, we compare and contrast approaches to patient distress from two very different systems: a community cancer center operating within a not-for-profit fee-for-service health care system and a VA medical center.

ADOPTION OF DISTRESS TOOLS IN THE COMMUNITY

To help patients such as Keith, St. Luke's Mountain States Tumor Institute (MSTI) in Boise, Idaho, has included psychosocial resources on site since 1968. Unlike most private community oncology clinics where referral to outside clinics would be required, there has been immediate access to psychosocial services in person or by phone. The timeline and the motivation behind the development of a structured distress detection system are outlined in Table 10C.1. Until 2009, MSTI did not consider screens for distress but made referrals by nursing or provider staff as questions arose, despite the importance of reliable screening for psychosocial needs.[5] By 2012, the National Comprehensive Cancer Network's (NCCN) Distress Management Tool (distress thermometer) had been implemented with the impetus of an National Cancer Institute (NCI) Community Cancer Centers Program grant and the accreditation requirements from the American College of Surgeons Commission on Cancer. The distress tool program included processes for staff education, tracking of screen positives, and assessments of the program's impact. Even those caregivers who were not directly involved in managing the distress tool were poised to call social work if patients expressed statements, actions, or even body language that suggested they needed psychosocial intervention.

Despite staff interest in using the distress screening tool, there was variation in the frequency

Table 10C.1. Timeline for the Adaptation of a Distress Screening Tool in a Community Clinic

YEAR	PSYCHOSOCIAL PROGRAM MILEPOSTS	INDIVIDUALS OR GROUPS RESPONSIBLE FOR INITIATING CHANGE
1968	Psychosocial services were initiated with the founding of MSTI, a multidisciplinary cancer treatment clinic.	Community hospitals, physicians, volunteers, clergy
2009	Exploration of distress screening, prompted by initiation of NCI Community Cancer Centers Programs participation.	NCI grant requirements, psychiatry and social work staff
2012	Implementation of NCCN Distress Management Tool.	NCI grant requirements, CoC requirements, psychiatry and social work staff
2013	Gaps in addressing patient reports of distress identified.	Psychiatry and social work staff
2014	Replacement of Distress Management Tool with PHQ-4, and implementation of process for triage of patients reporting distress.	Psychiatry and social work staff

CoC, American College of Surgeons, Commission on Cancer Accreditation Program; MSTI, Mountain State Tumor Institute; NCCN, National Comprehensive Cancer Network; NCI, National Cancer Institute; PHQ-4, Patient Health Questionnaire–4 for Depression and Anxiety.

of reporting elevated levels of patient distress. One medical assistant, Jayne, stood out. After just a few months at MSTI as a medical assistant, it became apparent that Jayne's approach to patients generated increased response rates to the Personal Health Questionnaire–4 (PHQ-4). She also made referrals to the social work staff that included additional information about the patient's behavioral/emotional presentation in the clinic. Jayne's early training in health care provided an explanation for Jayne's skills. Working as an emergency medical technician (EMT) in a rural community, Jayne had many opportunities to help patients cope with distress during the 1-hour ambulance ride to the nearest medical facility. On these long rides, Jayne was mentored by a seasoned EMT who had learned by trial and error how to assess anxiety, use distraction, and provide emotional support to help calm patients.

When Jayne joined MSTI, she recognized the similarity of the distress of cancer patients to the distress of the injured patients she had helped in the rural community. As she completed the distress tool, she would raise the issue of distress routinely but casually, and she would work to personalize every encounter. If the patient exhibited distress, then Jayne would gather collateral information about the patient's psychosocial stressors while expressing empathy for the patient's difficulties. These patients were offered the opportunity to talk with the clinic psychosocial staff. With any concerns, Jayne would approach clinic providers and offer to contact psychosocial support services if all agreed. Jayne recognized that delving into patient distress was difficult and uncomfortable. The screening tool provided support for what Jayne had recognized in her patient evaluation. Her ability to validate and normalize distress exemplified how staff could support the "whole person" and not just the cancer treatment. Jayne enhanced the value of the distress tool by utilizing it to fully assess patients and also using it to make sure the concerns were addressed.

THE VETERANS AFFAIRS INTEGRATED MENTAL HEALTH SYSTEM

Screening for distress in veterans with cancer may be more urgent than in a civilian population.[6] The Boise Veterans Administration Medical Center (BVAMC) had the advantage of employing the primary care–mental health integration programs of the VA. Utilizing the integrated VA medical record, the first VA oncology contact with a new referral was a phone call by a nurse to assess the needs of the veteran with a new diagnosis of cancer. The distress screening that had been done in primary care would be reviewed while the veteran was queried about any new distress, followed by discussions about lodging, transportation, and coordination of appointments. Although the value of this integrated approach is uncertain, addressing the weak links in care likely accounts for why VA outcomes for cancer treatment have been shown to be favorable compared to outcomes from other health care systems.[7]

WHICH SCREENING APPROACH IS MOST VALUABLE?

Although MSTI had integrated the distress thermometer into the clinic by 2012, multiple staff raised concerns about the impact of this tool. The screen queried both physical and emotional symptoms, leaving both the medical and the psychosocial staff responsible for all the reported symptoms. In a busy community oncology clinic, communication between teams could not be ensured to cover all complaints, so the original tool created confusion, with subsequent poor implementation. To remedy this problem, by 2014, the psychosocial support team determined that the optimal method to capture distress in patients suffering from cancer would require a tool covering both depression and anxiety. The PHQ-4 was the best fit. The clinic had departed from the initially recommended tool for distress screening but moved closer to the goal of providing psychosocial support to cancer patients.[8] With a new process, urgent concerns were addressed immediately by the social work clinicians. For less pressing issues, a social worker would contact a patient for further assessment within 5 days on any screens with a score of 6 or greater. However, screening was not uniform at MSTI because surgical oncology did not incorporate the PHQ-4. Instead, surgical services provided immediate access to psychosocial staff. With the surgeon's position on the front line after a new cancer diagnosis, there were frequent referrals.

In contrast, screening veterans for mental health conditions started with outreach and primary care efforts. Despite multiple entry points for mental health care not available in the community, VA practice-based screening may still miss substantial numbers of veterans with distress.[9] Although the VA oncology clinic had access to the primary care screening notes in the electronic medical records, the oncology clinic double-checked with the patient to make sure distress was managed.

SERIAL MEASUREMENT OF DISTRESS: WHAT INFORMATION CAN THIS PROVIDE?

Both MSTI and BVAMC have used distress screens on a serial basis. Data have suggested that outcomes are improved by this routine clinic exercise.[10] However, MSTI found the distress thermometer of limited assistance when the frequency of distress screening was increased to each patient visit without immediate on-site referral to psychosocial care. These observations were borne out in a recently completed prospective trial, in which only 56% of patients with concerns found in screening received further evaluation.[11] Although the VA collected distress information regularly in the primary care setting, this information is not obtained routinely in subspecialty care.

INFORMATION TRANSFER: HOW CAN THE CRITICAL HANDOFF BE OPTIMIZED?

The results of distress screening may not be prioritized in a busy clinic. Within MSTI, as noted with Keith's experience, transfer of information was enhanced if the person overseeing the distress tool was proactive. However, some screeners simply gathered the information and filed it for review. This meant psychosocial staff often had to make unsolicited calls and ask sensitive questions of distressed patients. In contrast, the surgical oncologist group could make a warm handoff to the embedded social worker, at the cost of more required personnel.

The VA has had a very different, multipronged approach to communicating information about distress. Both primary care and oncology staff have documented the distress results and verbally communicated with the provider. Importantly, all oncology team members have participated in the communication loop so that resources needed

to address concerns could be marshaled early as difficulties were identified.

BARRIERS TO TREATMENT

Distress screening implementation can only be called a success if treatment has improved the experience of illness. From stoicism and stigma against mental illness to availability and structural problems with access, many obstacles to receiving adequate treatment have been identified.

Stigma

One of the strongest barriers to patient care has been the stigma provoked by cancer-related distress. Despite regular MSTI meetings that emphasize addressing patient distress, patients still often fail to complete the distress score. Staff admit that they do not encourage completion of the distress score because they are uncomfortable addressing the screening questions. This avoidance behavior likely originated from stigmatization of patients who are struggling.[12]

Although the VA has a multifaceted approach to improving the mental health of veterans, small items can magnify stigma. To expedite complex services and limit infectious exposure, the BVAMC oncology clinic has asked cancer patients to go to the front of the queue for blood draws. The following is one veteran's view of this practice: "They send me to the front of the line; I guess they don't think I'll live that long." These observations point to the importance of addressing what appears to be discrimination, but evidence for reducing stigma remains sparse.[13]

Stoicism

The following case illustrates one of the unique challenges that health care givers face with veterans. A veteran's family called and voiced that the patient was depressed and potentially suicidal, but they believed that he would reject mental health intervention. Several visits with both oncology and mental health were required to break through this veteran's web of justifications for his irritability and depression. The VA integrated system allowed the care team to expand the focus of care from the cancer to this veteran's mental health.

MODEL OF CARE INFLUENCES AVAILABILITY AND ACCEPTABILITY OF DISTRESS TREATMENT

At MSTI, although in-house mental health staffing improved access, significant obstacles have remained for many patients with non-emergent problems. A practitioner who transitioned from the community to the VA noted, "In private practice, the insurance companies, and the mental health units made mental health access extremely difficult. For distressed patients, what takes 10 minutes in the VA, would take two or more hours in private practice." The VA system has emphasized mental health access and minimized payment barriers. This integration has allowed oncology patients to have distress addressed before the first visit to the oncology clinic. However, there have been limitations. None of the mental health professionals have oncology-specific training. In addition, when patients receive care outside the VA through the Choice program, they often lose access to the triggers for mental health intervention. Although Choice has matured and errors have decreased, fragmentation in communication through third-party oversight has remained.

CONCLUSION

There are significant cultural differences between cancer care in the private sector and that in the VA. The multiple obstacles to managing distress in cancer patients have been approached with a variety of tools in the community, but the approach has been fragmented. The VA integrated model has allowed a comprehensive approach to cancer patients. One summary from a practitioner that joined the VA after years in the community illustrates the difference: "The culture of the VA leads to an expectation that mental health will be addressed. There may be a concentration of patients needing mental health services, and this prevalence might help justify the provision of services." However, in the private sector, the lack of services or insurance coverage does not stem from rarity; even in the private world, the incidence of distress is approximately 40%.[14] Instead, the VA simply has a higher proportion of staff focused on patient distress.

REFERENCES

1. Hewitt ME, Simone JV; National Cancer Policy Board. *Ensuring Quality Cancer Care.* Washington, DC: National Academies Press; 1999. http://books.nap.edu/books/0309064805/html/index.html.

2. Greene F. *Cancer Program Standards 2012: Version 1.2.1.* Chicago: American College of Surgeons Commission on Cancer; 2012. https://www.facs.org/~/media/files/quality%20programs/cancer/coc/programstandards2012updates.ashx.

3. Zebrack B, Kayser K, Sundstrom L, et al. Psychosocial distress screening implementation in cancer care: An analysis of adherence, responsiveness, and acceptability. *J Clin Oncol.* 2015;33(10):1165–1170. https://www.ncbi.nlm.nih.gov/pubmed/25713427.

4. Walling AM, Tisnado D, Asch SM, et al. The quality of supportive cancer care in the Veterans Affairs health system and targets for improvement. *JAMA Intern Med.* 2013;123(22):2071–2079. https://www.ncbi.nlm.nih.gov/pubmed/24126685.

5. Passik SD, Dugan W, McDonald MV, et al. Oncologists' recognition of depression in their patients with cancer. *J Clin Oncol.* 1998;16(4):1594–1600. https://www.ncbi.nlm.nih.gov/pubmed/9552071.

6. Mulligan EA, Wachen JS, Naik AD, Gosian J, Moye J. Cancer as a criterion A traumatic stressor for veterans: Prevalence and correlates. *Psychol Trauma.* 2014;6(Suppl 1):S73–S81. https://www.ncbi.nlm.nih.gov/pubmed/25741406.

7. Zullig LL, Williams CD, Fortune-Britt AG. Lung and colorectal cancer treatment and outcomes in the Veterans Affairs health care system. *Cancer Manag Res.* 2015;7:19–35. https://www.ncbi.nlm.nih.gov/pubmed/25609998.

8. Stirman SW, Miller CJ, Toder K, Calloway A. Development of a framework and coding system for modifications and adaptations of evidence-based interventions. *Implement Sci.* 2013;8(4):65. https://www.ncbi.nlm.nih.gov/pubmed/23758995.

9. Yano EM, Chaney EF, Campbell DG, et al. Yield of practice-based depression screening in VA primary care settings. *J Gen Intern Med.* 2012;27(3):331–338. https://www.ncbi.nlm.nih.gov/pubmed/21975821.

10. Velikova G, Booth L, Smith AB, et al. Measuring quality of life in routine oncology practice improves communication and patient

well-being: A randomized controlled trial. *J Clin Oncol.* 2004;22(4):714–724. https://www.ncbi.nlm.nih.gov/pubmed/14966096.

11. Wagner LI, Pugh SL, Small W Jr, et al. Screening for depression in cancer patients receiving radiotherapy: Feasibility and identification of effective tools in the NRG Oncology RTOG 0841 trial. *Cancer.* 2017;123(3):485–493. https://www.ncbi.nlm.nih.gov/pubmed/27861753.

12. Campbell DG, Bonner LM, Bolkan CR, et al. Stigma predicts treatment preferences and care engagement among Veterans Affairs primary care patients with depression. *Ann Behav Med.* 2016;50:(4):533–544. https://www.ncbi.nlm.nih.gov/pubmed/26935310.

13. Griffith JL, Kohrt BA. Managing stigma effectively: What social psychology and social neuroscience can teach us. *Acad Psychiatry.* 2016;40(2):339–347. https://www.ncbi.nlm.nih.gov/pubmed/26162463.

14. Carlson LE, Waller A, Mitchell AJ. Screening for distress and unmet needs in patients with cancer: Review and recommendations. *J Clin Oncol.* 2012;30(11):1160–1177. https://www.ncbi.nlm.nih.gov/pubmed/22412146.

Case Study 10D

IMPLEMENTING LYNCH SYNDROME SCREENING IN THE VETERANS HEALTH ADMINISTRATION

Maren T. Scheuner, Marcia Russell, Jane Peredo, Alison B. Hamilton, and Elizabeth M. Yano

AN INTEGRATED health care delivery system promotes patient-centered care and better meets the health care needs of the populations served by striving for better quality at lower cost, with a focus on population health.[1] The Veterans Health Administration (VHA) is an example of an integrated health care system, providing care to more than 9 million enrolled veterans each year at more than 1,200 health care facilities, including 170 VA Medical Centers (VAMCs) and more than 1,000 outpatient sites.[2] The VHA has a common electronic health record (EHR) that can be accessed by providers throughout the system. VAMCs are located within regional Veterans Integrated Service Networks (VISNs) nationwide. Multiple VAMCs and their respective outpatient clinics are connected within each network, and each network is connected to the Central Office in Washington, DC. Resources for health care delivery are organized at the facility or network level. This case study of implementation science in cancer care delivery focuses on a population-based approach to Lynch syndrome (LS) screening that leverages the organizational structures and processes typically found in integrated health care systems.

LYNCH SYNDROME SCREENING: A CASE STUDY FOR IMPLEMENTATION SCIENCE

Diagnosing LS in patients with colorectal cancer (CRC) is key to ensuring high-quality care that has important patient and public health outcomes. Community-based estimates suggest 1 in every 35 individuals with CRC has LS.[3] LS is due to an inherited mutation in a mismatch repair gene (*MSH2, MLH1, MSH6,* or *PMS2*) or *8EPCAM* that predisposes to high lifetime risks for multiple primary CRCs and other cancers that develop at a younger age than typically expected.[4] Timely diagnosis of LS is critical to informing the extent of surgery at the time of CRC diagnosis and recommendations for enhanced cancer surveillance for early detection of new primary CRCs or their adenoma precursors, which can reduce CRC incidence and all-cause mortality in these high-risk individuals.[5] Moreover, diagnosing LS may have health benefits for at-risk family members through cascade testing, allowing for individualized cancer surveillance and prevention that can be life-saving.[5,6]

Lynch syndrome screening in a tumor specimen is performed by immunohistochemistry (IHC) staining to search for the absence of mismatch repair proteins or by molecular testing for evaluation of microsatellite instability (MSI). For individuals with a positive screen, the LS diagnosis is confirmed by detecting a pathogenic variant in germline DNA or if their family history meets clinical criteria. LS screening results in tumor tissue can also inform CRC treatment decisions. Tumors that have high MSI do not respond to fluorouracil-based chemotherapy,[7] but they do respond to treatment with programmed-death-1 (PD-1) blockade.[8]

Lynch syndrome is an exemplar case study for implementation science in integrated health care systems because of the population-based approach to screening; access to specialized screening and diagnostic tests; the need for specialized expertise; coordination of care between specialty clinicians and the laboratory; and transfer of knowledge to clinicians, the patient, and family that has implications for cancer surveillance, prevention, and treatment.

IMPLEMENTATION SCIENCE INFORMS LYNCH SYNDROME SCREENING IN THE VETERANS HEALTH ADMINISTRATION

The VHA Genomic Medicine Program Advisory Committee identified LS as a high-priority genetic condition relevant to the veteran population. In the following sections, we describe the pre-implementation, active implementation, and post-implementation activities of the LS Screening Program for VISN 22, which at the time included five VAMCs—four in Southern California and one in Las Vegas, Nevada. Our team was interdisciplinary, with expertise in medical genetics, genetic counseling, CRC care, medical anthropology, organizational theory, and implementation science. We also convened an advisory committee

composed of VA and non-VA stakeholders with LS expertise relevant to LS. Our advisors were instrumental in guiding the planning and execution of the LS Screening Program.

Pre-implementation Activities

We conducted 46 semi-structured interviews with key stakeholders in VISN 22 who might encounter patients with LS. We convened clinical and administrative leadership from the network to inform them of our findings. Upon review of the evidence and considering the needs of veterans, the network leadership agreed to support an LS screening protocol that targeted all newly diagnosed CRC cases aged 60 years or younger and also older CRC cases with a personal or family history of LS-associated cancer. The VISN 22 Clinical Genetics Program was selected to spearhead the effort, and a CRC surgeon emerged as a clinical champion of the program. Implementation strategies were selected that addressed challenges to implementation and leveraged the organizational structures and processes in the VHA, including a *registry* to identify all newly diagnosed CRC cases by extracting data from the data warehouse supporting the EHRs in the network; a *case manager* to track eligible CRC cases, monitor the LS screening process, and remind responsible clinicians to ensure LS screening and that screen-positive cases are to be referred for diagnostic evaluation; and *centralized technical assistance* from a VA laboratory to perform LS screening and from the VISN 22 Clinical Genetics Program to provide genetic services, monitor fidelity to the intervention, and assess observed versus expected results based on published experience of others.

Active Implementation Activities

After the launch of the VISN 22 LS Screening Program, we conducted (1) progress-focused activities to monitor impacts and indicators of progress toward the project goals and used data to inform need for modifying the original implementation strategies and (2) implementation-focused activities to assess discrepancies between implementation plan and execution; explore issues of fidelity, intensity, and exposure; and understand and document the nature and implications of local adaptation.

Progress-Focused Activities

With creation of the registry, we could assess uptake of LS screening according to the network protocol prior to and after implementation. In the 35 months preceding the launch of the program, there were 602 CRC cases (an average of 17 per month), 10.8% of which were screened for LS; 2.5% had positive LS screening results, and 0.8% were confirmed LS diagnoses. In the first 24 months of the LS Screening Program, there were 364 newly diagnosed CRC patients (an average of 15 per month), of which 145 were eligible for LS screening according to the protocol. Among the eligible cases, 90.3% were screened, with 6.7% having positive LS screening results and 0.9% were diagnosed with LS. Eligible cases not screened were in palliative care, deceased, or there was insufficient tissue to test. Thus, in the first 24 months of the LS Screening Program compared to pre-implementation, the overall screening rate among all CRC cases increased 2.9-fold, and the screen-positive rate increased 1.7-fold. However, LS diagnosis rates did not change.

The proportion of CRC tumors with positive LS screening results and confirmed LS was lower than expected compared to that of similar screening programs outside the VHA. We therefore had concerns about potential false-negative results from IHC screening performed by the centralized VA laboratory. To investigate, MSI testing was performed in a subset of tumors with normal IHC screening results. A minority had positive MSI results, which did not appreciably increase the screen-positive rate but provided evidence that MSI is a more sensitive screening method in the centralized VA laboratory. Given the low LS screen-positive rate, we concluded that veterans with CRC in VISN 22 were different from non-veteran patient populations. Likely reasons include an older patient population, with fewer CRC cases aged 40 years or younger, and higher prevalence of nongenetic risk factors for CRC, such as smoking, alcohol use, diabetes, and obesity. We found rare occurrences of problems with fidelity to the clinical intervention in the laboratory (i.e., simultaneous screening with both IHC and MSI).

Implementation-Focused Activities

We identified several challenges to execution of the implementation plan relating to procedures, personnel, and organizational issues.

Procedural issues arose when more than one CRC specimen was submitted to the laboratory for an eligible patient or when the screening results for two or more specimens from a single patient were discordant. To address these issues, we developed rules for the registry that distinguished a biopsy from a subsequent surgical resection from the same tumor and also a local recurrence from a second primary CRC. For discrepant screening results, diagnostic germline testing was always offered. There were also challenges when a specimen was received from an outside hospital. In these cases, there were substantial delays in receiving pathology reports and LS screening results when already performed or receiving specimens to perform LS screening.

Several challenges arose relating to *personnel issues*. After the first year of the LS Screening Program, one of the two genetic counselors acting as case managers for the registry resigned and was not replaced. Nonclinical staff were trained to perform the case management role; however, they were challenged to identify personal and family history eligibility criteria for older CRC cases. Thus, the remaining genetic counselor became solely responsible for case management of the registry, which was not ideal because interruptions in the tracking and monitoring schedule occurred primarily due to competing clinical demands. Another personnel issue arose 4 months after the launch of the LS Screening Program. At one of the VAMCs, the programmer responsible for entering structured data elements describing CRC pathology into the EHR retired and was not replaced for several months. Without these data, the registry could not capture newly diagnosed CRC cases from this facility. The facility's laboratory director submitted cases to the centralized VA laboratory for LS screening; however, we could not be sure all eligible cases were submitted. Another personnel issue relates to missing or limited documentation of cancer family history by clinicians caring for CRC patients. Without documentation of cancer family history, determining eligibility for older CRC cases was often not possible and an ineligible status was assigned.

Organizational issues also posed implementation challenges. Several months after implementation, consolidation of many VISNs occurred throughout the country, which directly affected the LS Screening Program because the Las Vegas VAMC was reassigned to another network. Data from the Las Vegas EHR were no longer available through the network data warehouse, and the LS registry could not identify CRC cases to enable monitoring of LS screening at that facility. Another organizational issue we identified was linked to inconsistent procedures at the centralized VA laboratory to manage receipt of specimens for LS screening, which was particularly problematic when there were staffing changes in the laboratory.

Implementation Fidelity, Intensity, and Exposure

Involvement of the case manager was necessary to ensure LS screening happened according to protocol for 63% of eligible CRC cases. The case manager prompted the responsible clinician every 2 weeks after a CRC diagnosis if screening had not occurred, which increased LS screening rates with variable success. If LS screening had not occurred after 6 weeks, the clinical geneticist requested screening; in the first 24 months, this occurred for 10% and 38% of eligible CRC cases aged 60 years or younger and those older than 60 years, respectively. There were no significant trends in LS screening rates, suggesting no change in behavior of responsible clinicians. In addition, there was substantial variability between VAMCs in reflexive LS screening of eligible CRC cases aged 60 years or younger by the laboratory (ranging from 37.5% to 83.3%) and among cases older than 60 years initiated by a gastroenterologist or surgeon (ranging from 0% to 52.9%). Feedback about screening variability was shared with network and facility leadership periodically throughout active implementation without an effect on performance.

We also observed CRC tumor screening performed when eligibility criteria were lacking. Among the 219 cases without eligibility criteria, 4.6% were screened; 1.4% had positive screening results, and none were diagnosed with LS. Tumor screening may have been requested to inform treatment options, or a family history of LS-associated cancers may have been elicited but not documented in the EHR.

Post-implementation Maintenance and Sustainability

We held two meetings with our advisory committee to review our progress after 12 and 24 months of implementation. We presented results from the progress- and implementation-focused activities to assess the usefulness and value of the VISN 22 LS Screening Program and to elicit recommendations for further intervention refinements. During each meeting, we asked whether the program should continue, given the low rates of positive screening results and LS diagnosis; there was unanimous agreement that the program was valuable and should continue. Yet, given staffing limitations in the centralized VA laboratory and the VISN 22 Clinical Genetics Program, there were concerns regarding sustainability.

After the 24-month meeting, several modifications to the LS Screening Program were recommended, including a change from IHC staining for mismatch repair proteins to MSI testing as the preferred LS screening method. This change was recommended given our experience with the performance of the two screening modalities in the centralized VA laboratory and the use of MSI results to inform other clinical decisions relating to treatment of CRC (5-fluorouracil for stage II cancers and PD-1 blockade for metastatic disease). In addition, our preliminary budget impact analysis found a similar cost for IHC and MSI screening. Last, MSI testing is an orderable item in the EHR laboratory menu, whereas IHC testing is not. As such, MSI test results are discrete data that are pulled into the LS registry from the EHR, which facilitates monitoring of the LS screening process.

Universal LS screening was also recommended to replace targeted screening by age and family history criteria. This was recommended in large part because of the evolving evidence for universal screening and the endorsement of universal screening from several professional organizations. The advisory committee also recognized the challenges of determining eligibility for older CRC cases (i.e., limited documentation of cancer family history in the EHR and the increased case management time needed to review the record to characterize eligibility). In addition, new clinical indications for screening CRC tumors for MSI emerged (i.e., PD-1 blockade for metastatic disease).[8]

Finally, we discussed the need to adapt the clinical intervention of LS screening as new technologies are developed. The VHA has initiated a Precision Oncology Program that utilizes next-generation sequencing (NGS) in DNA extracted from tumor tissue to identify gene variants that are the targets of specific cancer therapies. NGS testing of DNA extracted from normal tissue from a biopsy or resection specimen can directly inform a diagnosis of a hereditary cancer syndrome, such as LS. Thus, NGS of DNA from a CRC specimen could supplant the current recommendations for LS screening and diagnosis if the change were cost-neutral. However, this would pose additional implementation challenges that would need to be addressed.

CONCLUSION

Lynch syndrome screening provides a useful case study of the multilevel factors that influence implementation and sustainability of a cancer care program in an integrated health care system. We identified multiple implementation strategies that leveraged organizational structures and processes of the VHA that are characteristic of integrated health care systems and ensured successful LS screening of nearly all eligible CRC cases. However, the low prevalence of LS among the veterans in VISN 22 and the similar LS diagnosis rate before and after implementation of the LS Screening Program raised concerns about the value of a population-based approach to LS screening. This was compounded by implementation challenges of limited personnel with the necessary expertise, competing clinical priorities, and organizational changes. Last, with the evolving field of precision oncology, the clinical intervention of LS screening itself may be replaced by more comprehensive

diagnostic testing in tumor tissue, creating the need for a different implementation plan.

REFERENCES

1. Armitage GD, Suter E, Oelke ND, Adair CE. Health systems integration: State of the evidence. *Int J Integr Care*. 2009;9:e82.
2. About VHA. US Department of Veterans Affairs website. https://www.va.gov/health/aboutvha. asp. Accessed July 4, 2017.
3. Hampel H, Frankel WL, Martin E, et al. Feasibility of screening for Lynch syndrome among patients with colorectal cancer. *J Clin Oncol*. 2008;26(35):5783–5788.
4. Kohlmann W, Gruber SB. Lynch syndrome. *GeneReviews* [Internet] 2004. https://www.ncbi. nlm.nih.gov/books/NBK1211. Accessed July 4, 2017.
5. de Vos tot Nederveen Cappel WH, Järvinen HJ, Lynch PM, et al. Colorectal surveillance in Lynch syndrome families. *Fam Cancer*. 2013;12(2):261–265.
6. Hampel H. Genetic counseling and cascade genetic testing in Lynch syndrome. *Fam Cancer*. 2016;15(3):423–427.
7. Kawakami H, Zaanan A, Sinicrope FA. Microsatellite instability testing and its role in the management of colorectal cancer. *Curr Treat Options Oncol*. 2015;16(7):30.
8. Le DT, Uram JN, Wang H, et al. PD-1 blockade in tumors with mismatch-repair deficiency. *N Engl J Med*. 2015;372:2509–2520.

11

CANCER SURVIVORSHIP

OVERVIEW OF CASE STUDIES

Julia H. Rowland

SURVIVORSHIP SCIENCE, having secured its unique place on the cancer control continuum, is now well into its young adulthood.[1,2] The field's early years were spent largely mapping out the landscape of life after cancer for the millions living long term following their diagnosis. Descriptive and epidemiologic studies dominated in publications by survivorship researchers. The past decade has seen a steady shift in this pattern away from reports detailing the challenges post-treatment to more studies addressing them.[3] The body of literature on interventions to prevent when possible, or mitigate when not, the adverse effects of cancer and its treatment on individuals and their families is growing steadily.[4] As we advance into the new millennium, the emerging challenge for survivorship science is determining how best to translate what we already know into better care for those living with and beyond cancer.[5]

The three case studies included here illustrate well the unique barriers to bridging the implementation gap in survivorship science and potential solutions to address these barriers. The studies also reflect the spectrum of implementation readiness seen in today's interventions, from being "ready for prime time" to establishing metrics for success and identifying the right intervention for a known problem.

The benefits of continued physical activity among cancer survivors are well established (particularly among breast cancer survivors) and multiple, ranging from improved mood, lower fatigue, and better overall quality of life to enhanced tolerance for treatment, lower risk of other co-morbid conditions, and even longer survival.[6] A number of interventions to promote physical activity among survivors have proven effective in increasing rates of activity and reducing sedentary behavior.[6] Among these is the well-designed and studied Physical Activity and Lymphedema (PAL) program developed by Kathryn Schmitz and colleagues.[7]

When originally introduced, the PAL program was important in debunking the myth that breast cancer survivors experiencing lymphedema should avoid vigorous activity or use of the affected arm. Schmitz and colleagues' research found no increase in lymphedema among women participating in their carefully monitored program. Furthermore, data suggested a beneficial effect on reducing risk for subsequent onset of the condition.[7] The challenge then became how to encourage oncology care providers to recommend this care and women to engage in it. In their case study, Schmitz and Beidas, applying the Consolidated Framework for Implementation Research,[8] thoughtfully walk through the multilayered approach they followed to adapt their intervention for routine use. The strategy permitted them to examine what was needed to make their PAL intervention acceptable for women and their health care providers and readily implemented within the health care setting.

By comparison, the case study presented by Birken and colleagues tackles the implementation approach needed when the intervention is largely spelled out, but its impact—and hence potential buy-in for uptake—has yet to be determined. Use of survivorship care plans (SCPs) is recommended to help facilitate the transition for cancer survivors and their health care providers from active treatment to recovery and life beyond cancer.[9] Belief in the value of SCPs led to their use becoming a standard of quality cancer care.[10] Despite this, uptake of the practice of generating and delivering SCPs is variable at best and a target of considerable resistance at worst. As Birken and colleagues cogently argue, beyond the multiple practical barriers (demands on specific technology, time constraints, turnover in staff, lack of champions to promote use, and differing goals of care in diverse settings), a significant challenge to implementation of SCPs is the absence of proven benefit, with one notable exception,[11] to patient outcomes, or at least those studied to date. Some argue that we have yet to determine the appropriate outcomes that might be affected by the process of SCP implementation.[12] Improving satisfaction with care (already rated as high) or reducing distress (relatively low in patients completing therapy) are hard markers to move, especially if these documents are simply handed or sent to recipients without discussion, as happens in some settings. Importantly, interventions that demand not simply behavior but also culture change are doomed to failure if the fundamental question of "What's in it for me?" cannot be satisfactorily answered for all parties required for successful engagement—hence the emphasis in this case study on the need for incorporation of stakeholders' perspectives in any implementation process.

In the third case study, addressing cancer-related threats to employment status, we have a problem in search of a solution. In earlier decades, when survivors did not outlive their cancer diagnosis, concern about return to work was not a critical focus of attention. Now that most will live years and often decades after treatment, ensuring that these individuals can remain at or return to the workforce as needed or desired is becoming critical. The importance of employment not only as a source of income and often health insurance but also as a source of support and self-esteem is increasingly recognized.[13] As de Moor and colleagues note, however, few interventions currently exist to address this common challenge and the financial toxicity that often accompanies job loss, lock, or impairment.[14] They articulate the need for a process to identify those at risk, inform them about cancer's impact, and provide education regarding as well as access to resources to mitigate this risk as key next steps in implementing a program likely to change the picture for those affected.

An overarching theme across all three survivorship science case studies is the focus on cancer rehabilitation. Cancer has the potential to adversely affect all aspects of an individual's life, from physical (lymphedema and deconditioning) to financial. Finding and delivering interventions to reduce risk before treatment starts and planning for recovery when treatment ends (using SCPs) will be needed if we are to reduce the burden of cancer on individuals, families, and society. Toward this end, designing programs for successful implementation from the outset, while simultaneously acknowledging the diversity of the survivor population, their needs across the course of care, and the settings in which they are served and by whom,[15] will be critical to successfully realize this lofty goal.

REFERENCES

1. Rowland JH. Cancer Survivorship: New Challenge in Cancer Medicine. In: Bast RC, Croce CM, Hait WN, et al., eds. *Holland-Frei Cancer Medicine.* 9th ed. Hoboken, NJ: Wiley; 2017;909—916.
2. Rowland JH, Kent EE, Forsythe LP, et al. Cancer survivorship research in Europe and the United States: Where have we been, where are we going,

and what can we learn from each other? *Cancer.* 2013;119(11 Suppl):2094–2108.

3. Harrop JP, Dean JA, Paskett ED. Cancer survivorship research: A review of the literature and summary of current NCI-designated cancer center projects. *Cancer Epidemiol Biomarkers Prev.* 2011;20(10):2042–2047.

4. Stanton A, Rowland JH, Ganz PA. Life after diagnosis and treatment of cancer in adulthood. *Am Psychol.* 2015;70(2):159–174.

5. Alfano CM, Smith T, de Moor JS, et al. An action plan for translating cancer survivorship research into care. *J Natl Cancer Inst.* 2014;106(11);dju287.

6. Ligibel J. Lifestyle factors in cancer survivorship. *J Clin Oncol.* 2012;30(30):3697–3704.

7. Schmitz KH, Ahmed RL, Troxel A, et al. Weight lifting in women with breast-cancer-related lymphedema. *N Engl J Med.* 2009;361:664–673.

8. Damschroder LJ, Aron DC, Keith RE, Kirsh SR, Alexander JA, Lowery JC. Fostering implementation of health services research findings into practice: A consolidated framework or advancing implementation science. *Implement Sci.* 2009;4:50.

9. Hewitt M, Greenfield S, Stovall E, eds. *From Cancer Patient to Cancer Survivor: Lost in Transition.* Washington, DC: National Academies Press; 2006.

10. American College of Surgeons, Commission on Cancer. *Cancer Program Standards: Ensuring Patient-Centered Care (2016 Edition).* Chicago: American College of Surgeons; 2015 (Standard 3.3: Survivorship Care Plan, pp. 58–59).

11. Maly RC, Liang LJ, Liu Y, Griggs JJ, Ganz PA. Randomized controlled trial of survivorship care plans among low income, predominantly Latina breast cancer survivors. *J Clin Oncol.* 2017;35(16):1814–1821.

12. Parry C, Kent EE, Forsythe LP, Alfano CM, Rowland JH. Can't see the forest for the care plan: A call to revisit the context of care planning. *J Clin Oncol.* 2013;31(21):2651–2653.

13. Bradley CJ. Economic recovery: A measure of the quality of cancer treatment and survivorship? *Cancer.* 2015;12(24):4282–4285.

14. de Souza JA, Conti RM. Mitigating financial toxicity among US patients with cancer. *JAMA Oncol.* 2017;3(6):765–766.

15. Jacobsen PB, Rowland JH, Paskett ED, et al. Identification of key gaps in cancer survivorship research: Findings from the American Society of Clinical Oncology survey. *J Oncol Pract.* 2016;12(3):190–193.

Case Study 11A

IMPLEMENTING AN EVIDENCE-BASED EXERCISE PROGRAM FOR BREAST CANCER SURVIVORS

Kathryn H. Schmitz and Rinad Beidas

PROBLEMS THAT ARISE AFTER BREAST CANCER

Five-year disease-free survival is 89% for women diagnosed with breast cancer.[1] It is estimated that there are 3.5 million women living in the United States who have undergone treatment for breast cancer. Although increases in disease-free survival are certainly good news, the risk of recurrence remains a threat for the remainder of life after breast cancer. Furthermore, there are persistent adverse effects of breast cancer treatment that cause significant morbidity. Common adverse effects associated with treatment include loss of upper body strength and function, damage to the lymphatic system, fatigue, and weight gain.[2–4,5,6] These changes in upper body strength and function can then result in difficulties in fully returning to work and caring for self and family.[7]

EXERCISE BENEFITS FOR BREAST CANCER SURVIVORS

Exercise may be a low-cost, evidence-based intervention, with potential for scale-up, to address the challenge of recovering after breast cancer treatment. There have been hundreds of high-quality randomized controlled exercise trials in breast cancer survivors.[8–13] Benefits include improved upper body strength, physical function, lymphedema, quality of life, lessened fatigue, and reduced depression.[11,14–16]

Evidence of the benefits of exercise after breast cancer is provided by the Physical Activity and Lymphedema (PAL) trial, which led to significant and clinically meaningful improvements in lymphedema symptoms and reduced the need for therapist-delivered treatment among women who entered the study with a diagnosis of lymphedema.[20] Furthermore, the intervention also reduced the likelihood of increased arm swelling (the definition of lymphedema onset) by 70% among the subset of women who entered the study at elevated risk of lymphedema onset because they had had five or more lymph nodes removed.[14] In addition, the PAL intervention improved upper body strength compared to a no exercise comparison group.[14,20] Other documented benefits of the PAL protocol include improved physical function, lymphedema symptoms, body image, appendicular skeletal muscle mass, lower body strength, and body composition and reduced likelihood of lymphedema onset or worsening.[15,21,22] During the 7 years since completing the PAL trial, our colleagues and us have worked to translate this evidence-based intervention into a format that would facilitate implementation in breast cancer clinical practice.

We adapted the PAL intervention to implement it at Good Shepherd Penn Partners (the outpatient rehabilitation partner for the Abramson Cancer Center at the University of Pennsylvania). The Consolidated Framework for Implementation Research (CFIR)[23] was used to guide evaluation of the translation and implementation of the revised intervention in the new setting of the physical therapy clinic. We specifically focused on four of the five major domains from CFIR in our evaluation: intervention characteristics (e.g., complexity), outer setting (e.g., patients' needs), inner setting (e.g., needs of those referring patients and delivering the intervention), and the process used to implement the program (e.g., engagement of key stakeholders, fit within existing clinic structure, and adaptability). The effectiveness of the revised intervention with regard to upper body strength was statistically equivalent to the benefits of the PAL trial.[24]

Intervention Characteristics

The primary intervention characteristic that seemed to be problematic was the request of the developers to deliver the intervention in group physical therapy sessions. This is counter to how outpatient rehabilitation clinicians practice. Once we allowed for individual sessions, the physical therapists felt more comfortable with the implementation. Another implementation challenge was distance from patient to intervention location. We were able to open six locations, and this approach allowed more women to access Strength After Breast Cancer (SABC).

Outer Setting

Intervention cost was a major barrier for participation. After debating whether to seek third-party payer coverage or to proceed with a self-pay model, we opted for both. It seems that was wise. Many women had co-pays of $80 or more for a visit to outpatient rehabilitation. The self-pay cost per session was $37.50. For many women, the least expensive approach was to apply the evaluation to insurance (the self-pay cost of the evaluation was $229) but then to self-pay $37.50 for all subsequent sessions. However, the third-party coverage also enabled women for whom Medicare or Medicaid was their only coverage to attend the program for minimal cost. During the study (and since), no breast cancer survivor's insurance company refused payment for the SABC program. In addition, patients required home equipment to do the intervention. This posed a challenge for the outpatient rehabilitation clinicians and their patients due to the cost. Solutions included solicitation of donations from a manufacturer of adjustable dumb-bells and recommendations to purchase three to five pairs of light dumb-bells (3–15 pounds) at a local sporting goods store.

Inner Setting

Another major barrier to program implementation was the need for clinician referrals. Our first approaches to addressing this were the development and delivery of a clinician training for making referrals, as well as the creation of a "smart set" within the electronic health record system to ease logistical steps required for recruitment. The oncology providers had to print a hard-copy referral prescription for physical therapy evaluation and treatment and hand it to the patient, in addition to recording the referral in the electronic medical record. Despite making this process as simple as possible (three clicks of a mouse), in many cases it was too labor-intensive and confusing for busy clinicians to complete. One group of clinicians promised every patient in their clinic was referred into the program, yet none of these women made appointments to start the program. Further investigation revealed that these clinicians were unaware of the need to print the prescription for physical therapy and for the women to follow-up actively by calling the outpatient rehabilitation clinic to make an appointment. Because of how other referrals within that health system worked, the assumption was that the outpatient rehabilitation clinic would actively follow-up to call each woman for an appointment. This confusion led to the suggestion that the outpatient rehabilitation clinic make these active follow-up calls. Prior to making this change, 39% of referred women scheduled a pre-program assessment. After starting the active follow-up calls after clinician referrals, the outpatient rehabilitation clinic increased the proportion of referred women who scheduled a pre-program assessment to 65%. Future studies may want to explore the importance of the active follow-up to referral in implementing cancer rehabilitation and exercise programs.

The need for active follow-up calls was among several challenges that made clear the need for a champion in the outpatient rehabilitation setting. The champion acted as the chief problem-solver to implement a program that did not follow the usual pattern of clinical care offered in that setting. This champion was also essential to identifying necessary adaptations to the program implementation and assisting the research team in making those changes. First, adaptations were needed in the trainings for the physical therapists, principally explaining that they should adapt and individualize the SABC program to the needs of their patients. Second, we added a staff liaison in the oncology clinic to assist with referrals. Third, we started the active calls noted previously.

Provision of lymphedema education is crucial for breast cancer patients to understand the effects of their breast cancer treatment on their lymphatic systems, as well as what this means for their exercise program. To address this, we developed a power point presentation that outpatient rehabilitation clinicians could deliver to their patients. We provided training to outpatient rehabilitation clinicians to deliver the session.

We were aware that the training we provided to intervention staff was specialty training, not broadly available, and came at a cost (time away from usual job tasks). As such, we sought an implementation setting with relatively stable staff (to reduce the frequency with which training would need to be repeated at a given site). To minimize training time, we also sought a setting with relatively high educational levels regarding anatomy, physiology, injury prevention, and ability to follow protocols. We addressed these challenges by placing the intervention in an outpatient rehabilitation clinic. This setting also addressed the challenge of ensuring that all of the breast cancer survivors in the program would receive a high-quality pre-intervention evaluation to rule out those for whom the intervention would not be medically advisable. In the outpatient rehabilitation setting, a clinical pre-evaluation with a licensed physical therapist is required prior to any intervention.

Process to Implement the Program

To successfully implement the SABC program in a manner that would maximize safety and effectiveness, we needed to identify a setting that could provide supervised exercise with a low interventionist to patient ratio, the opportunity for ongoing re-evaluations in the event of symptom changes, and ongoing exercise adherence monitoring. To address each of these challenges, we chose to implement within an outpatient rehabilitation clinic. Doing so required some adaptations, including flexibility regarding group versus individual sessions.

CURRENT STATUS AND FUTURE STEPS OF THE STRENGTH AFTER BREAST CANCER PROGRAM IMPLEMENTATION

We continue to work on the implementation of SABC beyond the local efforts described previously. An online training is available to teach outpatient rehabilitation clinicians how to deliver the intervention (http://klosetraining.com/SABC). The training went live in spring 2014. More than 400 physical therapists had paid for the training by the summer of 2017. It is not currently known how many breast cancer survivors have received the SABC program. There is currently no system in place to evaluate whether these outpatient rehabilitation professionals are implementing SABC or whether they are delivering the program with fidelity to the training. Given that training is a necessary, but not sufficient, component of implementing a program,[25] there are clear opportunities for further research on the SABC program. Questions that remain include the following:

1. Would the implementation process work the same way in a community health system as it did in an academic health system?

2. What would be needed to create the conditions whereby the oncology clinicians make this referral as a part of the standard of care?

3. What are the characteristics of a successful champion for the program?

4. What happens when we alter the cost of the program? Is there a price point above/below which there is a marked change in uptake and/or referrals?

It is also vital that we better understand how clinic-based programs such as SABC will work in a setting with multiple options for exercise program referrals. One of the lessons learned during this study was that women did not view the SABC program as part of their treatment; they viewed it as a leisure time activity they could choose or dismiss. It was common for survivors to tell our staff liaison that they did want to exercise but that they preferred Pilates, Zumba, Curves, yoga, and many other popular forms of exercise. There is little research on the safety and efficacy of these more common community-based exercise programs, particularly for breast cancer survivors. Examination of the characteristics of programs that breast cancer survivors most prefer, and adaptation of SABC to those characteristics, could result in hybrid programs with promise of broad dissemination.

Our research team continues to seek funding to further study the best approaches to evaluate implementation of SABC, as well as other possible methods for scale-up of the PAL intervention (e.g., DVDs, personal trainers, and YMCA programs) for the general benefit of breast cancer survivors. There is little doubt that exercise has benefits worth pursuing for breast cancer survivors. The

Table 11A.1. Challenges and Approaches to Implementing a Strength Training Program for Breast Cancer Survivors

CHALLENGE	APPROACHES
Intervention Characteristics	
Original intervention delivered in group exercise sessions	To facilitate implementation in outpatient rehabilitation, a revision was made to allow for individual training sessions when needed.
Distance from patient to intervention location	Expanded from one to six sites around the metro region.
Outer Setting	
Payment for the program	Third party payer coverage (insurance and/or Medicaid/Medicare) with co-pays or self-pay.
Cost of home equipment for weightlifting	Donations or guidance where to buy multiple pairs of dumbbells.
Inner Setting	
Get oncology clinical staff to refer patients into the program	Place the program within an outpatient rehabilitation clinic partnered with the oncology clinic to increase clinician comfort with making the referral. Develop and deliver oncologist training to explain how to make referrals.
Need for a program champion in the outpatient rehabilitation clinic	Identification of a champion to do telephone follow-up with women referred by their oncologist.
Need for lymphedema education for patients	Creation of a slide deck and training for use by physical therapists.

Table 11A.1　Continued

CHALLENGE	APPROACHES
Staff training in ½ day or less	Place intervention within outpatient rehabilitation clinics, where staff training is high compared to community fitness facilities. This translates into greater background knowledge and reduced time required to complete training.
Staff stability to keep the frequency of staff training required to sustain the program low	Place intervention within outpatient rehabilitation clinics, where staff turnover is low compared to fitness facilities.
Pre-intervention assessments to ensure safety of participation	Physician referral required to undergo pre-intervention assessment. Physical therapists conducted assessments for all women regardless of lymphedema status.

Process for Program Implementation

Need for supervised exercise sessions to teach the program	Set the intervention within outpatient rehabilitation clinics.
Need for low ratio of supervisor to survivors in small group sessions	Require that clinics not exceed one physical therapist to seven or fewer survivors.
Need for ongoing safety assessments	Pre-evaluation, weekly by symptoms (self-monitoring), discharge evaluation, and recommendation that the patient return every 6 months for re-evaluation by physical therapists.
Method for follow-up if survivor needed help/assessment	Option to repeat elements of the program or assessments with physical therapists.
Exercise adherence monitoring	Self-reported on exercise logs completed by survivors.

unanswered questions include the format, setting, and cost that will maximize safety, efficacy, uptake, and maintenance on the part of the organizations that offer the program, as well as for survivors (Table 11A.1).

REFERENCES

1. American Cancer Society. *Cancer Facts and Figures 2016.* Atlanta, GA: American Cancer Society; 2016.
2. Schmitz KH, Speck RM, Rye SA, DiSipio T, Hayes SC. Prevalence of breast cancer treatment sequelae over 6 years of follow-up: The Pulling Through Study. *Cancer.* 2012;118(8 Suppl):2217–2225.
3. Verbelen H, Gebruers N, Eeckhout FM, Verlinden K, Tjalma W. Shoulder and arm morbidity in sentinel node-negative breast cancer patients: A systematic review. *Breast Cancer Res Treat.* 2014;144(1):21–31.
4. Rietman JS, Dijkstra PU, Debreczeni R, Geertzen JH, Robinson DP, De Vries J. Impairments, disabilities and health related quality of life after treatment for breast cancer: A follow-up study 2.7 years after surgery. *Disabil Rehabil.* 2004;26(2):78–84.
5. Smith SL. Functional morbidity following latissimus dorsi flap breast reconstruction. *J Adv Pract Oncol.* 2014;5(3):181–187.
6. de Haan AT, Hage JJ, Veeger HEJ, Woerdeman LAE. Function of the pectoralis major muscle after combined skin-sparing mastectomy and

immediate reconstruction by subpectoral implantation of a prosthesis. *Ann Plast Surg.* 2007;59:605–610.

7. Schmitz KH, Cappola AR, Stricker CT, Sweeney C, Norman SA. The intersection of cancer and aging: Establishing the need for breast cancer rehabilitation. *Cancer Epidemiol Biomarkers Prev.* 2007;16(5):866–872.

8. van Vulpen JK, Peeters PH, Velthuis MJ, van der Wall E, May AM. Effects of physical exercise during adjuvant breast cancer treatment on physical and psychosocial dimensions of cancer-related fatigue: A meta-analysis. *Maturitas.* 2016;85:104–111.

9. Cheema BS, Kilbreath SL, Fahey PP, Delaney GP, Atlantis E. Safety and efficacy of progressive resistance training in breast cancer: A systematic review and meta-analysis. *Breast Cancer Res Treat.* 2014;148(2):249–268.

10. Zou LY, Yang L, He XL, Sun M, Xu JJ. Effects of aerobic exercise on cancer-related fatigue in breast cancer patients receiving chemotherapy: A meta-analysis. *Tumour Biol.* 2014;35(6):5659–5667.

11. Brown JC, Huedo-Medina TB, Pescatello LS, Pescatello SM, Ferrer RA, Johnson BT. Efficacy of exercise interventions in modulating cancer-related fatigue among adult cancer survivors: A meta-analysis. *Cancer Epidemiol Biomarkers Prev.* 2011;20(1):123–133.

12. Speck RM, Courneya KS, Masse LC, Duval S, Schmitz KH. An update of controlled physical activity trials in cancer survivors: A systematic review and meta-analysis. *J Cancer Surviv.* 2010;4(2):87–100.

13. Schmitz KH, Holtzman J, Courneya KS, Masse LC, Duval S, Kane R. Controlled physical activity trials in cancer survivors: A systematic review and meta-analysis. *Cancer Epidemiol Biomarkers Prev.* 2005;14(7):1588–1595.

14. Schmitz KH, Ahmed RL, Troxel AB, et al. Weight lifting for women at risk for breast cancer-related lymphedema: A randomized trial. *JAMA.* 2010;304(24):2699–2705.

15. Brown JC, Schmitz KH. Weight lifting and physical function among survivors of breast cancer: A post hoc analysis of a randomized controlled trial. *J Clin Oncol.* 2015;33(19):2184–2189.

16. Brown JC, Huedo-Medina TB, Pescatello LS, et al. The efficacy of exercise in reducing depressive symptoms among cancer survivors: A meta-analysis. *PLoS One.* 2012;7(1):e30955.

17. Kushi LH, Doyle C, McCullough M, et al. American Cancer Society Guidelines on nutrition and physical activity for cancer prevention: Reducing the risk of cancer with healthy food choices and physical activity. *CA Cancer J Clin.* 2012;62(1):30–67.

18. Schmitz KH, Courneya KS, Matthews C, et al. American College of Sports Medicine roundtable on exercise guidelines for cancer survivors. *Med Sci Sports Exerc.* 2010;42(7):1409–1426.

19. Ligibel JA, Denlinger CS. New NCCN guidelines for survivorship care. *J Natl Compr Canc Netw.* 2013;11(5 Suppl):640–644.

20. Schmitz K, Ahmed, RL, Troxel, A, Cheville, A, Smith, R, Grant, LL, Bryan, CJ, Williams-Smith, CT, Greene QP. Weight lifting in women with breast cancer-related lymphedema. *N Engl J Med.* 2009;361:664–673.

21. Brown JC, Schmitz KH. Weight lifting and appendicular skeletal muscle mass among breast cancer survivors: A randomized controlled trial. *Breast Cancer Res Treat.* 2015;151(2):385–392.

22. Speck RM, Gross CR, Hormes JM, et al. Changes in the body image and relationship scale following a one-year strength training trial for breast cancer survivors with or at risk for lymphedema. *Breast Cancer Res Treat.* 2010;121(2):421–430.

23. Damschroder LJ, Aron DC, Keith RE, Kirsh SR, Alexander JA, Lowery JC. Fostering implementation of health services research findings into practice: A consolidated framework for advancing implementation science. *Implement Sci.* 2009;4:50.

24. Beidas RS, Paciotti B, Barg F, et al. A hybrid effectiveness–implementation trial of an evidence-based exercise intervention for breast cancer survivors. *J Natl Cancer Inst Monogr.* 2014;2014(50):338–345.

25. Edmunds JM, Beidas RS, Kendall PC. Dissemination and implementation of evidence-based practices: Training and consultation as implementation strategies. *Clin Psychol.* 2013;20(2):152–165.

Case Study 11B

USING AN IMPLEMENTATION SCIENCE APPROACH TO STUDY AND IMPROVE CANCER SURVIVORS' EMPLOYMENT OUTCOMES

Janet S. de Moor, Catherine M. Alfano, Erin E. Kent, Lynne Padgett, and Melvin Grimes

INTRODUCTION

A cancer diagnosis and treatment can lead to a broad range of symptoms and side effects that interfere with a survivor's ability to work. Common side effects of cancer treatment, such as fatigue, pain, lymphedema, mobility issues, bladder and bowel problems, cognitive dysfunction, and anxiety and depression, can force survivors to take prolonged sick leave, make changes to their schedule and workload, or withdraw from the labor force entirely.[1-4] A growing proportion of survivors are at risk for cancer-related work limitations. Approximately half of all people newly diagnosed with cancer are of working age, defined as ages 20–64 years, and older adults are increasingly working past the age of 65 years.[5,6] Although an estimated two-thirds of cancer survivors return to work at some point after diagnosis, rates of return to work range from 24% to 94%, underscoring the heterogeneity of cancer-related work outcomes.[2]

Employment outcomes are influenced by a complex interaction of factors, including a survivor's sociodemographic characteristics, his or her cancer treatment and functional limitations, and aspects of the work environment.[7,8] For example, older age, advanced disease, and intensive treatment are risk factors for poor work outcomes. Likewise, a physically demanding job and working in an environment that lacks supportive accommodations such as flexibility and access to paid sick leave are also associated with poor work outcomes.[2,9]

Cancer-related work limitations can adversely affect quality of life. Job loss and reduced productivity typically result in lost income, which exacerbates the financial burden of cancer and treatment. Likewise, employment changes can lead to the loss of employer-sponsored health insurance, which may interfere with access to timely and appropriate health care.[10-12] However, working during treatment or returning to work can have important psychosocial benefits, with a survivor's job being an important connection to "normal life" and a distraction from cancer.[13] Given the importance of work, interventions are needed to mitigate the impact of cancer on employment and optimize work outcomes after diagnosis.

CANCER-RELATED WORK LIMITATIONS

A small number of studies have evaluated the impact of "employment interventions," an umbrella term for a diverse set of patient education, psychosocial, physical training, and symptom management services.[14–17] This literature comprises interventions that were designed to improve work outcomes as well as interventions that affect employment by improving the functional limitations associated with cancer treatment. Although individual studies have demonstrated the efficacy of select intervention approaches,[14–17] there is a lack of consensus about the best way to mitigate cancer-related work limitations throughout treatment and recovery. Because cancer-related work limitations are influenced by factors operating at the patient, provider, and employer levels, efforts to optimize employment outcomes after cancer require a suite of multilevel and multidisciplinary strategies to support individuals as they co-navigate cancer treatment and work.[16,18]

CANCER REHABILITATION TO IMPROVE WORK OUTCOMES AFTER CANCER

Cancer rehabilitation is an example of a multidisciplinary approach to care with potential to improve work outcomes among cancer survivors. The goal of cancer rehabilitation is to maintain or restore a patient's functioning, reduce symptom burden, maximize independence, and improve quality of life.[19] The early identification of impairments and timely referral to rehabilitation providers who are trained to diagnose and treat the physical, psychological, and cognitive sequelae of cancer can be important for identifying and addressing functional limitations that may lead to poor work outcomes.[20] Although improvements in functioning should translate into improved ability to work, very few studies testing cancer rehabilitation interventions have included employment outcomes. Therefore, research is needed to simultaneously deliver evidence-based cancer rehabilitation to survivors and specifically evaluate rehabilitation services for their impact on work outcomes. The case presented in Box 11B.1 illustrates the benefits of a referral to

cancer rehabilitation and how a multidisciplinary approach to rehabilitation can improve the domains of functioning that are needed for work.

IMPLEMENTING REHABILITATION INTO CANCER CARE

Referrals to rehabilitation, initiated by the patient or the patient's oncologist, most often occur in response to the presence of debilitating symptoms that interfere with work, such as in Tammy's case. However, treatment planning should ideally include a conversation between oncologists and patients about how treatment will progress, what toxicities should be expected, and how these toxicities might interfere with work. By proactively anticipating symptoms that may occur, the oncology team can discuss how referrals to cancer rehabilitation can help treat these issues and preserve the ability to work.

Regardless of when the referral occurs, rehabilitation should begin with a comprehensive assessment of a person's employment status; the demands of his or her job; the person's organizational role and goals for working; as well as any accommodations to which he or she has access, such as worksite and schedule flexibility and access to paid sick leave. This assessment can help the rehabilitation provider and other members of the care team anticipate how treatment will impact aspects of the survivor's work life. This information can serve as the basis for a tailored plan to help patients navigate the anticipated or current challenges. In Tammy's case, breast cancer treatment had resulted in pain, mobility limitations, and cognitive dysfunction that interfered with her work life and other important roles and activities. Thus, an effective rehabilitation strategy had to be tailored to her symptoms as well as the demands of her job and goals for working.

Although rehabilitation services will vary depending upon a survivor's cancer, their current or anticipated limitations, and the nature of their job, all employed survivors should be provided with a tailored work management plan that includes both an assessment of symptoms that are likely to interfere with their job and either prevention or rehabilitation to address those symptoms. The tailored work management plan should also include education about survivors' legal rights and a list of resources in their communities. Importantly, the tailored work plan should be a tool that will educate and empower

Box 11B.1 Case Study

Tammy P (not her real name) is a 37-year-old woman with a history of stage 2A left breast invasive, poorly differentiated ductal carcinoma that was weakly ER-positive (5%), PR-negative, and HER2-negative. She was initially treated with neoadjuvant AC-T chemotherapy plus carboplatin. She then had a left breast lumpectomy and axillary lymph node dissection with 2 of 13 lymph nodes positive for carcinoma. Resection was followed by 6½ weeks of radiation therapy with 50 Gy in 25 fractions. Tamoxifen treatment was ongoing at the time of evaluation. Tammy self-referred to cancer rehabilitation for left arm pain, potentially secondary to cording or axillary web syndrome from her axillary lymph node dissection. She described her pain as 0/10 at rest and 2/10 with movement. She noted that although she had been a regular exerciser, she was unable to exercise currently.

She also reported irritability secondary to impaired memory and difficulty concentrating, particularly in situations requiring multitasking or attending to multiple stimuli. Her cognitive symptoms limited her ability to work full-time as a researcher. The combination of left arm pain and range-of-motion problems and cognitive dysfunction also limited her ability to care for her child and perform household chores as she had before her surgery. She was evaluated by a physiatrist, who noted axillary cording in her left axilla extending to the medial arm, post-surgical pain, early adhesive capsulitis (frozen shoulder) with splinting and restricted abduction of the left shoulder, intercostal brachial mononeuropathy without neuralgia, and mild cognitive impairment. She was prescribed physical therapy, lymphedema therapy, and cognitive rehabilitation. Physical therapy focused on myofascial release, neuromuscular re-education, range of motion, and strengthening. Comprehensive decongestive therapy targeted largely the chest wall and included manual lymphatic drainage, kinesio taping, and home exercises. Cognitive rehabilitation strategies included remediation and compensatory strategies, as well as cognitive–behavioral techniques and exercises to mitigate the stress of cognitive failures. As a result of these therapies and early detection of the adhesive capsulitis, Tammy's symptoms were improved at 6-week follow-up. She had increased range of motion in her left arm, limited pain, and improved cognition with improvements in both memory and concentration and decreased irritability. She reported restored ability to work full-time in her job, care for her child, and perform household chores. She had also returned to exercising approximately three times per week.

---

cancer survivors to effectively communicate with their employers.

Employers have a central role in either supporting or discouraging work sustainability or return to work following a cancer diagnosis.[6,21,22] Typically, the mode of communication between health care providers and employers is through the administration of paperwork. A health care provider documents the existence of a health-limiting disability or work limitation and sends this to the employer. However, for individuals who wish to keep working or return to work, rehabilitation providers can expand this interaction by providing documentation of the survivor's abilities and specific recommended work accommodations (informed by the comprehensive work assessment). This document can serve as an important communication tool, helping patients initiate conversations with their employer about cancer and a return to work or work sustainability plan.

IMPLEMENTATION CHALLENGES FOR IMPROVING CANCER SURVIVORS' WORK OUTCOMES

Implementation science is needed to overcome the following challenges to integrating rehabilitation into cancer care:

1. Routine screening for employment concerns and referral to cancer rehabilitation are not well-integrated into care. Data are lacking about the

effectiveness of different models of care for the screening and referral of patients to cancer rehabilitation and the collection of a comprehensive work assessment.

2. Patient-reported outcomes of symptoms that interfere with functioning and data on employment are not typically collected and archived in the electronic medical record, which constrains efforts to predict how specific treatments may impact a survivor's ability to be functional at work.

3. A minority of providers assess cancer survivors' concerns about working and actual work limitations as part of treatment decision-making and throughout the course of care. Provider- and system-level barriers to addressing employment concerns and limitations as part of clinical care need to be better understood and managed.

4. Survivors are typically responsible for translating complex medical information about their cancer into information that is salient to their employers. Employers must then act on this information to establish an appropriate set of accommodations to support work-related functioning. Efforts are needed to improve information sharing between survivors and their health care providers and between survivors and their employers. Research is currently lacking to support the different pieces of these interactions.

CONCLUSION

There is a critical need to implement better clinical pathways to identify, monitor, and mitigate the functional limitations that interfere with cancer survivors' ability to work. Information about work ability and employment status should be captured as part of clinical care and clinical trials for new treatments to develop the evidence base that providers can draw upon when advising their patients about the impact of different treatments on aspects of functioning. Research is also needed to evaluate the impact of different rehabilitation delivery approaches on work outcomes. As this body of evidence grows, important question will remain: What are the most effective methods to integrate these research findings into practice? How can these findings be most effectively disseminated to improve practice and thus patient outcomes? These are questions implementation science is uniquely qualified to answer.

REFERENCES

1. Stein KD, Syrjala KL, Andrykowski MA. Physical and psychological long-term and late effects of cancer. Cancer. 2008;112:2577–2592.
2. Mehnert A. Employment and work-related issues in cancer survivors. Crit Rev Oncol Hematol. 2011;77:109–130.
3. Stergiou-Kita M, Grigorovich A, Tseung V, et al. Qualitative meta-synthesis of survivors' work experiences and the development of strategies to facilitate return to work. J Cancer Surviv. 2014;8:657–670.
4. Islam T, Dahlui M, Majid HA, et al. Factors associated with return to work of breast cancer survivors: A systematic review. BMC Public Health. 2014;14(Suppl 3):S8.
5. Siegel RL, Miller KD, Jemal A. Cancer statistics, 2016. CA Cancer J Clin. 2016;66:7–30.
6. Adolescents and young adults with cancer. 2017. National Cancer Institute website. http://www.cancer.gov/types/aya.
7. Feuerstein M, Todd BL, Moskowitz MC, et al. Work in cancer survivors: A model for practice and research. J Cancer Surviv. 2010;4:415–437.
8. Mehnert A, de Boer A, Feuerstein M. Employment challenges for cancer survivors. Cancer. 2013;119(Suppl 11):2151–2159.
9. van Muijen P, Weevers NL, Snels IA, et al. Predictors of return to work and employment in cancer survivors: A systematic review. Eur J Cancer Care (Engl). 2013;22:144–160.
10. Kent EE, Forsythe LP, Yabroff KR, et al. Are survivors who report cancer-related financial problems more likely to forgo or delay medical care? Cancer. 2013;119:3710–3717.
11. Dusetzina SB, Winn AN, Abel GA, Huskamp HA, Keating NL. Cost sharing and adherence to tyrosine kinase inhibitors for patients with chronic myeloid leukemia. J Clin Oncol. 2014;32:306–311.
12. Nekhlyudov L, Madden J, Graves AJ, Zhang F, Soumerai SB, Ross-Degnan D. Cost-related medication nonadherence and cost-saving strategies used by elderly Medicare cancer survivors. J Cancer Surviv. 2011;5:395–404.
13. Blinder VS, Murphy MM, Vahdat LT, et al. Employment after a breast cancer diagnosis: A qualitative study of ethnically diverse urban women. J Community Health. 2012;37:763–772.
14. Bilodeau K, Tremblay D, Durand MJ. Exploration of return-to-work interventions for breast cancer patients: A scoping review. Support Care Cancer. 2017;25:1993–2007.

15. Tamminga SJ, de Boer AG, Verbeek JH, Frings-Dresen MH. Return-to-work interventions integrated into cancer care: A systematic review. *Occup Environ Med.* 2010;67:639–648.

16. de Boer AG, Taskila TK, Tamminga SJ, Feuerstein M, Frings-Dresen MH, Verbeek JH. Interventions to enhance return-to-work for cancer patients. *Cochrane Database Syst Rev.* 2015:Cd007569.

17. Fong CJ, Murphy K, Westbrook JD, Markle M. Behavioral, psychological, educational and vocational interventions to facilitate employment outcomes for cancer survivors: A systematic review. *Campbell Systematic Rev.* 2015;5.

18. Hunter EG, Gibson RW, Arbesman M, D'Amico M. Systematic review of occupational therapy and adult cancer rehabilitation: Part 2. Impact of multidisciplinary rehabilitation and psychosocial, sexuality, and return-to-work interventions. *Am J Occup Ther.* 2017;71:7102100040p710210004–7102100040p7102100048.

19. Silver JK, Raj VS, Fu JB, Wisotzky EM, Smith SR, Kirch RA. Cancer rehabilitation and palliative care: Critical components in the delivery of high-quality oncology services. *Support Care Cancer.* 2015;23:3633–3643.

20. Silver JK, Baima J, Newman R, Galantino ML, Shockney LD. Cancer rehabilitation may improve function in survivors and decrease the economic burden of cancer to individuals and society. *Work.* 2013;46:455–472.

21. Stergiou-Kita M, Pritlove C, van Eerd D, et al. The provision of workplace accommodations following cancer: Survivor, provider, and employer perspectives. *J Cancer Surviv.* 2016;10:489–504.

22. Stergiou-Kita M, Pritlove C, Kirsh B. The "Big C"—Stigma, cancer, and workplace discrimination. *J Cancer Surviv.* 2016;10:1035–1050.

Case Study 11C

THE CHALLENGE OF IMPLEMENTING SURVIVORSHIP CARE PLANS

Sarah A. Birken, Erin E. Hahn, Yan Yu, Emily Haines, Deborah K. Mayer, and Brian Mittman

SURVIVORSHIP CARE PLAN POLICY CONTEXT

The Institute of Medicine's publication, *From Cancer Patient to Cancer Survivor: Lost in Transition,*[1] recommends survivorship care plans (SCPs) as a method of improving post-treatment cancer survivorship care, individualized for cancer patients ending active curative-intent treatment. The publication describes the SCP as a written or electronic document that is meant to be a communication tool that summarizes diagnosis, treatment received, and any associated toxicities; includes a schedule of recommended post-treatment visits and services (e.g., imaging and laboratory tests); documents the oncology care team and contact information; and includes referrals and information for common issues, such as psychological distress. Akin to the hospital discharge summary, the SCP was conceptualized as a relatively simple way to guide cancer survivors, family members, and clinicians with respect to (1) what had happened

to the patient; (2) what the plan is going forward, including prevention of recurrent and new cancers and other late effects, surveillance for cancer and late effects, intervention for the consequences of cancer and its treatment, and coordination between cancer care providers and other follow-up care providers (e.g., primary care providers [PCPs]); and (3) contact information and resources for common issues.[1]

Evidence regarding SCPs' effectiveness in improving care quality and patient outcomes is mixed. Qualitative and observational work have found that survivors and PCPs benefit from SCPs,[2] but results of randomized controlled trials (RCTs) of SCPs' effectiveness have been null.[3–8] Despite lack of clear evidence of SCPs' effectiveness, several influential cancer organizations now recommend SCPs, including the American Society of Clinical Oncology and the National Comprehensive Cancer Network.[9,10] The American College of Surgeons Commission on Cancer accreditation program now requires accredited cancer programs to develop and deliver SCPs to the majority of their eligible cancer patients.[11] In addition, the Planning Actively for Cancer Treatment (PACT) Act was introduced in the US House of Representatives in 2015. The PACT Act would amend Medicare coverage to reimburse providers for cancer care planning and care coordination services, including SCPs.[12] Despite these recommendations for use, there has been little focus on SCP implementation planning and processes. Thus, policymakers have issued recommendations and requirements but have provided little guidance on how to effectively implement SCPs, and little knowledge exists of how to best adapt and tailor SCPs to fit local context and patient needs.

Indeed, evidence suggests that cancer care providers often do not develop SCPs; when SCPs are developed, they often lack recommended content and are seldom delivered to survivors and follow-up care providers, limiting their potential benefits.[13-17] Poor SCP implementation may be due in part to lack of guidance. For example, consensus is lacking regarding which cancer care providers are best suited to develop SCPs.[18] Evidence suggests that cancer care providers want to use SCPs but lack the resources and skills necessary to do so.[17] As a result, cancer programs often implement SCPs with the goal of maintaining accreditation rather than improving survivorship care;[19,20] including SCPs in patient health records is sufficient to confer accreditation, but SCPs must also be delivered with recommended content to benefit survivors and PCPs. Next, we describe the challenge of implementing SCPs in two equally reputable yet very different cancer programs.

UNIVERSITY-BASED CANCER HOSPITAL EXPERIENCE

The North Carolina Cancer Hospital (NCCH), part of the University of North Carolina Health Care System, is a tertiary academic National Cancer Institute (NCI)-designated comprehensive cancer center. NCCH has approximately 135,000 visits each year by patients from all of North Carolina's 100 counties. It features more than 100 cancer care providers, including physicians and nurse practitioners, serving patients in 13 tumor groups. Of note, like many other large cancer centers, NCCH coordinates efforts to promote SCP implementation with its affiliates, which include McCreary Cancer Center, Hayworth Cancer Center, and Rex Cancer Care.

Until 2009, SCP implementation at NCCH was limited to testicular cancer care providers, funded by a LIVESTRONG grant, and a single breast cancer care nurse practitioner—now the Director of Cancer Survivorship (Dr. Deborah Mayer). In 2014, as NCCH prepared to implement a new electronic health record (EHR), Mayer prepared to integrate into the EHR an SCP template based on that of the American Society of Clinical Oncology and her own research. Following EHR integration, Mayer led a quality improvement initiative intended to promote SCP implementation in three tumor groups that demonstrated readiness.[21] The initiative involved plan–do–check–act cycles in which tumor group staff offered feedback on an SCP template to meet its unique needs; integration of the revised template into the EHR; champions; and a process to promote SCP use among tumor group staff. In the near future, NCCH will integrate a best practice advisory to alert providers when a survivor is eligible for an SCP. Through these efforts, the time to develop an SCP was reduced from approximately 20 minutes to approximately 5 minutes, and SCP development and delivery increased.

Despite this improvement, like most US cancer programs, NCCH continues to struggle to implement SCPs. In 2016, 254 of 2,300 (11%) eligible cancer patients (stages 1–3 treated with curative intent) received an SCP, falling short of the Commission on Cancer's 2016 target of 25%. In 2017, the Commission on Cancer's target increased to 50%, and NCCH's report indicated that it also fell short of this goal. By the end of 2018, NCCH anticipates delivering SCPs to 50% of eligible patients, consistent with the Commission on Cancer's revised standards.[11]

NCCH has experienced multiple challenges to SCP implementation, including staff turnover and resistance, competing task demands, changing workflow, and technical difficulties. Some tumor groups have developed SCPs and delivered them to survivors but have not delivered them to their PCPs, whereas others have not completed documentation within the EHR to capture delivery. Strides that were made in other tumor groups have been diminished by turnover of key providers who were involved in SCP implementation. In other tumor groups, single providers develop and deliver SCPs, and their competing task demands limit SCP implementation. Some providers have resisted SCP implementation, asserting that the push to implement SCPs is driven by accreditation requirements and not evidence-based benefits to survivors. It has yet to be integrated into the oncology workflow and become as automatic as patient education before chemotherapy is administered.

Slow changes to EHR-integrated SCPs have also made implementation challenging; it may take several weeks for systems administrators to enact changes to templates or processes that tumor groups request. NCCH has also struggled to track SCP implementation in a valid and reliable manner. Initial reports over- or underestimated SCP delivery. Valid and reliable SCP implementation statistics would facilitate plan–do–study–act cycles that have driven improvements at NCCH in the past.

Perhaps most challenging at NCCH is the culture change required for SCP implementation. For many providers at NCCH, implementing SCPs requires shifting focus from diagnosis and treatment to follow-up care for survivors, including surveillance and prevention. This is made challenging by traditional visit schedules that might include newly diagnosed and metastatic cancer patients along with longer term survivors.

INTEGRATED HEALTH CARE SYSTEM EXPERIENCE

Kaiser Permanente (KP) is an integrated health care system providing comprehensive health care services to approximately 12 million members. KP operates in eight states and the District of Columbia, and it is divided into multiple regions. Oncology care within this system is typically delivered using a community model, with most oncologists treating most disease types. This contrasts with an academic/tertiary center model such as NCCH, which is typically highly specialized, although there is some specialization in oncology care delivery within KP.

At KP, there has been limited success in implementing systematic use of SCPs across the system and within regions and medical centers. Formal implementation strategies for SCPs have rarely been employed, and multiple barriers to implementation are present. We recently conducted qualitative interviews with cancer care clinicians, administrators, and patients in the Southern California region to explore SCP implementation processes.[19] As in most oncology care settings, addressing the rapidly changing treatment landscape is a priority, and the majority of resources are devoted to cancer diagnosis and treatment, including expanding access to novel therapies,

genomic testing, and supportive care services. Cancer survivorship is recognized as an important and distinct phase of the cancer care continuum; however, use of SCPs is not widespread. This may be due in part to a unique barrier within this integrated system: concern that SCPs may not substantially benefit patients in this setting. KP clinicians use a long-standing, comprehensive shared EHR with the ability to share information on cancer treatment and outcomes; patients have assigned primary care providers with a shared-care model with specialty care, and they have access to an online patient portal with pharmacy, labs, appointments, and other information.

In addition, not all regions or medical centers participate in external accreditation programs that require use of SCPs (e.g., National Accreditation Program for Breast Centers). This variation within the system greatly diffuses the potential impact of external credentialing and accreditation. Centers that maintain accreditation are striving to achieve the required use of SCPs but may not have system-wide support in their efforts. These issues, in addition to those common to other settings (e.g., staff turnover and resistance to change), have led to limited clinician championing of the SCP. However, we did find that a small number of clinicians within KP are advocating for systematic implementation of SCPs. These nascent efforts may be facilitated by health information technology solutions that are currently being developed and delivered by EHR vendors, such as the creation of auto-populated cancer treatment summaries (e.g., chemotherapy type and dose summary). However, just as with SCP implementation, these information technology solutions face implementation barriers. Multiple implementation strategies will be required for systematic implementation, including sustained engagement from clinical champions and operational leaders.

IMPLEMENTATION SCIENCE AS THE NEXT STEP TO PROMOTE SURVIVORSHIP CARE PLAN USE

As described previously, empirical and anecdotal evidence demonstrates the challenge of SCP implementation. Both qualitative and observational work have found that survivors and PCPs benefit from SCPs,[2] but results from RCTs of SCPs' effectiveness have largely been null. RCTs may be largely null because they have not taken into account the effect of implementation, a known determinant of intervention effectiveness.[13] The challenges associated with implementing SCPs are likely to influence SCPs' effectiveness, rendering results of extant RCTs of SCPs' effectiveness inconclusive.

Given the potential implications of implementation for SCPs' effectiveness, applying implementation science to SCP research is a critical next step for the field. Implementation science provides frameworks and strategies to help researchers look beyond the content of SCPs and focus on "revisiting the context" of SCP use to address barriers to widespread SCP implementation.[22] The integration of implementation science in SCP research can promote a deeper understanding of what works where and why with respect to SCPs. A critical first step in SCP implementation science would include the identification and specification of key implementation outcomes such as acceptability, feasibility, cost, and sustainability and also the identification and use of high-quality measures. Another key research need is to understand determinants of these implementation outcomes; knowledge regarding these determinants could help in the development of interventions to promote the implementation of SCPs in a way that is meaningful to survivors, cancer care providers, and follow-up care providers. Implementation science frameworks such as the Consolidated Framework for Implementation Research or the Theoretical Domains Framework may be helpful for conceptualizing determinants of SCP implementation. Until SCP implementation is optimized, SCPs' effectiveness cannot be fairly assessed. For example, SCPs cannot be effective in coordinating survivorship care if SCPs are developed but not delivered to survivors and their follow-up care providers.

SCPs' effectiveness may be best assessed using implementation science designs that allow for the simultaneous evaluation of clinical outcomes and implementation outcomes such as adoption and sustainability—that is, hybrid designs.[23] Curran et al.[24] described three types of hybrid designs that, to varying degrees, consider determinants of implementation. A type 1 hybrid approach would focus primarily on SCP effectiveness while simultaneously exploring factors and challenges in implementation. A type 2 hybrid design would place equal emphasis on SCP effectiveness and implementation. A type 3 hybrid study would focus primarily on evaluation of implementation strategies and outcomes while

secondarily measuring clinical effectiveness, and it might be especially useful for understanding the complexities of SCP delivery and tailoring SCP delivery to stakeholder (e.g., survivor and primary care provider) preferences. Using a type 3 hybrid study to test SCP implementation strategies[25] could allow researchers to identify the most feasible and effective strategies for implementing SCPs with fidelity as well as an eye toward stakeholder-centeredness (e.g., optimizing systems for implementing SCPs to minimize cancer care provider and maximize benefits to primary care providers, survivors, and caregivers).[26] Based on the two case studies discussed previously, SCP implementation may be facilitated by strategies such as clinician champions and reportable quality metrics. Future type 3 hybrid studies of SCP implementation could build off these strategies and other strategies to maximize implementation while simultaneously gathering evidence of SCP effectiveness.

CURRENT SURVIVORSHIP CARE PLAN IMPLEMENTATION RESEARCH

Currently funded, yet unpublished studies speak to the growth of SCP implementation science. Three of the six currently funded, in-progress studies that we identified aim to describe existing SCP implementation processes with the objective of leveraging findings to understand the influence of SCP implementation on SCP effectiveness. In a study conducted by the Institute for Patient-Centered Initiatives and Health Equity at the George Washington University Cancer Center, researchers will survey cancer care providers regarding their processes for SCP implementation with the long-term goal of identifying SCP implementation models that may be linked in future studies to improved communication and coordination among survivors, cancer care providers, and follow-up care providers.[27] In a Cancer Research Network-funded study, researchers are conducting semi-structured interviews to understand the outcomes that survivors, their caregivers, cancer care providers, hospital administrators, and primary care providers expect from SCP use and the extent to which existing implementation processes have promoted those outcomes; findings will be leveraged in a subsequent hybrid study that will assess the influence of SCP implementation on measures of SCP effectiveness that stakeholders have identified as relevant.[19] And in a North Carolina Translational and Clinical

Sciences Institute-funded study, researchers will use qualitative comparative analysis (QCA) to identify strategies that promote SCP implementation among cancer programs participating in the Quality Oncology Practice Initiative (QOPI).[20] QCA begins with interviews to identify SCP implementation strategies and then organizes interview data and QOPI performance data by using within-case analysis and logic-based cross-case analysis. Strategies found to promote SCP implementation will be assessed in a future comparative effectiveness trial.

The remaining studies that we identified aim to directly improve SCP implementation. In an RCT funded by the Patient-Centered Outcomes Research Institute, researchers will test three models of SCP implementation with the goal of identifying approaches that are feasible, patient-centered, and effective in increasing SCP development and delivery.[28] In an NCI-funded pilot study, researchers will assess the feasibility of the Head and Neck Survivorship tool (HN-STAR), an electronic survivorship care planning platform that aims to streamline the provision of personalized care for head and neck cancer survivors.[29] And in a pilot study funded by the Canadian Institutes of Health Research, researchers will assess the feasibility of integrating SCPs into routine cancer care.[30] Outcomes to be evaluated include the implementation processes and survivors' short-term clinical outcomes.

Currently funded yet unpublished SCP implementation studies are promising in several respects. First, several of these studies take into account stakeholders' perspectives on SCP implementation. This is critical because SCPs' effectiveness relies heavily on stakeholder engagement in SCP implementation (e.g., cancer care providers delivering SCPs in a way that effectively conveys their content). Second, several of these studies are being conducted with the explicit objective of leveraging findings for future studies in which implementation is examined as a determinant of SCP effectiveness. As we argued previously, this approach may produce more conclusive evidence of SCP effectiveness than has been obtained by extant RCTs.

We recommend that future research combine the strengths of current studies, using stakeholder preferences to develop systems for SCP implementation; effectiveness studies may be more conclusive following, or in conjunction with, optimized, stakeholder-informed implementation strategies. We also recommend that future studies investigate approaches to adapting and tailoring SCPs to fit cancer programs' unique contexts. This might involve identifying core components of SCPs by specifying their theory of change and major activities, adapting SCPs in a way that is consistent with theory of change and major activities, and evaluating adapted SCPs' effectiveness. In addition, future research should move beyond SCP implementation to investigate the implementation of survivorship care programs. SCPs represent just one component of what are ideally comprehensive survivorship care programs. These programs could be informed by existing care delivery models (e.g., the chronic care model).

REFERENCES

1. Institute of Medicine. *From Cancer Patient to Cancer Survivor: Lost in Transition*. Washington, DC: National Academies Press; 2006.
2. Shalom MM, Hahn EE, Casillas J, et al. Do survivorship care plans make a difference? A primary care provider perspective. *J Oncol Pract.* 2011;7(5):314–318.
3. Grunfeld E, Julian JA, Pond G, et al. Evaluating survivorship care plans: Results of a randomized clinical trial of patients with breast cancer. *J Clin Oncol.* 2011;29(36):4755–4762.
4. Hershman DL, Greenlee H, Awad D, et al. Randomized controlled trial of a clinic-based survivorship intervention following adjuvant therapy in breast cancer survivors. *Breast Cancer Res Treat.* 2013;138(3):795–806.
5. Brothers BM, Easley A, Salani R, et al. Do survivorship care plans impact patients' evaluations of care? A randomized evaluation with gynecologic oncology patients. *Gynecol Oncol.* 2013;129(3):554–558.
6. Grunfeld E, Pond G, Maunsell E, et al. Impact of survivorship care plans (SCP) on adherence to guidelines, health service measures, and patient-reported outcomes (PRO): Extended results of a multicenter randomized clinical trial (RCT) with breast cancer survivors. *Eur J Cancer.* 2012;48(Suppl):S147.
7. Ruddy KJ, Guo H, Baker EL, et al. Randomized phase 2 trial of a coordinated breast cancer follow-up care program. *Cancer.* 2016;122(22):3546–3554.
8. Emery JD, Jefford M, King M, et al. ProCare Trial: A phase II randomized controlled trial of shared care for follow-up of men with prostate cancer. *BJU Int.* 2017;119(3):381–389.
9. McCabe MS, Bhatia S, Oeffinger KC, et al. American Society of Clinical Oncology

statement: Achieving high quality cancer survivorship care. *J Clin Oncol.* 2013;31(5):631–640.

10. NCCN guidelines. National Comprehensive Cancer Network website. https://www.nccn. org/professionals/physician_gls/f_guidelines. asp#survivorship. Accessed August 17, 2017.

11. American College of Surgeons Commission on Cancer. *Cancer Program Standards: Ensuring Patient-Centered Care (2016 Edition).* Chicago: American College of Surgeons; 2016:58–59.

12. HR 2846: Planning Actively for Cancer Treatment (PACT) Act of 2015. 114th Congress; 2015–2016.

13. Birken SA, Deal AM, Mayer DK, et al. Determinants of survivorship care plan use in US cancer programs. *J Cancer Educ.* 2014;29(4):720–727.

14. Birken SA, Deal AM, Mayer DK, et al. Following through: The consistency of survivorship care plan use in United States cancer programs. *J Cancer Educ.* 2014;29(4):689–697.

15. Salz T, Oeffinger KC, McCabe MS, et al. Survivorship care plans in research and practice. *CA Cancer J Clin.* 2012;62(2):101–117.

16. Hahh EE, Ganz PA. Survivorship programs and care plans in practice: Variations on a theme. *J Oncol Pract.* 2011;7(2):70–75.

17. Klemanski DL, Browning KK, Kue J. Survivorship care plan preferences of cancer survivors and health care providers: A systematic review and quality appraisal of the evidence. *J Cancer Surviv.* 2016;10(1):71–86.

18. Keesing S, McNamara B, Rosenwax L. Cancer survivors' experiences of using survivorship care plans: A systematic review of qualitative studies. *J Cancer Surviv.* 2015;9(2):260–268.

19. Birken SA. Addressing stakeholders' perspectives on survivorship care plan implementation. Cancer Care Research Network (CRN15014), March 2016–February 2017.

20. Birken SA. Identifying strategies for the successful implementation of survivorship care plans in practice. North Carolina Translational and Clinical Sciences Institute, September 2016–August 2017.

21. Mayer DM, Taylor K, Gerstel AA, et al. How an expert approaches it: Implementing survivorship

care plans with an electronic health record in an academic medical center. *Oncology.* 2015;29(12):980–982, 989.

22. Parry C, Kent EE, Forsythe LP, et al. Can't see the forest for the care plan: A call to revisit the context of care planning. *J Clin Oncol.* 2013;13(21):2651–2653.

23. Landsverk J, Brown CH, Chamberlain P, et al. Design and analysis in dissemination and implementation research. In Brownson RC, Colditz GA, Proctor EK. *Dissemination and Implementation Research in Health: Translating Science to Practice.* New York: Oxford University Press; 2012:225–260.

24. Curran GM, Bauer M, Mittman B, et al. Effectiveness–implementation hybrid designs: Combining elements of clinical effectiveness and implementation research to enhance public health impact. *Med Care.* 2012;50:217–226.

25. Powell BJ, Waltz TJ, Chinman MJ, et al. A refined compilation of implementation strategies: Results from the Expert Recommendations for Implementing Change (ERIC) project. *Implement Sci.* 2015;10:21.

26. Selove R, Birken SA, Skolarus TA, et al. Using implementation science to examine the impact of cancer survivorship care plans. *J Clin Oncol.* 2016;34(32):3834–3837.

27. Birken SA, Chapman M, Raskin S, et al. A survey of survivorship care plan implementation processes among cancer care professionals. National Cancer Survivorship Resource Center, December 2015–July 2017.

28. Smith K. Simplifying survivorship care planning: Comparing the efficacy and patient-centeredness of three care delivery models. Patient-Centered Outcomes Research Institute, April 2015–October 2020.

29. Salz T. Simplifying care for the complex cancer survivor. Sloan-Kettering Institute for Cancer Research (5R21CA187441-02), April 2015–March 2018.

30. Howell DM, Jones JM. Transition to survivorship: Translating knowledge into action for testicular and endometrial cancer populations. Canadian Institutes of Health Research, October 2010–September 2013.

12

CANCER IN THE GLOBAL HEALTH CONTEXT

OVERVIEW OF CASE STUDIES

Sudha Sivaram

GLOBALLY, A shift in the pattern of disease from infectious etiology to chronic conditions is leading to an increased focus on the prevention and control of non-communicable diseases (NCDs). Recently, a 17% decrease in infectious diseases and deaths attributed to neonatal and maternal mortality has been reported; however, this decrease has been offset by an increase of 30% in deaths from NCDs including heart disease, stroke, and cancer.[1,2] In 2012, almost 80% of the 28 million deaths due to NCDs occurred in low- and middle-income countries (LMICs), with cancer being the leading cause of death among NCDs.[3] The primary risk factors for cancer in LMICs include exposure to tobacco, infectious agents, harmful alcohol use, poor diet and physical activity, as well as environmental carcinogens. More than 80% of world smokers live in LMICs, where the prevalence of smokeless tobacco use adds an additional burden of oral and nasopharyngeal cancers, which are more prevalent in these regions. Infectious agents such as human papilloma virus (HPV) and hepatitis

B and C viruses are preventable but remain major causes of public health burden. According to the World Health Organization,[2] in 2012, an estimated 15% of diagnosed cancers were attributed to infectious agents, including *Helicobacter pylori* (stomach cancer), HPV (present in all cervical cancers), hepatitis B virus, hepatitis C virus (liver cancer), and Epstein–Barr virus (Burkitt lymphoma). Alcohol is widely available and accessible, and increasing trends in harmful alcohol use such as binge drinking and alcohol dependence have been reported. A similar trend is seen in the prevalence of obesity. Data on diet and physical exercise in LMICs suggest a change in dietary patterns to include high-fat diet and an increase in obesity across the world, with reported high rates in children, women, and urban populations.[3,4] Recent analysis of global data shows that from 1980 to 2013, obesity rates in children in LMICs have risen from 8.1% to 12.9% in boys and from 0.4% to 13.4% in girls.[5] Environmental risk factor exposure is high in LMICs. Available figures, acknowledging variability between countries in exposure assessment, estimate that between 7% and 19% of cancers globally are attributable to environmental carcinogens. For ambient air pollution alone, the Global Burden of Disease 2010 project estimate for lung cancer is 223,000 attributable deaths.[6]

As we consider how to address these risk factors for cancer, the available evidence to prevent or deter the consequences of these exposures is encouraging.[7] Tobacco prevention and cessation strategies at community and clinic levels have highlighted specific approaches for intervention design. Vaccinations are available for HPV and hepatitis B virus. Early detection technologies for lung, breast, and cervical cancers that enable management of disease and improved survivorship are being implemented in many areas of the world. Interventions to educate and motivate behavior change among harmful alcohol users are moving from research realms to community settings. Several interventions to promote exercise have been developed, and national policies to reduce emissions as well as technological interventions, such as cook stoves, to reduce exposure to environmental carcinogens are examples of problem-solving in action.

However, there has been limited success in the implementation of cancer control in LMICs. Three factors may help explain this: social determinants of health, competing public health priorities, and the lack of context-specific evidence for cancer control approaches and strategies. Social determinants of health refers to the conditions in which people are born, grow, live, work, and age and also to social and economic factors other than medical care that affect health.[8] In cancer control, these factors include individual behaviors to limit exposure to risk factors and to seek care; efficiency of care delivery personnel, systems, and processes that help complete care and positively affect patients' outcomes; and the larger policy context that can often be either enabling or disabling to both the health care seeking as well as health care delivery process. For instance, in tobacco control, neighborhood access to tobacco and social influences such as peer use can influence and outweigh individual motivations to avoid use. Coupled with either poor availability or poor access to tobacco prevention or cessation services, this may disempower individuals from taking action. These multilevel and contextual factors influencing cancer control are poorly understood in LMICs.[9]

Another factor is competing health priorities. Although many governments are beginning to develop or strengthen national cancer control programs, cancer competes with other diseases such as malaria, HIV/AIDS, and tuberculosis. Coupled with increasing outbreaks of infections such as Zika and dengue hemorrhagic fever, cancer may not always be a funding priority.

The third factor is the lack of context-specific evidence for cancer control. There is little implementation science on cancer control in LMICs. Evidence from cervical cancer control—HPV vaccination and early detection—await widespread adoption because there is inadequate context-specific understanding of how to deliver them to communities. Systems for timely diagnosis of tumor specimens and linkage between physicians and patients to ensure completion of follow-up and treatment, which are the mainstay of cancer care in many high-income countries, are either absent or structured in a way that leads to patients being lost to follow-up or receiving incomplete care. Research studies under randomized conditions are limited in their generalizability to LMICs and in the knowledge they generate because intervention delivery settings are different, as are populations. The diversity of cancer in LMICs is a further case in point. For instance, liver cancer is the leading cause of death in Mongolia (97.8 deaths per 100,000 men with a 44.6% mortality rate compared to 9.8 per 100,000 and 4.4%, respectively, in the United States), and it is more prevalent in Asia and Africa and very rare in Latin America.[10] Gall bladder cancer is another regionally associated cancer with a unique geographical distribution. The highest rates of this cancer are seen among women in New Delhi, India (21.5 per 100,000); south Karachi, Pakistan; and Quito, Ecuador.[11] Remarkable differences also exist between urban and rural populations.[12] As such, research to identify strategies to develop cancer prevention and also early detection strategies for specific cancers is needed. Implementation science in LMICs that considers context, develops innovative strategies, and identifies quality improvement can generate knowledge that can potentially be applied anywhere. Innovations in the use of technology to improve cancer detection and treatment as well as limit loss to follow-up are emerging from LMICs, as are strategies to educate populations and increase efficiencies in care delivery.

In this chapter, three case studies illustrate the potential of implementation science in LMICs. The first seeks to understand the context of care seeking and caregiving for cervical cancer in India. This case highlights the social determinants of health, such as access to care, and factors within the health system, such as physician knowledge and attitudes toward cervical cancer screening. By understanding these factors at both the community level and the clinic level, this case illustrates how programs work with community resources and institutions to achieve cancer control goals. The second case presents more than a decade of work in El Salvador, a country with competing health priorities. The authors of this case study discuss how implementation science research was used to tailor evidence to the context of the country, and how these research findings informed national policy. Inasmuch as this research seeks to understand strategies in practical real-life settings, the case of El Salvador highlights how with investment in human and financial resources, a cervical cancer screening policy was established. The third case study describes how implementation science methods are being used in Vietnam to understand strategies to adopt tobacco cessation guidelines in community-based clinics.

REFERENCES

1. Dye, C. After 2015: Infectious diseases in a new era of health and development. *Philos Trans R Soc B Biol Sci.* 2014;369(1645):20130426. doi:10.1098/rstb.2013.0426
2. World Health Organization. *Global Status Report: Noncommunicable Diseases.* Geneva, Switzerland: World Health Organization; 2012.
3. Popkin BM. Nutrition transition and the global diabetes epidemic. *Curr Diab Rep.* 2015;15(9):64. doi:10.1007/s11892-015-0631-4
4. Gayathri R, Ruchi V, Mohan V. Impact of nutrition transition and resulting morbidities on economic and human development. *Curr Diabetes Rev.* 2017;13(5):452–460.
5. Ng M, Fleming T, Robinson M, et al. Global, regional, and national prevalence of overweight and obesity in children and adults during 1980–2013: A systematic analysis for the Global Burden of Disease Study 2013. *Lancet.* 2014;384(9945):766–781. doi:10.1016/S0140-6736(14)60460-8
6. Islam SM, Purnat TD, Phuong NT, Mwingira U, Schacht K, Fröschl G. Non-communicable diseases (NCDs) in developing countries: A symposium report. *Institute for Health Metrics and Evaluation. Global burden of disease cause patterns;* 2013. Available from: http://www.healthmetricsandevaluation.org/gbd/visualizations/gbd-cause-patterns
7. Farmer P, Frenk J, Knaul FM, et al. Expansion of cancer care and control in countries of low and middle income: A call to action. *Lancet.* 2010;376(9747):1186–1193. doi:10.1016/S0140-6736(10)61152-X
8. Braveman P, Gottlieb L. The social determinants of health: It's time to consider the causes of the causes. *Public Health Rep.* 2014; 129(Suppl 2):19–31.
9. Sivaram S, Sanchez MA, Rimer BK, Samet JM, Glasgow RE. Implementation science in cancer prevention and control: A framework for research and programs in low- and middle-income countries. *Cancer Epidemiol Biomarkers Prev.* 2014;23(11):2273–2284. doi:10.1158/1055-9965.EPI-14-0472
10. World Cancer Research Fund International. *Diet, Nutrition, Physical Activity and Liver Cancer.* London: World Cancer Research Fund International; 2015.
11. Randi G, Franceschi S, La Vecchia C. Gallbladder cancer worldwide: Geographical distribution and risk factors. *Int J Cancer.* 2006;118(7):1591–1602. doi:10.1002/ijc.21683
12. Rath GK, Gandhi AK National cancer control and registration program in India. *Indian J Med Paediatr Oncol.* 2014;35:288–290.

Case Study 12A

ADOPTING THE PREVENTABLE MODEL

A MULTISTEP APPROACH TO CHANGING A SECONDARY CERVICAL CANCER PREVENTION PARADIGM IN EL SALVADOR

Mauricio Maza, Karla Alfaro, Julia C. Gage, and Miriam Cremer

CERVICAL CANCER is one of the leading causes of cancer mortality in low- and middle-income countries (LMICs). El Salvador is no exception; incidence and mortality are 24.8 and 11.9 per 100,000, respectively,[1] well above the average rates of cancer in the Americas region of 14.9 and 5.9 per 100,000, respectively.[2] In recent years, there have been increased efforts in the region to reduce incidence rates through cervical cancer screening and treatment programs. The effectiveness of these efforts can be assessed using several parameters, including coverage, quality of the screening test, and follow-up of abnormal results. However, cancer prevention efforts in El Salvador do not meet these criteria. The country has one of the lowest reported screening rates in the region.[3] Although there are no studies measuring the quality of the Pap smear nationally, research conducted in Nicaragua and Honduras[3,4] has demonstrated that the Pap smear in those countries has very poor sensitivity. In addition, less than 50% of women with an abnormal Pap smear in this geographical area receive treatment.[5,6]

Poor sensitivity of Pap smear, low follow-up and treatment rates, and other economic and social barriers[7] are among the reasons why cervical cancer is often the leading cause of cancer deaths in resource-constrained settings.

Cervical cancer screening has traditionally relied on the Pap smear as the primary screening test, followed by colposcopy and biopsy for histological confirmation before proceeding to treatment. This necessitates a multi-visit approach and makes it difficult to implement in areas without proper infrastructure and trained personnel. Since the discovery that virtually all cervical cancer cases are due to persistent infections with the human papillomavirus (HPV), new methods of testing for HPV have been developed to screen at-risk women. Through DNA genotyping of the virus, these tests focus on HPV types most likely to cause cervical cancer. Currently, high-income countries such as the United States, Australia, and many European countries are transitioning from Pap smear to HPV testing. Mexico, Argentina, Honduras, Guatemala, and El

Salvador are also starting to adopt HPV DNA-based screening into their screening programs.[8]

BACKGROUND

In 2006, the non-profit organization Basic Health International (BHI) partnered with the El Salvador Ministry of Health (MOH) to address how best to increase the country's low cervical cancer screening coverage. At that time, many LMICs saw a potential solution in the use of visual inspection with acetic acid (VIA), an alternative method for cervical cancer screening. VIA is a cervical cancer screening test that consists of applying 3–5% concentrated acetic acid (vinegar) to the cervix, and if areas turn white (acetowhite lesion) after 1 minute, it is considered a positive test. Through the work conducted by MOH and BHI, more than 60 providers were trained and certified to conduct a *see and treat* strategy.[9,10] This strategy consisted of screening women in rural areas with VIA, followed by immediate cryotherapy treatment of eligible VIA-positive women. During this process, BHI identified critical barriers, such as resistance to change from health care professionals and medical societies when implementing a new technology or strategy such as VIA. After several meetings between key stakeholders (MOH, OB/GYN Society, colposcopists, cytologists, and BHI), technical guidelines for the use of VIA in El Salvador were established in 2008.

Although screening with VIA is used as an alternative to Pap smear in research settings, the scale-up of screening based on this method has proved to be challenging because it requires intense training to ensure high quality but the sensitivity of the test remains poor. As problems arose in the scale-up of VIA, BHI attempted to find viable alternatives for a good-quality test that was scalable for population-based screening and that would allow proper follow-up of screen-positive women. A key development occurred in 2009 with the introduction of a new, low-cost HPV screening tool, careHPV, developed through the combined efforts of the Bill and Melinda Gates Foundation, PATH, and Qiagen. As part of the QiagenCares program, the company committed to donating one million low-cost HPV tests to LMICs.[11] El Salvador was one of the first countries to be a recipient of this donation, which made the implementation of HPV primary screening a feasible option for the country.

This case study focuses on the evidence generated from our research experience in El Salvador during the change from a Pap-based screening paradigm to primary HPV DNA testing and with the planned scale-up of the program for national implementation. This information is presented using PREVENTABLE, a process of change model. PREVENTABLE is an acronym for *p*olitical will, *r*esearch *ev*aluation, *e*ducation/dissemination, *n*egotiation, *t*ransition, *a*dvocacy, *b*udget, and *l*egal frame work *e*vidence. The model consists of two primary pillars, two main drivers, and six secondary drivers. The primary and secondary driver contribute to the pillars of the model (Figure 12A.1).

THE PILLARS: POLITICAL WILL AND EVIDENCE

To accomplish a paradigm change, two components are essential: the political will of the current government and convincing scientific evidence. Political will can best be assessed from the initial stages of the evaluation of a country's readiness for change. In the case of El Salvador, a window of opportunity was created in 2009 due to a change in the governing political party. This was the first time the dominant party had changed since the peace accords that ended the country's civil war were signed in 1992. A similar phenomenon occurred in Mexico when the 71-year rule of the dominant party ended and the incoming administration strengthened the health reform process.[12] In El Salvador, the new government sought to effect substantial changes on regulations surrounding the health system. The previous government had worked on the Ley Sistema Nacional de Salud (Law of the National Health System),[13] and the new authorities introduced a health reform based on a new plan called Construyendo la Esperanza (Building Hope),[14] with the objective of reaching people with low medical coverage. To do this, MOH created *ECO teams*, community outreach groups consisting of a physician, a nurse, and a health promoter, and *Specialized ECOS*, which brought specialists to rural areas of the country.

In July 2009, a month after the new government came to power, the first meeting took place between BHI and the Vice Minister of Health. During that meeting, BHI explained to the Vice Minister that El Salvador could be eligible for a donation of low-cost HPV tests. After several more discussions and meetings between members of the US National Cancer Institute/National Institutes of Health (NCI/NIH), the technical team from the MOH,

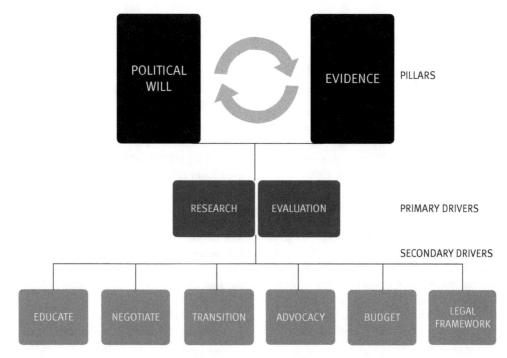

FIGURE 12A.1   PREVENTABLE: *p*olitical will, *r*esearch, *e*valuation, education/dissemination, *n*egotiation, *t*ransition, *a*dvocacy, *b*udget, and *l*egal frame work *e*vidence.

and the Vice Minister, a meeting with the Minister was scheduled in early 2010. At that meeting, BHI formally presented the evidence supporting the benefits of HPV testing, and the Minister and Vice Minister delegated the responsibility of exploring this possibility to their technical team. As a result, during the Latin America Sub-Regional Meeting on Cervical Cancer Prevention hosted by the Pan-American Health Organization (PAHO) in June 2010, the government of El Salvador proposed demonstration projects to phase in HPV screening within 2–5 years.[15]After various stakeholder meetings with local and international organizations, including the Association of Gynecology and Obstetrics of El Salvador, the Association of Colposcopists of El Salvador, PAHO, and NCI/NIH, a consensus was reached to proceed with the Cancer Prevention Program in El Salvador demonstration project (CAPE).

In 2011, MOH signed a memorandum of understanding (MOU) with BHI to formalize the role of BHI as a technical collaborator throughout the CAPE implementation process.[16] The following year, the MOH signed another MOU with QIAGEN to receive the donation of low-cost HPV tests. To create a more inclusive technical

and advocacy support group, MOH also formed the Alianza Interinstitucional e Intersectorial de Apoyo a la Salud Sexual y Reproductiva (The Interinstitutional and Intersectoral Alliance to support Sexual and Reproductive Health), which was later called the Interinstitutional and Intersectoral Alliance for Cancer Control. This alliance consists of both professional and community-based organizations that meet on a monthly basis to discuss issues regarding cancer control programs. The Salvadoran government demonstrated strong political will and commitment to improve the cancer policies of the country.

While a favorable political climate facilitated prioritization of cervical cancer control, the momentum to convene research, service delivery, and advocacy expertise was bolstered by a systematic process of presenting scientific evidence to policymakers. In El Salvador, NCI played a key role in this process by presenting recent evidence from cohort studies demonstrating the superior long-term reassurance against cervical cancer provided by a negative HPV test versus a negative Pap test.[17,18] In addition, a landmark international study suggested that primary HPV testing followed by treatment with cryotherapy effectively treated not only prevalent but also incident precursors of cervical cancer.[19,20]

THE MAIN DRIVERS: RESEARCH AND EVALUATION

In El Salvador, research and the evaluation of outcomes were two main drivers that helped reinforce the evidence that increased the political will of the decision-makers. The goal of research and evaluation was to demonstrate that a shift in the national cervical cancer screening program from conventional Pap smear to HPV screening was possible and to define the best algorithm for follow-up of HPV-positive women. Ultimately, MOH wanted a demonstration project that would provide it with an analysis of the country's current situation and locally derived evidence of the potential outcomes of a new intervention to motivate national-level implementation. With that goal in mind, a three-phase demonstration project among 30,000 women was defined as outlined in Table 12A.1.

The three phases of CAPE consisted of implementation of HPV screening followed by treatment with cryotherapy (a two-step approach) or a multiple-step approach of HPV testing, followed by colposcopy, followed by treatment. We referred to the screen-and-refer to colposcopy strategy as *colposcopy management* and the HPV testing followed by treatment strategy as *screen and treat*. We conducted the implementation of these two strategies followed by observational analysis of the results. Within these phases, we also nested studies to evaluate in more detail certain aspects of the implementation that would give us a better idea of acceptability, adherence to screening, and cost-effectiveness of each strategy.

Phase 1

RESEARCH

During the first phase of CAPE, which was launched in October 2012,[21] a total of 2,000 women were screened for HPV. Half of these women were referred to the colposcopy management arm, and the other 1,000 women were referred to the screen and treat arm. In this overall population, the HPV positivity rate was 10.6%. At 6-month follow-up, the implementation showed that it was significantly less likely for women in the colposcopy management cohort (68.8%) to have received treatment compared to women in the screen-and-treat cohort (98.3%).[22]

Two other projects were nested within this first phase. First, a study was conducted to evaluate the educational materials and workshops that had been developed for CAPE to assess the factors that affected a woman's decision to attend screening. The outcomes of the study showed that the educational sessions were effective in bringing women to screening appointments, although it remained difficult to convince women who had not been screened in more than 3 years or had never been screened to attend their appointment.[23] To reach this group, BHI decided to evaluate the acceptability of vaginal HPV self-sampling through a Fulbright-funded project. This second nested study showed that 38.8% of women preferred self-sampling compared to 31.9% who preferred sampling by a health provider and also that self-sampling had an overall acceptability

Table 12A.1. CAPE Phases and Goals of Project

CAPE PHASE	NO. OF WOMEN TO BE SCREENED	GOALS
Phase 1	2,000	*Introduction* of HPV testing and defining algorithm for management of HPV-positive women
Phase 2	8,000	*Scale-up* of HPV testing and defining algorithm for management of HPV-positive women
Phase 3	20,000	*Implementation* of HPV testing within the national cervical cancer prevention program

of 68.1%. The main reason for preferring self-sampling was a desire for privacy and/or embarrassment at being seen by a clinician. These results allowed us to consider self-sampling as a feasible option for those women who had a history of being under-screened.[24]

With the information gathered at the end of the first phase, a cost-effectiveness analysis was conducted in collaboration with the Harvard T. H. Chan School of Public Health (HSPH). The study compared the conventional Pap smear model against the colposcopy management and the screen-and-treat approach, and it concluded that the screen-and-treat strategy was the most cost-effective.[25]

EVALUATION

The second primary driver of the model is the evaluation of the research that has been conducted. CAPE outcomes were evaluated by MOH, BHI, HSPSH, and NCI/NIH, and the findings were presented to the Minister and the Vice Minister of Health. Both the behavioral and the clinical management studies led to major changes in how MOH decided to proceed with Phase 2 of CAPE. The cost-effectiveness analysis of the outcomes was crucial in increasing the political will of high-level officials at MOH. Considering the evidence required to change policy, this was one of the most important components in their decision to move forward with the second phase of CAPE.

Phase 2

RESEARCH

Because high-level authorities within the El Salvador government were satisfied with the accomplishments of Phase 1 of CAPE, they agreed to scale up the project to 8,000 women aged 30–49 years to be screened and treated in the same modalities. In this phase, self-sampling as well as provider sampling for HPV were employed as screening methods. At the end of the second phase, a total of 8,050 women were screened with both self and provider sampling. Of these, 4,087 women were placed in the screen-and-treat cohort and 3,963 women in the colposcopy management cohort. The overall HPV positivity rate was 11.9%. At 6-month follow-up, the implementation again showed that it was less likely for women in colposcopy management (44%) to have received treatment compared

to those in screen and treat (88%).[26] This cemented the decision that the screen-and-treat modality would be the best strategy moving forward.

After completing Phase 2, a small pilot study was conducted to further evaluate self-sampling as an option for those women who had not attended their HPV screening appointment. Results were similar to those of the Phase 1 study, with an acceptability rate of 68%, but in this small sample the prevalence of HPV was higher at 17% compared to 10.6% and 11.9% in Phase 1 and Phase 2, respectively.[27]

EVALUATION

Once the research outcomes were obtained and analyzed, a new meeting with the Minister of Health was arranged in July 2014. Since the start of CAPE, the government changed again in 2014, and the person appointed Minister of Health was the former Vice Minister of Health. Although many high-level authorities remained the same, there was a significant change in personnel of key technical staff within MOH. There was a need to obtain buy-in from a new team and present the data and lessons learned from the first two phases. The positive findings of the first two phases reinforced the political will from new senior officials who were in the middle of a transition. Preliminary cost-effectiveness data from Phase 2 showed the screen-and-treat strategy to once again be the most cost-effective, and this result was presented to the Minister by the HSPH and BHI team. After this discussion, the Minister instructed MOH's technical team to start working on new guidelines based on the evidence that was provided.

THE SECONDARY DRIVERS

As shown in Figure 12A.1, secondary drivers are crucial complements to the main drivers. They do not have to occur in a specific order, and some will be more relevant than others through the process of implementation. These include education and dissemination, negotiation, transition, advocacy, budget, and legal framework.

Education/Dissemination

Information gathered through research and evaluation must be disseminated and used to educate stakeholders. Between 2010 and 2017, three major symposia targeting health care providers, key stakeholders, and community leaders were conducted to present the latest evidence on cervical cancer screening.[28,29] Seminars were conducted by MOH throughout the country to educate its personnel and local community leaders on the outcomes of the project. The PAHO/World Health Organization (WHO) office in El Salvador, in partnership with the Centers for Disease Control and Prevention, the International Agency for Research on Cancer (IARC), and MOH, widely disseminated the new WHO guidelines for screening and treatment of precancerous lesions for cervical cancer prevention, which included the screen-and-treat modality as an option for women with an HPV-positive result.[30,31]

Negotiation

After the pertinent authorities made the decision to support the screen-and-treat modality, the evidence was presented to the Interinstitutional and Intersectoral Alliance for Cancer Control, which was responsible for developing the national guidelines for cervical cancer prevention. The evidence was evaluated critically among epidemiologists, colposcopists, pathologists, cytologists, primary care physicians, and representatives of civil society at several PAHO-guided monthly meetings. A consensus was reached to transition to primary HPV screening with the screen-and-treat approach for women between the ages of 30 and 59 years.

Legal Framework

In order to reinforce cancer control efforts, the central government elaborated a new policy for cancer control with a specific operational plan.[32,33] As part of this plan, new guidelines for cervical and breast cancer were created in 2015.[34] The policy change was completed by the Interinstitutional and Intersectoral Alliance for Cancer Control. Currently, HPV screening with a screen-and-treat approach is an approved clinical practice in the country.

Transition

Once new guidelines were established, a transition plan was required for a successful implementation. Large educational sessions and trainings for MOH staff in the region were required as part of this process. Educational material, paperwork, census information, registration and information systems, and monitoring and evaluation tools needed to be modified to incorporate the new guidelines. It was crucial that these systems were in place before starting implementation in a public program. When CAPE was initiated, MOH added cervical cancer monitoring and evaluation to its weekly meetings (in which other diseases, such as dengue fever and Zika virus, were discussed) in the target region.

Advocacy

Since the start of the campaign, media outlets have played a crucial role in spreading information about the CAPE project and its accomplishments both locally and internationally.[35,36] Many collaborators and MOH staff have been interviewed by newspaper, radio, and TV outlets. With the support of different local and international agencies, advocacy has been continuous in El Salvador. Symposia to inform and discuss HPV testing were held with the technical support of NCI, the American Society for Colposcopy and Cervical Pathology, and the University of Texas MD Anderson Cancer Center. During the Union for International Cancer Control's (UICC) World Cancer Day in 2016,[37] a symposium was held in El Salvador in which the new policies and guidelines were presented[38] and representatives from NCI/NIH, IARC, the Bill and Melinda Gates Foundation, and HSPH were present and showed strong support for the new national cervical cancer program. In addition, the Central America Cancer Control Leadership Forum was organized in Antigua, Guatemala, in 2016 by the Center for Global Health at NCI with the collaboration of the University of Texas MD Anderson Cancer Center, PAHO/WHO, and Vanderbilt University–Ingram Cancer Center. During this forum, the representatives/delegates from El Salvador developed an action plan that prioritized increasing advocacy to obtain more political support and financial resources for the cancer programs.

Budget

The initial two phases of CAPE were funded by UICC. Phase 3 received support from the Einhorn Family Charitable Foundation and from PATH through a grant awarded by the Bill and Melinda Gates Foundation.

Budget for implementation and evaluation is critical. In the cost-effectiveness analysis of

CAPE,[25] direct medical costs such as staff time, disposable supplies, equipment use, as well as patient time costs (travel to clinic and time to receive services) were particularly useful to understand how resources were allocated. There is a great need for studies that evaluate the initial implementation costs of programs. Throughout the phases of CAPE, financial support for MOH was crucial, but this diminished as the program was scaled up. In many circumstances, donations or loans will be necessary from international agencies while countries search for sustainable and innovative approaches to control non-communicable diseases such as cervical cancer. As the government continues to implement a national scale-up plan, funding sources are received from international loans and donations, which clearly indicates that long-term sustainability can only be attained if the program is included in the national MOH budget.

CONCLUSION

During the past few years in El Salvador, an LMIC, an important paradigm change in cervical cancer control has occurred. A combination of favorable political climate, evidence-based program implementation, and public and private partnerships has resulted in a shift from conventional screening methods that are not well-suited to resource-poor settings to HPV test-based screen-and-treat national guidelines that have the potential to significantly lower cervical cancer mortality. The key factors involved in this transition are identified in the PREVENTABLE model, which may be used as a reference for other developing countries that are considering implementing national cervical cancer control programs. With evidence from studies and strong political will as the main pillars, a change in paradigm can take place even in low-income settings. Since the CAPE project started, seven peer-reviewed studies have been published, with three more currently in development. In addition, a Spanish book chapter has been written describing the technologies and algorithms used in CAPE and enabling non-English-speaking stakeholders to access this information.[39] We hope that disseminating the data accumulated during CAPE helps decision-makers in other countries work toward the implementation of evidence-based policies that will reduce the cancer burden throughout the world.

REFERENCES

1. Ferlay J, Soerjomataram I, Dikshit R, et al. Cancer incidence and mortality worldwide: Sources, methods and major patterns in GLOBOCAN 2012. *Int J Cancer*. 2015;136(5):E359–E386
2. GLOBOCAN 2012: Estimated cancer incidence, mortality and prevalence worldwide in 2012. 2017. International Agency for Research on Cancer/World Health Organization website. http://globocan.iarc.fr/Pages/fact_sheets_population.aspx. Accessed June 30, 2017.
3. Murillo R, Almonte M, Pereira A, et al. Cervical cancer screening programs in Latin America and the Caribbean. *Vaccine*. 2008;26:L37-L48.
4. Jeronimo J, Bansil P, Lim J, Asthana S. A multicountry evaluation of careHPV testing, visual inspection with acetic acid, and Papanicolaou testing for the detection of cervical cancer. *Int J Gynaecol Cancer*. 2014;24(3):576-585. doi:10.1097/IGC.0000000000000084
5. Perkins RB, Langrish SM, Stern LJ, et al. Impact of patient adherence and test performance on the cost-effectiveness of cervical cancer screening in developing countries: The case of Honduras. *Womens Health Issues*. 2010;20(1):35-42. doi:10.1016/j.whi.2009.09.001. PMID:19944623
6. Maza M, Matesanz S, Alfaro K, et al. Adherence to recommended follow-up care after high-grade cytology in El Salvador. *Int J Healthcare*. 2016;2(2):31.
7. Arrossi S, Ramos S, Paolino M, Sankaranarayanan R. Social inequality in Pap smear coverage: Identifying under-users of cervical cancer screening in Argentina. *Reprod Health Matter*. 2008;16(32):50–58.
8. Jeronimo J, Holme F, Slavkovsky R, Camel C. Implementation of HPV testing in Latin America. *J Clin Virol*. 2016;76:S69–S73.
9. Masch R, Ditzian LR, April AK, et al. Cervical cancer screening and treatment training course in El Salvador: Experience and lessons learned. *J Women' Health*. 2011;20(9):1357–1361.
10. Estrategias de Prevención del Cancer Cervicouterino con Inspección Visual con Ácido Acético y Tratamiento con Crioterapia en América Latin y el Caribe. 2012. Organización Panamericana de la Salud website. http://www.paho.org/hq/dmdocuments/OPS_Estrategias_Prevencion_CC_2011.pdf. Accessed June 29, 2017.
11. The QIAGENcares program: Making improvements in life possible. QIAGENcares website. https://www.qiagen.com/us/

about-us/who-we-are/sustainability/ qiagencares. Accessed June 28, 2017.

12. Frenk J, González-Pier E, Gómez-Dantés O, et al. Comprehensive reform to improve health system performance in Mexico. *Lancet.* 2006;368(9546):1524–1534.

13. Ley de Creación del Sistema Nacional de Salud. *República de El Salvador en La America Central, Diario Oficial.* November 16, 2007. http://asp. salud.gob.sv/regulacion/pdf/ley/Ley_sistema_ nacional_salud.pdf. Accessed June 28, 2017.

14. Construyendo la Esperanza: Estrategias y Recomendaciones en Salud. 2009. Pan American Health Organization website. http:// www.paho.org/els/index.php?option=com_ docman&view=download&alias=658- politica-nacional-de-salud- construyendo-la-esperanza&category_ slug=documentacion-tecnica-1&Itemid=364. Accessed June 28, 2017.

15. Report of the Latin American subregional meeting on cervical cancer prevention: New technologies for cervical cancer prevention— From scientific evidence to program planning, 2010. 2010. Pan American Health Organization website. http://www1.paho.org/hq/ dmdocuments/2010/Panama_report_en.pdf. Accessed June 28, 2017.

16. Informe de Labores, Ministerio de Salud, 2010– 2011. 2011. Ministerio de Salud, El Salvador website. http://api.gobiernoabierto.gob.sv/ documents/98144/download. Accessed June 26, 2017.

17. Schiffman M, Glass AG, Wentzensen N, et al. A long-term prospective study of type-specific human papillomavirus infection and risk of cervical neoplasia among 20,000 women in the Portland Kaiser Cohort Study. *Cancer Epidemiol Prev Biomarkers.* 2011;20(7):1398–1409.

18. Sankaranarayanan R, Nene BM, Shastri SS, et al. HPV screening for cervical cancer in rural India. *N Engl J Med.* 2009;360(14):1385–1394.

19. Denny L, Kuhn L, De Souza M, et al. Screen-and-treat approaches for cervical cancer prevention in low-resource settings: A randomized controlled trial. *JAMA.* 2005;294(17):2173–2181.

20. Kuhn L, Wang C, Tsai WY, et al. Efficacy of human papillomavirus-based screen-and-treat for cervical cancer prevention among HIV-infected women. *AIDS.* 2010;24(16):2553–2561. doi:10.1097/QAD.0b013e32833e163e

21. Ministerio de Salud Junto a Basic Health International y Qiagen Realizarán 2 Mil Pruebas de Detección de Cáncer de Cérvix en San Vicente y Cuscatlán. 2012. Ministerio

de Salud de El Salvador website. http:// w2.salud.gob.sv/novedades/noticias/ noticias-ciudadanosas/209-octubre-2012/ 1562--16-10-2012-ministerio-de-salud-junto-a-basic-health-international-y-qiagen-realizaran-2-mil-pruebas-de-deteccion-de-cancer-de-cervix-en-san-vicente-y-cuscatlan.html. Accessed June 28, 2017.

22. Cremer ML, Maza M, Alfaro KM, et al. Introducing a high-risk HPV DNA test into a public sector screening program in El Salvador. *J Low Genit Tract Dis.* 2016;20(2):145–150. doi:10.1097/LGT.0000000000000188

23. Alfaro KM, Gage JC, Rosenbaum AJ, et al. Factors affecting attendance to cervical cancer screening among women in the paracentral region of El Salvador: A nested study within the CAPE HPV screening program. *BMC Public Health.* 2015;15(1):1058.

24. Rosenbaum AJ, Gage JC, Alfaro KM, et al. Acceptability of self-collected versus provider-collected sampling for HPV DNA testing among women in rural El Salvador. *Int J Gynaecol Obstet.* 2014;126(2):156–160.

25. Campos NG, Maza, M, Alfaro K, et al. The comparative and cost-effectiveness of HPV-based cervical cancer screening algorithms in El Salvador. *Int J Cancer.* 2015;137(4):893–902.

26. Cremer M, Maza M, Alfaro K, et al. Scale-up of an human papillomavirus testing implementation program in El Salvador. *J Low Genit Tract Dis.* 2017;21(1):26–32. doi:10.1097/LGT.0000000000000280

27. Laskow B, Figueroa R, Alfaro KM, et al. A pilot study of community-based self-sampling for HPV testing among non-attenders of cervical cancer screening programs in El Salvador. *Int J Gynaecol Obstet.* 2017;138(2):194–200. doi:10.1002/ijgo.12204

28. Segunda Jornada para la Prevención del Cáncer Cérvico Uterino. 2010. Ministerio de Salud de El Salvador website. http://w2.salud.gob.sv/ novedades/noticias/noticias-ciudadanosas/61- enero-2010/477--28-01-2010-segunda-jornada-para-la-prevencion-del-cancer-cervico-uterino. html. Accessed June 28, 2017.

29. Instituciones del Sector Salud Participan en Simposio sobre la Atención Integral del Cáncer. 2015. Ministerio de Salud de El Salvador website. http://w2.salud.gob.sv/novedades/noticias/ noticias-ciudadanosas/344-noviembre-2015/ 3168--03-11-2015-instituciones-del-sector-salud-participan-en-simposio-sobre-la-atencion-integral-del-cancer.html. Accessed June 28, 2017.

30. Presentan Nueva Guía para el Tamizaje y Tratamiento del Cáncer Cervicouterino. 2017. Organización Panamericana de la Salud-Organización Mundial de la Salud website. http://www.paho.org/els/index. php?option=com_content&view=article&id=8 94:presentan-nueva-guia-tamizaje-tratamiento-cancer-cervicouterino&Itemid=291. Accessed June 28, 2017.

31. WHO Guidelines: Screening and Treatment of Precancerous Lesions for Cervical Cancer Prevention. 2013. World Health Organization website. http://apps.who.int/iris/bitstream/ 10665/94830/1/9789241548694_eng.pdf. Accessed June 28, 2017.

32. Politica Nacional para la Prevención y Control del Cancer. *Republica de El Salvador en la America Central, Diario Oficial.* September 16, 2015. http://asp.salud.gob.sv/regulacion/pdf/ politicas/politica_prevencion_y_control_del_ cancer.pdf. Accessed June 28, 2017.

33. Plan de Implementación de la Política Nacional para la Prevención y Control del Cancer. 2017. Ministerio de Salud de El Salvador website. http://asp.salud.gob. sv/regulacion/pdf/politicas/politica_ prevencion_y_control_del_cancer.pdf. Accessed June 28, 2017.

34. Lineamientos Técnicos para la Prevención y Control del Cáncer Cérvico Uterino y de Mama. 2015. Ministerio de Salud de El Salvador website. http://asp.salud.gob.sv/regulacion/ pdf/lineamientos/lineamientos_prevencion_ cancer_cervico_uterino_y_de_mama_v3.pdf. Accessed June 28, 2017.

35. McNeil DG Jr. Cervical cancer: El Salvador gets a screening test that women can administer at home. *The New York Times,* September 24, 2012. http://www.nytimes. com/2012/09/25/science/cervical-cancer-el-salvador-gets-a-screening-test-that-women-can-administer-at-home.html?_r=4&adxn nl=1&ref=health&adxnnlx=1348754605-AOwb2TAFkSR06t+AatG1DA&. Accessed June 28, 2017.

36. Cáncer Cérvico, Primera Causa de Muerte. *elsalvador.com.* October 28, 2014. http://www. elsalvador.com/noticias/nacional/138392/ cancer-cervico-primera-causa-de-muerte/ Published. Accessed June 29, 2017.

37. Actualización para la Prevención del Cáncer Cervicouterino. 2012. Ministerio de Salud de El Salvador website. http://w2.salud.gob.sv/ component/content/article/208-octubre-2012/ 1563--18-10-2012--inauguracion-del-simposio-qactualizacion-para-la-prevencion-del-cancer-cervico-uterinoq-y-firma-del-memorando-de-entendimiento-entre-basic-health-la-universidad-de-texas-y-el-ministerio-de-salud.html. Accessed June 28, 2017.

38. El Salvador Conmemora el Día Mundial de la Lucha Contra el Cáncer. 2016. Ministerio de Salud de El Salvador website. http://www.salud. gob.sv/04-02-2016-el-salvador-conmemora-el-dia-mundial-de-la-lucha-contra-el-cancer. Accessed June 28, 2017.

39. Tatti S, Fleider L, Tinnirello MA, Caruso R, eds. *Enfoque Integral de las Patologías Relacionadas con el Virus del Papiloma Humano.* Mexico City, Mexico: Editorial Medica Panamericana; 2017.

Case Study 12B

IMPLEMENTING EVIDENCE-BASED TOBACCO USE TREATMENT IN COMMUNITY HEALTH CENTERS IN VIETNAM

Mark Parascandola and Donna Shelley

EACH YEAR, 7 million people die as a result of tobacco use. It is responsible for 1 in 10 deaths globally, and costs governments more than $1 trillion in health care expenditure and lost productivity annually.[1,2] Although tobacco use has been declining in most high-income countries (HICs), it has remained constant or increased in other areas of the world, shifting to low- and middle-income countries (LMICs). A disproportionate share of the global tobacco burden falls on LMICs, where 84% of the world's 1.3 billion current smokers reside.[3] Although smoking prevalence remains comparatively low in some regions, such as sub-Saharan Africa, use is likely to increase because of increased economic development and marketing of manufactured cigarettes, among other factors, if strong tobacco control measures are not implemented.

During the past decade, there has been tremendous progress in adopting evidence-based tobacco control measures in many countries. Progress has been driven by the Framework Convention on Tobacco Control (FCTC), an international treaty that was adopted by the 56th World Health Assembly in 2003 and went into force in 2005.[2] As of 2017, 181 countries were parties to the treaty. The FCTC imposes a range of tobacco control provisions, including increased tobacco taxes, protection from second-hand smoke, warning labels, advertising and sponsorship restrictions, product regulation, restrictions on sales to minors, and support for tobacco cessation. The United Nation's (UN) 2030 Agenda for Sustainable Development also recognizes the importance of addressing tobacco use in LMICs. Sustainable Development Goal (SDG) 3, to "ensure healthy lives and promote well-being for all at all ages," includes Target 3A to "strengthen the implementation of the WHO FCTC in all countries, as appropriate" as a means of reaching the SGDs by 2030.[4] Numerous evidence-based tools and guidelines exist to assist countries in adopting effective tobacco control measures. Notably, the WHO's MPOWER measures (monitor, protect from tobacco smoke, offer help to quit, warn about dangers, enforce bans on promotions, and raise taxes) provide a package of evidence-based tobacco control measures for countries to implement. Although substantial room for progress remains, two-thirds of countries, covering 63% of the world's population, currently have at least one MPOWER measure in place at the recommended level.[2]

For these measures to be effective in practice, they must be successfully implemented. Adoption of laws or policies does not necessarily ensure full implementation. For example, although comprehensive smoke-free legislation is in place in 55 countries (covering almost 20% of the world's population), data show that only 22 (40%) of these countries have high compliance rates. Data further suggest that enforcing smoke-free laws is particularly challenging in cafés, pubs, and bars, for which only 25% of countries report high compliance.[2] In addition, even measures such as raising tobacco taxes, arguably the most consistently effective measure for reducing tobacco use, require effective tax structures and administration to ensure they have the intended effect.[5] Implementation may be especially challenging for LMICs. Many LMICs currently have limited capacity for implementing tobacco control programs, dealing with the health and economic burdens of tobacco use, and addressing challenges from the tobacco industry. In addition, until recently, much of the evidence base for tobacco control measures has come from HICs, and this experience may not be directly applicable to low-resource environments. Guidelines for tobacco cessation treatment, for example, must be responsive to the availability of medications and the structure and capacity of the local health care setting.

Implementation science can play a critical role in supporting ongoing progress in tobacco control. Factors on multiple levels impact tobacco use. In addition to individual-level factors and peer influences on tobacco use, broader economic, social, and political conditions can influence patterns of tobacco use and efforts to control it. The global tobacco control environment is also changing rapidly because of new technologies and mass media channels, the introduction of new tobacco products, and economic and policy developments. In addition, the ongoing activities of the tobacco industry to promote their products and oppose stronger tobacco control measures can impede the success of proven interventions. Thus, an intervention that has been "proven" in one setting may not necessarily have the same effect elsewhere if these factors are not taken into account.

The FCTC requires countries to monitor tobacco use and related measures through regular surveillance to assess the impact of tobacco control efforts. The Global Tobacco Surveillance System (https://www.cdc.gov/tobacco/global/gtss/gtssdata/index.html) and research endeavors such as the International Tobacco Control Policy Evaluation Project (http://www.itcproject.org) have provided a wealth of data to track progress in tobacco control. On a local scale, tobacco control advocates have used air quality measurements in restaurants and bars to bring attention to lack of enforcement of smoke-free laws.[6] However, beyond monitoring, in-depth research is needed to identify and understand factors that influence the successful implementation of tobacco control policies and interventions.

To date, there has been limited application of implementation science theories and methods to tobacco control, especially in LMICs. A handful of recent examples appear in the literature, particularly focused on increasing health care provider engagement in tobacco dependence assessment and treatment across a variety of settings, including challenges faced in rural and low-resource environments.[7-12] Other studies have evaluated the dissemination and use of surveillance tools to assess point-of-sale advertising and promotions and the tobacco retail environment.[13,14] Yet, implementation science methods remain underutilized, leaving a major gap in addressing the complexity of real-world factors that influence how a tobacco control policy or intervention behaves in practice. The following case study provides a key example of how implementation science methods can address challenges in implementing the FCTC in LMICs.

IMPLEMENTING EVIDENCE-BASED TOBACCO USE TREATMENT IN COMMUNITY HEALTH CENTERS IN VIETNAM

Article 14 of the FCTC requires parties to implement effective strategies to "promote cessation of tobacco use and adequate treatment for tobacco dependence."[15] In 2010, WHO released guidelines to assist parties in meeting their obligations under Article 14.[15] Despite this guidance, and a large body of evidence supporting the effectiveness and affordability of a range of health care interventions,[16] progress in providing access to evidence-based cessation services has been slow. A 2014 WHO assessment of FCTC implementation found that one-third of countries still had minimal or no cessation programs, with gaps in service highest among low-income countries.[3,17]

The multilevel barriers to implementing tobacco use treatment in health care settings are well documented and similar across high- and low-income countries. These include a lack of health care provider training, individual- and organizational-level norms and priorities that do not support adoption of treatment, and a lack of systems to facilitate routine screening and referral to population-based resources.[18-22] There is also an extensive literature on effective strategies for overcoming these barriers, including clinical reminder systems, audit and feedback, and referral systems that allow providers to delegate more intensive counseling.[23-27] However, these studies have been conducted exclusively in HICs. Policy and system approaches that are effective in HIC health care systems are likely to require adaptations to local contexts in LMICs.[16,28] Implementation science offers methods for conducting research that can guide large-scale adaptation and adoption of promising strategies for implementing tobacco use treatment guidelines in health system in LMICs.

This case uses formative evaluation (FE) to identify and address the multilevel factors that may facilitate or hinder implementation of Article 14 guidelines in the public health system in Vietnam.[29] Stetler et al.[29] describe FE as key to the "success, interpretation, and replication of results of implementation projects" (p. S7). In collaboration with the Institute for Social Medical Studies, a research institute in Hanoi, Vietnam, we are using a cluster-randomized design to compare the cost-effectiveness of two strategies that are hypothesized to increase implementation of evidence-based tobacco use treatment interventions in community health centers (CHCs) in Vietnam: (1) training, clinical reminder, and documentation systems and toolkit (TCT) and (2) TCT + referral to a village health worker (VHW) for three in-person counseling sessions.[30] The implementation strategies draw on evidence-based approaches and a growing literature that supports the effectiveness of leveraging lay health workers to improve access to preventive services.[23,25-27,31-34] We adapted a staged approach to FE that included developmental, implementation, and progress-focused and interpretive FE.[29] Here, we describe the goals, our use of mixed

methods, and a brief overview of findings for each stage of FE.

Stage 1: Developmental FE

There were two phases of the developmental FE.

PHASE 1

Goals: The purpose of the first phase was to (1) to understand the primary care workforce in Vietnam, including the role of clinicians and VHWs who work in CHCs; (2) to explore current practices and barriers related to delivering tobacco use treatment (e.g., frequency of screening and offering brief advise to quit, attitudes, and norms); and (3) to assess the acceptability and feasibility of integrating a system in CHCs in which VHWs served as a population-based referral resource for more intensive counseling.

Methods: To obtain this information, we conducted four focus groups with VHWs and a survey of 129 clinicians who worked in CHCs in Thai Nguyen, the province where we planned to conduct the study.[19,20] Focus groups were informed by Bowen et al.[35] model for assessing the feasibility of implementing evidence-based interventions or new care processes (e.g., acceptability, practicality, and adaptation). The clinician survey assessed current practices and attitudes, norms, and self-efficacy related to tobacco use treatment.[36,37] We also met with the director of the Vietnam Committee on Smoking and Health (VINACOSH) to ensure that the proposed model for implementing Article 14 guidelines in CHCs was aligned with the tobacco control program's policy agenda for increasing access to cessation assistance.

Findings and implications: Focus group and survey findings supported the proposed implementation strategies and confirmed gaps in training and cessation service delivery.[19] VHWs fully supported the feasibility and acceptability of serving as a referral resource for providers in local CHCs.[19] One VHW stated, "We have the responsibility to protect the public health. This program is not outside that goal." The most frequently cited barrier to offering cessation services was the lack of prioritization by the Ministry of Health (MOH). Despite enacting a National Tobacco Control Action plan, cessation was not one of the national prevention priorities. As a result, VHWs have not been "assigned" to help smokers quit by MOH. Clinician-reported barriers included a lack of training, time constraints, and a lack of referral resources and staff support to counsel patients.[20] However, like VHWs, clinicians agreed that cessation assistance was well within their scope of work.[19,20]

PHASE 2

Goals and methods: We conducted (1) key informant interviews (KIs) with leaders in the public health sector responsible for developing and implementing policy in Vietnam to assess contextual factors (e.g., MOH and district-level policy priorities) that may influence implementation and dissemination; (2) study site observations to inform necessary adaptations to the proposed system changes (i.e., reminder, documentation, and referral systems) to increase "fit" in the local delivery system context;[38] and (3) guided by the Consolidated Framework for Implementation Research, KIs with clinicians and VHWs ($n = 40$) in 8 of the 26 CHCs enrolled in the study to inform further modifications to the implementation strategies that may be necessary to translate a model of care delivery from an HIC to the local context of an LMIC.[39]

Findings and implications: Site observations revealed that there was no chart system to use for the reminder and documentation system. Therefore, we designed a poster to prompt clinicians to ask about tobacco use, offer brief advice, and, in Arm 2, refer to the VHW. We also created two forms— one for clinicians to document screening, smoking status, and delivery of brief advice to quit and a separate referral form. Finally, we worked with the sites and local partners to develop a new workflow for integrating tobacco use screening, treatment, and referral. Key informant interviews with VINACOSH leadership indicated that MOH was beginning to build infrastructure to implement Article 14, but only in provincial hospitals and not in CHCs, which serve as the front line for primary care services. These interviews confirmed the need for data to support cost-effective models for disseminating cessation services system-wide, including CHCs.

The KIs with VHWs and clinicians pointed to several potential facilitators and barriers to implementing a new model of collaborative care that includes VHWs to optimize integration of tobacco use treatment in CHCs.[21] In summary, potential facilitators

of the intervention included the relative advantage of the intervention given the complete lack of cessation training and resources currently available (e.g., one CHC staff member stated, "We have no knowledge to give them advice. We need to get the proper training"), MOH-driven policies (e.g., smoke-free air laws and media campaigns) that have led to a growing awareness of the burden of tobacco use in the population, CHC leadership engagement, and a strong sense of collective efficacy that was illustrated by the following comment from a CHC director: "VHWs and CHC staff support each other in each task. To me they are like my long arm and whether health care at grassroots is good or not mainly depends on the VHWs."

Potential barriers included the perception that the intervention was more complex and not necessarily compatible with current workflows and staffing that were historically designed to address infectious disease prevention and control rather than chronic disease prevention. However, a model that shifted primary responsibility for counseling to VHWs was viewed as consistent with their role and an appropriate solution to reducing clinician burden. Additional perceived barriers included competing priorities that are determined by MOH and the lack of autonomy to make local changes. A WHW stated, "We do not decide by ourselves about what to do," and a CHC director noted, "The program's implementation still depends on the support of authorities."

Stage 2: Implementation and Progress-Focused FE

Goals: The purpose was to (1) identify modifiable barriers to implementing the intervention components with fidelity, (2) use the data to make needed refinements to the intervention, and (3) obtain data relevant to future scale-up (e.g., the amount of training and monitoring needed).[29] There were several sources of data in this stage of the evaluation; however, we focus here on the on the FE related to assessing the VHW referral and counseling component.

Methods: VHWs were trained to use a three-session counseling manual.[30] Research assistants (RAs) were trained to observe a random sample of sessions and used a standard form to assess VHW adherence to the goals of each session. VHWs also used a tracking form to document each session. Finally, we collected referral forms at each site and used these to confirm that patients who were referred were enrolled in counseling. Three months after the initial training, we conducted an additional 2-day training that specifically addressed barriers identified by reviewing these data sources and in further discussions with the VHWs.

Findings and implications: The tools proved useful for tracking and providing feedback to the VHWs on their performance. They also allowed us to rapidly identify VHWs who were struggling with delivering the intervention and to intervene to increase confidence and skills through the additional training. A similar "booster" training was conducted with clinicians from the CHCs during which we elicited challenges with the documentation and referrals systems that resulted in some adjustments to the workflow and reinforced screening and counseling skills.

Stage 3: Interpretative FE

Goal and methods: The purpose of this stage of FE was to (1) gain a deeper understanding of the impact and value of the intervention; and (2) assess if the barriers described in the developmental and implementation stages were addressed through refinement of the intervention components or if they required further adaptation to improve implementation effectiveness and potential for sustainability and system-wide scale-up. We conducted post-intervention KIs with clinicians and VHWs in 16 sites (*n* = 42).[40]

Findings and implications: Contrary to initial concerns about the complexity and time demands of the intervention, providers reported that screening and offering brief advice were feasible and appropriate (i.e., fit into workflow): One provider stated, "The screening and counseling are integrated into our work. It only takes a few minutes, so it's ok." These interviews also confirmed the value of the ask (screen all patients), advise, refer model in shifting responsibility for counseling to a trained health care worker and the feasibility, acceptability, and perceived effectiveness of a model that integrates tobacco use treatment into routine workflow. A CHC staff member commented, "I think when patients are referred to the VHWs, the effectiveness of the program is very high." In this stage of evaluation, we elicited several recommendations for improving the approach. VHWs noted that many smokers do not access the CHC, an important fact that was not described in the development FE

stage, and suggested integrating tobacco cessation with other community-based VHW-led prevention programs to increase the reach of cessation support. One VHW stated, "We should not sit and wait for patients coming to the CHC." Both VHWs and clinicians were highly satisfied with the educational materials and training, but they also emphasized the need for ongoing training to maintain skills. Finally, VHWs and clinicians emphasized their lack of autonomy to make local changes in care processes and the need for MOH to prioritize tobacco cessation to ensure sustainable change. A CHC staff member noted, "If we want the program to be continued, this program should be handled the same way as other national health programs."

CONCLUSION

This case demonstrates the value of conducting FE at several stages across a study timeline to complement the randomized controlled trial outcome data, and it highlights challenges associated with applying this methodology. One that has been well described is the need to balance fidelity and adaption when modifying implementation strategies (interventions).[29,41] Our approach to achieving this balance was to maintain the core elements of the intervention that were hypothesized to produce the main effect while allowing tailoring to local context (e.g., the chart reminder system became a poster reminder), providing implementation support through feedback and booster training, and concurrently conducting a rigorous assessment of fidelity.[42,43] Using a framework, like the one proposed by Stirman et al.,[43] to systematically capture the rationale, nature, and number of adaptations and the process by which they were achieved will help address the challenge of interpreting the impact of these changes on study outcomes .[41,43]

Our qualitative interviews with health care professionals and VINACOSH in the first and final stages of FE were particularly important for elucidating the significant impact that the political context of this LMIC has on implementation efforts. The centralization of decision-making authority makes it difficult for CHCs and VHWs to innovate locally and to sustain interventions without MOH approval and support. In this political context, we developed a process and infrastructure for early and ongoing engagement with key stakeholders across all four levels of the health care system in Vietnam (i.e., national, provincial, district, and community). Meetings focused on aligning the project with national tobacco control priorities for expanding access to cessation services, sharing data, and obtaining feedback on modifications needed to disseminate the implementing strategies more widely. We continue to meet with VINACOSH to build on our recommendations from the final stage of FE and to provide additional assistance with other plans for implementing Article 14.

Finally, countries such as Vietnam, which ratified the FCTC in 2004, are making progress in implementing the full range of MPOWER recommendations.[44] However, to accelerate and optimize implementation effectiveness and inform decisions about optimal system-wide scale-up, partnerships with local institutions and MOHs are needed to build local research capacity, with a specific focus on applying implementation science methods to monitoring and evaluation efforts. This case study provides an example of how implementation science methods can aid the dissemination and implementation of tobacco control interventions, particularly in a low-resource setting.

REFERENCES

1. National Cancer Institute/World Health Organization. *The Economics of Tobacco and Tobacco Control*. National Cancer Institute Tobacco Control Monograph 21; NIH Publication No. 16-CA-8029A. Bethesda, MD: US Department of Health and Human Services, National Institutes of Health, National Cancer Institute; and Geneva, Switzerland: World Health Organization; 2016.

2. World Health Organization. WHO report on the global tobacco epidemic, 2017: monitoring tobacco use and prevention policies. 2017. http://www.who.int/tobacco/global_report/2017/en.

3. World Health Organization. WHO report on the global tobacco epidemic, 2015. 2015. http://apps.who.int/iris/bitstream/10665/178574/1/9789240694606_eng.pdf?ua=1.

4. UN Inter-Agency Task Force on the Prevention and Control of NCDs. How NCDs are reflected in governing body policies, strategies and plans. 2016. http://www.who.int/ncds/un-task-force/NCDs-governingbodypolicies-feb2016.pdf

5. Gao S, Zheng R, Hu TW. Can increases in the cigarette tax rate be linked to cigarette retail prices? Solving mysteries related to the cigarette pricing mechanism in China. *Tob Control*. 2012;21(6):560–562.

6. Jackson-Morris A, Bleymann K, Lyall E, et al. Low-cost air quality monitoring methods to assess compliance with smoke-free regulations: A multi-center study in six low- and middle-income countries. *Nicotine Tob Res*. 2016;18(5):1258–1264.

7. Bartlem KM, Bowman J, Freund M, et al. Effectiveness of an intervention in increasing the provision of preventive care by community mental health services: A non-randomized, multiple baseline implementation trial. *Implement Sci*. 2016;11:46.

8. Duffy SA, Ronis DL, Ewing LA, et al. Implementation of the Tobacco Tactics intervention versus usual care in Trinity Health community hospitals. *Implement Sci*. 2016;11(1):147.

9. Elsey H, Khanal S, Manandhar S, Sah D, Baral SC, Siddiqi K, Newell JN. Understanding implementation and feasibility of tobacco cessation in routine primary care in Nepal: A mixed methods study. *Implement Sci*. 2016;11:104.

10. Slattery C, Freund M, Gillham K, Knight J, Wolfenden L, Bisquera A, Wiggers J. Increasing smoking cessation care across a network of hospitals: An implementation study. *Implement Sci*. 2016;11:28.

11. Eaves ER, Howerter A, Nichter M, Floden L, Gordon JS, Ritenbaugh C, Muramoto ML. Implementation of tobacco cessation brief intervention in complementary and alternative medicine practice: Qualitative evaluation. *BMC Complement Altern Med*. 2017;17(1):331.

12. Knudsen HK. Implementation of smoking cessation treatment in substance use disorder treatment settings: A review. *Am J Drug Alcohol Abuse*. 2017;43(2):215–225.

13. Cantrell J, Ganz O, Ilakkuvan V, et al. Implementation of a multimodal mobile system for point-of-sale surveillance: Lessons learned from case studies in Washington, DC, and New York City. *JMIR Public Health Surveill*. 2015;1(2):e20.

14. Henriksen L, Ribisl KM, Rogers T, et al. Standardized Tobacco Assessment for Retail Settings (STARS): dissemination and implementation research. *Tob Control*. 2016;25(Suppl 1):i67–i74.

15. World Health Organization Conference of the Parties. Guidelines for implementation of Article 14 of the WHO Framework Convention on Tobacco Control. 2010. http://www.who.int/fctc/Guidelines.pdf. Accessed January 26, 2017.

16. West R, Raw M, McNeill A, et al. Health-care interventions to promote and assist tobacco cessation: A review of efficacy, effectiveness and affordability for use in national guideline development. *Addiction.* 2015;110(9):1388–1403.

17. Raw M, Regan S, Rigotti NA, McNeill A. A survey of tobacco dependence treatment guidelines in 31 countries. *Addiction.* 2009;104(7):1243–1250.

18. Yan J, Xiao S, Ouyang D, Jiang D, He C, Yi S. Smoking behavior, knowledge, attitudes and practice among health care providers in Changsha City, China. *Nicotine Tob Res.* 2008;10:737–744.

19. Shelley D, Nguyen L, Pham H, VanDevanter N, Nguyen N. Barriers and facilitators to expanding the role of community health workers to include smoking cessation services in Vietnam: A qualitative analysis. *BMC Health Serv Res.* 2014a;14:606. doi:10.1186/s12913-014-0606-1

20. Shelley D, Tseng TY, Pham H, Nguyen L, Keithly S, Stillman F, Nguyen N. Factors influencing tobacco use treatment patterns among Vietnamese health care providers working in community health centers. *BMC Public Health.* 2014b;14:68.

21. VanDevanter N, Zhou S, Katigbak C, Naegle M, Sherman S, Weitzman M. Knowledge, beliefs, behaviors, and social norms related to use of alternative tobacco products among undergraduate and graduate nursing students in an urban U.S. university setting. *J Nurs Scholarsh.* 2016;48(2):147–153.

22. Thomas D, Abramson MJ, Bonevski B, George J. System change interventions for smoking cessation. *Cochrane Database Syst Rev.* 2017;2017(2):CD010742. doi:10.1002/14651858.CD010742.pub

23. Bentz CJ, Bayley KB, Bonin KE, et al. Provider feedback to improve 5A's tobacco cessation in primary care: A cluster randomized clinical trial. *Nicotine Tob Res.* 2007;9(3):341–349.

24. Fiore MC, Jaén C, Baker T, et al. *Treating Tobacco Use and Dependence: 2008 Update. Clinical Practice Guideline.* Rockville, MD: US Department of Health and Human Services, Public Health Service; 2008.

25. Rothemich SF, Woolf SH, Johnson RE, Burgett AE, Flores SK, Marsland DW, Ahluwalia JS. Effect on cessation counseling of documenting smoking status as a routine vital sign: An ACORN study. *Ann Fam Med.* 2008;6(1):60–68.

26. Shelley D, Cantrell J. The effect of linking community health centers to a state-level smoker's quitline on rates of cessation assistance. *BMC Health Serv Res.* 2010;10:25.

27. Sheffer MA, Baker TB, Fraser DL, Adsit RT, McAfee TA, Fiore MC. Fax referrals, academic detailing, and tobacco quitline use: A randomized trial. *Am J Prev Med.* 2012;42(1):21–28.

28. McRobbie H, Raw M, Chan S. Research priorities for Article 14 demand reduction measures concerning tobacco dependence and cessation. *Nicotine Tob Res.* 2013;15 (4):805–816.

29. Stetler CB, Legro MW, Wallace CM, Bowman C, Guihan M, Hagedorn H, Kimmel B, Sharp ND, Smith JL. The role of formative evaluation in implementation research and the QUERI experience. *J Gen Intern Med.* 2006;21(Suppl 2):S1–S8.

30. Shelley D, VanDevanter N, Cleland CC, Nguyen L, Nguyen N. Implementing tobacco use treatment guidelines in community health centers in Vietnam. *Implement Sci.* 2015 Oct 9;10:142. doi:10.1186/s13012-015-0328-8. PMID:26453554.

31. Rosenthal EL, Brownstein JN, Rush CH, et al. Community health workers: part of the solution. *Health Aff (Millwood).* 2010;29(7):1338–1342.

32. Landers SJ. Community health workers—Practice and promise. *Am J Public Health.* 2011;101:2198.

33. Singh P, Chokshi DA. Community health workers—A local solution to a global problem. *N Engl J Med.* 2013;369:894–896.

34. Jeet G, Thakur JS, Prinja S, Singh M. Community health workers for non-communicable diseases prevention and control in developing countries: Evidence and implications. *PLoS One.* 2017;12(7):e0180640. doi:10.1371/journal.pone.0180640

35. Bowen DJ, Kreuter M, Spring B, et al. How we design feasibility studies. *Am J Prev Med.* 2009;36(5):452–457.

36. Ajzen I. The theory of planned behavior. *Organ Behav Hum Decis Process.* 1991;50:179–211.

37. Francis JJ, Eccles MP, Johnston M, Whitty P, Grimshaw JM, Kaner EF, Smith L, Walker A: Explaining the effects of an intervention designed to promote evidence-based diabetes care: A theory-based process evaluation of a pragmatic cluster randomised controlled trial. *Implement Sci.* 2008,3:50. doi:10.1186/1748-5908-3-50

38. Proctor EK, Silmere H, Raghavan R, et al. Outcomes for implementation research: Conceptual distinctions, measurement challenges, and research agenda. *Adm Policy*

Ment Health. 2011;38(2):65–76. doi:10.1007/s10488-010-0319-7

39. Damschroder LJ, Aron DC, Keith RE, Kirsh SR, Alexander JA, Lowery JC. Fostering implementation of health services research findings into practice: A consolidated framework for advancing implementation science. *Implement Sci.* 2009;4:50.

40. Shelley D, et al. SRNT annual conference presentation, Florence, Italy, 2017.

41. Stirman SW, Kimberly J, Cook N, Calloway A, Castro F, Charns M. The sustainability of new programs and innovations: A review of the empirical literature and recommendations for future research. *Implement Sci.* 2012;7(17):1–19.

42. Bosworth H B, Almiral, D, Weiner BJ, et al. The implementation of a translational study involving a primary care based behavioral program to improve blood pressure control: The HTN-IMPROVE study protocol (01295). *Implement Sci.* 2010;5:54. doi:10.1186/1748-5908-5-54

43. Stirman, SW, Miller, CJ, Toder, K, Calloway A. Development of a framework and coding system for modifications and adaptations of evidence-based interventions. *Implement Sci.* 2013;8(65):1–12.

44. Minh HV, Ngan TT, Mai VQ, et al. Tobacco control policies in Vietnam: Review on MPOWER implementation progress and challenges. *Asian Pac J Cancer Prev.* 2016;17(Suppl):1–9.

Case Study 12C

ASSESSING THE COMMUNITY CONTEXT WHEN IMPLEMENTING CERVICAL CANCER SCREENING PROGRAMS

Prajakta Adsul and Purnima Madhivanan

ACCORDING TO estimates by the World Health Organization, in 2016 there were approximately 122,844 new cases of cervical cancer and 67,544 deaths due to cervical cancer in India.[1] With 38% of the cervical cancer cases occurring among women between the ages of 15 and 45 years, the economic and social impact of the disease in India is substantial.[2] Studies using visual inspection methods (such as Visual Inspection using Acetic Acid (VIA),for cervical cancer screening have demonstrated significant decreases in incidence and mortality.[3,4] Cancer screening, however, presents a challenge for implementation because a successful screening program requires the coordination of a series of steps beyond initial testing, including appropriate diagnostic follow-up and adequate treatment. In addition, uptake of cancer screening among asymptomatic populations can be affected by several individual- and system-level contextual factors, such as economic status, place of residence, facility resources, and stakeholder support. More important, for "evidence-based"

decision-making, there is a critical need to understand and report the context and implementation information for interventions such as cancer screening in different populations. This contextual information is lacking in the existing literature.[5] The objective of this case study is to demonstrate the use of qualitative, community-based, participatory research in order to understand the context in which cervical cancer screening programs are implemented in rural India, thereby enabling not just successful implementation but also future sustainability of the program in the community.

This study is based on the experience of the Public Health Research Institute of India (PHRII), a nongovernmental organization located in Mysore, India. PHRII was established in 2007 with a goal to improve the health of Indian women through research and health care on issues that affect women's lives from birth through old age. To carry out its work, PHRII has more than 23 full-time employees, including physicians, nurses, administrators, laboratory

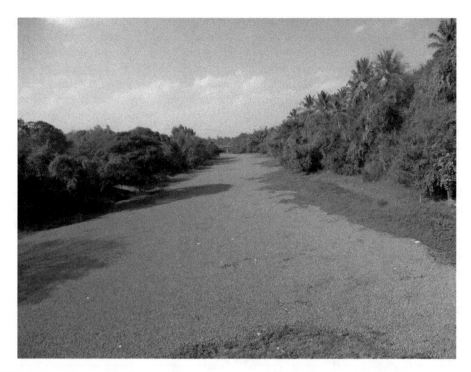

FIGURE 12C.1   Photograph of an algal bloom due to river pollution taken by a 31-year-old female participant.

personnel, health counselors, and community outreach workers. What makes PHRII unique is that most of the employees are women from within the community that PHRII serves. The institute also operates the Prerana Reproductive Health Clinic, which offers free outpatient services for family planning, reproductive health care, cervical cancer screening, and HIV prevention to low-income communities in and near Mysore. In addition, it operates mobile clinics that provide reproductive health care in a rural catchment of more than 144 rural villages in the Mysore District. Through this clinical work, PHRII has been able to establish unique networks with the primary, secondary, and tertiary public health and private health care organizations serving this community. Despite these community–clinical linkages and providing access to free services, most women in the community have not participated in cervical cancer screening programs. In addition, understanding the views of the providers (both clinicians and community health workers) seemed essential to capture a comprehensive understanding of the community context.

The projects described in this case study were conducted as part of the primary author's Fogarty Global Health Equity Fellowship based with PHRII as the training site. A series of studies were undertaken to understand the cervical cancer screening program in its current state and provide information for the implementation of future programs. These studies included (1) qualitative interviews with physicians delivering cervical cancer care in the private and public sector, (2) focus group discussions with healthcare workers in primary health care clinics, and (3) a photovoice study with women residing in the communities. We discuss these studies from a socioecological perspective (Figure 12C.1) to reveal the context in which cervical cancer screening takes place in this community. We follow up with a discussion on the lessons learned through these studies as relevant to the implementation of a national program for cervical cancer screening in India.

INDIVIDUAL KNOWLEDGE AND BELIEFS

At the individual level, women at risk for cervical cancer could be influenced to participate in the screening programs based on their personal knowledge and misinformation about cancer and cancer screening tests and their personal beliefs of stigma associated with cancer in the community.

To explore these perceptions, we recruited 14 women aged 30–60 years residing in rural villages around Mysore, Karnataka, India, to participate in a photovoice project. Each participant was provided with a digital camera and asked to photo document her everyday realities that reflected the perceived barriers toward cervical cancer screening. During the photo collection, participants met individually with the researchers to discuss the meaning of their photographs. Discussions were primarily based on a set of questions using the mnemonic "SHOWED": What do you see here? What is really happening? How does this relate to our lives? Why does this problem exist? and What can we do about it? Group discussions were conducted on the action steps required to address these barriers. Themes that emerged from these data are presented below. t.

Information and Misinformation About Cancer Screening

In the photovoice study, several women reported lack of information about cancer and its prevention. One participant clicked a picture (Figure 12C.1) of an algal bloom in a river due to pollution and stated:

> Women in my community always say they are okay and don't need to go for any test. Just like this river, when you look at the river you think this is beautiful but what they don't know is that underneath all the grass is a polluted river.

Discussions around this picture highlighted that many women do not understand the concept of cancer prevention because they believe that cancer is a fatal disease. Other women reported several instances of misinformation about the cervical cancer screening test. Some reported hearing about physicians and nurses who were not gentle with patients during the pelvic exam, whereas others stated that women experience pain and itching after the pelvic exam, which prevented them from seeking screening services.

Fear Associated with Cancer Diagnosis

Many women reported strong perceptions of fearing a cancer diagnosis. Several women in the study reported hearing of women in their community who

had died due to cancer despite seeking medical care and investing significant financial resources. They believed that no medical intervention could prevent death and thus convinced themselves not to avail of any preventive services. When probed further, women reported that they did not know cancer could be identified early and treated to prevent death.

FAMILY AND PEER SUPPORT

Interactions with family members and peer community groups had important influences on women participating in the cervical cancer screening programs.

Role of Family

In India, marriage and family dominate a woman's life.[6] After the wedding ceremony, women are required to leave their parents' home and reside in their husband's and in-laws' home. Within the family context, women in our study reported being at a disadvantage as follows: When a woman in their community was diagnosed with a life-threatening disease (cancer, stroke, or cardiac), the husband and in-laws often shrugged their financial responsibility toward her treatment. Thus, the woman would be left with no other option but to return to the home of her parents, who were likely already living in poverty and could not afford to pay for her treatment. Consequently, many women reported not wanting to find out a cancer diagnosis so as not to burden their families with their health and financial issues.

In addition, many women also reported the belief that their personal time and health were not respected by the members of their family, especially their husband and mother-in-law. One of the women in the study described her feelings of helplessness when she spoke about a picture she clicked showing the entrance gate to her house:

> I feel like I don't have the right to take a decision for myself. If I want to go for screening, I have to explain why it is important for my health to everyone in the household and finally it is their choice whether to let me go for it or not.

Mother-in-laws usually did not support the women participating in preventive services for their health, stating that they themselves were alive and well despite not getting screened.

Role of Community-Based Peer Groups

Several participants provided pictures of Mahila Sangha ladies associations during their meetings in the community Although these associations were created with the purpose of empowering women via financial programs in the community, they could serve as avenues for perpetuating negative experiences and false information. The participant that clicked a picture of one of these meetings (Figure 12C.2), stated, "I have heard from other women in my group that pelvic exams involved doctors putting their entire hands in the vagina. That scared me and other women in the group too!" Some women, however, reported that these groups could also serve as good avenues for delivering group-based health education to increase peer support. Such peer support could be instrumental in

motivating women to participate in preventive services such as cervical cancer screening programs.

HEALTH CARE SERVICES AND PROVIDERS

To provide comprehensive information about the context of women in the Mysore community, we conducted a qualitative inquiry to explore the perceptions of medical professionals actively providing care to women in the community who were eligible for cervical cancer screening. Our informants were gynecologists practicing in the community, radiation and medical oncologists from both private and public hospitals, pathologists, and primary care physicians practicing in public hospitals. We restricted our sample to physicians who were practicing in the rural and urban areas surrounding Mysore to better understand the local context of implementation within this community. PHRII is one of the key stakeholders and an organization with a decade of expertise in providing

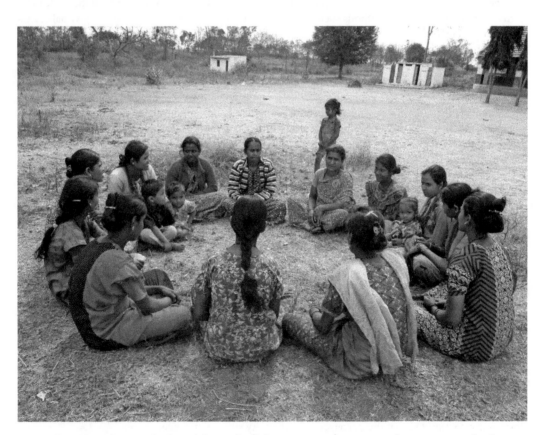

FIGURE 12C.2 Photograph of a Mahila Sangha (ladies association) meeting in the community taken by a 41-year-old participant.

cervical cancer screening for at-risk women in this community.

Perceptions from the Physicians

With regard to cervical cancer prevention in their communities, several physicians stated that vaccinations were the best way to reduce the cervical cancer burden because they believed that women in their communities would not come for screening. When queried further, several gynecologists reported that women in the community lacked knowledge that cervical cancer could be prevented using screening, feared positive screening results, and lacked financial resources for follow-up and treatment, thus leading them not to seek screening. Almost all stakeholders mentioned Pap smears as the most commonly used screening methodology and did not use visual inspection methods. Physicians in our study were not aware of the HPV DNA testing option.

When probed, almost half the stakeholders reported that visual inspection methods such as VIA would be acceptable to them and the women in their communities, and they would be feasible to implement within their resource-limited settings. Although providers believed in the importance of preventive services such as screening, they were unable to provide these services to all patients due to two specific reasons: (1) the current practice needs demanded attention to secondary care and required them to focus on treatment rather than prevention, and (2) they believed that patients were not aware of the concept of prevention and only seek care when symptomatic. As front-line workers providing care to the community, the providers expressed the need for more public–private partnerships that could help balance the lack of resources in the public sector and the need for additional human resources, specifically nurses and patient navigators.

The perceptions of the health care providers reported in this study align with perceptions about primary prevention reported in previous studies. Mirand and colleagues[7] found that delivery of non-reimbursed but critical health behavior counseling services was conceptually important to the physicians but encountered barriers by the predominant clinical emphasis on secondary care. Physicians also reported that the perceived role of a doctor is one that "diagnoses and provides an immediate answer to a patient's problem."[8] Physicians, however, remain the most trusted source for health or medical information.[9] Along with the need for system-wide changes (payers and practice organizations) to increase the rewards for preventive behavior, there is a need for physicians to fully utilize their unique positions to deliver preventive care.

Perceptions from the Health Care Workers

In the rural health care system in India, auxiliary nurse midwives (ANMs), or more recently known as female/male health workers (F/MHWs), are key field-level personnel who interact directly with the community and act as liaisons between the public health care system and the people served.[10] Traditionally, FHWs are appointed to primary care clinics after obtaining a 2-year clinical associate's degree, and their role has primarily focused on family planning and preventive services.[11] However, the operational guidelines for the National Program for Prevention and Control of Cancer, Diabetes, CVD and Stroke (NPCDCS) may expand their role to include cervical cancer screening using visual examination methods.[12]

The delegation strategy to realign human resources in health systems has been used in many settings in India and indicates moving particular tasks up or down a traditional role ladder.[13] Indeed, several studies reporting cervical cancer screening delivery have evaluated the role of community health care workers.[14,15] Two information gaps exist in this context: (1) the traditional use of health workers to deliver maternal and child health care but not cancer-related services and (2) the health workers' perceptions toward cervical cancer control and prevention because they are usually the first point of contact between the health care systems and women in the community. Therefore, we decided to focus our qualitative inquiry on evaluating the perceptions of health workers who currently work in primary health care centers in the community. Specifically, we wanted to collect information on cancer-related services that are provided to the women in the community, community perceptions about cancer, health policies for cancer care, and barriers to delivering and accessing cancer care in the community. We also inquired about their perceived role in supporting women in the community who are at risk for cancer.

The FHW's in the primary care clinics reported adequate understanding regarding cancer prevention; however, they could not provide information on specific screening methods for cervical cancer. In some cases, health care workers brought up misconceptions around the causes of cervical cancer. Many workers reported hearing about cancer cases in the community that were usually fatal. Although most workers shared the belief that cancer could be prevented, they reported not having enough training or knowledge to provide community members with cancer prevention-related information. In addition, they did not have access to information materials at their government clinics that could help educate the communities within their reach. The most important barrier for implementing cervical cancer prevention programs highlighted by the health workers was the lack of knowledge regarding cervical cancer, its prevention, and the facilities where cervical cancer screening was provided in their communities.

POLICIES SUPPORTING CERVICAL CANCER PREVENTION AND CONTROL

At the time of this work, the government was offering no cervical cancer screening programs in this community. Many participants reported that Pap tests were not currently delivered in primary care clinics. The health workers in the community reported several financial resources for the treatment of chronic diseases, but none of these were specific to cancer. Some workers reported private hospitals conducting screening programs for heart and eye disease but not for cancer, and none of these programs collaborated with primary care centers. Based on their knowledge of the health care systems, the health care workers reported that no government health care organizations in their communities dealt with cancer-related issues. The nearest facility that could diagnose and treat cancer was the District Level Hospital in Mysore, located 35–50 kilometers away from their communities.

CONCLUSION

Using community-based research helped identify elements of the social and cultural context of rural communities that provided information on several contextual factors that could be integrated into pre-intervention capacity development in the future. We captured data from three different sources—women at risk for cervical cancer in the community, physicians and other providers providing health care to women in the community, and the health workers—allowing us to portray a comprehensive context of implementing cervical cancer screening programs in this community.

Research

The work conducted within the photovoice project was instrumental in developing an in-depth understanding of the specific barriers for women participating in screening programs. Integrating these barriers into interventions that target at-risk women can be important as primary health care settings deliver cervical cancer prevention programs in their communities. Our work also suggests that the role of family and peer support for women in rural communities needs emphasis in health education-based communication strategies for cervical cancer prevention programs. As cervical cancer prevention programs are scaled up to different communities, it will be crucial to conduct pre-implementation science among key stakeholders and address the challenges upfront. More research focused on implementation and context is needed in conducting a formative assessment of the community that is being targeted and, more important, to evaluate the programs throughout implementation to ensure sustainability.

Policy

To reduce the burden of cervical cancer, the Government of India has instituted NPCDCS, which includes an algorithm for how cervical cancer screening should occur within India's public health infrastructure.[12] Our qualitative research suggests that as cervical cancer screening programs are implemented in various setting across India, there is a need to provide intensive training to clinicians in the public health care system, which has traditionally focused on maternal and child health, to reorient and focus on cancer prevention. The success of the policy and the programs at primary care clinics will depend on community workers, who are often the first point of contact for women in the community. It will also be necessary to reorient the education and training of health workers to meet the health needs of the community as awareness about cervical cancer and prevention grows and to achieve high participation rates from women within the community. Last, if women are to participate in the screening programs, there is a critical need for treatment coverage either through government policies (as they currently exists for chronic diseases) or through employee insurance coverage.

Practice

The work in the Mysore community, although not widely generalizable, has important practice implications. Women in the underserved communities need to be provided with opportunities through health communication campaigns to improve their knowledge about cervical cancer and the important fact that it can be prevented by early detection through screening exams. Survivor stories in this context were reported to be one strategy that may influence women's beliefs and motivate them to participate in screening programs. For a health care system that has primarily relied on symptomatic individuals seeking health care, program implementers will need to be creative in choosing strategies that can motivate asymptomatic women to undergo preventive care services.

Health workers in our study described being overburdened with work. Offering appropriate packages of monetary and nonmonetary incentives to encourage qualified health workers to serve in rural, remote, and underserved areas will need to be a focus as cancer screening and prevention programs are integrated into primary health care settings. Implementing national cancer control programs will also be a valuable intersection to integrate specific strategies to improve quality of services, self-efficacy for providers delivering both medical and paramedical cancer care, and strategies for motivating the at-risk but asymptomatic women in the community.

Advancing knowledge on implementation of evidence based interventions has become critical because low- and middle-income countries share the highest burden of cervical cancer. Studies that use community-based participatory research principles provide researchers with an opportunity to understand the context in which interventions are delivered and utilized, ultimately contributing to the much-needed field of implementation science.

ACKNOWLEDGMENT

Research reported in this publication was supported by the Fogarty International Center of the National Institutes of Health (under training grant TW009338). The content is solely the responsibility of the authors and does not necessarily represent the official views of the National Institutes of Health.

REFERENCES

1. Bruni L, Barrionuevo-Rosas L, Albero G, et al. *Human Papillomavirus and Related Diseases in India.* Barcelona, Spain: ICO Information Centre on HPV and Cancer (HPV Information Centre); 2016.
2. Krishnan S, Madsen E, Porterfield D, Varghese B. Advancing cervical cancer prevention in India: Implementation science priorities. *The Oncologist.* 2013;18(12):1285–1297.
3. Kishor S, Gupta K. Gender equality and women's empowerment in India. National Family Health Survey (NFHS-3) India 2005-06. 2009.
4. Sankaranarayanan R, Esmy PO, Rajkumar R, et al. Effect of visual screening on cervical cancer incidence and mortality in Tamil Nadu, India: A cluster-randomised trial. *Lancet.* 2007;370(9585):398–406.
5. Luoto J, Shekelle PG, Maglione MA, Johnsen B, Perry T. Reporting of context and implementation in studies of global health interventions: A pilot study. *Implement Sci.* 2014;9:57–57.
6. Sharma I, Pandit B, Pathak A, Sharma R. Hinduism, marriage and mental illness. *Indian J Psychiatry.* 2013;55(Suppl 2):S243–S249.
7. Mirand AL, Beehler GP, Kuo CL, Mahoney MC. Physician perceptions of primary prevention: Qualitative base for the conceptual shaping of a practice intervention tool. *BMC Public Health.* 2002;2(1):16.
8. Mirand AL, Beehler GP, Kuo CL, Mahoney MC. Explaining the de-prioritization of primary prevention: Physicians' perceptions of their role in the delivery of primary care. *BMC Public Health.* 2003;3(1):15.
9. Hesse BW, Nelson DE, Kreps GL, et al. Trust and sources of health information: The impact of the internet and its implications for health care providers: Findings from the first Health Information National Trends Survey. *Arch Intern Med.* 2005;165(22):2618–2624.
10. Mavalankar D, Vora KS. The changing role of auxiliary nurse midwife (ANM) in India: Implications for maternal and child health (MCH). Working paper No. 2008-03-01. Indian Institute of Management; 2008.
11. Rao M, Rao KD, Kumar AS, Chatterjee M, Sundararaman T. Human resources for health in India. *Lancet.* 2011;377(9765):587–598.

12. Operational framework: Management of common cancers. 2016. Ministry of Health and Family Welfare website. http://www.ncdc.gov.in/writereaddata/mainlinkFile/File643.pdf. Accessed March 1, 2017.

13. Krupp K, Madhivanan P. Leveraging human capital to reduce maternal mortality in India: Enhanced public health system or public–private partnership? *Hum Resour Health.* 2009;7(1):18.

14. Shastri SS, Mittra I, Mishra G, Gupta S, Dikshit R, Badwe RA. Effect of visual inspection with acetic acid (VIA) screening by primary health workers on cervical cancer mortality: A cluster randomized controlled trial in Mumbai, India. Paper presented at the ASCO Annual Meeting Proceedings, 2013.

15. Basu P, Mittal S, Banerjee D, et al. Diagnostic accuracy of VIA and HPV detection as primary and sequential screening tests in a cervical cancer screening demonstration project in India. *Int J Cancer.* 2015;137(4):859–867.

SECTION III

EMERGING ISSUES IN IMPLEMENTATION SCIENCE ACROSS THE CANCER CONTROL CONTINUUM

13

USING PRECISION MEDICINE TO IMPROVE HEALTH AND HEALTHCARE

THE ROLE OF IMPLEMENTATION SCIENCE

Mindy Clyne, Amy Kennedy, and Muin J. Khoury

PRECISION MEDICINE (PM) is "an innovative approach to disease prevention and treatment that takes into account individual differences in people's genes, environments, and lifestyles," as defined in the US Precision Medicine Initiative (PMI), which was announced by President Barack Obama during his 2015 State of the Union Address.[1] Similarly, precision public health applies to improvements in disease prevention and treatment through the identification of these differences at the population level. At both the individual level and the population level, incorporating evidence-based practices and programs using rigorous implementation science (IS) methods and study designs will be critical for the success of PM and precision public health. Precision medicine goes beyond genomic data (DNA and RNA) to include other "omics"[2]—transcriptomics (RNA transcripts), proteomics (proteins), metabolomics (metabolites present within an organism),[3] and epigenomics (epigenetic

modifications)—as well as environmental and lifestyle factors ("the exposome"[4]). Research is underway to identify biomarkers spanning these "omics technologies"—a promising area for future cancer care.

Cancer has emerged at the forefront of PM,[5] and it has been identified in the Precision Medicine Initiative as a "near-term focus" for population health impact.[6] Precision medicine spans the cancer care continuum, from risk assessment to primary prevention, detection, diagnosis, precursor and cancer treatment, post-treatment survivorship, and end-of-life care. A multilevel approach to cancer care, introduced by Taplin and Rodgers,[7] is necessary for implementation of PM.[8] This approach addresses PM application along the care continuum, as well as transitions between them. It also addresses the multilevel influences, which include individual, family/social support, provider/team, organization and/or practice setting, local community environment, and health policy environment at both state and national levels.[9]

A recent review of the literature on IS in genomic medicine revealed many scientific gaps and areas requiring improvement, including (1) utilization of IS frameworks, models, and/or theories; (2) expansion to a wider range of clinical and public health contexts; (3) incorporation of experimental studies (i.e., the majority of studies were observational); and (4) collaborative processes (i.e., approach not multilevel).[10] Similar findings were identified in a review of the National Institutes of Health's (NIH) portfolio of awarded grants on IS in genomic medicine.[11] A model for convergence of IS, PM, and the Learning Health Care System (LHCS) was proposed as a means to help with integration of genomics and other PM interventions (e.g., behavioral).[12] Discoveries identified through the PMI can be integrated into LHCS to bring these findings and breakthroughs into cancer patient care.

Two major elements of the PMI are being led by the NIH, with the PMI Oncology component driven by the National Cancer Institute (NCI).[13,14] To advance the field of precision oncology, NCI received $70 million in 2016 to accelerate research to discover unique therapies that treat a patient's cancer based on the genomic characteristics of the tumor. The four focal areas for the PMI Oncology component are expanding genomics-based clinical trials, understanding and overcoming drug resistance, developing new laboratory models for research, and developing a national cancer database to integrate genomic and clinical information and outcomes.[14] The NCI-MATCH (Molecular Analysis for Therapy Choice) trial is designed for patients to receive treatment based on the specific abnormalities of their tumor, with the primary goal to determine how many patients have a complete or partial response to these tailored treatments. The trial is open to patients who have advanced tumors, lymphomas, or myelomas or rare cancers without standard treatment.[15] In the summer of 2017, the NCI-COG Pediatric MATCH trial, which is cosponsored by the Children's Oncology Group (COG), was launched to enroll children and adolescents to test the use of PM in pediatric cancers that are not responding to standard treatment and have an actionable genetic mutation in their tumor.[16]

The All of Us research program, the second component of the PMI led by the NIH, received $130 million in fiscal year 2017 to build a national research cohort of volunteers to better understand health and disease.[17] This million-person cohort will enable a new era of medicine, in which data-driven research is heavily influenced by participant engagement, and the convergence of the fields of personal genomics, data science, an individual's environment, lifestyle, and social behavior, and basic human biology will unearth new advances in precision prevention and treatment. Individualized care is the underlying goal of creating such a powerful research resource.[18]

This chapter explores PM across the cancer care continuum and describes IS challenges and opportunities. Although the focus is on genomic medicine, defined by the National Human Genome Research Institute (NHGRI) as "using an individual patient's genotypic information in his or her clinical care,"[19] we recognize other PM areas of intervention development and implementation (i.e., other 'omics' areas, environmental and lifestyle factors). Research to move the field of PM forward, throughout the cancer care continuum, can be accomplished by (1) including IS methods to identify and address the dynamic processes involved (advances in genomics, changes in health care systems, innovative technology, etc.) and (2) improving upon the integration of IS methods as we develop the PM evidence base.

MULTILEVEL APPROACH TO IMPLEMENTATION OF PRECISION MEDICINE ACROSS THE CANCER CONTINUUM

Across the cancer care continuum, beginning with risk assessment, followed by prevention, detection, diagnosis, treatment, survivorship, and end-of-life care, there are examples of how the introduction of PM and precision public health can help improve cancer care at both patient and population levels. Examples of PM along the cancer care continuum are provided in Table 13.1.

The need for a multilevel approach to implementation of PM interventions is evident by reviewing the example of the US Preventive Services Task Force's "Risk Assessment, Genetic Counseling, and Genetic Testing for BRCA-Related Cancer in Women."[20] The recommendation calls for primary care providers to screen women with a family history of breast or ovarian or other related cancer and also for subsequent genetic counseling and testing if risk criteria are met. Within this context, at the patient level, there needs to be an understanding of the purpose for genetic counseling (patient–primary care interaction) and, once in the genetic counseling

Table 13.1. Examples of Precision Medicine Across the Cancer Care Continuum

CANCER CARE CONTINUUM	PRECISION MEDICINE EXAMPLES
Risk assessment	BRCA1/2 germline testing for hereditary breast and ovarian cancer risk assessment
Primary prevention	Chemoprevention or risk-reducing surgery for women with BRCA1 or BRCA2 mutation
Detection	Lynch syndrome mutation carriers undergo more frequent colorectal cancer screenings for early detection of cancer
Diagnosis	Multigene next-generation sequencing panel for diagnosing malignancy of thyroid nodules
Cancer or precursor treatment	Pharmacogenomic therapy using dabrafenib, trametinib, or vemurafenib for melanoma with BRAF V600E mutation
Post-treatment survivorship	Analysis of circulating tumor cells for monitoring metastasis in lung cancer
End-of-life care	OPRM1 AG genotype cancer patients requiring higher dose of morphine to be effective and enhance their quality of life

setting, an understanding of what testing will and will not reveal, as well as post-test result interpretation and a thorough understanding of options to take based on test results (patient–genetic counselor interaction). Family and social support systems can impact patient support, as well as potential caregiving issues. Risk to other family members due to the hereditary nature of the condition must also be considered. The health care organization, or referral system, requires standardized procedures for ensuring patients are referred for counseling and subsequent patient follow-up for those who agree to genetic testing. These organizations are also responsible for complying with policies established at the local, state, and national levels, which adds a layer of interaction between the agencies enforcing the policies and the health care organization. Community-based interventions can benefit women identified within populations in which primary care screening for BRCA-related cancers is low. Community-based interventions can be effective, for example, when education is provided by members of the community who share the same cultural background as those receiving the intervention. An evaluation of a culturally tailored breast cancer education and navigation program in North Carolina found that using lay breast health educators from the community helped improve awareness of and access to breast cancer screening.[21]

LHCS are model systems for integrating PM interventions while also incorporating IS.[12] Characteristics of an LHCS include, but are not limited to, the following: (1) patients as part of the learning care team, (2) care experience captured digitally for real-time generation and application of knowledge, (3) a leadership commitment to teamwork, and (4) collaboration and adaptability.[22] All of these facilitate the utilization of IS methods. For example, the implementation of a clinical decision support tool for genetic testing referral of individuals at risk for hereditary breast cancer could utilize a mixed method approach for quantitative and qualitative feedback to measure the implementation processes and outcomes. In this scenario, support from administrators, informatic technology for data linkage with electronic health records (EHR), and the ability to evaluate both patient and provider experience are inherent within the LHCS.

STATUS OF PRECISION MEDICINE IMPLEMENTATION IN CANCER CONTROL

In 2015, a systematic review of genomic test recommendations for cancer screening, diagnosis, prognosis, and treatment identified 45 tests that were evaluated for clinical test use. Of these, 9 and 14 received strong and moderate recommendations for use, respectively, and 22 were not recommended for use.[23] Those receiving a strong recommendation included tests for five common cancers (non-small cell lung, colon, chronic lymphocytic leukemia, breast, and melanoma) and two rare cancers (glioma and thyroid), and more than half of the tests were pharmacogenomic in nature, although screening, diagnostic, and prognostic testing purposes were also represented within this group. From discovery (gene–disease association or multigene assay development) to final recommendation of clinical use, overall the 45 tests took 14.7 median years, and the subset of those given a strong recommendation took 15.7 median years. These results are not unlike those published in 2000, reporting that original clinical research takes 17 years, on average, to convert to patient care, with a step along the pathway (i.e., evidence reported in reviews, publications, and textbooks) taking between 7.4 and 14.4 years.[24]

Identifying the evidence-based applications ready for implementation is the first step moving forward with implementation within cancer care settings. Evidence-based applications in cancer PM can be identified using an implementation classification system developed by the Centers for Disease Control and Prevention's Office of Public Health and Genomics in collaboration with the NCI's Epidemiology and Genomics Research Program.[25,26] The applications ready for implementation (Tier 1) are those with an evidence base supporting implementation in practice, which incorporates evidence derived from US Food and Drug Administration (FDA) labeling information, Centers for Medicare & Medicaid Services coverage decisions, clinical practice guidelines, and systematic reviews. Applications with insufficient evidence supporting their implementation (Tier 2)—for example, a test having systematic review support but without a clinical practice guideline—may be useful for informing selective use through individual clinical or public health policy decision-making. Finally, those applications identified in Tier 3 include (1) evidence supporting recommendations against or discouraging use or (2) no evidence currently available.

Currently, there are more than 50 cancer-related applications that fall under Tier 1.[27] Nineteen Tier 1 applications for risk prediction and/or assessment exist, all specific to hereditary breast and ovarian cancer (HBOC) or other BRCA-related cancers, including one that also applies to informed decision-making on chemoprevention. Two Tier 1 applications exist relating to Lynch syndrome for (1) diagnostic and screening of individuals with positive family history of Lynch syndrome[28] and (2) screening and cascade testing of relatives in patients with newly diagnosed colorectal cancer.[29,30] Two additional Tier 1 applications are prognostic, identifying tumor markers in breast cancer and in invasive colorectal cancer.[31-33] The majority of Tier 1 applications ($n = 29$) involve pharmacogenomics for treatment use, identified by the FDA as "Phamacogenomic Biomarkers in Drug Labeling,"[34] and include treatment for breast, ovarian, colorectal, melanoma, non-small cell lung, and gastrointestinal cancers, along with leukemia and lymphoma.

To accelerate translation of PM-related efforts at the system level, such as the integration of family history into EHR[35] and utilization of tumor boards for successful guidance of PM[36] have been proposed. An example of integration at the health system level is the launch of the Precision Medicine Alliance at Dignity Health and Catholic Health Initiatives in Denver, Colorado. The Precision Medicine Alliance offers patients from both health care systems faster and more accurate diagnostic and treatment protocols based on their genetic and molecular profile information.[37] There are also academic centers focusing on both PM and IS through an NIH-funded network, Implementing GeNomics In pracTicE (IGNITE).[38] In addition, prominent cancer centers are implementing PM strategies, for example, MD Anderson and Memorial Sloan Kettering Cancer Centers.[39,40]

CHALLENGES OF IMPLEMENTATION ACROSS THE CONTINUUM

Challenges in implementation of PM exist at the clinical and public health levels, across all disease areas, including cancer, and specific to different areas along the care continuum. Basic research in cancer genomics is progressing rapidly, and there is an urgent need to translate this into clinical validity and utility. Furthermore, the multilevel nature of implementation presents its own challenges: patient and family burden; provider-level capacity issues; system-level limitations; and, at the policy and health care payer levels, the need to address coverage and reimbursement of tests. A shortage of and lack of access to genetic counselors within the workforce have also been identified. Options for improving access include telehealth counseling, and the demand for counseling may be satisfied by allowing non-genetic specialists to provide counseling and by increasing the number of certified genetic counseling training programs. Within the LHCS, the means of storage, sharing, and other management issues relating to data become highly technical, and related costs factor in. Ethical, legal, and social issues (ELSI) associated with implementation of PM applications must be addressed at multiple levels, including ethics of professional care, organizational ethics including LHCS, and ethics of public health.[41] In a systematic review, the following 11 ELSI topic areas in genomic medicine were identified: consent, data sharing, disclosure, groups with different cultural perspectives or social or political interests, privacy, ethics committees and institutional review board oversight, specimen ownership, use of racial categories, benefits and harms of genetic engineering, justice and fairness related to health disparities, and genetic discrimination.[42] Unique challenges specific to cancer PM regarding molecular profiling and targeted therapy exist, such as issues related to heterogeneity between primary and metastatic tumors and clonal evolution of metastatic tumors affecting treatment effectiveness. In addition, there is a need for standardization across laboratories performing tumor profiling and development and implementation of clinical practice guidelines.[43]

Data on challenges identified through six NHGRI-funded IGNITE- network projects were synthesized, resulting in three overarching challenges identified by all projects:[44] (1) the integration of genomics within the EHR, (2) increasing clinicians' knowledge and beliefs about genomic medicine, through education and training, development of expertise, providing information on how to access testing, and identifying means for the investment in time and money for training, and (3) engaging patients in the genomic medicine projects, through mass media efforts, active involvement in the implementation process, and preparing patients to be active participants in health care decisions. Increasing genomic literacy, the awareness and understanding of genomics, among the general public as well as at the system and clinic levels is also necessary. Assuming educational needs are met, management at the clinical or system level associated with assaying, reporting, intervening, and follow-up presents challenges that may require organizational changes and/or modifications to the care delivery model.

Challenges exist relating to reporting of genomic test results, including addressing the psychological burden of receiving test results at the patient level, reporting practices at the laboratory level, interpretation of tests by the ordering provider, and accessibility at the community level of genetic counseling services. Test results that reveal a previously unknown risk to an individual carry a psychological burden. A systematic review of eight studies involving BRCA1/2 testing identified the potential for short-term psychological distress, although study results on longer term distress, anxiety, and depression were mixed, with some studies reporting long-term effects and in others no long-term effects were identified.[45] Further research to include more diverse populations and improved screening instruments was suggested, and an urgent need for implementation of coping strategies for disease management in clinical practice was called for. Patients may receive results reporting variants of unknown/uncertain significance (VUS), defined as gene variants identified through testing but for which it cannot be determined whether they are deleterious or benign. In a recent study, patients who received VUS results for Lynch syndrome genetic testing were recruited to participate in telephone interviews to identify types of uncertainty experienced, assessment of the implications of uncertainty (appraisal), and coping strategies.[46] Many participants identified VUS results as a health threat and reported concern about relaying results to family members. Strategies at the provider level (including primary, specialty, and genetic counseling and others involved in direct patient care) to help patients understand and cope with newly identified genetic risk for cancer and results reporting VUS are critical. In addition, there needs to be system-level monitoring and protocols established for contacting at-risk individuals who are eligible for extended genetic testing that may further refine risk and also individuals whose original VUS results are modified based on new findings that may inform diagnostic or treatment guidance.

An individual who undergoes genetic testing for cancer risk assessment is given the onus of reporting his or her results to potential at-risk family members. This may be part of an organized cascade screening process, which systematically identifies and tests at-risk relatives. Multilevel challenges exist, ranging from the communication of results by an affected family member to other family members[47] to professional guidelines and higher level policy regarding the duty to warn balanced with privacy issues regarding disclosure and mid-level involvement of practitioners,[48] who are faced with the ethical responsibility to inform while at the same time respecting patient privacy and Health Insurance Portability and Accountability Act of 1996 privacy rule.

To avoid unintended health disparity/inequity issues, caution must be exercised for any PM activity being introduced. Inclusion of minorities in preliminary research on the prevalence of risk-related genetic variants is necessary if PM interventions are to be informative across all individuals and populations. Equal access to testing and related costs/coverage must also be addressed. The monitoring should not just be at the patient level but also at the provider, system, and public health levels.

Challenges within an LHCS are not necessarily unique to PM; however, challenges regarding data capture, completeness, quality, storage and access, and interoperability[49,50] are expected due to an abundance of information collected from next-generation sequencing and the potential for other omics-level data. It is expected that advances in PM will take place by integrating big data from all "omics" and other collected data (e.g., environmental and lifestyle). The amount of data resulting from genomic outcomes (e.g., next-generation sequencing data and array-based data) alone is becoming big data in and of itself, and when combined with other types of data, such as measurements of physical activity, ambient air exposures, and neighborhood environmental data, it becomes extremely complex. This requires corresponding advances in the field of bioinformatics.

Challenges at the public health level include the level of readiness among various health departments to include population-level PM applications (e.g., population screening), addressing increased costs involved with implementing and managing cancer registries that are incorporating additional genomic and/or family history detail, and the structural reorganization required for bidirectional reporting between cancer registries and reporting providers or hospitals. The investment of effort at the intersection of public health and health care systems to improve monitoring and reporting of hereditary cancers and standardization of genetic testing must be a priority for PM to be successful.

OPPORTUNITIES FOR IMPLEMENTATION ACROSS THE CONTINUUM

Moving forward, it is critical to integrate IS methods into PM across the cancer care continuum at every level. Tsimberidou et. al.[43] propose modifications to existing paradigms of clinical research and health care delivery, requiring both scientific and technological breakthroughs as well as changing the way practitioners work together (e.g., cross-disciplinary). In addition, they suggest changes in regulatory standards for drugs and devices, modifications in coverage at the policy level, and patient data collection and analysis through EHR with linkage to registries and learning systems. Identifying implementation strategies for these proposed modifications and changes will enable the necessary adaptations at the appropriate levels.

Identifying socioecologic factors related to a PM application at multiple levels will be useful. For IS purposes, this can provide the basis for integration of existing knowledge and identify gaps that need to be addressed. Using HBOC referral for risk prediction through genetic counseling and testing, previously highlighted in the section titled "Challenges of Implementation Across the Continuum" describing the need for a multilevel approach, offers an opportunity to formulate an implementation science agenda. Table 13.2 identifies some multilevel socioecologic factors specific to HBOC.

The best way to incorporate IS in PM is to follow the path being taken by LHCS. These systems are (1) committed to active leadership, with engagement across the system; (2) adaptable to changes in patient and clinical management; and (3) open to innovative technologies enabling the expedition of genomic findings into clinical use.[22] They are poised for EHR enhancement, including the integration of family history and patient-reported outcomes. Clinic staff can systematically document what has been learned from previous implementation efforts so that future efforts are more resource efficient, culturally appropriate, and effective. The open access capture system, provision of access to clinical groups for test results interpretation, and research functionality are all part of the infrastructure. Preemptive testing is facilitated through EHR integration and present at point of care, thus minimizing delays and costs, lack of follow-up, and avoiding of duplicate testing. Patients can be placed in control of their own genetic information, in contrast to control at the system/institution level. Capturing data within a LHCS provides the opportunity to gather knowledge systematically for future benefit at multiple levels. The American Society of Clinical Oncology (ASCO) created the

Table 13.2. Examples of Multilevel Factors Influencing Implementation of Genetic Counseling and Testing Referral of Hereditary Breast and Ovarian Cancer

SOCIOECOLOGIC LEVEL	EXAMPLES OF SOCIOECOLOGIC LEVEL FACTORS
Individual with family history of hereditary breast or ovarian cancer	Individual's access to health care; willingness to seek regular medical check-ups; subsequent willingness to undergo counseling and testing if risk exists; capacity to understand the familial risk; adherence to recommended screening; ability to access counseling and testing services. In individual with positive *BRCA* results, ability to understand post-test result interpretation and recommended screening uptake; preventive options for consideration (including risk-reducing prophylactic surgeries and chemoprevention); communication of risk to relatives; cost coverage and reimbursement
Relatives of individual	Unique characteristics of different families; proximity of relatives for support; interpersonal interaction
Provider	Assessment of knowledge regarding genetic testing; ability to communicate risk and recommendations to patient; incentives for referral of high-risk individuals; identification of at-risk relatives; ability to coordinate among genetic counselors, laboratory personnel, screening radiologists, and surgeons
Health care organization	Standardized referral process/policy for genetic counseling; reminder system in place for screening reminders; leader-initiated support for following guidelines; integration of guidelines into EHR; availability of decision support tools; interorganizational communication capacity
Community	Community mass media campaigns addressing family history collection and *BRCA* risk-related cancers; issues unique within culture of community that affects decision-making regarding genetic testing
State and national health policy	Coverage and reimbursement for counseling and tests; guidelines for incorporating *BRCA* status in medical records and cancer registries if applicable; efforts at state level to promote adoption of guidelines; national policies and oversight and regulation of genomic tests and performance of laboratories; ELSI issues regarding testing addressed at policy level

BRCA, one of two DNA repair genes (*BRCA1* and *BRCA2*); EHR, electronic health record; ELSI, ethical, legal, and social issues.
Source: Information for this table was obtained from References 51–67.

CancerLinQ initiative, which incorporates LHCS characteristics into an oncology setting.[68] Within the PM arena, there is potential for CancerLinQ to readily examine the clinical utility of genetic tests and identify exceptional responders based on germline or other individual factors, which can further be utilized for research on understanding underlying cancer cause.

Critical, yet lacking, in cancer PM translational research is the need to incorporate IS theories, models, and frameworks to guide implementation efforts.[10] As explained by Skolarus et al. in Chapter 3 of this volume, selection of appropriate models is critical to successful implementation of interventions. Across the cancer care continuum, models for PM applications can be selected to

Table 13.3. Examples of Implementation Science Questions Across the Cancer Care Continuum with Associated Target of Implementation

CANCER CARE CONTINUUM	TARGET OF IMPLEMENTATION	EXAMPLES OF IMPLEMENTATION SCIENCE QUESTIONS
Risk assessment	Clinic/health system	How can an existing hereditary breast cancer risk decision aid be implemented with ongoing adaptation in a rural health care system?
	Community	What are the optimal methods to utilize a faith-based cancer family history educational campaign to improve uptake of an online family health history tool?
Primary prevention	Health care provider	What are the barriers and facilitators of incorporating an obesity management program for women with *BRCA1* or *BRCA2* mutations into counseling sessions?
	Clinic/health system	How can a multidisciplinary educational program for clinicians and staff on the use of tamoxifen to protect against breast cancer be sustained within health systems over time?
Detection	Health care provider	How does a decision support tool help primary care providers increase appropriate referrals for genetic testing for hereditary cancer?
	Community/public health	How can the implementation of a partnering program between a health department and a community-based organization improve uptake of screening for hereditary cancers?
Diagnosis	Clinic/health system	What strategies can be used to improve quality management of an oncology program to increase the number of colorectal cancer patients who are referred for Lynch syndrome testing?
	Public health	How can financing policies improve cascade screening for genomic testing of hereditary cancer following diagnosis?
Cancer or precursor treatment	Health care provider	What strategies can be developed over time that might inform provider treatment selection when next-generation sequencing of patient's tumors has been performed?
	Clinic/health system	What are the barriers and facilitators of implementing a molecular tumor board into a community oncology clinic for standardization of treatment based on tumor genomic profiling?

Table 13.3   Continued

CANCER CARE CONTINUUM	TARGET OF IMPLEMENTATION	EXAMPLES OF IMPLEMENTATION SCIENCE QUESTIONS
Post-treatment survivorship	Health care provider	What training modalities for clinic staff are effective in supportive ongoing care of cancer survivors with genetic test results pertaining to ongoing cancer risk?
	Clinic/health system	How do system-level guidelines for expanded genetic testing impact provider referral for cancer survivors?
End-of-life care	Health care provider	What are the barriers and facilitators of implementing a pharmacogenomic-guided pain management program into end-of-life palliative care?

answer the relevant IS question(s). Examples of IS questions related to PM applications across the cancer care continuum are presented in Table 13.3.

Although the number of evidence-based applications within the PM field is still small, it is possible to integrate IS as the evidence base is developed. Effectiveness of applications can be evaluated alongside IS efforts through effectiveness–implementation hybrid design studies. This design was used in a program for primary care called the Genomic Medicine Model, which employed a web-based family health history tool and clinical decision support program, MeTree, along with provision of educational materials (for patient and provider).[69] The analysis included measures of the effectiveness of the MeTree tool in identifying relevant guidelines, such as cancer risk management for hereditary cancer syndromes, based on the reporting of positive family history. In addition, implementation feasibility was measured in relation to the increase in resource demand resulting from non-routine recommendations identified through the MeTree tool.

SUMMARY

Genomics represents the leading edge of PM in cancer. Opportunities for IS in genomics and cancer exist throughout the cancer care continuum. The translation of genomics into clinical applications and public health programs to reduce the burden of cancer in populations requires a robust IS agenda. The intersection of the fields of IS and genomic

medicine is currently sparse, and the existing studies reflect gaps in methodological rigor in study design and conduct. Moving forward, a multilevel, multidisciplinary approach to PM implementation is necessary. Using LHCS represents an ideal model to accelerate the promise of PM in cancer and beyond.

REFERENCES

1. Fact sheet: President Obama's Precision Medicine Initiative. 2015. The White House website. https://obamawhitehouse.archives.gov/the-press-office/2015/01/30/fact-sheet-president-obama-s-precision-medicine-initiative. Accessed October 14, 2017.
2. Chen R, Snyder M. Promise of personalized omics to precision medicine. *Wiley Interdiscip Rev Syst Biol Med.* 2013;5(1):73–82.
3. Beger RD, Dunn W, Schmidt MA, et al. Metabolomics enables precision medicine: "A white paper, community perspective." *Metabolomics.* 2016;12(10):149.
4. Wild CP. Complementing the genome with an "exposome": The outstanding challenge of environmental exposure measurement in molecular epidemiology. *Cancer Epidemiol. Biomarkers Prev.* 2005;14(8):1847–1850.
5. Clyne M, Schully SD, Dotson WD, et al. Horizon scanning for translational genomic research beyond bench to bedside. *Genet Med.* 2014;16(7):535–538.
6. Collins FS, Varmus H. A new initiative on precision medicine. *N Engl J Med.* 2015;372(9):793–795.

7. Taplin SH, Rodgers AB. Toward improving the quality of cancer care: Addressing the interfaces of primary and oncology-related subspecialty care. *J Natl Cancer Inst Monogr*. 2010;2010(40):3–10.

8. Khoury MJ, Coates RJ, Fennell ML, et al. Multilevel research and the challenges of implementing genomic medicine. *J Natl Cancer Inst Monogr*. 2012;2012(44):112–120.

9. Taplin SH, Anhang Price R, Edwards HM, et al. Introduction: Understanding and influencing multilevel factors across the cancer care continuum. *J Natl Cancer Inst Monogr*. 2012;2012(44):2–10.

10. Roberts MC, Kennedy AE, Chambers DA, Khoury MJ. The current state of implementation science in genomic medicine: Opportunities for improvement. *Genet Med*. 2017;19(8):858–863.

11. Roberts MC, Clyne M, Kennedy AE, Chambers DA, Khoury MJ. The current state of funded NIH grants in implementation science in genomic medicine: A portfolio analysis. *Genet Med*. 2017. [Epub ahead of print]

12. Chambers DA, Feero WG, Khoury MJ. Convergence of implementation science, precision medicine, and the learning health care system: A new model for biomedical research. *JAMA*. 2016;315(18):1941–1942.

13. White House Precision Medicine Initiative. 2017. The White House website. https://obamawhitehouse.archives.gov/node/333101. Accessed October 31, 2017.

14. NCI and the Precision Medicine Initiative. 2017. National Cancer Institute website. https://www.cancer.gov/research/areas/treatment/pmi-oncology. Accessed October 31, 2017.

15. NCI-MATCH trial. 2017. National Cancer Institute website. https://www.cancer.gov/about-cancer/treatment/clinical-trials/nci-supported/nci-match. Accessed October 31, 2017.

16. NCI-COG Pediatric MATCH. 2017. National Cancer Institute website. https://www.cancer.gov/about-cancer/treatment/clinical-trials/nci-supported/pediatric-match. Accessed October 31, 2017.

17. About the All of Us research program. 2017. National Institutes of Health website. https://allofus.nih.gov/about/about-all-us-research-program. Accessed October 31, 2017.

18. Scientific opportunities. 2017. National Institute of Health website. https://allofus.nih.gov/about/scientific-opportunities. Accessed October 31, 2017.

19. Manolio TA, Chisholm RL, Ozenberger B, et al. Implementing genomic medicine in the clinic: The future is here. *Genet Med*. 2013;15(4):258–267.

20. Moyer VA. Risk assessment, genetic counseling, and genetic testing for BRCA-related cancer in women: U.S. Preventive Services Task Force recommendation statement. *Ann Intern Med*. 2014;160(4):271–281.

21. Torres E, Richman AR, Schreier AM, Vohra N, Verbanac K. An evaluation of a rural community-based breast education and navigation program: Highlights and lessons learned. *J Cancer Educ*. 2017. [Epub ahead of print]

22. Smith MD. *Best Care at Lower Cost: The Path to Continuously Learning Health Care in America*. Washington, DC: Institute of Medicine; 2012.

23. Chang CQ, Tingle SR, Filipski KK, et al. An overview of recommendations and translational milestones for genomic tests in cancer. *Genet Med*. 2015;17(6):431–440.

24. Balas E, Boren S. Managing clinical knowledge for health care improvement. In: vanBemmel J, McCray A, eds. *Yearbook of Medical Informatics*. Stuttgart, Germany: Schattauer Verlagsgesellschaft; 2000:65–70.

25. Dotson WD, Douglas MP, Kolor K, et al. Prioritizing genomic applications for action by level of evidence: A horizon-scanning method. *Clin Pharmacol Therap*. 2014;95(4):394–402.

26. Khoury MJ, Coates RJ, Evans JP. Evidence-based classification of recommendations on use of genomic tests in clinical practice: Dealing with insufficient evidence. *Genet Med*. 2010;12(11):680–683.

27. Public health genomics knowledge base (v2.0): Tier table database. 2017. Centers for Disease Control and Prevention website. https://phgkb.cdc.gov/PHGKB/topicFinder.action;jsessionid=7A382F41E9C1A0797B5B3C6EFFE52729?Mysubmit=init&query=tier+1. Accessed November 1, 2017.

28. Provenzale D, Gupta S, Ahnen DJ, et al. Genetic/familial high-risk assessment: Colorectal version 1.2016, NCCN clinical practice guidelines in oncology. *J Natl Compr Canc Netw*. 2016;14(8):1010–1030.

29. EGAPP Working Group. Recommendations from the EGAPP Working Group: Genetic testing strategies in newly diagnosed individuals with colorectal cancer aimed at reducing morbidity and mortality from Lynch syndrome in relatives. *Genet Med*. 2009;11(1):35–41.

30. Palomaki GE, McClain MR, Melillo S, Hampel HL, Thibodeau SN. EGAPP supplementary

evidence review: DNA testing strategies aimed at reducing morbidity and mortality from Lynch syndrome. *Genet Med.* 2009;11(1):42–65.

31. NICE Diagnostics Guidance (DG10): Gene expression profiling and expanded immunohistochemistry tests for guiding adjuvant chemotherapy decisions in early breast cancer management: MammaPrint, Oncotype DX, IHC4 and Mammostrat. 2013. National Institute for Health and Care Excellence website. https://www.nice.org.uk/guidance/dg10.

32. Febbo PG, Ladanyi M, Aldape KD, et al. NCCN Task Force report: Evaluating the clinical utility of tumor markers in oncology. *J Natl Compr Canc Netw.* 2011;9(Suppl 5):S1–S32; quiz S33.

33. Locker GY, Hamilton S, Harris J, et al. ASCO 2006 update of recommendations for the use of tumor markers in gastrointestinal cancer. *J Clin Oncol.* 2006;24(33):5313–5327.

34. Table of pharmacogenomic biomarkers in drug labeling. 2017. US Food and Drug Administration website. https://www.fda.gov/Drugs/ScienceResearch/ucm572698.htm. Accessed October 14, 2017.

35. Levenson D. Electronic family health history records draw attention: Proposed federal regulation and new tool emphasize digital conversion. *Am J Med Genet A.* 2012;158a(6):ix–x.

36. Harada S, Arend R, Dai Q, et al. Implementation and utilization of the Molecular Tumor Board to guide precision medicine. *Oncotarget.* 2017;8(34):57845–57854.

37. Precision Medicine Alliance. 2017. Catholic Health Initiatives website. http://www.catholichealthinitiatives.org/precision-medicine-alliance. Accessed October 14, 2017.

38. Weitzel KW, Alexander M, Bernhardt BA, et al. The IGNITE network: A model for genomic medicine implementation and research. *BMC Med Genom.* 2016;9:1.

39. Hyman DM, Solit DB, Arcila ME, et al. Precision medicine at Memorial Sloan Kettering Cancer Center: Clinical next-generation sequencing enabling next-generation targeted therapy trials. *Drug Discov Today.* 2015;20(12):1422–1428.

40. Meric-Bernstam F, Farhangfar C, Mendelsohn J, Mills GB. Building a personalized medicine infrastructure at a major cancer center. *J Clin Oncol.* 2013;31(15):1849–1857.

41. Wolf SM, Burke W, Koenig BA. Mapping the ethics of translational genomics: Situating return of results and navigating the research–clinical divide. *J Law Med Ethics.* 2015;43(3):486–501.

42. Callier SL, Abudu R, Mehlman MJ, et al. Ethical, legal, and social implications of personalized genomic medicine research: Current literature and suggestions for the future. *Bioethics.* 2016;30(9):698–705.

43. Tsimberidou AM, Ringborg U, Schilsky RL. Strategies to overcome clinical, regulatory, and financial challenges in the implementation of personalized medicine. *Am Soc Clin Oncol Educ Book.* 2013:118–125.

44. Sperber NR, Carpenter JS, Cavallari LH, et al. Challenges and strategies for implementing genomic services in diverse settings: Experiences from the Implementing GeNomics In pracTicE (IGNITE) network. *BMC Med Genom.* 2017;10(1):35.

45. Ringwald J, Wochnowski C, Bosse K, et al. Psychological distress, anxiety, and depression of cancer-affected BRCA1/2 mutation carriers: A systematic review. *J Genet Couns.* 2016;25(5):880–891.

46. Solomon I, Harrington E, Hooker G, et al. Lynch syndrome limbo: Patient understanding of variants of uncertain significance. *J Genet Couns.* 2017;26(4):866–877.

47. Daly MB, Montgomery S, Bingler R, Ruth K. Communicating genetic test results within the family: Is it lost in translation? A survey of relatives in the randomized six-step study. *Fam Cancer.* 2016;15(4):697–706.

48. Dheensa S, Fenwick A, Shkedi-Rafid S, Crawford G, Lucassen A. Health-care professionals' responsibility to patients' relatives in genetic medicine: A systematic review and synthesis of empirical research. *Genet Med.* 2016;18(4):290–301.

49. Building Blocks: Healthcare data. 2018. The Learning Healthcare Project website. http://www.learninghealthcareproject.org/section/building-blocks/healthcare-data. Accessed October 16, 2017.

50. Foley T, Fairmichael F. The potential of learning healthcare systems. 2015. The Learning Healthcare Project website. http://www.learninghealthcareproject.org/LHS_Report_2015.pdf. Accessed October 16, 2017.

51. Buchanan AH, Voils CI, Schildkraut JM, et al. Adherence to recommended risk management among unaffected women with a BRCA mutation. *J Genet Couns.* 2017;26(1):79–92.

52. Cragun D, Besharat AD, Lewis C, Vadaparampil ST, Pal T. Educational needs and preferred methods of learning among Florida practitioners who order genetic testing for hereditary breast and ovarian cancer. *J Cancer Educ.* 2013;28(4):690–697.

53. Febbraro T, Robison K, Wilbur JS, et al. Adherence patterns to National Comprehensive Cancer Network (NCCN) guidelines for referral to cancer genetic professionals. *Gynecol Oncol.* 2015;138(1):109–114.

54. George R, Kovak K, Cox SL. Aligning policy to promote cascade genetic screening for prevention and early diagnosis of heritable diseases. *J Genet Couns.* 2015;24(3):388–399.

55. Kelly KM, Sturm AC, Kemp K, Holland J, Ferketich AK. How can we reach them? Information seeking and preferences for a cancer family history campaign in underserved communities. *J Health Commun.* 2009;14(6):573–589.

56. Klabunde CN, Haggstrom D, Kahn KL, et al. Oncologists' perspectives on post-cancer treatment communication and care coordination with primary care physicians. *Eur J Cancer Care.* 2017;26(4).

57. Kne A, Zierhut H, Baldinger S, et al. Why is cancer genetic counseling underutilized by women identified as at risk for hereditary breast cancer? Patient perceptions of barriers following a referral letter. *J Genet Couns.* 2017;26(4):697–715.

58. Mays D, Sharff ME, DeMarco TA, et al. Outcomes of a systems-level intervention offering breast cancer risk assessments to low-income underserved women. *Fam Cancer.* 2012;11(3):493–502.

59. Morgan D, Sylvester H, Lucas FL, Miesfeldt S. Perceptions of high-risk care and barriers to care among women at risk for hereditary breast and ovarian cancer following genetic counseling in the community setting. *J Genet Couns.* 2010;19(1):44–54.

60. Nycum G, Avard D, Knoppers BM. Factors influencing intrafamilial communication of hereditary breast and ovarian cancer genetic information. *Eur J Hum Genet.* 2009;17(7):872–880.

61. Pal T, Cragun D, Lewis C, et al. A statewide survey of practitioners to assess knowledge and clinical practices regarding hereditary breast and ovarian cancer. *Genet Test Mol Biomarkers.* 2013;17(5):367–375.

62. Quillin JM, Krist AH, Gyure M, et al. Patient-reported hereditary breast and ovarian cancer in a primary care practice. *J Community Genet.* 2014;5(2):179–183.

63. Sturm AC, Sweet K, Schwirian PM, Koenig C, Westman J, Kelly KM. Lessons learned while developing a cancer family history campaign in the Columbus, Ohio metropolitan area. *Community Genet.* 2008;11(5):304–310.

64. Trepanier AM, Supplee L, Blakely L, McLosky J, Duquette D. Public health approaches and barriers to educating providers about hereditary breast and ovarian cancer syndrome. *Healthcare (Basel).* 2016;4(1):19.

65. Wang G, Beattie MS, Ponce NA, Phillips KA. Eligibility criteria in private and public coverage policies for BRCA genetic testing and genetic counseling. *Genet Med.* 2011;13(12):1045–1050.

66. Whitworth P, Beitsch P, Arnell C, et al. Impact of payer constraints on access to genetic testing. *J Oncol Pract.* 2017;13(1):e47–e56.

67. Zapka J, Taplin SH, Ganz P, Grunfeld E, Sterba K. Multilevel factors affecting quality: Examples from the cancer care continuum. *J Natl Cancer Inst Monogr.* 2012;2012(44):11–19.

68. Sledge GW, Hudis CA, Swain SM, et al. ASCO's approach to a learning health care system in oncology. *J Oncol Pract.* 2013;9(3):145–148.

69. Orlando LA, Wu RR, Beadles C, et al. Implementing family health history risk stratification in primary care: Impact of guideline criteria on populations and resource demand. *Am J Med Genet C Semin Med Genet.* 2014;166c(1):24–33.

14

HARNESSING BIG DATA-BASED TECHNOLOGIES TO IMPROVE CANCER CARE

Gurvaneet S. Randhawa and Edwin A. Lomotan

INTRODUCTION

Big data has the potential to tap knowledge from vast databases to support the delivery of care and to conduct research at an unprecedented scale and speed.[1] To help place big data in the context of implementation science and cancer care, we begin with a scenario.

Scenario

The chief executive officer (CEO) of a health care delivery system wants to use a recently installed electronic health record (EHR) system in a new program to prevent colon cancer. The chief medical officer (CMO) advises the CEO to use two US Preventive Services Task Force (USPSTF) recommendations—aspirin use to prevent colorectal cancer and screening for colorectal cancer—as the foundation for the program.[2,3] The chief information officer (CIO) plans to use big data-based methods to implement this program.

We briefly enumerate the clinical and data-specific issues to be considered in implementing a big data-based program based on these two USPSTF recommendations:

1. Aspirin use to prevent disease: It is important to understand the balance between the benefits and risks of regular aspirin use for a patient. The benefit of reducing a patient's risk of colon cancer, and of heart disease, must be balanced against the risk of bleeding caused by aspirin. Therefore, the relevant clinical and family history data must be obtained to ascertain the potential benefits and risks of aspirin use for a patient.

2. Colorectal cancer screening: It is important to provide a reminder to the clinician and the patient to start screening for colorectal cancer at 50 years of age. Several tests, such as direct visualization tests (e.g., colonoscopy and sigmoidoscopy) and stool-based tests (e.g., fecal occult blood tests and fecal immunochemical tests), can be used to screen

for colorectal cancer. It is important to ascertain a patient's preferences and circumstances before selecting the appropriate screening test. It is also important to ensure the colorectal screening program facilitates appropriate follow-up based on the test results. Finally, it is important to provide reminders to rescreen the patient at an appropriate interval, which depends on the screening test. Therefore, the implementation program needs analytic and decision support tools that can analyze data from the relevant clinical databases to ascertain when a patient is eligible for screening and remind the clinician or the patient when the patient needs to be screened (or rescreened), communicate the results of the screening to the primary care provider and the patient, facilitate appropriate referral, and close the communication loop so that the primary care clinician knows the outcome of the referral.

This new colorectal cancer prevention program will need to access the relevant patient-specific data from diverse sources—EHR, prescription, billing and claims, and diagnostic databases (containing data from laboratory and radiology tests)—to understand the potential risks and benefits to the patient and to help with patient follow-up. The program will need to use analytic and visualization tools to rapidly analyze the relevant data and present the information in a timely and user-friendly manner to facilitate shared decision-making between the clinician and the patient during a clinical encounter to select the appropriate preventive service. The program also needs a well-designed decision support system that provides appropriate reminders for screening and follow-up, including referrals, that are integrated smoothly in the clinical workflow. Finally, the program needs to monitor the success in the delivery of preventive services, which will help the CEO and CMO make appropriate program adjustments to improve the delivery of the preventive services to the patient population served by the health system.

Next, we provide an overview of big data and its applications in health care delivery, especially in cancer care delivery, before returning to this scenario and considering its implications for implementation science.

BIG DATA

Big data has been defined as an information asset characterized by such a high volume, velocity, and variety that it requires specific technology and analytical methods for its transformation into value.[4] We will explain the four V's—volume, velocity, variety, and value—of big data in the context of health care delivery. Veracity is a fifth attribute of big data; we address it in the discussion of data quality

Volume refers to the scale of big data and the enormous amount of information that is potentially available for aggregation and analysis. One reason for the large increase in digital health care information has been the sharp rise in adoption of EHRs. For example, adoption of a basic EHR by non-federal acute care hospitals increased from 9% in 2008 to 84% in 2015.[5] In addition to the rapid increase in electronic records for clinical documentation of hospital stays and progress notes, the digitization of other forms of medical information (e.g., laboratory and radiologic data) contributes not only to the different types of data but also to the sheer volume of data associated with each file or study (e.g., radiologic images such as those obtained by magnetic resonance imaging).

Velocity refers to the rapidity by which big data are being generated. In health care, data are being rapidly generated from routine care, basic and applied clinical research, and quality improvement activities. The velocity challenge of big data in health care refers not only to the pace at which data are generated but also to the pace at which data must be exchanged and analyzed to become useful.

Variety refers to the multitude of types of data that are becoming available. Clinical data are no longer simple electronic renditions of progress notes, laboratory data, prescription information, or other data traditionally included in a patient's medical chart. Rather, clinical data encompass a wide array of structured data, unstructured or "free text" data, data within data (e.g., descriptions of findings on a radiologic study separate from the conclusion or result), and data about data (metadata). Patient-generated data obtained from mobile sensors and other sources add to the heterogeneity of data types.

Value refers to the need to transform the data into meaningful, usable, and actionable information that organizations can then use to further their mission. In health care, this usually means improved patient outcomes, better health for individuals and communities, improved provider outcomes, and lowered cost.

HEALTH CARE DELIVERY DATA

A large volume of data is generated during the routine delivery of health care. Although these data can be used for research, it is useful to keep in mind that the data were created for the purposes of delivering health care to the patient and meeting the operational needs of the health care delivery organization, not for the purpose of conducting research. Hence, the quality and comprehensiveness of the data often do not meet the needs of a researcher.

Data relevant to health care delivery have been categorized into five types:[6]

1. Administrative data: Data primarily used for administration of health care (e.g., reimbursement) and secondarily for assessing outcomes and quality of care
2. Clinically generated data: Data recorded by clinicians for health maintenance, diagnosis, and treatment
3. Patient-generated data, clinically directed: Data requested by the clinician or delivery organization, reported by the patient
4. Patient-generated data, individually directed: Data recorded by the patient for self-monitoring, social networking, or peer support
5. Machine-generated data: Data automatically generated by sensors, medical devices, and so on to monitor patients

Although this categorization is conceptually useful, it masks the complexity of data sources and types that can occur within each category. For example, clinically generated data for diagnosis may include radiology images and studies, pathology reports, laboratory tests (including genomic tests), and clinical observations recorded in EHRs. Similarly, data on treatments can be obtained from electronic prescriptions, clinical notes and treatment summaries in EHRs, and pharmacy information systems. It is a challenging task to link and aggregate patient-specific information across diverse databases that may reside in different organizations while maintaining patient privacy and protecting the security and integrity of information systems.

It is useful to keep in mind that the health care delivery data are created from patients served by the health care system. Data on persons (whether healthy or sick) who do not interact with the health care delivery system are absent. Also typically missing in health care delivery data are data from a patient's daily life, such as environmental and psychological stressors in homes and workplaces; details on dietary intake, exercise, and other health-related behaviors; and details on a patient's caregiver and social support system. This imperfect representation of a person's lived experience has been termed the "data shadow" of the person.[6] This limitation should be kept in mind when conducting research using health care delivery data.

HEALTH CARE APPLICATIONS OF BIG DATA

Big data has several applications in delivery of health care, including safety surveillance, understanding the burden of disease, efficient conduct of large-scale observational research, quality improvement, designing safer health information technology (IT), and support of care delivery. All of these contribute to the ongoing need to implement optimal interventions to maximize patient benefit.

Safety Surveillance

One example of the use of big data for safety surveillance is the US Food and Drug Administration (FDA)'s Sentinel Initiative, which was launched in 2008.[7] The Sentinel is a national electronic system that monitors the safety of FDA-regulated products, including drugs, vaccines, biologics, and medical devices. Through the Sentinel, the FDA can rapidly and securely access information from large amounts of electronic data obtained from diverse data sources, such as EHRs, insurance claims, and registries. The first phase of this initiative was called the mini-Sentinel pilot, which informed the development of the Sentinel System. The Sentinel System was formally launched in February 2016. The Sentinel System uses a distributed data infrastructure to access data from more than 193 million patients in collaboration with 18 data partners.

Understand Burden of Disease

The Surveillance, Epidemiology, and End Results (SEER) program of the National Cancer Institute is an authoritative source of information on cancer incidence and survival in the United States.[8] It collects and publishes data from population-based cancer registries that cover approximately 28% of the US population. It collects data on patient demographics, primary tumor site, tumor morphology, first course of treatment, and follow-up for vital status. The mortality data reported by SEER are provided by the National Center for Health Statistics. The SEER data are helpful in clarifying geographic variations in the burden of cancer and the changes over time.

Large-Scale Observational Research

The Observational Health Data Sciences and Informatics (OHDSI) program is a multistakeholder, interdisciplinary collaborative that brings out the value of health data through large-scale analytics.[9] This program is committed to open, collaborative science, and its solutions are in the public domain. It has an international network of researchers and observational databases with a central coordinating center housed at Columbia University. In 2016, OHDSI published an analysis of treatment pathways, using EHR and administrative claims data obtained from approximately 250 million patients across four countries, to understand the variations in the sequence of medications taken over 3 years by patients with diabetes, hypertension, or depression.[10]

Quality Improvement

The Pediatric Emergency Care Applied Research Network is a national network for research on pediatric emergencies and emergency medical services for children.[11] One of its projects is to develop an emergency care visit data registry for pediatric patients that merges data from four hospitals within the network and contains data representing more than 1.2 million pediatric emergency department visits.[12] The registry is being used to collect and report performance measures to each emergency department as well as their individual practitioners.

Designing Safer Health Information Technology

Health IT needs to be properly designed and implemented to avoid introducing new types of errors or unintended consequences. One example is the work being done by the National Center for Human Factors in Healthcare at MedStar Health to identify safety gaps in current health IT systems through a retrospective analysis of safety event reports and to use these findings to inform the development of design and implementation guidelines.[13] These researchers are using machine learning and natural language processing on large sets of patient safety event data (containing more than 100,000 events) to develop automated solutions that can reliably identify health IT-related safety events without the need for manual abstraction.

Support Care Delivery

One way big data can support care delivery is by transforming the data into actionable knowledge in the form of clinical decision support (CDS). Often framed as the "Five Rights," CDS can bring the right information to the right audience in the right channel and in the right format at the right time during workflow.[14] The right information may be from clinical practice guidelines, laboratory results, decision aids, or any other information that is patient specific and aimed at improving care. The right audience for CDS has traditionally been clinicians as target audiences for computer-enabled alerts and reminders, but it could also be others on the clinical team (e.g., coordinators and administrators) or patients and their caregivers. The right channel and the right format refer to the ways in which the CDS could be delivered, such as through well-designed alerts or dashboards implemented through the EHR or through other software or technology. The right time for CDS is critical; the CDS must be sensitive to the target audience's work flow and cognitive load and must be delivered at a time that makes sense for the intended response and decision-making at hand. A framework has been proposed to construct usable, useful, and effective CDS based on the lessons learned during the conduct of a trial to efficiently integrate clinical prediction rules into workflow.[15]

The Agency for Healthcare Research and Quality (AHRQ) has long supported research to transform data into actionable knowledge through CDS.[16] AHRQ has launched a new CDS initiative that aims to accelerate the implementation of research evidence into practice through CDS and to make CDS more shareable, health IT standards based, and publicly available.[17] One part of this initiative is a Learning Network to engage a community of stakeholders and to advance the concept of patient-centered CDS.[18] A second part of this initiative is CDS Connect, which is building digital infrastructure for sharing CDS resources, including a publicly available national repository of CDS "artifacts."[19]

TRANSFORMING BIG DATA INTO KNOWLEDGE

A significant promise of big data is that it can be used to fuel "learning health systems" in which the data are transformed into knowledge that then drives continuous learning and improvement of the overall system. The National Academy of Medicine has described a learning health system in which science and informatics, patient–clinician partnerships, incentives, and culture are aligned to promote continuous and real-time improvement in effectiveness and efficiency of care.[20] Infrastructure—both technological and human—needs to support the collection, use, and reuse of the data for the learning health system to work. There are several steps in the path to transform big data into knowledge: manual collection or automatic generation of patient-specific data, data extraction, data harmonization and aggregation, data analysis, and presentation of data to inform decision-making and clinical actions. IT-based tools can help in each of these steps, as described next.

Person-level data collection is an entry point for data about individuals that can be gathered either during the delivery of clinical care or during research. The data can be collected manually (e.g., data recorded by a patient, caregiver, or a researcher; or a patient's data entered in the EHR by a clinician) or automatically by a device (e.g., an implantable cardioverter defibrillator recording the heart rhythm or a smartphone application recording the physical activity).

Data extraction includes data access and exchange. Data access refers to the authorization and process of storing, retrieving, or transferring data housed in a database. One example is the DataMart Client of the PopMedNet, which acts as an inbox for data partners to receive, review, and respond to queries distributed from a network portal.[21] The data partner may choose to execute the query, hold it for further review, or reject it. Extract, transform, and load processes (ETLs) are used to combine, translate, and integrate data residing in different data sources. The Reusable OMOP and SAFTINet Interface Adaptor (ROSITA) is an example of a packaged data tool that transforms EHR and claims data to the OMOP common data model.[22]

Data harmonization and aggregation are critical steps in the path to make sense of the big data collected during health care delivery. It is important to have a common terminology that provides uniform definitions and descriptions of clinical observations and data. A lack of common terminology can hinder research.[23] One useful resource for researchers is the National Institutes of Health's (NIH) Common Data Elements (CDE) Repository, a platform for identifying related data elements in use across diverse areas, for harmonizing data elements, and for linking CDEs to other existing standards and

terminologies.[24] A common data model (CDM) enables researchers to standardize the format and vocabularies used across different data sources and types. Several CDMs are used for clinical research: The OMOP CDM is well suited for supporting data sharing for longitudinal, EHR-based studies.[25] Data transformation to a CDM is time-consuming and needs substantial resources, but once that is achieved, the CDM minimizes the effort to develop cohorts and analyze results across sites.[26]

Data analysis tools can range from relatively simple query tools to complex distributed analytic tools. The Shared Health Research Information NEtwork (SHRINE) custom workbench and the Research Data Explorer (RedX) are examples of query tools that can answer queries on the feasibility of conducting research within a set of databases.[27,28] The Grid Binary LOgistic REgression (GLORE) tool is an example of a complex analytic tool that can build shared models without sharing the data; it can be used to perform distributed research on data residing in diverse organizations.[29] The data analytic tools can help researchers rapidly answer population-level queries, and they are essential to turn data into knowledge.

Decision support tools, which can be provider-, patient-, or researcher-facing, help turn knowledge into action. A recent example is the Stroke Prevention in Healthcare Delivery Environments (SPHERE) tool, which is an EHR-based CDS visualization to enhance patient–provider communication around cardiovascular health in a primary care outpatient setting.[30] This tool is provider- and patient-facing; it is designed as a user-friendly tool that minimally impacts clinical workflow. Other examples of decision support tools are automated reports that support pre-visit planning, population management, and quality improvement in a pediatric network-based learning health system.[31]

Finally, it is important to consider *trust* and *governance* issues that have an impact on the use of big data to create knowledge and inform patient-specific actions. Several federal and state laws and regulations, aimed at protecting the privacy and security of health information, govern the access to and use of identifiable health information for research.[32] Proprietary and cybersecurity concerns of care delivery organization are additional constraints on access to data stored by these organizations. Meaningful stakeholder engagement is needed to develop good governance policies and build trust, which in turn is helpful in building electronic data infrastructure to conduct research.[33]

Transparent and user-friendly policies that adhere to all applicable laws and regulations are needed to govern the flow and use of data in a network to foster trust within a data network. The data governance requirements for distributed research networks are beginning to be specified.[34] Multi-institution collaborations are needed to conduct big data-based research. However, increasing the number of institutions in a data network can increase the risk of delays in starting or executing research projects, which can slow the pace of research. Innovative approaches developed collaboratively by research, administrative, and regulatory staff across participating organizations can prevent delays and accelerate regulatory progress in multi-institutional research.[35]

BIG DATA, NEW TECHNOLOGIES, AND THE CANCER CARE CONTINUUM

There is a continuum in the delivery of cancer care, which includes the following: primary prevention (e.g., smoking cessation or human papillomavirus vaccination), secondary prevention (e.g., screening for breast or colorectal cancer), diagnosis, treatment, survivorship, and end-of-life care. Here, we provide examples to demonstrate how big data and new technologies can be used to implement interventions that improve delivery of care across the cancer care continuum.

Primary Prevention

Cessation of tobacco smoking can prevent cancer. Approximately 69% of smokers report an interest in quitting.[36] Many smokers visit their primary care provider each year; however, too few leave their visit with an evidence-based treatment. An EHR-based referral mechanism integrated into the clinical workflow and designed to close the loop between a quitline service and primary care increased the number of smokers who accepted the quitline service.[37]

Big data and health IT can also be used for understanding the burden and trends in tobacco use. Traditional surveillance systems that monitor tobacco use have several limitations, including cost. EHRs have the potential to be used as a surveillance system within health care delivery systems.

A study has shown the feasibility of using EHRs from six health care delivery organizations to assess trends in tobacco cessation in diverse patient populations.[38] This study was able to electronically create and follow a cohort of nearly 35,000 patients over 4 years.

Secondary Prevention

Early detection of disease, in the presence of effective treatments for screen-detected diseases, can improve outcomes. The USPSTF evaluates the evidence on the benefits and harms of screening for many diseases, including several cancers, and makes recommendations based on its assessment of the net benefit of screening.

Breast Cancer Screening

The USPSTF recommends biennial screening mammography for women between the ages of 50 and 74 years.[39] There have been two digital innovations in mammography: digital mammography, which has become the predominant method for mammography, and computer-aided detection (the use of computer algorithms) to assist radiologists screen women for breast cancer. Computer-aided detection (CAD) rapidly diffused into practice, increasing from nearly 4% of mammograms in older women in 2001 (when Congress extended Medicare coverage to CAD) to more than 60% in 2006.[40] Despite its popularity, it has been shown that CAD does not improve diagnostic accuracy of mammography; in fact, it may reduce sensitivity of mammography.[41] This example illustrates the need for outcomes research to better understand the balance between benefits and harms prior to implementing new technologies in practice.

Health IT can be used to implement preventive services in practice. AHRQ has designed an application called Electronic Preventive Services Selector (ePSS) to help primary care clinicians identify USPSTF-recommended preventive services appropriate for their patients.[42] Another example is an informatics tool called CareManager, which provides CDS through EHRs for USPSTF-recommended preventive services delivered within a physician organization called Providence Medical Group.[43] The cancer screening module within this tool was initially used to screen for cervical and breast cancer. Data from one provider showed that this module led to an improvement in the cervical cancer screening rate from 26% to 46%.[43]

Diagnosis

The increased availability of smartphones equipped with cameras has facilitated the ability of patients to capture and send images, which can be used for clinical purposes such as diagnosis of skin cancer. One study evaluated the accuracy of four commercially available applications (apps) to diagnose melanoma from archived images of skin lesions.[44] Three apps used an automated analysis algorithm for diagnosis, and the fourth sent the images to a dermatologist to make a diagnosis. Of the three apps using algorithms, one had poor sensitivity (~7%) and high specificity (~94%), and the other two had higher sensitivity (69–70%) and lower specificity (37–40%). The fourth app, which sent the images to a dermatologist, had the highest sensitivity (98%) and the lowest specificity (~30%). However, it took approximately 24 hours to receive feedback for this app compared to almost immediate feedback for the other three apps (<1 minute on average). This app also cost the most at $5 per lesion, compared to the other three, which ranged in cost from free to $4.99 for an unlimited number of lesions. The authors concluded that the apps are highly variable, and reliance on them has the potential to delay diagnosis and cause harm to patients.

Machine learning is a method that uses computers to learn from data. It is of two types: supervised learning, which has the goal of predicting a known output or target, and unsupervised learning, which tries to find naturally occurring patterns or groupings within data and has no outputs to predict. Both approaches have been used in medicine.[45] One example of machine learning that may assist cancer diagnosis is the Computational Pathologist (C-Path) system, which used 6,642 features from breast cancer epithelium and stroma to construct a prognostic model strongly associated with overall survival; this model is an improvement over the traditional model that grades breast cancer based only on epithelial features.[46]

Treatment

Tumor boards are used to obtain multidisciplinary input for cancer treatment planning. Information technology can support virtual tumor boards. A study has shown that a virtual tumor board program improved the quality and timeliness of the multidisciplinary evaluation process while avoiding the travel burden.[47]

Big data-based approaches can be used to evaluate treatment outcomes. It takes considerable effort to obtain data on long-term treatment outcomes, especially from patient subgroups excluded from clinical trials. One example of the promise of big data is the approach taken by the OHDSI collaborative to harmonize and analyze data from several large databases to characterize the variations in the sequence of treatments given to patients with diabetes, depression, or high blood pressure.[10] This approach can be extended to understand treatment outcomes in cancer and in different patient subgroups over long periods of times. Machine learning is another approach that can be used to understand the outcomes of cancer treatments. Big data-based approaches can make it easier, faster, and cheaper to do large-scale research on cancer therapeutics.

Survivorship

The increased effectiveness of cancer treatments has increased the life expectancy of many patients diagnosed with cancer. Based on data obtained from the SEER program and population projections from the US Census Bureau, it is estimated there will be 18 million cancer survivors by 2022.[48] Of this population, 64% have survived at least 5 years, 40% have survived at least 10 years, and 15% have survived at least 20 years. It is estimated that 63% of cancer survivors will be at least 65 years of age by 2020.[49] Older cancer patients are likely to have other comorbid conditions, which necessitates coordination of their care between the oncologist, primary care provider, and other relevant specialists. Here, we discuss depression in cancer patients and care coordination for cancer survivors as two examples to illustrate how big data and IT can support care delivery in cancer survivorship.

DEPRESSION IN CANCER

Depression is common in cancer; its prevalence ranges from 8% to 24%.[50] Depression worsens quality of life, decreases adherence to treatments, and contributes to increased mortality in cancer patients.[51,52] Due to the availability of accurate screening and diagnostic tests and also effective treatments, USPSTF recommends screening all adults for depression.[53] USPSTF also recommends that depression screening should be implemented with adequate systems in place to ensure accurate diagnosis, effective treatment, and appropriate follow-up. Because such systems are seldom in place in health care delivery organizations, it is not surprising that a large, population-based study found that 73% of cancer patients with depression were not receiving any effective treatment for depression and that only 5% of the cancer patients with depression visited a mental health professional.[54] A recent trial showed that a collaborative care treatment program of multidisciplinary clinicians was more effective than enhanced usual care in treating depression in cancer patients: 62% of patients in the intervention arm responded to treatment compared to 17% in the enhanced usual care arm.[55] Although effective, this care delivery model is resource-intensive, and it needs a high level of coordination among several providers—oncologists, oncology nurses, general nurses, psychiatrists, psychologists, and primary care providers (PCPs)—which limits the adoption of this delivery model in under-resourced areas such as rural community oncology practices. It is worth noting that the low response rate in the enhanced usual care arm of this trial occurred even though the patients, oncologists, and PCPs were informed of the depression diagnosis, which demonstrates the need for a system-level intervention, such as IT, to support the treatment and follow-up of cancer patients diagnosed with depression.

One IT-based approach to improve management of depression is the use of apps for monitoring depression. A study evaluated a patient-facing app using the Patient Health Questionnaire–9 (PHQ-9) to aid the self-assessment of depression symptoms.[56] This study found an adherence of 78% and showed that the app-collected results correlated well with traditionally administered PHQ-9s.

However, it is not easy to select a useful depression-specific app. A recent study found 243 unique depression apps; 34% of these apps focused on providing treatment, 32% focused on psychoeducation, 17% focused on medical assessment, and 8% focused on symptom management.[57] This study found that a search for depression apps yielded three times as many non-depression-specific apps as depression-specific apps. In addition, inadequate reporting of organizational affiliation and content source made it difficult to assess the credibility and reliability of many apps. Only the medical assessment apps adequately described their sources. This demonstrates the need for standardized reporting in app stores to help consumers select appropriate tools.

Health IT can also be used to deliver psychological interventions to either prevent or treat major depression. A recent randomized controlled trial demonstrated that a web-based guided self-help intervention can prevent major depression in adults with subclinical depression.[58] This study used a multimedia, interactive online tool consisting of six 30-minute sessions and an online trainer who provided support but not therapeutic advice. Only 27% of the participants in the intervention group experienced depression compared to 41% in the control group. Although this result is encouraging, further research is needed to understand whether the effects are generalizable to both the onset of depression and the recurrence of depression and the efficacy of web-based interventions without the use of an online trainer.

CARE COORDINATION IN CANCER SURVIVORS

Care for cancer survivors needs to be coordinated between their PCP and cancer specialists. A recent review found inadequacies in the frequency, content, style, and mode of communication from the cancer specialists to PCPs.[59] This review found little evidence on the extent and quality of ongoing communication from PCPs to cancer specialists regarding a patient's overall condition. PCPs often ask patients for information or use re-referral as a strategy to overcome difficulty in directly communicating with cancer specialists; these are inefficient and inaccurate communication strategies. This review also found that the use of a shared EHR system (such as that used by clinicians within the Veterans Administration) enhanced communication between cancer providers and PCPs. It was noted that outside of integrated delivery systems, cancer specialists do not typically have access to primary care records. Intervention strategies aimed to improve and facilitate the communication between PCPs and cancer specialists may improve patient and provider satisfaction while reducing duplication or omission of services.

Health Information Technology in Support of Collaborative Care

Collaborative care is used to treat depression and improve care coordination. A review identified five principles of collaborative care: patient-centered care; evidence-based care; measurement-based care; treat-to-target, population-based care; and accountable care.[60] The following are examples of how health IT can support these principles:

1. Patient-centered care: Patient education and self-management tools delivered through internet, mobile web, and apps; patient portals; secure email; and sharing of care plans and patient outcomes across providers and with patients

2. Evidence-based care: Electronic education materials and decision aids for patients; EHRs and registries in conjunction with electronic decision support tools and treatment algorithms for providers; and technology-enabled delivery of evidence-based psychosocial interventions

3. Measurement-based care: Improved data collection coupled with electronic triggers to alert providers

4. Population-based care: Electronic registry that tracks patients and highlights those patients who may need more clinical support; telemedicine assessments and remote delivery of behavioral interventions for difficult-to-reach patients

5. Accountable care: Registry with electronic data analytic capability to aggregate and analyze data on processes and outcomes at the provider, practice, and organizational level to help with quality improvement activities

ADVANCED CANCER AND END-OF LIFE CARE

Advanced care patients receiving palliative care only and those in underserved areas report the most severe symptoms due to their tumor burden, limited access to treatment, and infrequent contact with clinicians, particularly after the curative treatment is ended. A trial examined the efficacy of a collaborative care intervention to reduce the symptom burden in patients with advanced cancer.[61] The intervention included access to a psychoeducational website and to a care coordinator trained in cognitive–behavioral therapy and in psycho-oncology. Compared to patients in the enhanced usual care arm, patients in the intervention arm reported reductions in depression, pain, and fatigue. This study also found a reduction in stress and depression in caregivers of cancer patients randomized to the intervention arm.

EXISTING BARRIERS AND POTENTIAL SOLUTIONS

The growing availability of big data in health care delivery poses both an opportunity and a challenge in our quest to turn data into knowledge that supports timely, evidence-based, and patient-centered clinical decisions and actions. Better integration of the diverse types of data requires tools and approaches that improve interoperability while protecting the privacy and confidentiality of the patient's information. In addition, these tools need to be designed to provide value to the end-users and have the capability of supporting care delivery at multiple levels: patient, teams, and systems. Here, we provide an overview of these issues.

Interoperability

Health information interoperability is a broader concept than the traditional view of syntactic (data can be read across systems) and semantic (the meaning of data can be understood across systems) interoperability. An EDM Forum report identified four levels of information interoperability: syntactic, semantic, technical, and process.[62] This report found more than 75 health IT standards in use, most of which support technical, syntactic, and semantic interoperability. Only 2 standards address process interoperability. This is not surprising because process interoperability is difficult: It requires input and buy-in from the end-users, it is difficult to harmonize workflows and processes across different settings of care and in different geographic areas, and there is a lack of market incentives to encourage process interoperability. Three specific opportunities to improve process interoperability were identified in this report: (1) better integration of EHRs (and other health IT) into clinical workflows, (2) creating the right market incentives, and (3) ensuring the security and privacy of health information as it flows through and between health IT systems.

Developing Useful Informatics Tools

Widespread adoption of smartphones has enabled the rapid growth in the development and use of new mobile apps. Because not all mHealth apps provide clinical value (as described previously), it is difficult for the end-users (clinician, patient, or caregiver) to know whether an app can satisfactorily meet their needs. Apps of questionable quality have been called the "digital snake oil" of the 21st century.[63] A greater standardization in the app development process, including meaningful involvement of end-users during all stages of development, better validation, and standardized reporting, will help produce useful and effective apps.

Increased availability of EHR data has facilitated the development and use of electronic predictive analytics to forecast clinical events in real time to improve clinical decision-making and patient outcomes. A recent consensus statement on electronic health predictive analytics pointed to the urgent need for a systematic framework to guide the development and application of predictive analytics to ensure the field develops in a scientifically sound, ethical, and efficient manner.[64] This statement provided a framework that included developing an oversight strategy and standards for transparency, privacy, risk–benefit analysis, data availability, and workforce training and education. A similar approach can be adopted in development of other health IT tools.

UNDERSTANDING SYSTEM-LEVEL HUMAN–INFORMATION TECHNOLOGY INTERACTIONS

Achieving greater information interoperability and creating useful informatics tools to support individual decision-making are necessary but not sufficient to ensure the optimal use of IT to improve health care delivery. The movement toward team-based care and the rapid growth in cognitive technologies (e.g., unsupervised machine learning) mean that we need to shift our traditional focus on how IT can support information processing in an individual to how it can support information processing in an extended care delivery team embedded in one or more health care delivery systems.

Distributed cognition is a theory of human cognition that describes how information processing is distributed across people and their workplace, their

technologies, and their social organization and its influences over time.[65] The distributed cognition framework has been used to study and evaluate the use of health care technologies in a few health care delivery settings, such as infusion administration in intensive care units.[66] Distributed cognition is a promising approach to understand and improve the human–IT interactions from a systems perspective. The National Cancer Institute has commissioned a project to create a framework that applies the concepts of distributed cognition to cancer care delivery.

Situation awareness is another concept that can be used to understand human–IT interaction. Situation awareness is described as the ability of actors to become and remain coupled to the dynamics of their environment or, more simply, as "having the big picture"; it can be studied at the level of an individual, a team, or a system.[67] The system model of situation awareness considers both human and non-human agents and uses a system as its unit of analysis.

Both distributed cognition and system awareness are systems-based conceptual frameworks that can be applied to study and improve cancer care delivery systems. Systems-based cancer care delivery research can improve cancer care delivery and patient outcomes. However, systems-based health care delivery research is still in its infancy, and it will be a while before we can reap the benefits of this research.

BIG DATA AND IMPLEMENTATION: ISSUES TO CONSIDER

Given the challenges and opportunities presented by big data, we offer a few considerations on issues that the CEO, CMO, and CIO will face in using a big data-based approach to implement USPSTF recommendations to prevent colon cancer in the scenario outlined at the start of this chapter.

Incomplete Clinical Information

Big data-based approaches can use data from numerous and disparate data sources to provide an accurate and comprehensive clinical picture of the patient. Information about current aspirin use and about risks for bleeding may derive from structured and unstructured data in the EHR, from the patient portal, or from consumer billing data from pharmacies and grocery stores (because aspirin is an over-the-counter drug, the traditional pharmacy claims databases will not have information on aspirin use). One needs to be mindful of the fact that data in EHRs and patient portals may be incomplete or inaccurate, which may result in erroneous conclusions.

Improving Data Quality

It is important to detect and address issues that affect data quality. This is especially important when combining data from disparate databases. It will be useful to adopt, and adapt, the ongoing work of a collaborative that has recently harmonized the data quality assessment terminology and created a framework for the secondary use of EHR data.[68] Individual data elements that support determination of whether patients fit inclusion or exclusion criteria for aspirin use and for colon cancer screening need to be validated.

Human-Centered, System-Minded Design

The end-users (e.g., clinicians, patients, and caregivers) need to be involved in the design, testing, and implementation of the relevant informatics components of the colorectal cancer prevention program. This will lead to enhanced usability and user experience while undertaking a rapid product development life cycle analogous to the design approaches recently used for connected health systems.[69] It is important to be cognizant of the multiple levels of human interactions with the IT: individual, team, and system. A systems-minded design approach will facilitate distributed cognition and help in the delivery of timely and coordinated care.

Enhancing Care at the Individual Level

The ability to connect and extract data from disparate databases allows for machine learning and similar techniques to enhance detection methods and algorithms that can (1) drive clinical decision support to implement the recommendations to prescribe aspirin use or screen for colon cancer, (2) assess whether recommendations were implemented, and (3) provide a higher level of support to patients who may need additional support to help implement the recommendations. Big data can empower patients through patient-facing technologies that can both capture data and deliver knowledge directly to patients.

Enhancing Care at the Population Level

We can envision techniques for data capture, machine learning, and quality reporting not just for a single patient but also for all the patients within the health care delivery system. A population-level focus will allow the system to direct interventions to all members of the care teams (e.g., physicians, nurses, and physician assistants), deliver interventions over time (i.e., beyond a single patient visit), and use multiple technologies (e.g., EHRs, mobile apps, and quality management dashboards).

IT is rapidly transforming the way in which data are collected, aggregated, processed, and displayed, and it is affecting all facets of health care delivery. The growth of big data, and its applications, is a natural extension of the ongoing rapid technological progress. Big data provides an opportunity to analyze data from disparate databases to understand the trajectory of a person's health, the modifiable factors that influence a person's health, and a person's experience with a health care delivery system. Although IT has the potential to dramatically improve health care delivery, especially for the cancer care continuum, we need to cross several technical, evidentiary, and usability hurdles before we can fully harness IT to transform health care delivery.

REFERENCES

1. Weil AR. Big data in health: A new era for research and patient care. *Health Aff.* 2014;33:1110.
2. Bibbins-Domingo K; US Preventive Services Task Force. Aspirin use for the primary prevention of cardiovascular disease and colorectal cancer: US Preventive Services Task Force recommendation statement. *Ann Intern Med.* 2016;164:836–845.
3. US Preventive Services Task Force; Bibbins-Domingo K, Grossman DC, et al. Screening for colorectal cancer: US Preventive Services Task Force recommendation statement. *JAMA.* 2016;315:2564–2575.
4. De Mauro A, Greco M, Grimaldi M. A formal definition of big data based on its essential features. *Library Rev.* 2016;65:122–135.
5. Non-federal acute care hospital electronic health record adoption. Office of the National Coordinator for Health Information Technology

website. https://dashboard.healthit.gov/quickstats/pages/FIG-Hospital-EHR-Adoption.php. Accessed September 8, 2017.

6. Deeny SR, Steventon A. Making sense of the shadows: Priorities for creating a learning healthcare system based on routinely collected data. *BMJ Qual Saf*. 2015;24:505–515.

7. FDA's Sentinel initiative. US Food and Drug Administration website. https://www.fda.gov/Safety/FDAsSentinelInitiative/ucm2007250.htm. Accessed September 8, 2017.

8. Surveillance, Epidemiology, and End Results program. National Cancer Institute website. https://seer.cancer.gov/about/overview.html. Accessed September 8, 2017.

9. Welcome to OHDSI! OHDSI Observational Health Data Sciences and Informatics website. http://www.ohdsi.org. Accessed September 8, 2017.

10. Hripcsak G, Ryan PB, Duke JD, et al. Characterizing treatment pathways at scale using the OHDSI network. *Proc Natl Acad Sci USA*. 2016;113:7329–7336.

11. Welcome to the Pediatric Emergency Care Applied Research Network. Pediatric Emergency Care Applied Research Network website. http://www.pecarn.org. Accessed September 8, 2017.

12. Improving the quality of pediatric emergency care using an electronic medical record registry and clinician feedback (Illinois). US Department of Health and Human Services, Agency for Healthcare Research and Quality, Health Information Technology website. https://healthit.ahrq.gov/ahrq-funded-projects/improving-quality-pediatric-emergency-care-using-electronic-medical-record. Accessed September 8, 2017.

13. Developing evidence-based, user-centered design and implementation guidelines to improve health information technology usability (Maryland). US Department of Health and Human Services, Agency for Healthcare Research and Quality, Health Information Technology website. https://healthit.ahrq.gov/ahrq-funded-projects/developing-evidence-based-user-centered-design-and-implementation-guidelines. Accessed September 8, 2017.

14. Osheroff J, Teich J, Levick D, Saldana L, Velasco F, Sittig D, Rogers K, Jenders R. *Improving Outcomes with Clinical Decision Support: An Implementer's Guide*. 2nd ed. Chicago: Healthcare Information and Management Systems Society; 2012.

15. Kannry J, McCullagh L, Kushniruk A, Mann D, Edonyabo D, McGinn T. A framework for usable and effective clinical decision support: Experience from the iCPR Randomized Clinical Trial. *EGEMS*. 2015;3:1150.

16. Clinical decision support (CDS). US Department of Health and Human Services, Agency for Healthcare Research and Quality, Health Information Technology website. https://healthit.ahrq.gov/ahrq-funded-projects/clinical-decision-support-cds. Accessed September 8, 2017.

17. Clinical decision support. US Department of Health and Human Services, Agency for Healthcare Research and Quality website. http://cds.ahrq.gov. Accessed September 8, 2017.

18. Patient-Centered Clinical Decision Support Learning Network. https://pccds-ln.org. Accessed September 8, 2017.

19. Clinical decision support. US Department of Health and Human Services, Agency for Healthcare Research and Quality website. https://cds.ahrq.gov/cdsconnect. Accessed September 8, 2017.

20. National Academy of Medicine. *Best Care at Lower Cost: The Path to Continuously Learning Health Care in America*. Washington, DC: National Academies Press; 2013.

21. Davies M, Erickson K, Wyner Z, Malenfant J, Rosen R, Brown J. Software-enabled distributed network governance: The PopMedNet experience. *EGEMS*. 2016;4:1213.

22. Schilling LM, Kwan BM, Drolshagen CT, et al. Scalable Architecture for Federated Translational Inquiries Network (SAFTINet) technology infrastructure for a distributed data network. *EGEMS*. 2013;1:1027.

23. Kahn MG, Bailey LC, Forrest CB, Padula MA, Hirschfeld S. Building a common pediatric research terminology for accelerating child health research. *Pediatrics*. 2014;133:516–525.

24. NIH CDE repository. National Institutes of Health, National Library of Medicine website. https://cde.nlm.nih.gov/home. Accessed September 11, 2017.

25. Garza M, Del Fiol G, Tenenbaum J, Walden A, Zozus MN. Evaluating common data models for use with a longitudinal community registry. *J Biomed Inform* 2016;64:333–341.

26. FitzHenry F, Resnic FS, Robbins SL, et al. Creating a common data model for comparative effectiveness with the Observational Medical Outcomes Partnership. *Appl Clin Inform*. 2015;6:536–547.

27. McMurry AJ, Murphy SN, MacFadden D, et al. SHRINE: Enabling nationally scalable multi-site disease studies. *PLoS One.* 2013;8:e55811.

28. Wilcox A, Vawdrey D, Weng C, Velez M, Bakken S. Research Data Explorer: Lessons learned in design and development of context-based cohort definition and selection. *AMIA Jt Summits Transl Sci Proc.* 2015;2015:194–198.

29. Wu Y, Jiang X, Kim J, Ohno-Machado L. Grid Binary LOgistic REgression (GLORE): Building shared models without sharing data. *JAMIA.* 2012;19:758–764.

30. Foraker RE, Kite B, Kelley MM, et al. EHR-based visualization tool: Adoption rates, satisfaction, and patient outcomes. *EGEMS.* 2015;3:1159.

31. Marsolo K, Margolis PA, Forrest CB, Colletti RB, Hutton JJ. A digital architecture for a network-based learning health system: Integrating chronic care management, quality improvement, and research. *EGEMS.* 2015;3:1168.

32. Kim KK, McGraw D, Mamo L, Ohno-Machado L. Development of a privacy and security framework for a multistate comparative effectiveness research network. *Med Care.* 2013;51:S66–S72.

33. Randhawa GS. Building electronic data infrastructure for comparative effectiveness research: Accomplishments, lessons learned and future steps. *J Comp Eff Res.* 2014;3:567–572.

34. Kim KK, Browe DK, Logan HC, Holm R, Hack L, Ohno-Machado L. Data governance requirements for distributed clinical research networks: Triangulating perspectives of diverse stakeholders. *JAMIA.* 2014;2:714–719.

35. Paolino AR, Lauf SL, Pieper LE, et al. Accelerating regulatory progress in multi-institutional research. *EGEMS.* 2014;2:1076.

36. Centers for Disease Control and Prevention. Quitting smoking among adults—United States, 2001–2010. *MMWR Morb Mortal Wkly Rep.* 2011;60:1513–1519.

37. Adsit RT, Fox BM, Tsiolis T, et al. Using the electronic health record to connect primary care patients to evidence-based telephonic tobacco quitline services: A closed-loop demonstration project. *Transl Behav Med.* 2014;4:324–332.

38. Stevens VJ, Solberg LI, Bailey SR, et al. Assessing trends in tobacco cessation in diverse patient populations. *Nicotine Tob Res.* 2016;18:275–280.

39. Siu AL; US Preventive Services Task Force. Screening for breast cancer: US Preventive Services Task Force recommendation statement. *Ann Int Med.* 2016:164:279–296.

40. Fenton JJ, Xing G, Elmore JG, et al. Short-term outcomes of screening mammography using computer-aided detection: A population-based study of Medicare enrollees. *Ann Int Med.* 2013;158(8):580–587.

41. Lehman CD, Wellman RD, Buist DS, Kerlikowske K, Tosteson AN, Miglioretti DL; Breast Cancer Surveillance Consortium. Diagnostic accuracy of digital screening mammography with and without computer-aided detection. *JAMA Inter Med.* 2015;175:1828–1837.

42. Electronic Preventive Services Selector. US Department of Health and Human Services, Agency for Healthcare Research and Quality website. https://epss.ahrq.gov/PDA/index.jsp. Accessed September 11, 2017.

43. Impact case studies. US Department of Health and Human Services, Agency for Healthcare Research and Quality website. http://www.ahrq.gov/policymakers/case-studies/cp31311.html. Accessed September 11, 2017.

44. Wolf J, Moreau J, Akilov O, et al. Diagnostic inaccuracy of smart phone applications for melanoma detection. *JAMA Dermatol.* 2013;149:422–426.

45. Deo RC. Machine learning in medicine. *Circulation.* 2015;132:1920–1930.

46. Beck AH, Sangoi AR, Leung S, et al. Systematic analysis of breast cancer morphology uncovers stromal features associated with survival. *Sci Transl Med.* 2011;3:108ra113.

47. Salami AC, Barden GM, Castillo DL, et al. Establishment of a regional virtual tumor board program to improve the process of care for patients with hepatocellular carcinoma. *J Oncol Pract.* 2015;11:e66–e74.

48. De Moor JS, Mariotto AB, Parry C, et al. Cancer survivors in the United States: Prevalence across the survivorship trajectory and implications for care. *Cancer Epidemiol Biomarkers Prev.* 2013;22(4):561–570.

49. Parry C, Kent EE, Mariotto AB, Alfano CM, Rowland JH. Cancer survivors: A booming population. *Cancer Epidemiol Biomarkers Prev.* 2011;20:1996–2005.

50. Krebber AMH, Buffart LM, Kleijn G, et al. Prevalence of depression in cancer patients: A meta-analysis of diagnostic interviews and self-report instruments. *Psycho-Oncology.* 2014;23:121–130.

51. Colleoni M, Mandala M, Peruzzotti G, Robertson C, Bredart A, Goldhirsch A. Depression and degree of acceptance of adjuvant cytotoxic drugs. *Lancet.* 2000;356:1326–1327.

52. Satin JR, Linden W, Phillips MJ. Depression as a predictor of disease progression and mortality

in cancer patients: A meta-analysis. *Cancer* 2009;115:5349–5361.

53. Siu AL; US Preventive Services Task Force; Bibbins-Domingo K, et al. Screening for depression in adults: US Preventive Services Task Force recommendation statement. *JAMA.* 2016;315:380–387.

54. Walker J, Hansen CH, Martin P, Symeonides S, Ramessur R, Murray G, Sharpe M. Prevalence, associations, and adequacy of treatment of major depression in patients with cancer: A cross-sectional analysis of routinely collected clinical data. *Lancet Psychiatry.* 2014;1:343–350.

55. Sharpe M, Walker J, Holm Hansen C, et al. Integrated collaborative care for comorbid major depression in patients with cancer (SMaRT Oncology-2): A multicentre randomised controlled effectiveness trial. *Lancet.* 2014:384:1099-1108.

56. Torous J, Staples P, Shanahan M, et al. Utilizing a personal smartphone custom app to assess the Patient Health Questionnaire–9 (PHQ-9) depressive symptoms in patients with major depressive disorder. *JMIR Mental Health.* 2015;2:e8.

57. Shen N, Levitan M-J, Johnson A, et al. Finding a depression app: A review and content analysis of the depression app marketplace. *JMIR Mhealth Uhealth.* 2015;3(1):e16.

58. Buntrock C, Ebert DD, Lehr D, et al. Effect of a web-based guided self-help intervention for prevention of major depression in adults with subthreshold depression: A randomized clinical trial. *JAMA.* 2016;315:1854–1863.

59. Dossett LA, Hudson JN, Morris AM, et al. The primary care provider (PCP)–cancer specialist relationship: A systematic review and mixed methods meta-synthesis. *CA Cancer J Clin.* 2017;67:156–169.

60. Bauer AM, Thielke SM, Katon W, Unützer J, Areán P. Aligning health information technologies with effective service delivery models to improve chronic disease care. *Prev Med.* 2014;66:167–172.

61. Steel JL, Geller DA, Kim KH, et al. A web-based collaborative care intervention to manage cancer-related symptoms in the palliative care setting. *Cancer.* 2016;122:1270–1282.

62. Padgham D, Edmunds M, Holve E; Academy Health. Toward greater health information interoperability in the United States health system: EDM Forum. May 13, 2016. http://www.academyhealth.org/files/Toward%20Greater%20Health%20Information%20Interoperability.pdf.; Accessed September 12, 2017.

63. Hall S. AMA's James Madara: Healthcare must separate "digital snake oil from the useful" tools. June 13,2016. FierceHealthcare website. http://www.fiercehealthcare.com/it/ama-s-madara-healthcare-must-separate-digital-snake-oil-from-useful-tools. Accessed September 12, 2017.

64. Amarasingham R, Audet A-MJ, Bates DW, et al. Consensus statement on electronic health predictive analytics: A guiding framework to address challenges. *EGEMS.* 2016;4:1163.

65. Hazlehurst B. When I say distributed cognition. *Med Educ.* 2015;49:755–756.

66. Rajkomar A, Blandford A. Understanding infusion administration in the ICU through distributed cognition. *J Biomed Inform.* 2012;45:580–590.

67. Stanton NA, Salmon PM, Walker GH, Salas E, Hancock PA. State-of-science: Situation awareness in individuals, teams and systems. *Ergonomics.* 2017;60:449–466.

68. Kahn MG, Callahan TJ, Barnard J, et al. A harmonized data quality assessment terminology and framework for the secondary use of electronic health record data. *EGEMS.* 2016;4:1244.

69. Harte R, Glynn L, Rodríguez-Molinero A, et al. A human-centered design methodology to enhance the usability, human factors, and user experience of connected health systems: A three-phase methodology. *JMIR Hum Factors.* 2017;4:e8.

15

SCALING-UP CANCER CONTROL INNOVATIONS

Nancy C. Edwards, Barbara L. Riley, and Cameron D. Willis

THERE IS an expanding literature and practitioner interest in examining how innovations can be made more accessible to those who might benefit from them. In part, this is due to increasing recognition that despite the development of innovative products, practices, and programs, we have often fallen short of realizing their full potential impact due to scaling-up challenges.[1–3]

Evidence and experience on how to scale up come from health and other sectors, such as agriculture, education, and business. Much has been learned from resource-constrained settings in which deliberate, longer term, and concerted efforts to scale-up interventions have been used to address major health gaps. Local, national, and transnational examples of scale-up in these settings are prominent in the gray and published literature. They reflect a wide gamut of innovations ranging from primary prevention to diagnostic and treatment strategies. Examples include immunizations, micronutrient food supplements, potable water supplies, family planning, cataract surgery, antiretrovirals for HIV/ AIDS, and malaria prevention.

This chapter considers scaling-up issues that are pertinent to the field of cancer control—from prevention to treatment and survivorship. Its goal is to inform and accelerate scaling-up innovations for cancer control and to identify a timely and relevant research agenda to guide future efforts. Following a review of what is meant by scaling-up, the chapter presents a typology that can help guide scaling-up approaches.[1] It then illustrates application of the typology to two cancer control innovations for which scale-up has been

---

1. An earlier version of the typology on scale-up presented in this chapter was included in the report titled "Scaling-Up Health Innovations and Interventions in Public Health: A Brief Review of the Current State-of-the-Science." This commissioned paper was authored by Nancy C. Edwards and prepared for the 2010 Conference to Advance the State of the Science and Practice on Scale-Up and Spread Effective Health Programs.

Table 15.1. Illustrative Definitions of Scale-Up

REFERENCE	DEFINITION
Hanson et al. (2010)[9]	"The term 'scaling-up' is widely used as shorthand to describe the objective or process of expanding service delivery. It can refer to the outcome, in terms of increased coverage, or the inputs required, whether financial, human or capital resources. Similarly, scaling-up can also refer to a policy, strategy or the process of expansion" (p. 1).
International Institute of Rural Reconstruction (2000)[6]	Scaling-up involves "efforts to bring more quality benefits to more people over a wider geographical area more quickly, more equitably and more lastingly" (p. iv).
Mangham and Hanson (2010)[1]	Scaling-up is a process requiring "a strategy and implementation plan that considers the policy context, delivery mechanisms and resource requirements, as well as the pace of change, sequencing of activities, areas for prioritization and monitoring and evaluation" (p. 87).
Milat et al. (2013)[10]	Scale-up is "the ability of a health intervention shown to be efficacious on a small scale and or under controlled conditions to be expanded under real world conditions to reach a greater proportion of the eligible population, while retaining effectiveness" (p. 285).
Reis et al. (2016)[7]	Successful scale-up is achieved "when an intervention outgrows the research setting and becomes embedded in a system, thereby ensuring maintenance and sustainability of its health benefits" (p. 1337).
Simmons et al. (2007)[4]	Scaling-up involves "efforts to increase the impact of innovations successfully tested in pilot or experimental projects so as to benefit more people and to foster policy and program development on a lasting basis" (p. viii).
Victora et al. (2004)[8]	Going to scale is "a policy that builds on one or more interventions with known effectiveness and combines them into a program delivery strategy designed to reach high, sustained, and equitable coverage, at adequate levels of quality, in all who need the interventions" (p. 1541).
WHO (2010)[11]	Scaling-up entails "deliberate efforts to increase the impact of successfully tested health innovations so as to benefit more people and to foster policy and program development on a lasting basis" (p. 2).

prominent, namely tobacco control and the human papillomavirus (HPV) vaccine. Efforts to scale up other innovations, especially cancer screening (particularly for cervical and breast cancer) and other vaccination programs (hepatitis B and C), are also used as examples. The chapter concludes by proposing a research agenda on scaling-up in the field of cancer control.

WHAT IS SCALING-UP?

Scaling-up involves approaches to introduce innovations with demonstrated effectiveness through a program delivery structure and with the aim of improving coverage and population access to the innovation(s) and its intended benefits. Although definitions of scale-up consistently refer to the spread, reach, or coverage of an innovation or intervention, they vary considerably on three other dimensions: equity (equitable access and outcomes), lasting effects, and synergistic effects (for a comparison of illustrative definitions on these dimensions, see Table 15.1). Some definitions emphasize reach and coverage but without explicitly addressing equity.[4] Others emphasize equity considerations, suggesting that equitable reach is a fundamental aim of scale-up in health and other sectors.[5,6] Lasting effects or benefits[6] occur when an effective intervention is sustained or becomes embedded in a system.[7] Synergistic processes are reflected in several definitions. Victora et al.[8] suggest that the combined impact of innovations in a program delivery strategy results from synergistic effects, whereas Mangham and Hanson[1] make reference to both internal program planning synergies achieved through sequencing and attending to resources needed and external synergies occurring because of the policy context.

A PROPOSED TYPOLOGY FOR SCALING-UP

A vast literature has helped describe features of innovations and approaches that may influence scale-up. Enduring contributions are from Rogers'[12] earlier work on the diffusion of innovations. His work focused on both the innovation and those who adopted an innovation. He described several characteristics of an innovation that influence its rate of diffusion within a population, including its affordability, compatibility, transferability, and usability. Extensive research in health, agriculture, and technology sectors has demonstrated the predictive value of these innovation characteristics.

More recent work has considered the complexity of innovations, how innovations are delivered, the context for delivery, and a wide range of factors enabling and constraining scale-up efforts. Gericke et al.[13] described four dimensions of complex interventions that determine their technical complexity and may influence their uptake. Similar to Rogers,[12] they identified characteristics of the intervention that affected diffusion but noted that features of intervention delivery, government capacity requirements to deliver the intervention, and characteristics of use also affect rates of uptake. Greenhalgh et al.'s framework[14] described inner and outer organizational factors that affect scale-up. This framework presents a comprehensive set of contextual factors, and it describes how they intersect with both the innovation itself and those scaling-up an innovation. Other recent additions to the scaling-up literature focus on different directions (e.g., vertical and horizontal) for scaling-up[4,11] and different pathways (e.g., linear and iterative) for expanding the delivery and benefits of innovations.[15] The typology we propose integrates this diverse literature into a basic classification structure to guide scaling-up practice and research. Table 15.2 shows the proposed typology with its five dimensions, subgroups within these dimensions, and illustrative examples.

Dimension 1: The Object of Scaling-Up

The typology we propose includes what Hanson et al.[9] refer to as the "object" of scaling-up to distinguish different types of innovations. *Discrete innovations* have also been called direct interventions.[16] They are considered simple or complicated rather than complex interventions. They are ready for scale-up because of demonstrated effectiveness and may be packaged for ease of delivery.[17] Although these interventions are simple or complicated, they often are being introduced into complex delivery systems that are not necessarily well understood.[8,17] Indeed, Victora et al.[18] called into question the assumption that "the intervention delivered through RCTs can be replicated under routine conditions" (p. 400), in part because many system pathways are involved for the successful scale-up of discrete interventions such as HPV vaccines or Pap tests.[19,20]

Complex innovations involve many interacting elements (i.e., multistrategy) targeted at more than one system level (i.e., multilevel).[21] These innovations have components that must act synergistically to yield their intended benefits. Elements of these complex innovations need to be adjusted to characteristics of target populations and to dynamic implementation contexts while retaining the active ingredients of the intervention. The effective scale-up of these innovations depends on the relationships and interactions among intervention elements, understood within a socioecological framework that makes explicit the interactions among multilevel mechanisms for change.[22] With this subgroup of innovations, there may be considerable blurring between what is the innovation and what is the implementation context and also uncertainty about the active ingredients of interventions.[23,24]

Table 15.2. Typology for Scale-Up

DIMENSION	SUBGROUPS	EXAMPLES
Object of scaling-up	Discrete innovations Complex innovations	Vaccines; mobile phone apps Comprehensive tobacco control; Integrated service delivery models for cervical cancer screening, diagnosis, and treatment; comprehensive sun protection initiatives
Adaptations of innovations for scaling-up	Incremental changes Disruptive changes	Updating media and educational materials to reflect new public norms about cancer prevention behaviors Provision of the HPV vaccine to boys as well as girls
Directions of scaling-up	Vertical scale-up Horizontal scale-up	State/provincial policy to support local smoke-free bylaws Expansion of primary care offices offering brief interventions for smoking cessation
Pathways for scaling-up	Linear pathway Nonlinear pathway	Replicating cancer screening programs across hospitals Changes to professional and legislative regulations permitting task-shifting for cervical cancer screening
Factors influencing scaling-up	Localized influence Systemic influence	Hospital-based champions for cancer screening programs Nonsmoking becomes the social norm

The effective scale-up of both discrete and complex innovations depends on their dynamic interplay with contextual influences both within and across systems levels (e.g., interpersonal, community, and policy) and sectors (e.g., private and public; or health, agriculture, and transportation). Factors such as organizational policies, legislation and regulations, political support, levels of community engagement, leadership, demand for services, accountability systems, and social networks have been shown to influence the scale-up of both types of innovations.[1,16,25-27]

Dimension 2: Adaptations to Innovations for Scaling-Up

Although we describe only two subgroups of adaptations (incremental or disruptive), in reality this adaptation exists on a continuum. *Incremental changes* reflect minor adjustments to the innovation adhering as much as possible to the original innovation. In contrast, *disruptive changes* to innovations involve fundamental shifts to the objects of scale-up that may substantially alter or be altered by options

for service delivery. For instance, in a resource-constrained Zambian program for cervical cancer screening, having nurses visually inspect samples in the clinic, rather than sending samples to a lab for histological processing, enabled a much larger segment of the population to be reached.[28]

Disruptive innovations may also arise from a fundamental rethink of the causal pathways underlying the problem, which in turn shifts thinking about the target group or the delivery modality. For example, when environmental tobacco smoke was identified as a carcinogen, a new era of tobacco control policies was launched. Also, when the HPV vaccine was identified as efficacious for boys and girls, the vaccine (and the discourse about HPV) shifted to include both sexes, providing a means to more rapidly halt transmission of the virus.[29,30]

Dimension 3: Directions of Scaling-Up

Types of scaling-up are variably described (e.g., spontaneous, vertical, horizontal, diagonal, and functional).[15] A key source of debate about the scale-up of programs concerns the optimal direction of scale-up, that is required to achieve intended outcomes. There is increasing recognition that both horizontal and vertical scale-up strategies must be implemented in order to achieve equitable coverage and lasting benefits.[15,31]

Vertical scale-up (also known as political, legal, or institutional scale-up) involves the adoption of an innovation at an organizational, regional, or national level, whereby policy change, legal action, and/or systemic and structural modifications are made to support sustainable implementation of the innovation.[4] Vertical scale-up requires linkages among system levels. For instance, increasing the uptake of vaccines at the primary health care level involves a supply chain that gets vaccines, with potency maintained by a functional cold chain, from the manufacturer to the client in the right dose and at the right time. It also requires policies, procedures, and capacities at each system level that enable delivery. For instance, a national plan is required that includes vaccines on the essential drug list, capacity and infrastructure are needed to roll out the initiative, and a monitoring and reporting system needs to be in place that transfers information from community to district and national levels. Vertical programs are often disease specific and centrally managed in isolation from general health services.[1] In a review of case studies of large-scale vertical programs,[32,33] technical innovation, realistic financing arrangements, effective management, and strong leadership were all identified as reasons for success. However, vertical programs have come under substantial criticism because they are not necessarily well integrated within health systems.[34,35]

Horizontal scale-up (sometimes also called expansion, replication, or spread) involves expanding the reach of a successful innovation to other sectors or settings or extending it to larger or different target groups.[4,36] Horizontal scale-up refers to the uptake of an intervention at the same level of the system, such as across government departments or community organizations. An example is getting front-line providers working in acute care, long-term care, and community health sectors to assess all clients for their smoking status and offering brief interventions for those identified as smokers or recent quitters. A horizontal approach to scale-up may be selected to respond to increases in local demand or funding, to fulfill the agenda of an organization and/or champion, or to fill gaps or unmet needs.[37] Horizontal scale-up can increase efficiency and cost-effectiveness by replicating successful innovations. This approach is used when an innovation is both transferable and adaptable to new implementation contexts.[37]

Horizontal and vertical scale-up may also be achieved in combination with functional scale-up, which involves piggybacking a newer innovation to another that has already achieved wide acceptance and coverage within a population.[15] A functional scale-up approach has been used for many years with discrete interventions such as vaccination programs for children, when additional vaccines are added to those already being delivered. Examples of functional scale-up in the field of cancer prevention include reminding women of the importance of mammography screening during routine annual visits or offering fecal immunochemical testing to eligible patients when they come in for their annual flu shot.[38]

Dimension 4: Pathways for Scaling-Up

Three recent reviews[2,17,39] identified conceptual models for scale-up. Two models, scaling-up management[40] and ExpandNet,[15] were identified in all three reviews. Both models emphasize the need to take the political context and program management factors into account when planning scale-up,[17] considering the scalability potential of innovations,[11,15,39] and determining what would be a "scalable unit" for testing.[2]

There has been a tendency to address scale-up as a sequential, mechanistic, and linear process, reflected in descriptors such as early versus mature expansion.[41] More recent frameworks for scale-up emphasize the importance of nonlinear and iterative processes[2,42,43] and the necessity of learning by doing.[2,17]

Thus, essentially two pathways for scaling-up are evident in the literature. The first is linear, involving a deliberate stepwise approach to expand the coverage of an innovation. The second is nonlinear, wherein steps to scale-up are leapfrogged and large improvements in scale-up may be achieved more quickly. Nonlinear pathways are evident in approaches such as task-shifting,[28] or using an existing supply chain in another sector.

Dimension 5: Factors Influencing Scaling-Up

An understanding of what can support the scale-up of innovations comes from an examination of both failed and successful scaling-up efforts. Previous analyses[5] reveal both localized and systemic factors that influence scale-up. *Localized factors* exert their influence on parts of systems or groups only, whereas *systemic factors* spread throughout a group or a system as a whole. In this section, we describe six main challenges, which focus primarily on systemic factors.

UNDERESTIMATING THE TYPE AND QUANTITY OF RESOURCES REQUIRED FOR SCALE-UP

The scale-up of innovative programs involves human, financial, and infrastructural resources. Such resource constraints have limited scaling-up responses in many fields, including mental health,[44] cervical cancer screening,[28] communicable disease control,[27,45] hepatitis B prevention,[46] and the distribution of antiretroviral drugs.[47] Estimating the resources required for wide scale-up requires more than a mere multiplication of resources needed for pilot programs. Relative to the pilot introduction of an innovation, scaling-up may allow for per capita savings due to economies of scale. However, these costs may exponentially increase when one takes into consideration the cost of reaching late rather than early adopters of an innovation.[12] Furthermore, a differential distribution of who bears direct or indirect costs of scale-up is likely when issues of geographic access, population density, sources of income, and regional deprivation are in play.[48,49]

Importantly, the capacity needed for scale-up requires far more than health human resources and strong leadership. Numerous authors have described scale-up failures that resulted from either underestimating or ignoring capacities in other areas, including governance, legal, administrative, supervisory, management, accountability, and financial systems.[50]

POLITICAL AND POLICY NAIVETY

Scaling-up requires political commitment and policy support.[51] Several authors have described failures to understand the actors involved in successfully scaling-up and the underlying dimensions of power, authority, and vested interests that may adversely impact scale-up efforts. Policy is socially constructed, and policy actors differ in their values and interests and also in their views about the content and goals of policy.[52] Resolutions such as that passed by the World Health Organization (WHO)[53] regarding hepatitis B vaccine point to the types of political support required for national policy change. This hepatitis B resolution called for national strategies and surveillance systems, global targets for vaccine distribution, lowering prices for treatment and prevention, integrating the vaccination program within health care systems, and public–private partnerships.[53]

LACK OF ATTENTION TO ISSUES OF SUSTAINABILITY AND SCALING-UP IN INITIAL EFFORTS TO TEST THE INNOVATION

There is a growing consensus that conditions for sustainability and scale-up should be considered early in the process of introducing an innovation.[2,15,54] Often, however, these conditions are not taken into account until the post-pilot project phase, resulting in boutique interventions that are not scalable. Scaling-up strategies that are pertinent to earlier project phases include appraising institutional capacity for scaling-up and developing networks and partnerships that reflect pathways to scaling-up from the grassroots to end users.[55,56] When insufficient attention is paid to scaling-up at the outset of a program, key opportunities for organizational learning about ways in which the innovation may need to be adapted for wider scale-up will also be lost.[2]

OVEREMPHASIS ON EITHER THE VERTICAL OR THE HORIZONTAL SPREAD OF INNOVATIONS

An overemphasis on either horizontal or vertical elements of scaling-up has proven problematic. In a call for "diagonal programs," Ooms et al.[57] noted that "a vertical approach works for a while, and then hits the ceiling of insufficient health workers and dysfunctional health systems" (p. 3), citing the example of AIDS treatment in resource-poor settings. Similar challenges have been observed in efforts to scale up cervical cancer screening programs in some low- and middle-income countries (LMICs).[28] Failed efforts to expand the introduction of nurse practitioners in Canada illustrate inattention to vertical scale-up. It was not until the 1990s that the provincial-level regulatory structures and financing structures that were required to support implementation of nurse practitioners in the health care system were finally addressed.[58] These changes enabled nurse practitioners to work under a broader scope of practice, including functions such as performing Pap smears for cervical cancer screening.

UNEVEN ATTENTION TO SPATIAL AND TEMPORAL DIMENSIONS OF SCALING-UP

The public health and health services literature has concentrated on the spatial dimension of scale-up with a focus on coverage, reach, availability, and accessibility of services.[1,59–62] In contrast, the temporal dimension is less often described. Temporality takes into account the differential rate of change at each level of the system and the conditions that are required to initiate, sustain, or alter change processes both within and between system levels.[63] This temporal dimension is an inherent characteristic of complex adaptive systems, explaining the adaptive processes of revolt (representing a systems change) and remembering (representing a tendency to revert back to the status quo) that underlie how innovations take hold within and across system levels.[58,63] Interorganizational networks and strategic alliances may strengthen vertical connections, providing the inter-system social matrix that is required for scale-up.[6,64,65] Tobacco control provides an excellent example of what networks and alliances can achieve (see Scaling-Up Tobacco Control).

INATTENTION TO THE DEMAND SIDE OF SCALE-UP

Tackling the supply side of scale-up involves putting in place strategies to make the innovation readily accessible to targeted populations. The demand side of scale-up refers to building demands and expectations for the innovation among targeted populations. Pokhrel[66] and others[67] have posited that we pay more attention to the supply side than the demand side of service delivery, reminding us that both are essential for successful scale-up. A similar emphasis on the supply side of scale-up is reflected in the literature on costing,[49,68] in which the government perspective on the cost of supplying services is paramount while the societal cost of seeking care is often ignored. Johns and Torres[48] have called for a more thorough and rigorous set of methods to be used for costing scale-up. Such procedures would better inform priority options for scale-up.

When the supply side is weak, uneven, or erratic, this may further reduce public demand for the innovation.[20] Intermediaries, such as the media, can play a pivotal role in shifting demand. For instance, the media can inadvertently decrease the demand for HPV vaccines through its coverage of reported side effects or favorably increase the demand for HPV vaccine through public service announcements showing the consequences of cervical cancer. Strategies for orchestrating the best quotients of supply and demand need to be implemented within health and other sectors.

APPLYING THE TYPOLOGY TO CANCER CONTROL INNOVATIONS

In this section, experiences in scaling-up tobacco control and the HPV vaccine are discussed. These two illustrations are used to highlight some of the dimensions within the typology for scaling-up, along with instructive lessons from these scaling-up experiences.

Scaling-Up Tobacco Control

Tobacco control is arguably the most well-known public health and cancer control success story of the 20th century, and the efforts, successes, and challenges continue today. As the single greatest preventable risk factor for cancer and other chronic diseases,[69] and with tobacco-related deaths projected to increase to 8 million people worldwide each year by 2030,[70] there is an urgent need to continue scaling-up effective tobacco control innovations. A comprehensive approach to tobacco control is most effective and an excellent example of a complex innovation—a coordinated, interdependent set of interventions that includes multiple strategies (e.g., media, education, policy, monitoring, and evaluation) and targets multiple levels within a socioecological system (e.g., individual, interpersonal, community, and societal) while addressing multiple goals (e.g., prevention, cessation, protection, and denormalization of the tobacco industry). Although discrete interventions are nested within this comprehensive approach, we focus on scaling-up comprehensive tobacco control in this illustration. We also emphasize scaling-up globally.

Impressive scaling-up of comprehensive tobacco control has been achieved both vertically and horizontally. In the vertical direction, the creation of the Framework Convention on Tobacco Control (FCTC) is the first public health treaty on an international scale. The FCTC was formally adopted by WHO in 2003, with key provisions including sales bans to minors, advertising bans, tax increases, package labeling, smoke-free environments, and finding alternatives to tobacco production.[71,72] Horizontal scaling-up has been achieved through progressive adoption of the FCTC by 92% of the 191 member countries of WHO.[72]

The pathway for scaling-up tobacco control can generally be described as nonlinear—stimulated and constrained by both localized and systemic factors such as the opening and closing of policy windows, shifts in public opinion, and the emergence of tobacco control champions. However, it is also possible to characterize distinct and sequential phases of scaling-up of tobacco control, characteristic of a linear pathway. Globally, Reubi and Berridge[73] identified three main stages in the history of global tobacco control. They described Stage 1 (mid-1960s to late 1970s) as International Conferences and Exchanges that solidified tobacco use as a public health and cancer control priority. This stage is akin to "building the base" in the early stages of a social movement,[74] with leadership primarily from North America and Europe. They described Stage 2 (late 1970s to early 1990s) as Smoking and the Third World, which enhanced global exchanges and resulted in international authorities (WHO and the Union of International Cancer Control) establishing their first permanent tobacco control programs. Stage 3 (early 1990s to late 2000s) was referred to as Globalisation and Tobacco, with the creation of the FCTC and other global initiatives that recognized the increased and disproportionate burden of tobacco use among LMICs. This account of scaling-up tobacco control provides a macro-level narrative of the movement over many decades.

A major contribution from more than 40 years of scaling-up comprehensive tobacco control is lessons about how to overcome major challenges to scaling-up (factors influencing scaling-up in the typology). Scale-up of tobacco control at a global level was possible by overcoming systemic challenges at other jurisdictional levels. First, government commitment at municipal, provincial/state, and federal levels was essential to resource a comprehensive tobacco control strategy involving multifaceted interventions over an extended period of time.[75] Second, the work of coalitions and alliances was critical to maintain momentum toward tobacco reduction goals and to direct media and public attention toward changes, such as reductions in tobacco tax, that would have weakened key strategy elements. These alliances helped build a groundswell of support from the public for stronger tobacco control measures and enhanced recognition of that public support among politicians working at municipal, provincial/state, and federal levels. Alliance members also worked across political jurisdictions, using a systems approach to address tobacco control.[76] Furthermore, they addressed the temporal dimensions of scale-up, providing continuity and momentum for a social movement on tobacco control that transcends borders and spans changes in political leadership. Third, monitoring and evaluation systems were put in place to inform decisions about steady or failing progress in tobacco control. These systems used nationally and internationally agreed upon indicators, and they provided data on a wide range of shorter to longer term outcomes that helped identify shifts in patterns of tobacco use signaling scaling-up successes and challenges. Fourth, comparative epidemiological and policy analyses provided a means to examine the most salient elements of policy strategies and the differential impact of these policy elements on population subgroups. Fifth, constant scanning and vigilance within the tobacco control community helped identify countermeasures by the tobacco industry, including shifting marketing strategies to target youth, cross-border advertising, and strategic efforts to delay and weaken the content and scope of legislation.[77–82] These countermeasures by the tobacco industry represent efforts to decrease implementation of tobacco control programs with the aim of scaling-up market share of tobacco products.

An important present-day frontier for global tobacco control is a greater focus on equitable scale-up. Tobacco use disproportionately affects the poorest people: More than 80% of the world's smokers live in LMICs.[69] Within high-income countries, although the proportion of smokers has halved during the past two decades, certain subgroups have disproportionately high smoking rates.[83,84] Smoking rates among Canada's Aboriginal populations, for example, are twice as high as those of non-Aboriginal Canadians.[85] People with a mental illness also have significantly higher rates of smoking compared to the general population, with rates reported as high as 88%.[83] These disproportionate smoking rates among subgroups have been known for some time, yet there are few examples of equity considerations incorporated into scaling-up strategies. More common are examples of inequitable access to and benefits from tobacco control interventions.[86]

At the global level, uneven adoption of the FCTC is a case in point, with higher adoption among countries in the Pacific or Southeast Asian regions and those that are democratic, have lower male smoking prevalence, have a lower rate of female participation in the labor force, belong to the same GLOBALink subscription groups, and do comparatively less trading with other countries.[71,72] Dialogue about "end-game" strategies for tobacco control[87] may be setting the stage for some upcoming disruptive changes that ideally will achieve more equitable scale-up in global tobacco control efforts.

Scaling-Up the Human Papillomavirus Vaccine

The vaccine against HPV is an example of a discrete intervention (the object of scale-up), which involves multiple doses given over a 6-month period. The HPV vaccine was developed to prevent cervical cancer, which is the fourth most frequent cancer in women, with an estimated 530,000 new cases per year, representing 7.5% of all female cancer deaths.[82] As infection with HPV is the main cause of cervical cancer.[88] Multiple vaccines have been developed to prevent different types of HPV infection.[89,90]

The HPV vaccine was first licensed for use in 2006. Currently, various forms of the HPV vaccine are available in more than 100 countries,[91] with the United States, Australia, Canada, and the United Kingdom among the first to introduce the HPV vaccine into their national immunization programs. Despite its availability in these countries, uptake of the vaccine in many jurisdictions remains low.[88,90,92] Vaccine utilization is a multifactorial phenomenon influenced by the vaccine's acceptability and an individual's perceived disease susceptibility, perceived benefit of vaccination, and intention to receive the particular vaccine.[93] Barriers to increasing the uptake of HPV vaccination relate to the object of scale-up (i.e., features of the innovation such as use of a two- or three-dose schedule, distrust of combination vaccines, and delayed effects) and a range of factors negatively influencing scale-up, including parents (lack of knowledge and views about teenage sexuality), providers (inconsistent recommendations to patients and insufficient knowledge about or support for the vaccine), and the delivery system (lack of primary care provider, failure to track vaccine coverage, inadequate reminder capabilities for notifying patients of which vaccines are needed and when they are due, and vaccine cost coupled with lack of insurance coverage).[88]

The history of scaling-up the HPV vaccine illustrates vertical and horizontal directions of scaling-up, a nonlinear pathway for scaling-up, as well as an adaptation to the innovation that would be classified as disruptive. Vertically, HPV vaccination programs have been incorporated into regional and national efforts, both school-based and clinic-based. This has required influencing the perceptions of policymakers and legislators so they perceive cervical cancer as a problem and the HPV vaccination as a solution meriting policy action, identifying and working with political forces and interest groups that both facilitate and impede vaccine adoption, and understanding those factors influencing the attention given to different policy options.[94] The results of these efforts have included federal approval for the vaccine such as by the US Food and Drug Administration in 2006 and the introduction of state-level legislation regarding vaccine coverage in more than 40 US states by 2007.[94,95]

With respect to horizontal scale-up, the HPV treatment regimen has been replicated in multiple jurisdictions and has been expanded for use among boys. This expansion to a different beneficiary represents a disruptive adaptation of the innovation because this adaptation challenges perceptions of risk (because boys do not have a cervix), and it questions where responsibility should be placed for sexual transmission of disease (e.g., family planning measures are primarily aimed at women).

A key question facing HPV vaccine scaling-up efforts is whether this disruptive change is preferable to increasing the vaccination rate only or primarily among girls.[96] In some jurisdictions, such as the province of Prince Edward Island in Canada, the answer to this question may be seen in school-based programs that provide the vaccine to both girls and boys.[97] A number of contextual factors have enabled this shift, including a high level of support from leading Canadian health agencies; an existing public health immunization program, which has seen much success in the implementation of new vaccines in the province;[98] and local public health nurses with established relationships with schools, parents, and students.[97]

Experiences with the HPV vaccine provide insights into the broad range of actions that are needed to scale up even discrete innovations, and the highly nonlinear pathway that often characterizes such scaling-up efforts. For the HPV vaccine, scaling-up actions have included deliberate shifts in policy, financing models, and communication strategies; incorporation into existing public health delivery programs; and intentional efforts to increase acceptance of HPV programs by the public.[91] These actions have been iterative, reshaping contexts in which other actions take place. Specific actions within these broad domains have included the following:

- Defining and redefining the primary (and secondary) target populations[30]
- Developing links among diverse stakeholders involved in implementation and scale-up[99]
- Understanding and incorporating important sociocultural barriers to the equitable vaccination of young adolescents in particular settings[100]
- Identifying measures and indicators for tracking performance over time[45]

Undertaking these activities requires a range of associated scaling-up actions that involve different working groups of existing health and non-health infrastructures, including innovative public–private governance models such as partnerships and networks. Integrating an HPV vaccination program into existing service delivery structures is also an important action, as is developing and communicating clear guidance on who, where, how, and why population groups should be vaccinated.

PROMISING DIRECTIONS FOR FUTURE RESEARCH

Although insights about scaling-up are accumulating, many questions remain unanswered that could strengthen scaling-up practice. We propose a forward-looking research agenda on scaling-up in cancer control, highlighting key areas for future research investments. Specific examples of priority research questions are listed in Box 15.1. Overall, more emphasis is needed on scaling-up complex cancer control interventions, examining the conditions for scaling-up actions that increase or decrease health equity, and discerning and removing systemic barriers to scaling-up. Evidence requirements for scaling-up are poorly understood: Future studies must examine what evidence and what types of research designs are needed to inform various phases of scale-up and the iterative nature of the process. The costs of scale-up are a critical consideration for decision-makers. Further work is required to delineate the parameters for costing the scale-up of different types of discrete and complex interventions, taking into account governmental (health and other sectors) and societal perspectives.

There are some useful and promising systems-oriented models emerging to guide scale-up approaches.[2] These have largely been applied to health issues other than those related to cancer control. Their utility in the cancer control area is a priority for study.

SUMMARY

Scaling-up generally involves processes to introduce innovations with demonstrated effectiveness through a delivery structure and with the aim of improving coverage and equitable population access to the innovation(s) and its intended benefits. Although cited in some definitions of scaling-up, a focus on equity is underdeveloped in scale-up efforts.

This chapter proposes a typology for better understanding and improving scaling-up of cancer control, which highlights five key dimensions:

1. The object of scaling-up: discrete or complex

Discrete innovations: simple or complicated interventions that often appear straightforward yet are introduced into complex delivery systems

Complex innovations: less prescriptive and less structured than discrete innovations, and involve multiple interacting elements targeting more than one system level

2. Adaptations to innovations for scaling-up: incremental or disruptive

Incremental adaptations: relatively minor changes or adjustments to the innovation

Disruptive adaptations: fundamental changes to innovations that may substantially shift options for delivery and scale-up

3. Directions for scaling-up: horizontal or vertical

Horizontal scale-up: the uptake of an intervention at the same level of the system, such as across departments, organizations, and/or sectors

Vertical scale-up: specifically focuses on the linkages among system levels and generally includes organizational, policy, and other system changes

4. Pathways for scaling-up: linear or nonlinear

Linear pathway: considers scaling-up as a sequential, mechanistic, and linear process, including concepts of early and mature intervention scale-up

Nonlinear pathway: iterative, cyclical, or organic processes that may leapfrog some typical steps involved in scaling-up

5. Factors influencing scaling-up: localized or systemic

Localized influence: factors that exert their influence on parts of systems or groups only, and whose effects may be short term

Systemic influence: factors that spread throughout a group or a system as a whole, and normally have more enduring effects than isolated factors

Six main systemic challenges for scaling-up are highlighted: (1) underestimating the resources required for scale-up, (2) political and policy naivety, (3) lack of attention to issues of sustainability and scale-up during early efforts to test or implement innovation uptake, (4) an overemphasis on either the vertical or the horizontal spread of innovations, (5) inattention to temporal elements of scaling-up, and (6) inattention to the demand side of scale-up.

The experiences of scaling-up tobacco control and the HPV vaccine illustrate various aspects of the typology. Both experiences illustrate a dynamic interplay of all dimensions of the typology, nonlinear pathways for scale-up, and the need to emphasize equity across populations and jurisdictions in scaling-up goals and strategies. Comprehensive tobacco control is a complex innovation with a 40-year history of scaling-up, and this innovation uniquely illustrates how the tobacco control community addressed major challenges to scaling-up using strategies such as creating a social movement, monitoring and averting competing agendas, and sustaining a strong political and policy agenda. The HPV vaccine is a discrete innovation and uniquely illustrates a disruptive adaptation to the innovation by targeting boys in addition to girls and by the introduction of a discrete intervention into a complex delivery system.

Advancing both the theory and the practice of scaling-up in cancer control may benefit from a strategic research agenda that examines a subset of priority domains (e.g., conditions for scaling-up actions that increase or decrease health equity and ways for discerning and removing systemic barriers to scaling-up) and informs practitioner efforts to make cancer control and other innovations more accessible to those who might benefit from them.

REFERENCES

1. Mangham LJ, Hanson K. Scaling up in international health: What are the key issues? *Health Policy Plan*. 2010;25(2):85–96.

2. Barker PM, Reid A, Schall MW. A framework for scaling up health interventions: Lessons from large-scale improvement initiatives in Africa. *Implement Sci*. 2016;11:12.

3. Paina L, Peters DH. Understanding pathways for scaling up health services through the lens of complex adaptive systems. *Health Policy Plan*. 2012;27(5):365–373.

4. Simmons R, Fajans P, Ghiron L. *Scaling Up Health Service Delivery: From Pilot Innovations to Policies and Programmes*. Geneva, Switzerland: World Health Organization; 2007.

5. Edwards N, Barker PM. The importance of context in implementation research. *J Acquir Immune Defic Syndr*. 2014;67(Suppl 2):S157–S162.

6. International Institute of Rural Reconstruction, Global Forum for Agricultural Research. *Going to Scale: Can We Bring More Benefits to More People More Quickly?* Silang, Cavite, Philippines: International Institute of Rural Reconstruction; 2000.

7. Reis RS, Salvo D, Ogilvie D, Lambert EV, Goenka S, Brownson RC. Scaling up physical activity interventions worldwide: Stepping up to larger and smarter approaches to get people moving. *Lancet*. 2016;388(10051):1337–1348.

8. Victora CG, Hanson K, Bryce J, Vaughan JP. Achieving universal coverage with health interventions. *Lancet*. 2004;364(9444):1541–1548.

9. Hanson K, Cleary S, Schneider H, Tantivess S, Gilson L. Scaling up health policies and services in low- and middle-income settings. *BMC Health Serv Res*. 2010;10(Suppl 1):I1.

10. Milat AJ, King L, Bauman AE, Redman S. The concept of scalability: Increasing the scale and potential adoption of health promotion interventions into policy and practice. *Health Promot Int*. 2013;28(3):285–298.

11. World Health Organization. *ExpandNet: Nine Steps for Developing a Scaling-Up Strategy*. Geneva, Switzerland: World Health Organization; 2010.

12. Rogers EM. *Diffusion of Innovations*. 4th ed. New York: Free Press; 1995.

13. Gericke CA, Kurowski C, Ranson MK, Mills A. Intervention complexity—A conceptual framework to inform priority-setting in health. *Bull World Health Organ*. 2005;83(4):285–293.

14. Greenhalgh T, Robert G, Macfarlane F, Bate P, Kyriakidou O. Diffusion of innovations in service organizations: Systematic review and recommendations. *Milbank Q*. 2004;82(4):581–629.

15. World Health Organization. *Practical Guidance for Scaling Up Health Service Innovations*. Geneva, Switzerland: World Health Organization; 2009.

16. Scaling up nutrition: A framework for action. *Food and Nutrition Bulletin*. 2010;31(1):178–186.

17. Subramanian S, Naimoli J, Matsubayashi T, Peters DH. Do we have the right models for scaling up health services to achieve the Millennium Development Goals? *BMC Health Serv Res*. 2011;11:336.

18. Victora CG, Habicht JP, Bryce J. Evidence-based public health: Moving beyond randomized trials. *Am J Public Health*. 2004;94(3):400–405.

19. Yothasamut J, Putchong C, Sirisamutr T, Teerawattananon Y, Tantivess S. Scaling up cervical cancer screening in the midst of human papillomavirus vaccination advocacy in Thailand. *BMC Health Serv Res*. 2010;10(Suppl 1):S5.

20. McCree R, Giattas MR, Sahasrabuddhe VV, et al. Expanding cervical cancer screening and treatment in Tanzania: Stakeholders' perceptions of structural influences on scale-up. *Oncologist*. 2015;20(6):621–626.

21. Craig P, Dieppe P, Macintyre S, et al. Developing and evaluating complex interventions: The new Medical Research Council guidance. *Br Med J*. 2008;337:a1655.

22. Edwards N, Davison C. Strengthening communities with a socio-ecological approach: Local and international lessons in whole systems. In: Hallstrom LK, Guehlstorf N, Parkes M, eds. *Ecosystems, Society and Health: Pathways Through Diversity, Convergence and Integration*. Montreal, Quebec, Canada: McGill–Queen's University Press; 2015:Chapter 2, 33–67.

23. Hawe P, Shiell A, Riley T. Theorising interventions as events in systems. *Am J Community Psychol*. 2009;43(3–4):267–276.

24. Hawe P. Lessons from complex interventions to improve health. *Annu Rev Public Health*. 2015;36:307–323.

25. Merzel C, D'Afflitti J. Reconsidering community-based health promotion: Promise, performance, and potential. *Am J Public Health*. 2003;93(4):557–574.

26. Riley BL, Edwards NC, d'Avernas JR. People and money matter: Investment lessons from the Ontario Heart Health Program, Canada. *Health Promot Int.* 2008;23(1):24–34.

27. Simmonds S. Institutional factors and HIV/ AIDS, TB and malaria. *Int J Health Plan M.* 2008;23(2):139–151.

28. Parham GP, Mwanahamuntu MH, Kapambwe S, et al. Population-level scale-up of cervical cancer prevention services in a low-resource setting: Development, implementation, and evaluation of the cervical cancer prevention program in Zambia. *PLoS One.* 2015;10(4):e0122169.

29. Sinisgalli E, Bellini I, Indiani L, et al. HPV vaccination for boys? A systematic review of economic studies. *Epidemiol Prev.* 2015;39(4 Suppl 1):51–58.

30. Schmeler KM, Sturgis EM. Expanding the benefits of HPV vaccination to boys and men. *Lancet.* 2016;387(10030):1798–1799.

31. Hartmann A, Linn J. *Scaling-Up: A Framework and Lessons for Development Effectiveness from Literature and Practice.* Washington, DC: Brookings Institution; 2008.

32. Levine R. *Millions Saved: Proven Successes in Global Health.* Washington, DC: Centre for Global Development; 2004.

33. Medlin CA, Chowdhury M, Jamison DT, Measham A. Improving the health of populations: Lessons of experience. In: Jamison DT, Breman JG, Measham AR, et al., eds. *Disease Control Priorities in Developing Countries.* 2nd ed. Washington, DC: World Bank; 2006:Chapter 8, 165–180.

34. Tudor Car L, Van Velthoven MH, Brusamento S, et al. Integrating prevention of mother-to-child HIV transmission programs to improve uptake: A systematic review. *PLoS One.* 2012;7(4):e35268.

35. Atun RA, Bennett S, Duran A. *Policy Brief: When Do Vertical (Stand-Alone) Programmes Have a Place in Health Systems?* Geneva, Switzerland: World Health Organization; 2008.

36. Uvin P, Miller D. Paths to scaling-up: Alternative strategies for local nongovernmental organizations. *Hum Organization.* 1996;55:344–354.

37. Goldman KD. Planning for program diffusion: What health educators need to know. *Californian J Health Promot.* 2003;1(1):123–139.

38. FluFIT. 2017. University of California San Francisco website. http://flufit.org. Accessed May, 2017.

39. Milat AJ, Bauman A, Redman S. Narrative review of models and success factors for scaling up public health interventions. *Implement Sci.* 2015;10:113.

40. Kohl R, Cooley L. *Scaling Up—A Conceptual and Operational Framework.* Washington, DC: Management Systems International; 2003.

41. Smith JM, de Graft-Johnson J, Zyaee P, Ricca J, Fullerton J. Scaling up high-impact interventions: How is it done? *Int J Gynaecol Obstet.* 2015;130(Suppl 2):S4–S10.

42. Peters DH. The application of systems thinking in health: Why use systems thinking? *Health Res Policy Syst.* 2014;12:51.

43. Massoud MR, McCannon CJ. *Options for Large-Scale Spread of Simple, High-Impact Interventions.* Bethesda, MD: USAID Health Care Improvement Project; 2010.

44. Lancet Mental Health Group. Scale up services for mental disorders: A call for action. *Lancet.* 2007;370(9594):1241–1252.

45. World Health Organization. *Preparing for the Introduction of HPV Vaccines: Policy and Programme Guidance for Countries.* Geneva, Switzerland: World Health Organization; 2006.

46. Wang S, Smith H, Peng Z, Xu B, Wang W. Increasing coverage of hepatitis B vaccination in China: A systematic review of interventions and implementation experiences. *Medicine (Baltimore).* 2016;95(19):e3693.

47. World Health Organization. *Scaling Up Health Workforce Production: A Concept Paper Towards the Implementation of World Health Assembly Resolution WHA59.23.* Geneva, Switzerland: World Health Organization; 2007.

48. Johns B, Torres TT. Costs of scaling up health interventions: A systematic review. *Health Policy Plan.* 2005;20(1):1–13.

49. Wafula CO, Edwards N, Kaseje DC. Contextual variations in costs for a community health strategy implemented in rural, peri-urban and nomadic sites in Kenya. *BMC Public Health.* 2017;17(1):224.

50. Fokom-Domgue J, Vassilakos P, Petignat P. Is screen-and-treat approach suited for screening and management of precancerous cervical lesions in sub-Saharan Africa? *Prev Med.* 2014;65:138–140.

51. Goss PE, Strasser-Weippl K, Lee-Bychkovsky BL, et al. Challenges to effective cancer control in China, India, and Russia. *Lancet Oncol.* 2014;15(5):489–538.

52. Shiffman J, Smith S. Generation of political priority for global health initiatives: A framework

and case study of maternal mortality. *Lancet.* 2007;370(9595):1370–1379.

53. *World Health Assembly Resolution 67.6, Hepatitis.* Geneva, Switzerland: World Health Organization; 2014.

54. Pluye P, Potvin L, Denis JL, Pelletier J. Program sustainability: Focus on organizational routines. *Health Promot Int.* 2004;19(4):489–500.

55. Gundel S, Hancock J, Anderson S. *Scaling-Up Strategies for Research in Natural Resources Management: A Comparative Review.* Chatham, UK: Natural Resources Institute; 2001:1–61.

56. Gilson L, Schneider H. Commentary: Managing scaling up: What are the key issues? *Health Policy Plan.* 2010;25(2):97–98.

57. Ooms G, Van Damme W, Baker BK, Zeitz P, Schrecker T. The "diagonal" approach to Global Fund financing: A cure for the broader malaise of health systems? *Global Health.* 2008;4:6.

58. Edwards N, Rowan M, Marck P, Grinspun D. Understanding whole systems change in health care: The case of nurse practitioners in Canada. *Policy Polit Nurs Pract.* 2011;12(1):4–17.

59. Bryce J, Victora CG, Habicht JP, Vaughan JP, Black RE. The multi-country evaluation of the integrated management of childhood illness strategy: Lessons for the evaluation of public health interventions. *Am J Public Health.* 2004;94(3):406–415.

60. Glasgow RE, Klesges LM, Dzewaltowski DA, Estabrooks PA, Vogt TM. Evaluating the impact of health promotion programs: Using the RE-AIM framework to form summary measures for decision making involving complex issues. *Health Educ Res.* 2006;21(5):688–694.

61. Murray CJL, Evans DB. *Health Systems Performance Assessment: Debates, Methods and Empiricism.* Geneva, Switzerland: World Health Organization; 2003.

62. Verma R, Shekhar A, Khobragade S, et al. Scale-up and coverage of Avahan: A large-scale HIV-prevention programme among female sex workers and men who have sex with men in four Indian states. *Sex Transm Infect.* 2010;86(Suppl 1):i76–i82.

63. Gunderson LH, Holling CS. *Panarchy: Understanding Transformations in Human and Natural Systems.* Washington, DC: Island Press; 2001.

64. De Souza R-M. *Scaling Up Integrated Population, Health and Environment Approaches in the Philippines: A Review of Early Experiences.* Washington, DC: World Wildlife Fund and the Population Reference Bureau; 2008.

65. Gallardo J, Goldberg M, Randhawa B. Strategic alliances to scale up financial services in rural areas. World Bank Working Paper No. 76. Washington, DC: World Bank; 2006.

66. Pokhrel S. Scaling up health interventions in resource-poor countries: What role does research in stated-preference framework play? *Health Res Policy Syst.* 2006;4:4.

67. Ensor T, Cooper S. Overcoming barriers to health service access: Influencing the demand side. *Health Policy Plan.* 2004;19(2):69–79.

68. Cleary S, McIntyre D. Financing equitable access to antiretroviral treatment in South Africa. *BMC Health Serv Res.* 2010;10(Suppl 1):S2.

69. World Health Organization. *WHO Report on the Global Tobacco Epidemic, 2015: Raising Taxes on Tobacco.* Geneva, Switzerland: World Health Organization; 2015.

70. World Health Organization. *Beginning with the End in Mind: Planning Pilot Projects and Other Programmatic Research for Successful Scaling Up.* Geneva, Switzerland: World Health Organization. 2011.

71. Wipfli HL, Fujimoto K, Valente TW. Global tobacco control diffusion: The case of the Framework Convention on Tobacco Control. *Am J Public Health.* 2010;100(7):1260–1266.

72. Valente TW, Dyal SR, Chu KH, Wipfli H, Fujimoto K. Diffusion of innovations theory applied to global tobacco control treaty ratification. *Soc Sci Med.* 2015;145:89–97.

73. Reubi D, Berridge V. The internationalisation of tobacco control, 1950–2010. *Med Hist.* 2016;60(4):453–472.

74. Masters B, Osborn T. Social movements and philanthropy: How foundations can support movement building. *Foundation Rev.* 2010;2(2).

75. Pierce JP. Tobacco industry marketing, population-based tobacco control, and smoking behavior. *Am J Prev Med.* 2007;33(6 Suppl):S327–S334.

76. Davis RM, Wakefield M, Amos A, Gupta PC. The hitchhiker's guide to tobacco control: A global assessment of harms, remedies, and controversies. *Annu Rev Public Health.* 2007;28:171–194.

77. Assunta M, Chapman S. "The world's most hostile environment": How the tobacco industry circumvented Singapore's advertising ban. *Tob Control.* 2004;13(Suppl 2):ii51–ii57.

78. Landman A, Glantz SA. Tobacco industry efforts to undermine policy-relevant research. *Am J Public Health.* 2009;99(1):45–58.

79. MacKenzie R, Collin J, Sriwongcharoen K. Thailand—Lighting up a dark market: British

American tobacco, sports sponsorship and the circumvention of legislation. *J Epidemiol Community Health.* 2007;61(1):28–33.

80. Nakkash R, Lee K. The tobacco industry's thwarting of marketing restrictions and health warnings in Lebanon. *Tob Control.* 2009;18(4):310–316.

81. Pierce JP, Messer K, James LE, et al. Camel No. 9 cigarette-marketing campaign targeted young teenage girls. *Pediatrics.* 2010;125(4):619–626.

82. World Health Organization. *Estimated Cancer Incidence, Mortality and Prevalence Worldwide.* Geneva, Switzerland: World Health Organization; 2012.

83. Metse AP, Wiggers J, Wye P, et al. Uptake of smoking cessation aids by smokers with a mental illness. *J Behav Med.* 2016;39(5):876–886.

84. Quinn EC, Sacks R, Farley SM, Thihalolipavan S. Development of culturally appropriate support strategies to increase uptake of nicotine replacement therapy among Russian- and Chinese-speaking smokers in New York City. *J Community Health.* 2017;42(3):431–436.

85. Physicians for a Smoke-Free Canada. Factsheets: Smoking among Aboriginal Canadians; 2013.

86. Brown T, Platt S, Amos A. Equity impact of European individual-level smoking cessation interventions to reduce smoking in adults: A systematic review. *Eur J Public Health.* 2014;24(4):551–556.

87. McDaniel PA, Smith EA, Malone RE. The tobacco endgame: A qualitative review and synthesis. *Tob Control.* 2016;25(5):594–604.

88. Bratic JS, Seyferth ER, Bocchini JA Jr. Update on barriers to human papillomavirus vaccination and effective strategies to promote vaccine acceptance. *Curr Opin Pediatr.* 2016;28(3):407–412.

89. Immunization, vaccines and biologicals: School-based immunization. 2016. World Health Organization website. http://www.who.int/immunization/programmes_systems/policies_strategies/school_based_immunization/en.

90. Forster AS, Waller J. Taking stock and looking ahead: Behavioural science lessons for implementing the nonavalent human papillomavirus vaccine. *Eur J Cancer.* 2016;62:96–102.

91. Markowitz LE, Tsu V, Deeks SL, et al. Human papillomavirus vaccine introduction—The first five years. *Vaccine.* 2012;30(Suppl 5):F139–F148.

92. Peterson CE, Dykens JA, Brewer NT, et al. Society of Behavioral Medicine supports increasing HPV vaccination uptake: An urgent opportunity for cancer prevention. *Transl Behav Med.* 2016;6(4):672–675.

93. Das JK, Salam RA, Arshad A, Lassi ZS, Bhutta ZA. Systematic review and meta-analysis of interventions to improve access and coverage of adolescent immunizations. *J Adolesc Health.* 2016;59(4 Suppl):S40–S48.

94. Abiola SE, Colgrove J, Mello MM. The politics of HPV vaccination policy formation in the United States. *J Health Polit Policy Law.* 2013;38(4):645–681.

95. Markowitz LE, Dunne EF, Saraiya M, et al. Quadrivalent human papillomavirus vaccine: Recommendations of the Advisory Committee on Immunization Practices (ACIP). *MMWR Recomm Rep.* 2007;56(RR-2):1–24.

96. Stanley M, O'Mahony C, Barton S. HPV vaccination. *Br Med J.* 2014;349.

97. McClure CA, MacSwain MA, Morrison H, Sanford CJ. Human papillomavirus vaccine uptake in boys and girls in a school-based vaccine delivery program in Prince Edward Island, Canada. *Vaccine.* 2015;33(15):1786–1790.

98. Zelman M, Sanford C, Neatby A, et al. Implementation of a universal rotavirus vaccination program: Comparison of two delivery systems. *BMC Public Health.* 2014;14.

99. Tung IL, Machalek DA, Garland SM. Attitudes, knowledge and factors associated with human papillomavirus (HPV) vaccine uptake in adolescent girls and young women in Victoria, Australia. *PLoS One.* 2016;11(8):e0161846.

100. Ferrer HB, Audrey S, Trotter C, Hickman M. An appraisal of theoretical approaches to examining behaviours in relation to human papillomavirus (HPV) vaccination of young women. *Prev Med.* 2015;81:122–131.

16

SUSTAINABILITY OF CANCER PRACTICES AND PROGRAMS

Shannon Wiltsey Stirman and James W. Dearing

AS THE field of implementation science has matured, increasing attention has been paid to whether and how newly implemented interventions and programs can be sustained over time. Questions regarding the extent to which innovations in cancer prevention and care can best be sustained to provide desired benefits are essential to consider because many practices and programs require a substantial upfront investment of time and resources. Stakeholders make this investment with the expectation that the interventions will be delivered and that the intended recipients will benefit from them over the long term, but there is increasing evidence that sustainability of evidence-based programs and interventions remains precarious.[1] Consider the case of the Comprehensive Health Enhancement Support System (CHESS), an online social support tool for cancer survivors developed at the University of Wisconsin, tested for efficacy and effectiveness in multiple health care delivery systems, and then subjected to implementation study in two Colorado delivery systems. CHESS had been

the object of multiple randomized controlled trials that documented its effectiveness. Nevertheless, Colorado decision makers engaged in a lengthy introduction, review, and redesign process before it was approved for implementation. Even after this substantial groundwork was in place, continued reminders and checks were needed to sustain its visibility and use by providers and patients.[2] Clearly, evidence of effectiveness can be insufficient even for the sustained use of effective cancer prevention and care innovations, let alone for sustained benefit to patients.

Sustainability has been defined as the continued use of program components and activities for the continued achievement of desirable program and population outcomes.[3] Sustainability has sometimes been distinguished from the term *sustainment*, defined as the continued use of an intervention within practice,[4] meaning that sustainability then refers to the extent to which an evidence-based intervention can deliver its intended benefits over an extended period of time after external support is terminated.[4]

In this view, sustainment equates with normalization; when organizational delivery staff continue to offer programs and engage in practices and no longer perceive them to be new, the sustainment of programs and practices has occurred, and sustainability encompasses whether the program and its intended benefits are maintained. A recent review of the sustainability literature suggested that a program or intervention may be considered to be sustained at a given point in time if, after initial implementation support has been withdrawn, core elements are maintained (e.g., remain recognizable or delivered at a sufficient level of fidelity or intensity to yield desired health outcomes) and adequate capacity for continuation of these elements is maintained.[5] Arguably more important, however, is whether a program's or an intervention's *impact* is sustained— that is, if desired health benefits remain at or above the level achieved during implementation and this increase can be attributed to continuation of the program.[5] Thus, in considering sustainability, it is useful to consider a number of potential outcomes.

SUSTAINABILITY OUTCOMES

In addition to listing sustainability as an important implementation outcome, Proctor and colleagues[6] identify several other implementation outcomes that are also relevant to sustainability: acceptability, appropriateness, costs, feasibility, fidelity, and penetration. Depending on the nature of the program or intervention, appropriate outcomes to assess may include consumer-, patient-, or recipient-level outcomes (e.g., health outcomes); fidelity; modifications or adaptations to the intervention; capacity to administer or deliver the program or intervention; and maintenance of necessary collaborations between key stakeholders or coalitions. To inform research and assessment of sustainability outcomes, Scheirer[7] recommends differentiating six types of interventions according to their structure—who and what are required for continued delivery—rather than to their health content area. As indicated in Table 16.1, the different forms of programs and interventions have implications for planning, selecting strategies to promote sustainment, and determining whether the program or intervention is sustained. The programmatic outcomes that will be most relevant will be determined by the type of program.[7] For example, interventions delivered by individual providers may include a focus on sustained provider skill or

fidelity, the number of providers available to provide the intervention, penetration (proportion of eligible consumers who receive the intervention), and clinical outcomes. Interventions that focus on partnerships and coalition building may instead evaluate communication patterns, coalition activities, member engagement, and other indicators that the partnership remains active. Stakeholder goals should also inform evaluations of sustainability to ensure that outcomes that are relevant to key partners and decision makers are reflected in evaluations. In every case, however, a critical outcome to examine is whether the desired health benefits for intended beneficiaries have been maintained or improved upon.[4,5,7]

In addition, there will be circumstances under which discontinuation or reinvention of an existing practice or program, or adoption and implementation of a more effective, efficient, or better fitting intervention, is desirable. All of these considerations should factor into planning and evaluation of long-term sustainment.

SUSTAINABILITY FRAMEWORKS

A number of frameworks have been put forth to conceptualize sustainability, either in the context of a broader implementation framework or as a separate consideration.[1,8] Table 16.2 lists 27 frameworks that describe processes or factors related to sustainment. These frameworks have been developed in a number of areas, such as mental or physical health, prevention, and public health. The majority of the frameworks describe factors that are also highlighted in implementation frameworks discussed in previous chapters of this book, classified broadly as follows: *outer context* (e.g., sociopolitical context), *inner context* (e.g., organization-level factors, including climate, culture, leadership, and resources), *provider level* (e.g., training backgrounds and attitudes), and *intervention or program characteristics* (e.g., relative advantage, complexity, compatibility, and cost). Some conceptualizations of sustainability emphasize the likelihood of mutual influence between factors at the different levels.[9,10] For example, policy related to health care financing is likely to influence the level of leadership support that a program receives within a health care organization. The relative influence of these different factors on sustainment may be different than that during the post-adoption implementation phase. Although organizations may find ways to absorb

Table 16.1. Key Sustainability Outcomes by Program Type

PROGRAM TYPE	EXAMPLES OF INTERVENTIONS	SUSTAINABILITY OUTCOME IN ADDITION TO DESIRED HEALTH BENEFITS
Intervention delivered by individual providers	Health education, psychotherapy (e.g., Project HEAL[36])	Whether, and to what extent, the core elements (the elements most closely associated with desired health benefits) are maintained
Intervention requiring coordination between multiple providers	Community–academic cancer prevention programs, surgical procedures (e.g., short-stay program after breast cancer surgery[39])	Continuation of program elements or activities, particularly those most closely linked to desired health benefits
New technologies, policies, or procedures	Screening, electronic reminders, smoking bans (e.g., CHESS program[2])	Continued availability and use of the technology; continued adherence to the policy or procedure
Interventions that build capacity or infrastructure	Leadership training, board development, strategic planning (e.g., national or local Cancer Prevention Coalitions)	Maintenance or expansion of capacity and infrastructure and resources
Collaborative partnerships or coalitions	Community-based smoking cessation programs	Maintenance or expansion of partnerships
Broad-scale system change	Comprehensive cancer programs, integrated medical and behavioral health	Changes in the ways that organizations, practitioners, financial sources, and other factors interact to impact problem area; culture change

initial costs of implementation activities such as training and purchasing equipment or materials that contribute to initial implementation success, ongoing cost–benefit assessments may determine whether a program or intervention is sustainable. As Scheirer[7] notes, the nature of the program or intervention will factor in to the relative salience of potential influences, as well as the outcomes when considering sustainability. As illustrated in Table 16.2, the frameworks that attend to sustainability span a number of domains and fields, and they may therefore emphasize different factors and processes depending on the field and context from which it

originated. Thus, selection of a framework to guide planning or evaluation should be informed by the type of program, the goals, and the complexity of the intervention.

Although the concept of sustainability has implied a static, rather than evolving, form of ongoing implementation, a more dynamic concept of sustainability has recently been proposed as the Dynamic Sustainability Framework.[4] This framework explicitly addresses the importance of considering the fact that programs and interventions are implemented in rapidly changing contexts and that mechanisms for adapting to these changes to

Table 16.2. Sustainability Frameworks

AUTHORS	FOCUS	HOW SUSTAINABILITY IS DEFINED		INTERVENTION				SETTING TYPE
		EXPLICIT DEFINITION	SUSTAINABILITY OUTCOMES CONSIDERED	TYPE	DOMAIN	INTENT		
Aarons et al.[56]	Conceptualizing implementation	No	Intervention activities	Individual providers	Mental health/ substance abuse	Treatment		Organization
Adelman and Taylor[57]	Conceptualizing sustainability	Yes	Intervention activities, organizational policies, replication	Individual providers, multiple staff	Education	Treatment		Community, organization
Akerlund[58]	Conceptualizing sustainability	Yes	Intervention activities, replication	Policies/procedures/ technologies	Mental health/ substance abuse	Prevention		Organization
Altman[59]	Conceptualizing sustainability	Yes	Intervention activities, community partnerships, organizational policies	Individual providers, multiple staff, policies/procedures/ technologies, capacity/ infrastructure building	Public health	Prevention, treatment		Community
Beery et al.[60]	Evaluation/ measurement	No	Consumer benefits, Intervention activities	Individual providers, multiple staff, policies/procedures/ technologies, capacity/ infrastructure building	Public health	Promotion		Community

(continued)

Table 16.2 Continued

AUTHORS	FOCUS	HOW SUSTAINABILITY IS DEFINED		INTERVENTION			
		EXPLICIT DEFINITION	SUSTAINABILITY OUTCOMES CONSIDERED	TYPE	DOMAIN	INTENT	SETTING TYPE
Chambers et al.[4]	Conceptualizing sustainability	Yes	Intervention activities, benefits	Individual providers, multiple staff, policies/procedures/technologies, capacity/infrastructure building	Health care	Prevention, treatment	Organization, community
Feldstein et al.[61]	Conceptualizing implementation	No	Intervention activities	Individual providers, multiple staff	Health and human services	Treatment	Organization
Glaser[62]	Conceptualizing sustainability	Yes	Intervention activities	Individual providers	Mental health/substance abuse	Treatment	Organization
Goodman and Steckler[63]	Conceptualizing sustainability	Yes	Intervention activities, organizational policies	Individual providers, multiple staff, policies/procedures/technologies	Public health	Promotion	Organization
Gruen et al.[10]	Conceptualizing sustainability	No	Intervention activities	Individual providers, multiple staff, policies/procedures/technologies, capacity/infrastructure building, collaborative partnerships, broad-scale system change	Public health	Unspecified	Unspecified

Author							
Han and Weiss[64]	Conceptualizing implementation	Yes	Intervention activities	Individual providers	Mental health/substance abuse	Prevention, treatment	Individual, organization
Johnson et al.[65]	Conceptualizing sustainability	Yes	Intervention activities, organizational policies	Policies/procedures/technologies, capacity/infrastructure building	Mental health/substance abuse	Prevention	Community, government/municipality, organization
Mancini and Marek[51]	Evaluation/measurement	Yes	Client benefits, intervention activities	Individual providers, multiple staff, policies/procedures/technologies	Health and human services	Unspecified	Community
Miles[66]	Conceptualizing sustainability	No	Intervention activities, organizational policies	Individual providers, multiple staff	Education	Unspecified	Organization
Nilsen et al.[67]	Conceptualizing sustainability	Yes	Client benefits, intervention activities	Policies/procedures/technologies, capacity/infrastructure building	Public health	Prevention	Government/municipality
Olsen[68]	Conceptualizing sustainability	Yes	Intervention activities, organizational policies	Individual providers, multiple staff	Health and human services	Unspecified	Community
Pluye et al.[13]	Conceptualizing sustainability	Yes	Intervention activities, organizational policies	Policies/procedures/technologies, capacity/infrastructure building	Public health	Promotion	Community, organization
Racine[69]	Conceptualizing sustainability	Yes	Client benefits	Individual providers, multiple staff, policies/procedures/technologies	Health and human services	Unspecified	Organization

(continued)

Table 16.2   Continued

AUTHORS	FOCUS	HOW SUSTAINABILITY IS DEFINED		INTERVENTION			
		EXPLICIT DEFINITION	SUSTAINABILITY OUTCOMES CONSIDERED	TYPE	DOMAIN	INTENT	SETTING TYPE
Rosenheck[70]	Conceptualizing implementation	No	Intervention activities	Individual providers	Mental health/ substance abuse	Treatment	Organization
Sarriot et al.[71]	Evaluation/ measurement	Yes	Community partnerships, organizational policies, broader attention	Multiple providers, policies/procedures/ technologies	Public health	Prevention	Community
Savaya et al.[72]	Conceptualizing sustainability	Yes	Client benefits, intervention activities, organizational policies		Mental health/ substance abuse	Prevention, treatment	Organization
Scheirer and Dearing[3]	Research agenda	Yes	Client benefits, intervention activities	Policies/procedures/ technologies	Public health	Unspecified	Organization
Schell et al.[49]	Conceptualizing sustainability	Yes	Client benefits, intervention activities, organizational policies	Individual providers, multiple staff, policies/procedures/ technologies, capacity/ infrastructure building	Public health	Unspecified	Community, organization

Shediac-Rizkallah and Bone[73]	Conceptualizing sustainability	Yes	Client benefits, intervention activities, community partnerships, organizational policies	Individual providers, multiple staff, policies/procedures/ technologies, capacity/ infrastructure building	Public health	Unspecified	Community
Shelton et al.[76]	Conceptualizing Sustainability	Yes	Client benefits, intervention activities, community partnerships, organizational policies	Individual providers, multiple staff, policies/procedures/ technologies, capacity/ infrastructure building	Public health, medicine, mental health.	Multiple	Multiple
Swerissen and Crisp[74]	Conceptualizing sustainability	Yes	Client benefits, intervention activities, organizational policies	Policies/procedures/ technologies, capacity/ infrastructure building	Public health	Promotion	Community, government/ municipality, individual, organization
Yin et al.[75]	Conceptualizing sustainability	Yes	Intervention activities, organizational policies	Policies/procedures/ technologies	Health and human services	Unspecified	Organization

Source: Sarah Behler, PhD, and Amber Calloway, MA, contributed to the development of this summary of sustainability frameworks.

promote sustainment may increase the likelihood that programs are sustained in a manner that meets stakeholder needs. Rather than emphasizing fidelity to an intervention as originally developed, this framework suggests that an intervention should not be considered optimized until it has been delivered, tested, and adapted in the setting in which it will ultimately be deployed, and implementers in delivery organizations continue to attend to opportunities to further fine-tune the program as the organizational external and internal contexts evolve. Especially with programs and interventions that rely on people to deliver them to prospective beneficiaries, a tension exists between maintaining fidelity to the intervention as previously tested and adapting it as needed to an evolving environment to ensure compatibility between the context and intervention, although the degree of control necessary or desired will vary depending on the intervention in question and the objectives of the original source organization and the delivery organization.[11] Although changes to core components have the potential to erode the impact of the intervention, there is the possibility that certain adaptations by program staff can both provide greater benefits and be more compatible with the delivery organization, thus promoting sustainability. The Dynamic Sustainability Framework suggests that adaptation should be an expected part of the implementation process, although it should occur in a manner that allows stakeholders to ensure that the changes have a positive impact on the desired program outcomes. This framework suggests the use of quality improvement methods such as plan–do–study–act cycles that delivery staff themselves design, manage, observe, and assess to optimize fit in response to changes within a particular context while carefully evaluating the impact of adaptations. For example, if budget cuts lead to shortages in delivery personnel, rapid tests of change may be used to determine whether adaptations such as changes in mode of delivery (e.g., shifts from individual- to group-level interventions, delivery by paraprofessionals, or delivery by web or app), induction strength (fewer hours in group sessions or fewer meetings), or a reduced number of program components (keeping a weekly group meeting and social media reminders but eliminating an online discussion forum and quarterly check-up) are feasible and result in acceptable levels of desired outcomes.

The importance of considering and planning for sustainability during initial intervention design and throughout the conduct of formative evaluation has been called for in program planning processes, partly by emphasizing "pull" strategies for attracting, engaging, and rewarding implementation staff in health delivery organizations. Comprehensive program planning can help surface a variety of factors important to program effectiveness and sustainability, including the identification of aspects of the intervention that are necessary to promote the desired outcomes and that can guide design and/or implementation decisions about whether and how to make adaptations. Furthermore, research suggests the importance of considering the decisions or events that have the potential to influence the sustainability of program-related activities from the very early stages of implementation.[12] This approach departs from linear stage models of implementation, in which sustainability is only considered after programs are implemented.[13]

Rather than thinking of sustainment as maintaining what had been implemented, consideration of how the same decision may have different effects over the long term versus the short term may aid in planning for sustainability.[13] For example, devoting substantial, nonrecurring resources to a program by hiring special staff to deliver an intervention may positively impact implementation in the short term by increasing penetration throughout the community or system. However, over the longer term, it may not be feasible to continue to allocate limited resources to a dedicated staff position, and failure to integrate the program into the existing workforce and personnel structures may lead to the disappearance of the program when that position is cut. Thus, as Pluye and colleagues[13] warn, too many external resources may actually be unfavorable to sustainability. Consistent with the notion that sustainability should be planned for and considered prior to and throughout the process of implementation, Lynge and colleagues[14] emphasize the importance of planning, feasibility testing, and piloting before scaling-up cancer screening programs. These steps allow potential threats to sustainability to be discovered and addressed before large-scale implementation. Key indicators that Lynge et al. recommend assessing include societal acceptance, local ownership, evidence-based practice, and verification of adequate performance in each phase of implementation. Qualitative investigation can identify events and vulnerabilities that may have implications for sustainability, which should be addressed before continuing to scale.

A DEEP AND LASTING CHANGE?

Concepts such as embedding and changing the culture and routines of an organization have been studied in relation to implementation and sustainability.[15,16] Researchers who develop and test educational interventions both in the kindergarten through 12th grade and higher education contexts have studied practice and program sustainability for years, most commonly by studying what teachers do in classroom settings and what students learn as a result, over time.[17] Thus, they are frequently studying organizations that embed multiple layers of authority and approval (district school boards, superintendents, principals and teachers, and students and their families) that share certain commonalities with health care systems in terms of degree of complexity.

In an influential 2003 article, Coburn[18] conceptualized sustainability primarily in terms of time and the extent to which districts and schools institutionalized support for changed teacher practice, but she also argued for the primacy of depth of the changed behavior and the shift of felt ownership as key determinants of whether a practice or program and its effects would persist. Depth, in this sense, meant not just changes in materials, classroom organization, or activities with students but, more important, altered teacher beliefs, norms of interaction among teachers and students, and underlying pedagogical principles. Shift meant whether an intervention eventually became understood by teachers as being generated internally versus coming from an external source. Other subsequent educational researchers have also come to view sustainability as being dependent on depth and shift.[19] Both depth and shift relate to the intrinsic motivation and sense of personal responsibility on the part of delivery staff to best help their potential beneficiaries, whether they be students or patients. In the literature on health intervention sustainability, this shift is often characterized as a culture shift, and although there has been less research on culture change in organizations that deliver cancer interventions and programs, some research findings in other areas of health care suggest that organizational culture has the potential to influence sustainability, which may in fact need to shift to facilitate positive long-term outcomes.[5]

RESEARCH ON SUSTAINABILITY OF CANCER INTERVENTIONS AND PROGRAMS

In the area of cancer control, attention to sustainability has increased in recent years. A recent review of grants awarded by the National Cancer Institute indicated that although only 38% examined sustainability explicitly, approximately half of grant awards proposed cost indicators and other considerations relevant to sustainability.[20] Research and evaluation projects that focus on sustainability illustrate some of the previously described concepts that are relevant to sustainability. In this section, we consider research on a number of different program types, such as prevention programs, screening programs, and tobacco control. In doing so, we highlight concepts from implementation frameworks and consider findings related to implementation success and factors that influence these outcomes.

Community-Based Prevention Programs

The sustainability of skin cancer prevention programs has been examined in multiple studies. The programs that have been studied, such as the Pool Cool Program[21,22] and Go Sun Smart,[23] are multicomponent in nature and include resources such as toolkits that describe how to implement the program, lesson cards, visual aids and posters, sunscreen dispensers, and tip signs. Enhanced implementation strategies that have been tested in research on these programs have included additional sun safety items for distributions, tip sheets, reinforcement, incentives and feedback, and supplementary materials with guidance to promote implementation and sustainability. Research conducted several years after initial implementation of Go Sun Smart indicated that the organizations that received the enhanced support were more likely to yield desired long-term outcomes, such as fewer sunburns among staff.[23] Consistent with previous evaluation of the Pool Cool program that found that a majority of pools maintained the program over several years,[21] a recent study found that organizations that received enhanced implementation support demonstrated evidence of sustained program implementation.[22] Glanz and colleagues[22] found that the organizations that received enhanced implementation support had significantly greater overall maintenance of the program over three summers of participation.

Furthermore, organizations that received enhanced support established and maintained significantly more sun-safety policies and supportive environments over time. Collectively, these findings suggest that enhanced implementation support, ease of use and accessibility of necessary supplies and program components, and ability to integrate program activities into routines are associated with sustainability of prevention programs of this nature.

Community-Based Screening and Health Promotion Programs

Other sustainability research has focused on cancer screening programs, including the use of lay health advisors (LHAs), or community health advisors, to promote cancer screening behaviors among underrepresented populations. A number of potential barriers to sustainability of these programs have been identified, including factors in the outer context such as lack of funding, lack of national standards and policies to guide program implementation, and difficulty conducting program evaluation to provide data to support program continuation.[24–26] In addition, intervention factors, such as costs of implementing programs, and inner context factors, including availability of time and resources required for training, dissemination of materials, space, and resources for program evaluation, have been identified.[26] At the provider level, recruitment and retention of LHAs have been challenging, particularly when, as is often the case, health advisors are volunteers who receive little, if any, compensation.[24,27] These factors can lead to high turnover and low retention and also limited activity among health advisors, which in turn impacts the sustainability of programs that rely on LHAs. Thus, although there has been increased interest in non-professional delivery of interventions, attention must be paid to the potential for sustainment of such programs.

Shelton and colleagues[24] recently investigated retention among LHAs for the National Witness Project (NWP), one of the National Cancer Institute's "Research Tested Intervention Programs."[28] The NWP is an evidence-based program that has been found to be effective in increasing breast and cervical cancer screening among African American women.[29] The NWP has been implemented in more than 40 sites throughout the United States. During group-based meetings in community settings, trained African American LHAs provide education, support, and resources to African American women.[30] In the NWP model, at least half of the LHAs are African American breast and cervical cancer survivors who serve as "role models" and deliver testimonials to empower women to get screened for cancer and engage in healthy behaviors.[29,31] These LHAs work together with project directors from their sites to organize meetings and recruit participants.

Because one factor that reduces the impact and sustainability of the programs is turnover among LHAs,[32,33] Shelton and colleagues[24] examined whether differences across NWP programs were associated with LHA retention. There is some variation in the ways in which NWP is implemented, including the type of host institution and compensation for LHAs and project directors. Findings suggested that LHAs based at non-academic sites such as churches were less likely to remain engaged in the program. Duration of involvement in the program also predicted retention, with LHAs who had been involved in the program longer being less likely to remain involved over the follow-up. Greater role clarity and commitment among LHAs were associated with a greater likelihood of retention. After adjustment for self-reported baseline LHA activity status, however, only affiliation with an academic site was significantly associated with increased odds of LHA retention.[24] Factors such as educational background, paid versus voluntary positions, and breast cancer survivorship were not associated with retention. These findings provide some guidance that is relevant to efforts to plan for sustainability in programs of this nature. First, affiliations with academic institutions (which may have access to resources that are not available in other settings) may promote sustainment of programs that rely on LHAs. Second, rather than selecting LHAs based on certain characteristics, building commitment and increasing role clarity may increase retention rates. Finally, the finding that LHAs who had been involved with the program for longer periods of time were less likely to be retained suggests that planning for turnover and developing mechanisms to rapidly identify and train new LHAs when needed may be an important step to promote sustainability.

Another recent study involving LHAs examined the issue of training LHAs.[34,35] Project HEAL (Health through Early Awareness and Learning) is a community-based participatory research project that relies on LHAs to improve cancer screening among African Americans.[36] Traditional classroom and online approaches to training LHAs were compared, with the 14 churches that participated in this project randomly assigned to training format. Although Project HEAL resulted in changes in knowledge across both conditions, participants expressed greater satisfaction with workshops from the online training approach, with greater increases in knowledge about prostate cancer at a 12-month follow-up among men taught by online-trained LHAs. The results of this evaluation suggest that in light of the turnover inherent in LHA-led cancer programs, online training can be used successfully to train new LHAs and may yield additional benefits at the consumer level. Sustainability is a focus for Project HEAL, which is ongoing, and future results will provide additional insight into factors associated with continued program activities and outcomes.[34]

Prevention and Treatment Interventions in Health Care Settings

As Scheirer indicates, research on processes and outcomes related to sustainability can vary greatly depending on the intervention type.[7,37] Whereas LHA programs are delivered by individuals outside of a health care setting, other cancer control programs are delivered within health care organizations. A qualitative evaluation of tobacco treatment services in Massachusetts was undertaken to assess sustainability after funding for the Massachusetts Tobacco Control Program was substantially reduced in 2002.[38] The study focused on 77 sites, which included hospitals, community health centers, mental health and substance abuse treatment agencies, and other agencies that had received funding. One-third of these sites reported no sustainment of tobacco treatment services, and approximately one-third reported minimal tobacco treatment services. Only 5% of the agencies were able to sustain their programs at the same level after external funding was removed. Consistent with other research on sustainment,[5] these findings illustrate how significantly changes in funding can impact sustainability. In general, the results of the qualitative aspect of the evaluation suggested that creative use of resources and creation of demand were critical to sustainment. Five general strategies were identified as positively influencing sustainability: alignment of services with organizational goals, selecting acceptable and affordable services, locating alternative funding, changing staffing patterns, and assigning

resources to create demand for services.[38] The study also illustrated how, consistent with the Dynamic Sustainability Framework,[4] efforts were made at low and moderate sustaining sites to adapt and retain some of their services. However, sites did not appear to use the quality improvement strategies suggested by the framework to rapidly evaluate and refine efforts to sustain the programs.

Research on cancer care programs has varied in approaches and findings related to sustainability. One study of a short-stay program after breast cancer surgery[39] found high rates of sustainability (82%) 5 years after an implementation effort that used implementation strategies which were tailored to the needs of each individual setting.[40] These penetration rates were comparable to the proportion in short stay after initial implementation. In addition, compliance to the key recommendations to facilitate short stay after breast cancer surgery increased from 65% directly after implementation to 78% 5 years after implementation. At least two key factors may have contributed to these promising findings. First, there are substantial economic incentives and reinforcers to short-stay programs within the financing structure of the health care system in which the program was implemented, and cost savings for the program have been documented.[41] High levels of patient satisfaction and findings of no reductions in quality of life associated with the program further suggest that benefits of the program were experienced by stakeholders at multiple levels. Second, the use of tailored implementation strategies allowed potential barriers at each hospital to be carefully targeted and addressed, which may have had positive implications for long-term sustainability.[39,40]

IMPLICATIONS OF RESEARCH ON CANCER PROGRAM SUSTAINABILITY

Facilitators

The previously mentioned research points to several implications for future research. First, enhanced implementation strategies that include attention to the specific needs and contexts of organizations that will deliver cancer prevention or interventions to their local communities appear to enhance sustainability. Second, as the Massachusetts Tobacco Control Program evaluation and studies in other areas of health care indicate,[1,38] funding is an important influence on sustainability. It is important to develop a funding model that involves sustainable financing (e.g., reimbursement for services from insurance companies) or diversification of funding sources (e.g., grants and in-kind donations) unless financial benefits (e.g., reduced need for subsequent, costly intervention or decreased length of stay) can directly offset costs related to long-term implementation. It is likely necessary to plan for scarcity of resources to support long-term implementation by integrating programs into existing staffing and workflow models, identifying technology-based modes of delivery,[42] or identifying sustainable approaches for training and supporting non-professional health workers to deliver interventions. In the case of the latter suggestion, identification of structures and processes to support these individuals and address workforce turnover appears to be especially critical.

Adaptation

Planning for and adapting to the dynamic contexts in which programs and interventions are implemented is another key implication from the current review. As the Tobacco Control evaluation illustrated, interventions and programs can be particularly vulnerable to reductions in funding and shifts in policy.[38] Identifying creative, scalable ways to continue to deliver interventions and to rapidly adapt them to cuts in funding may be necessary for sustainment. In so doing, it is important to evaluate the impact of these adaptations on the key outcomes that have been identified by stakeholders, even if those assessments are based in localized improvement cycles managed by program delivery staff. For example, if changes in resource availability require a reduction in the number of program components that are delivered, the impact of the adapted intervention on key health behaviors or outcomes should be carefully evaluated.

Categorizing the types of adaptations that are made to programs and interventions can yield more specific information about which types of adaptations result in desired outcomes. Forms of adaptation can include changes to the mode of delivery (e.g., group vs. individual, and web or app vs. practitioner-delivered), personnel who deliver the interventions (e.g., trained medical professionals vs. lay workers), the target audience (e.g., translating an intervention developed for African Americans for delivery to Latinos), the intervention content (e.g., cultural adaptations and changes to core or peripheral aspects of the intervention), and altering

the strength of the intervention (e.g., holding fewer group sessions or sending out fewer encouraging messages to a patient's social network contacts).[43,44] Within the category of intervention content, potential adaptations include changes to the duration or pacing of the intervention, removal of elements, addition of elements, integration of other intervention elements, tailoring of content (e.g., changing terminology or language, adaptation of intervention materials), reordering of elements, or substitution of elements. By identifying the nature of the adaptions that are made and examining program evaluation data (e.g., clinical outcomes and penetration), the impact of the adaptation can be explored.[43] In the context of quality improvement methodologies, organizations or communities can plan and test adaptations to learn fairly rapidly how adaptations might improve or erode fit, recipient-level outcomes, and penetration, and they can refine or plan accordingly.[4]

Future Directions

The literature on sustainability of interventions and programs in health care settings has expanded rapidly during the past several years.[1] Researchers are increasingly examining questions related to sustainability in many topical domains within health, education, and specifically in the area of cancer prevention and control.[20] Over time, the sophistication of research on cancer prevention and control has expanded from published reports of program evolution to include prospective and experimental designs. Although progress is being made in identifying some factors associated with sustainability in this topical domain and within the broader literature on sustainability, very little research has been undertaken to identify and prioritize strategies to promote sustainability. Implementation researchers have identified 73 distinct implementation strategies that may hold promise for promoting sustainability.[45] This may be too much for busy health care systems. Methods such as intervention mapping can be used to identify promising strategies and, in particular, packages of strategies that can be tested prospectively as plausible and cost-effective alternatives to one another.[46] Furthermore, methodologies such as concept mapping or Delphi studies can be used to identify the broad categories of strategies that are most promising for different types of cancer control programs or interventions.[47] Last, there is considerable potential to flip conventional study designs on their heads and conduct observational studies of those interventions and programs for individuals at risk of cancer, cancer patients, and cancer survivors that have sustained for long periods of time in the operations of delivery organizations. Why do these long-running programs persist? What interests of their delivery organizations and/or patients are these sustained programs serving? Is their sustainability best explained by how they rank in a profile of innovation characteristics, because they satisfy organizational mission or well address organizational care priorities, because they demonstrate the desired health benefits, or is their sustained availability due more to consistency in the extraorganizational environment? Certainly, well-funded topical domains such as breast cancer have the resources to continue the delivery of breast cancer prevention and care programs. Is that what explains their persistence? If so, what combination of factors led to decisions to fund these programs at higher levels?

An important future direction for research in sustainability is the advancement of measurement. Although some tools have been developed to assess potential determinants of sustainability[48,49] and some aspects of sustainability,[50,51] comprehensive assessments of sustainability that include the full range of potential indicators[3,5] have not been developed. The following considerations for identifying and developing measures and reporting findings can lead to more rigorous measurement and greater convergence in terminology:

- It remains necessary to determine whether unique measures of determinants of sustainability are needed or whether existing implementation measures are sufficient.
- Validated measures that include comprehensive assessments of all determinants included in sustainability frameworks can streamline assessment.
- Measures should be developed for administration at multiple time points.
- Measures of sustainability outcomes should include multiple indicators and allow projects to operationalize how each indicator is assessed but provide guidance regarding appropriate data sources and well-defined benchmarks (e.g., full, partial, or not sustained).
- When objective measures are not feasible (e.g., if observation of fidelity is not possible due to the size and spread of a program), triangulation between sources of information and measurement recipient-level impact should be employed.

- Consistency of language for characterizing processes, strategies, and adaptations that may lead to sustainability remains necessary. Interview guides, measures, and reports should clearly define each construct.

Implications for the Implementation of Cancer Interventions and Programs

Based on findings and recommendation from both the cancer literature and the broader literature on sustainability, we recommend the following to promote and study sustainment:

1. Plan for sustainability at the outset by designing low-cost, simple, and adaptable interventions and programs.[12,13,52] Anticipate decreases in resources and build processes into existing structures, particularly in the absence of evidence that the intervention or program will have a cost-neutral impact.

2. Choose an implementation framework to guide an initial needs assessment; identify potential barriers and facilitators to long-term sustainment in addition to initial implementation; and assess the readiness of the program, delivery organization, and potential beneficiaries.[1,53]

3. Design interventions for compatibility with implementation sites; provide guidance to implementers, showing them how to responsibly adapt the intervention so that customization maximizes beneficial effects for patients and residents; and evaluate the impact of these adaptations.[4,54] Make and evaluate adaptations as changes in the broader context require them, using quality improvement strategies.

4. Identify a set of adaptations that are associated with desired outcomes and those that result in diminished outcomes to inform ongoing and future implementation efforts. Communicate these results back to implementers to further guide their future adaptations.[1,43]

5. Use intervention mapping or system dynamics modeling approaches to identify strategies to address potential barriers to implementation or sustainability.[46]

6. Use a process-oriented framework to guide the implementation program.[14,55]

7. Conduct program evaluation with heavy emphasis on formative evaluation or quality improvement performed by front-line staff, and include outcomes that are relevant to key stakeholders. Use

models of implementation and sustainability to inform the evaluation.[4,5]

SUMMARY

The existing research on sustainability suggests that for some interventions and programs, the potential for long-term sustainment is fairly high.[1,8] For other interventions, particularly those that are complex and multifaceted, or those that require increased personnel or resources, sustainability is more precarious and may always be at risk. Without careful planning and attention to relevant drivers of sustainability, programs may not be continued over the long term.[8] In such cases, research on strategies to promote sustainability is necessary. Still, as indicated previously, the broader literature provides some guidance for those who seek to implement cancer programs and interventions with an eye toward sustainment. Practice-based research networks, prospective research, and reports of evaluation and quality improvement projects can all contribute to the growing literature on the sustainability of cancer programs. As the literature on sustainability, particularly in the area of cancer control,[20] expands, we can look forward to additional guidance and innovative methods to achieve long-term implementation of effective programs and interventions.

REFERENCES

1. Stirman SW, Kimberly J, Cook N, Calloway A, Castro F, Charns M. The sustainability of new programs and innovations: A review of the empirical literature and recommendations for future research. *Implement Sci.* 2012;7:17.
2. Rahm AK, Hawkins RP, Dearing JW, et al. Implementing an evidence-based breast cancer support and communication tool to newly diagnosed patients as standard care in two institutions. *Transl Behav Med.* 2015;5(2):198–206.
3. Scheirer MA, Dearing JW. An agenda for research on the sustainability of public health programs. *Am J Public Health.* 2011;101(11):2059–2067.
4. Chambers DA, Glasgow RE, Stange KC. The Dynamic Sustainability Framework: Addressing the paradox of sustainment amid ongoing change. *Implement Sci.* 2013;8(1):117.
5. Stirman SW, Kimberly JR, Calloway A, Cook N, Castro F, Charns MP. The sustainability of new programs and interventions: A review of the empirical literature and recommendations for future research. *Implement Sci.* 2012;7:17.
6. Proctor E, Silmere H, Hovmand P, et al. Outcomes for implementation research: Conceptual distinctions, measurement challenges, and research agenda. *Adm Policy Mental Health.* 2011;38(2):65–67.
7. Scheirer MA. Linking sustainability research to intervention types. *Am J Public Health.* 2013;103(4):e73–e80.
8. Scheirer MA. Is sustainability possible? A review and commentary on empirical studies of program sustainability. *Am J Eval.* 2005;23:320–347.
9. Gutner C, Barlow D, Sloan D, Stirman SW, Ametaj A. *Supporting EBP Implementation in Routine Care: An Examination of Fidelity and Its Relationship to Clinical Outcomes.* Philadelphia, PA: Anxiety and Depression Association of America.
10. Gruen RL, Elliott JH, Nolan ML, et al. Sustainability science: An integrated approach for health-programme planning. *Lancet.* 2008;372(9649):1579.
11. Sezgi F, Mair J. To control or not control: A coordination perspective to scaling. In: Bloom P, Skloot E, eds. *Scaling Social Impact.* New York: Palgrave Macmillan; 2010:29–44.
12. Pluye P, Potvin L, Denis J-L, Pelletier J, Mannoni C. Program sustainability begins with the first events. *Eval Program Plann.* 2005;28(2):123–137.
13. Pluye P, Potvin L, Denis J-L. Making public health programs last: Conceptualizing sustainability. *Eval Program Plann.* 2004;27(2):121–133.
14. Lynge E, Törnberg S, von Karsa L, Segnan N, van Delden JJ. Determinants of successful implementation of population-based cancer screening programmes. *Eur J Cancer.* 2012;48(5):743–748.
15. Schneider B, Brief AP, Guzzo RA. Creating a climate and culture for sustainable organizational change. *Organizational Dynamics.* 1996;24(4):7–19.
16. Martin GP, Weaver S, Currie G, Finn R, McDonald R. Innovation sustainability in challenging health-care contexts: Embedding clinically led change in routine practice. *Health Serv Manage Res.* 2012;25(4):190–199.
17. Looi CK, Teh LW, eds. *Scaling Educational Innovations.* Singapore: Springer; 2015.
18. Coburn CE. Rethinking scale: Moving beyond numbers to deep and lasting change. *Educational Researcher.* 2003;32(6):3–12.

19. Lagemann EC, Dede C, Honan JP, Peters LC. *Scaling Up Success: Lessons from Technology-Based Educational Improvement.* New York: Wiley; 2015.

20. Neta G, Sanchez MA, Chambers DA, et al. Implementation science in cancer prevention and control: A decade of grant funding by the National Cancer Institute and future directions. *Implement Sci.* 2015;10(1):1.

21. Escoffery C, Glanz K, Hall D, Elliott T. A multi-method process evaluation for a skin cancer prevention diffusion trial. *Eval Health Professions.* 2009;32(2):184–203.

22. Glanz K, Escoffery C, Elliott T, Nehl EJ. Randomized trial of two dissemination strategies for a skin cancer prevention program in aquatic settings. *Am J Public Health.* 2015;105(7):1415–1423.

23. Walkosz BJ, Buller DB, Andersen PA, Scott MD, Cutter GR. The sustainability of an occupational skin cancer prevention program. *J Occup Environ Med.* 2015;57(11):1207–1213.

24. Shelton RC, Dunston SK, Leoce N, et al. Predictors of activity level and retention among African American lay health advisors (LHAs) from the National Witness Project: Implications for the implementation and sustainability of community-based LHA programs from a longitudinal study. *Implement Sci.* 2016;11(1):41.

25. Koskan A, Friedman DB, Messias DKH, Brandt HM, Walsemann K. Sustainability of promotora initiatives: Program planners' perspectives. *J Public Health Manag Pract.* 2013;19:E1–E9.

26. Twombly EC, Holtz KD, Stringer K. Using promotores programs to improve Latino health outcomes: Implementation challenges for community-based nonprofit organizations. *J Soc Serv Res.* 2012;38:305–312.

27. Strachan DL, Källander K, Asbroek AH, et al. Interventions to improve motivation and retention of community health workers delivering integrated community case management (iCCM): Stakeholder perceptions and priorities. *Am J Trop Med Hyg.* 2012;87:111–119.

28. The Witness Project: Products. National Cancer Institute website. http://rtips.cancer.gov/rtips/productDownloads.do?programId=270521. Accessed September 15, 2015.

29. Erwin DO, Ivory J, Stayton C, et al. Replication and dissemination of a cancer education model for African American women. *Cancer Control.* 2003;10.

30. Erwin DO, Spatz TS, Stotts RC, Hollenberg JA, Deloney LA. Increasing mammography and breast self-examination in African American women using the Witness Project model. *J Cancer Educ.* 1996;11:210–215.

31. Erwin DO. The Witness Project: Narratives that shape the cancer experience for African American women. In: McMullin J, Weiner D, eds. *Confronting Cancer: Metaphors, Advocacy, and Anthropology.* Sante Fe, NM: School for Advanced Research Press; 2009:125–146.

32. Bhattacharyya K, Winch P, LeBan K, Tien M. *Community Health Worker Incentives and Disincentives: How They Affect Motivation, Retention and Sustainability.* Arlington, VA: USAID-BASICS II; 2001.

33. Yiu C, Au WT, Tang CS. Burnout and duration of service among Chinese voluntary workers. *Asian J Soc Psychol.* 2001;4:103–111.

34. Santos SLZ. Involve, engage, and retain: Retention techniques from Project HEAL, a cancer-focused implementation project in African American churches. Paper presented at the 2015 APHA Annual Meeting & Expo, October 31–November 4, 2015.

35. Holt CL, Santos SLZ, Tagai EK, et al. Using technology for improving population health: Comparing classroom vs. online training for peer community health advisors in African American churches. *Implement Science.* 2015;10(1):1.

36. Holt CL, Tagai EK, Scheirer MA, et al. Translating evidence-based interventions for implementation: Experiences from Project HEAL in African American churches. *Implement Sci.* 2014;9(1):1.

37. Scheirer MA, Dearing JW. An agenda for research on the sustainability of public health programs. *Am J Public Health.* 2011;101:2059–2067.

38. LaPelle NR, Zapka J, Ockene JK. Sustainability of public health programs: The example of tobacco treatment services in Massachusetts. *Am J Public Health.* 2006;96:1363–1369.

39. Ament S, Gillissen F, Maessen J, et al. Sustainability of short stay after breast cancer surgery in early adopter hospitals. *The Breast.* 2014;23(4):429–434.

40. De Kok M, van der Weijden T, Voogd A, et al. Implementation of a short-stay programme after breast cancer surgery. *Br J Surg.* 2010;97(2):189–194.

41. de Kok M, Dirksen CD, Kessels AG, et al. Cost-effectiveness of a short stay admission programme for breast cancer surgery. *Acta Oncol.* 2010;49(3):338–346.

42. Kulchak Rahm A, Morse EF, McDowell H, et al. Implementation of an evidence-based breast cancer support tool for newly diagnosed breast cancer patients as standard care at two institutions: Use and sustainability. *J Patient-Centered Res Rev.* 2015;2(2):109–110.

43. Stirman SW, Miller CJ, Toder K, Calloway A. Development of a framework and coding system for modifications and adaptations of evidence-based interventions. *Implement Sci.* 2013;8(65).

44. Chambers DA, Norton WE. The adaptome: Advancing the science of intervention adaptation. *Am J Prev Med.* 2016;51(4):S124–S131.

45. Powell BJ, Waltz TJ, Chinman MJ, et al. A refined compilation of implementation strategies: Results from the Expert Recommendations for Implementing Change (ERIC) project. *Implement Sci.* 2015;10:21.

46. Powell BJ, Beidas RS, Lewis CC, et al. Methods to improve the selection and tailoring of implementation strategies. *J Behav Health Serv Res.* 2017;44(2):177–194.

47. Waltz TJ, Powell BJ, Matthieu MM, et al. Use of concept mapping to characterize relationships among implementation strategies and assess their feasibility and importance: Results from the Expert Recommendations for Implementing Change (ERIC) study. *Implement Sci.* 2015;10:109.

48. Maher L, Gustafson D, Evans A. *Sustainability Model and Guide.* London: NHS Institute for Innovation and Improvement; 2007.

49. Schell SF, Luke DA, Schooley MW, et al. Public health program capacity for sustainability: A new framework. *Implement Sci.* 2013;8(1):1.

50. Goodman RM, McLeroy KR, Steckler AB, Hoyle RH. Development of level of institutionalization scales for health promotion programs. *Health Educ Q.* 1993;20:161–178.

51. Mancini JA, Marek LI. Sustaining community-based programs for families: Conceptualization and measurement. *Fam Relat.* 2004;53(4):339–347.

52. Dearing JW, Kreuter MW. Designing for diffusion: How can we increase uptake of cancer communication innovations? *Patient Educ Couns.* 2010;81:S100–S110.

53. Dearing JW, Smith DK, Larson RS, Estabrooks CA. Designing for diffusion of a biomedical intervention. *Am J Prev Med.* 2013;44(1 Suppl 2):S70–S76.

54. Aarons GA, Green A, Palinkas LA, et al. Dynamic adaptation process to implement an evidence-based child maltreatment intervention. *Implement Sci.* 2012;7:32.

55. Kilbourne AM, Neumann MS, Pincus H, Bauer MS, Stall R. Implementing evidence-based interventions in health care: Application of the replicating effective programs framework. *Implement Sci.* 2007;2:42.

56. Aarons G, Hurlburt M, Horwitz SM. Advancing a conceptual model of evidence-based practice implementation in public service sectors *Adm Policy Ment Health.* 2011;38(1):4–23.

57. Adelman HS, Taylor L. On sustainability of project innovations as systemic change. *J Educ Psychol Consult.* 2003;14(1):1–25.

58. Akerlund KM. Prevention program sustainability: The state's perspective. *J Community Psychol.* 2000;28(3):353–362.

59. Altman DG. Sustaining interventions in community systems: On the relationship between researchers and communities. *Health Psychol.* 1995;14(6):526–536.

60. Beery WL, Senter S, Cheadle AD, et al. Evaluating the legacy of community health initiatives: A conceptual framework and example from the California Wellness Foundation's Health Improvement Initiative. *Am J Eval.* 2005;26:150–165.

61. Feldstein AC, Glasgow RE, Smith DH. A Practical, Robust Implementation and Sustainability Model (PRISM) for integrating research findings into practice. *Jt Comm J Qual Patient Saf.* 2008;34(4):228–243.

62. Glaser EM. Durability of innovations in human service organizations. *Sci Commun.* 1981;3(2):167–185.

63. Goodman RM, Steckler AB. A model for the institutionalization of health promotion programs. *Fam Community Health.* 1987;11:63–78.

64. Han SS, Weiss B. Sustainability of teacher implementation of school-based mental health programs. *J Abnormal Child Psychol.* 2005;33(6):665–679.

65. Johnson K, Hays C, Center H, Daley C. Building capacity and sustainable prevention innovations: A sustainability planning model. *Eval Progr Plan.* 2004;27:135–149.

66. Miles MB. Unraveling the mystery of institutionalization. *Educ Leadership.* 1983;41(3):14–19.

67. Nilsen P, Timpka T, Nordenfelt L, Lindqvist K. Towards improved understanding of injury prevention program sustainability. *Saf Sci.* 2005;43(10):815.

68. Olsen IT. Sustainability of health care: A framework for analysis. *Health Policy Plan.* 1998;13(3):287.

69. Racine DP. Reliable effectiveness: A theory on sustaining and replicating worthwhile innovations. *Adm Policy Ment Health.* 2006;33(3):356–387.

70. Rosenheck R. Stages in the implementation of innovative clinical programs in complex organizations. *J Nerv Ment Dis.* 2001;189(12):812–821.

71. Sarriot EG, Winch PJ, Ryan LJ, et al. A methodological approach and framework for sustainability assessment in NGO-implemented primary health care programs. *Int J Health Plann Manage.* 2004;19(1):23–41.

72. Savaya R, Spiro S, Elran-Barak R. Sustainability of social programs: A comparative case study analysis. *Am J Eval.* 2008;29(4):478.

73. Shediac-Rizkallah MC, Bone LR. Planning for the sustainability of community-based health programs: Conceptual frameworks and future directions for research, practice and policy *Health Educ Res.* 1998;13(1):87–108.

74. Swerissen H, Crisp BR. The sustainability of health promotion interventions for different levels of social organization. *Health Promot Int.* 2004;19(1):123–130.

75. Yin RK, Quick SK, Bateman PM, Marks EL. *Changing Urban Bureaucracies: How New Practices Become Routinized.* Santa Monica, CA: RAND; 1978.

76. Shelton RC, Brittany Rhoades Cooper, Shannon Wiltsey Stirman. The sustainability of evidence-based interventions and practices in public health and health care. *Annual Review of Public Health.* 2018.

17

OVERUSE AND DE-IMPLEMENTATION OF INAPPROPRIATE CANCER SCREENING, DIAGNOSIS, AND TREATMENT PRACTICES

Maryam Doroudi, Barnett S. Kramer, and Paul F. Pinsky

IN ITS 1998 consensus statement, "The Urgent Need to Improve Health Care Quality," the Institute of Medicine National Roundtable on Health Care Quality coined the term "overuse." It reads "overuse occurs when a health care service is provided under circumstances in which its potential for harm exceeds the possible benefit."[1] A recent Institute of Medicine (now the National Academy of Medicine) report estimated that approximately $210 billion per year in the United States is wasted due to unnecessary health care services, including medical overuse. Overuse has been estimated to represent approximately 30% of the provided health care services offered in the forms of screening, diagnostic tests, and treatment.[2] Despite the high prevalence, financial toxicity incurred, and harm to patients of medical overuse,[3,4] it has been a remarkably slow process to get physicians, patients, payers, and policymakers to give attention to this issue and implement effective strategies to reduce its burden. However, the recent formation of organizations and initiatives such as Right Care Alliance, Proven Best

Choices, and Choosing Wisely, whose goals are reducing overuse in our health care system, is a testimony to increasing awareness.

In the past four decades, increasingly sensitive screening technologies have prompted the medical community to put a great emphasis on early detection of cancer. Although clinical trials and secular trends indicate that these efforts have successfully reduced the rate of late-stage malignancies and cancer-specific mortalities in a few cancer types, overuse of such technologies has also substantially increased the incidence of indolent and early stage tumors in other cancer types without proportionally reducing the incidence of late-stage tumors and related mortalities, creating a reservoir of patients at risk for overdiagnosis and overtreatment. Overuse in cancer screening and diagnostic tests occurs when individuals undergo procedures that do not meaningfully change the treatment success probability, and outcomes or harms caused by the procedure may outweigh benefits. Overtreatment is often "rooted in outmoded habits, supply-driven behaviors, and ignoring science," as described by Drs. Donald M. Berwick and Andrew D. Hackbarth in their report, "Eliminating Waste in US Health Care."[4] In the literature, overuse in screening, diagnostic tests, and treatment may be referred to as overdetection, overutilization, or overmedicalization.[5] The concepts related to outcomes of medical overuse are described using terminologies such as low-value care and overdiagnosis.[5,6] Worldwide, there are no established programs of research to identify and quantify medical overuse, and thus its frequency of occurrence in each field of medicine remains mostly unknown. In recent years, a small but growing body of literature has focused on identifying medical services currently used in our health care system that lack proven evidence of benefit or that incur greater harm than benefit. The goal of this chapter is to elucidate the issue of overuse in the cancer control continuum by highlighting the current literature and identifying areas ripe for future research on de-implementation.

First, we present some specific examples of overuse in cancer screening and diagnostic tests and cancer treatment. We define overuse as application of intervention for which there is no reliable evidence of a meaningful benefit in important health outcomes compared to the previous standard of care. Overuse is often associated with opportunity costs—diverting resources that are better spent on more effective strategies to improve health. Next, we discuss factors promoting overuse, including those at the patient, provider, and systems levels. Finally, we review strategies to mitigate overuse, summarizing the current research in the area and examining potential future research directions.

EXAMPLES OF OVERUSE IN DIAGNOSTIC AND SCREENING TESTS

Thyroid Cancer Screening in the Republic of South Korea: Ultrasonography Test

In 1999, the Republic of South Korea started a national screening program that provided multiphasic screening, free of charge or for a small copayment, under its national health insurance program. In addition to the offered screening services for detection of colorectal, gastric, cervical, breast, and hepatic cancers,[7] South Korean providers frequently offered additional low-priced screening services, including ultrasonography, to detect thyroid cancer. In 2014, Dr. Hyeong Sik Ahn and colleagues[7] reported the effect of such large-scale thyroid cancer screening using South Korea's vital statistics and cancer registry data. Over the span of almost 8 years, the rate of papillary thyroid cancer diagnosis increased 15-fold, from less than 5 (in 1993) to approximately 70 (in 2011) cases per 100,000 individuals, placing thyroid cancer among the most common types of cancer diagnosed in South Korea.[7] This compared to an estimated 11 cases per 100,000 individuals throughout the rest of the world by the end of the study period.[8]

Until the turn of the century, thyroid cancer was considered an uncommon type of cancer, and its incidence rates varied by country, ranging from 0.5 to 10 per 100,000 individuals.[9] Histologically, papillary thyroid carcinomas comprised approximately 40–70% of all diagnosed thyroid cancer cases.[9] In a previously published systematic review,[10] more than one-third of adults had autopsy-detected papillary thyroid cancer, indicating that the "vast majority" of cases remain asymptomatic and do not cause harm during the patient's lifetime. In South Korea, despite a dramatic increase in the incidence of thyroid cancer associated with screening effort, thyroid cancer mortality rates remained virtually unchanged. Screening for thyroid cancer appeared to detect primarily clinically insignificant lesions, resulting in substantial overdiagnosis of thyroid cancer, with little or no apparent benefit but with all the attendant harms of unnecessary surgery.[7]

Evidence shows that most of these screen-detected thyroid cancer cases received treatment. In 2011, more than 60% of thyroid cancer cases received radical thyroidectomy, with most of the remainder undergoing subtotal thyroidectomy.[7] The 1995–2011 trends in surgical management of thyroid cancer indicated a fourfold increase in surgery rates among patients diagnosed with tumors less than 1 cm in diameter.[7] Moreover, Ahn and colleagues[7] found that nearly 25% of thyroid cancer surgeries were performed on patients harboring tumors less than 0.5 cm in diameter, which went against then recommended guidelines. Furthermore, insurance claims indicated substantial surgical morbidity: More than 10% of patients developed hypoparathyroidism, and approximately 2% reported paralysis of one or both vocal folds.[7]

In 2014, a group of South Korean physicians responded by forming an assembly called "The Coalition of Doctors to Prevent Overdiagnosis of Thyroid Cancer" with the goal of educating the public and policymakers on the issue of overdiagnosis. Soon after its inception, the organization penned an open letter to the Korean public recommending against ultrasonography screening for thyroid cancer. It also facilitated several hearings and held broadcasted public debates on the subject of thyroid cancer overdiagnosis. These efforts were strongly supported by the media industry. At approximately this time, television stations started running short investigative reports and newspapers published columns with catchy titles such as "What Caused Jump in Thyroid Cancer Cases?"[11] and "Why Is Thyroid Cancer So Common Here?"[12] A 2015 follow-up report indicated a 35% reduction in the number of operations for thyroid cancer between 2013 and 2015.[13]

Prostate Cancer Screening in the United States: Prostate-Specific Antigen Test

Prostate cancer is the most common non-skin cancer and the second leading cause of cancer deaths among men in the United States.[14] In 1986, the US Food and Drug Administration (FDA) approved a blood test for prostate-specific antigen (PSA), a glycoprotein enzyme secreted by the epithelial cells of the prostate, to monitor prostate cancer treatment response and tumor recurrence. Subsequently, the potential of this test as a prostate cancer screening tool gained the medical community's attention, leading to its approval by the FDA as an aid, in conjunction with digital rectal exam, for the diagnosis of prostate cancer in 1994. By then, the PSA test had become the most commonly prescribed test by physicians to help diagnose, as well as screen for, prostate cancer. From 1973 through the late 1980s, the incidence rates of prostate cancer gradually increased, likely due in large measure to incidental findings at transurethral resections of the prostate for benign prostatic enlargement causing symptoms of lower urinary tract obstruction. However, during the late 1980s and early 1990s, in a span of less than 6 years, the rate of prostate cancer diagnosis increased approximately twofold in both White men, increasing from 86 (in 1986) to 179 (in 1992) cases per 100,000 men per year, and Black men, increasing from 124 (in 1986) to 250 (in 1993) cases per 100,000 men per year, in concert with increasing prevalence of PSA testing in asymptomatic men.[15]

In 2008, the US Preventive Services Task Force (USPSTF) released a recommendation discouraging PSA screening for men aged 75 years or older.[16] In 2012, the Task Force released another guideline recommending against PSA screening for all average-risk men.[17] This recommendation was primarily based on the results of two large randomized controlled trials (RCTs), one conducted in the United States and one in Europe, which compared prostate cancer-specific mortality rates between men randomized to PSA screening and those randomized to a no-screening control arm and failed to demonstrate a clear mortality benefit from PSA screening.[18,19] Since the release of the recommendation, two studies have investigated its impact on PSA screening rates.[20,21] The first study used data from the 2005, 2010, and 2013 National Health Interview Survey (NHIS) to estimate PSA screening rates among men aged 40 years or older following the release of the 2012 USPSTF recommendation. Whereas study findings indicated no change in PSA screening rates among American men aged 40–49 years from 2010 to 2013, a significant decline in rates of screening was observed in men 50 years of age or older in the same time frame.[20] The second study used the 2005, 2008, 2010, and 2013 NHIS data to estimate PSA screening rates among all men (no exclusion by age). In American men 50 years of age or older, investigators reported an approximate 10% increase and 18% decrease in screening rate ratios between 2005 and 2008 and between 2010 and 2013, respectively.[21] Both studies concluded that PSA screening rates declined after USPSTF released its 2012 guideline recommending against PSA screening. In addition, two studies have examined the impact of the 2012 USPSTF guideline on prostate cancer incidence rates.[21,22] Both studies reported a reduction in the incidence of early stage prostate cancer following the release of the 2012 guideline recommending against PSA screening for men.

The harms associated with PSA testing are related to choices a patient and his physician make based on the test result. These choices usually include further diagnostic testing, as well as treatment options for prostate cancer if so diagnosed. The harms associated with further testing, which often includes multiple prostate biopsies, are mainly pain, bleeding, and infection. The harms associated with false-positive test results include complications related to biopsy procedures and anxiety. In addition, side effects from prostate cancer treatment—namely urinary dysfunction, bowel dysfunction, and erectile dysfunction—can severely and permanently affect components of a patient's quality of life.[23] If radiation is part of the management, the risk for secondary cancers increases.

Cervical Cancer Screening in the United States: Pap Test

Whereas in developing nations, cervical cancer remains the leading cause of cancer-related deaths for women, in the United States remarkable success has been achieved in reducing cervical cancer incidence and mortality rates in the past 40 years. This reduction is largely attributable to cervical cancer screening with cytology, also referred to as the Papanicolaou (Pap) test. It has been more than a decade since USPSTF and several US medical organizations first published their guidelines recommending that average-risk women older than age 30 years receive cervical cytology screening every 3 years as part of routine preventive services rather than annually.[24-26] Women who undergo yearly screening experience more unnecessary follow-up evaluations, psychological distress, and economic burden related to false-positive smears (rate = 20%) compared to those who undergo this screening in 3-year intervals, without evidence of meaningful incremental benefit.[27-30] Annual screening with Pap test therefore constitutes overuse. In 2012, several organizations, including USPSTF, the American Cancer Society, the American Society for Colposcopy and Cervical Pathology, and the American Society for Clinical Pathology, published another guideline recommending average-risk women aged 30–65 years should be screened with Pap testing every 3 years or co-tested with the Pap test plus human papillomavirus testing every 5 years if both are normal.[31,32] Between 2002 and 2013, studies showed that physicians continued to perform annual screening without clinical indication: Approximately 40–60% of women received Pap smears at intervals of less than 3 years.[33-36]

The annual and triennial Pap smear tests generate major differences in cost burden on the US health care system. A 2003 study using the National Breast and Cervical Cancer Early Detection Program projected that an additional 69,665 Pap smears and 3,861 colposcopic examinations in women aged 30–44 years and 209,324 Pap smears and 11,502 colposcopic examinations in women

aged 45–59 years would be needed to prevent one case of cervical cancer by screening 100,000 women annually instead of triennially.[29] A later study using the National Ambulatory Medical Care Survey estimated that adoption of cytology-based screening once every 3 years would decrease the annual number of Pap tests by 6.3 million and would save $403.8 million in health care costs.[37]

Recently, the Institute for Clinical and Economic Review conducted a qualitative study to identify major drivers of such overuse. Its interviews of clinical and policy experts from the fields of obstetrics and gynecology and family practice identified several patient, physician, and payer factors driving medical overuse. When describing potential patient-related factors contributing to overuse of Pap testing, experts highlighted patient demand, lack of copayments for this test under the Affordable Care Act, and an absence of patient education on the harms associated with receiving it on the annual basis.[36] Physician-related factors that potentially drive overuse in Pap testing included "reluctance from clinicians to stop performing Pap tests when it motivates women to attend their annual visit," "difficulty of changing behavior of clinicians trained to perform annual Pap tests," "automatic scheduling of Pap tests as part of women's annual pelvic exams," "lack of knowledge of current guidelines due to history of conflicting recommendations," and "transient patient populations making it difficult to track long-term screening history."[36] Payer-related factors included "administrative challenges for payers to distinguish when Pap tests are medically necessary."

Colorectal Cancer Screening in the United States: Colonoscopy for Colorectal Cancer Screening and Polyp Surveillance

Colorectal cancer (CRC) is the third most common non-skin cancer and the third leading cause of cancer deaths in the United States.[14] Screening for CRC using fecal occult blood testing, sigmoidoscopy, or colonoscopy is effective in reducing CRC-related mortality and, in the case of the latter two interventions, incidence, and it has been recommended by USPSTF.[38-40] Currently, USPSTF and the US Multi-Society Task Force on Colorectal Cancer (MSTF) recommend colonoscopy every 10 years for average-risk individuals from ages 55 to 75 years.[40,41] Shorter surveillance intervals are recommended in those with neoplasia.[41] Repeating colonoscopies more frequently than recommended by current guidelines represents a case of overuse that may increase costs and harms without benefiting individuals.

Several studies have investigated overuse in colonoscopy. A 2015 retrospective observational study using 2008 administrative claims, physician databases, and electronic medical records evaluated the rate of physicians' non-adherence to MSTF recommendations for colorectal cancer screening and polyp surveillance in 1,455 patients aged 50–64 years who received colonoscopy in the Veterans Affairs (VA) health care system. The rate of non-adherence to MSTF recommendations ranged from 3% to 80% among 25 VA medical facilities. The non-adherence rate was 28% and 45–52% for physicians with patients undergoing normal screening and physicians with patients diagnosed with hyperplastic or adenomatous polyps, respectively.[42] The calculated follow-up colonoscopy interval was shorter in 34% of patients and longer in 2% of patients compared with MSTF guidelines.[42] Shorter follow-up was associated with identification of hyperplastic or high-risk adenomatous polyps, geographic region, and bowel preparation quality.[42] A 2016 study of participants in the Veterans Health Administration study reported that 16% of patients with no adenomas and 26% of patients with low-risk adenomas received follow-up colonoscopies earlier than recommended.[43] Similar to these findings, an ancillary study on surveillance colonoscopy use undertaken in 2008 among participants in the Prostate, Lung, Colorectal, and Ovarian Cancer (PLCO) screening trial also found considerable overuse of surveillance colonoscopy among relatively low-risk subjects.[44] Approximately one-third of those with one or two non-advanced adenomas received surveillance colonoscopy within 4 years, even though the MSTF recommended interval is 5–10 years.[45] A 2014 retrospective cohort study using electronic health record data for patients aged 50–65 years reported colonoscopy overuse, with more than half of screening or surveillance colonoscopies performed at least 1 year earlier than recommended.[46]

In recent years, health care systems have proposed platforms to identify and reduce overuse. Of note is the Veterans Affairs Health Care System's recent progress in developing an electronic performance measure of overuse of screening colonoscopy.[44]

Ovarian Cancer Screening in the United States

Ovarian cancer represents 1.3%[47] of all new non-skin cancer cases in the United States, and in 2016 it ranked fifth[14] among the leading causes of cancer-related death in women.

Carbohydrate antigen 125 (CA-125), the most widely used marker, is a cell-surface glycoprotein expressed in tissues derived from coelomic epithelia, including, but not limited to, ovaries and fallopian tubes. This biomarker is approved by the FDA as an aid in either detecting recurrent ovarian cancer in patients who have received first-line therapy or in monitoring ovarian cancer patients' responses to the therapy. Although this protein has long been used as a marker for ovarian cancer detection, recent studies have demonstrated low specificity, as elevated levels of CA-125 in women with active cervical or endometrial cancer, those with acute pelvic inflammatory disease, pregnant women, and individuals with symptoms of heart failure have been reported.[48–50] Because many non-ovarian cancer conditions are associated with increased levels of CA-125, the marker has triggered a substantial burden of unnecessary follow-up testing in women. In addition, this test has poor sensitivity for early stage (50% for stage I) ovarian cancer; sensitivity increases at more advanced stages, for which cure is less likely.

Currently, the American Cancer Society and USPSTF do not recommend screening for ovarian cancer in average-risk women. Despite the lack of recommendations, there is evidence that physicians are continuing to prescribe CA-125 for ovarian cancer screening. A 2012 survey study of 1,088 family physicians, general internists, and obstetrician–gynecologists about non-adherence to ovarian cancer screening recommendations (defined as sometimes or almost always ordering screening with transvaginal ultrasound or CA-125 or both) indicated a considerable number of physicians reported non-adherence to guidelines for low-risk (1.5% lifetime ovarian cancer risk, defined as a woman with a mother with breast cancer at age 70 years) and medium-risk (4.0–5.0% lifetime ovarian cancer risk, defined as a woman with a mother who died of ovarian cancer at age 65 years) women for ovarian cancer, respectively.[51] Approximately 18% of physicians believed that CA-125 was an effective ovarian cancer screening test, and they were more likely to report non-adherence to guidelines when their patient requested screening.[51]

This non-nationally representative sample of the US physician population indicated potential CA-125 overuse. However, a 2016 study using 2008–2013 Truven Health MarketScan Commercial Claims and Encounters Database exhibited a downward trend in CA-125 overuse, from 4.7 to 3.3 per 1,000 women who did not have a diagnosis of ovarian cancer or other relevant clinical indicators.[52]

Since its original design, the CA-125 test has been adapted into several forms of tests, including the Risk of Ovarian Cancer Algorithm (ROCA), which estimates a woman's risk of having ovarian cancer by integrating age risk with longitudinal CA-125 values. ROCA is currently manufactured by Abcodia, which has its US headquarters in Boston. Although ROCA has not been shown to reduce ovarian cancer-specific incidence or mortality, Abcodia's website claims that

the ROCA Test is a simple blood test that when added to your annual exam assesses your risk of having ovarian cancer on a routine basis. The test is for postmenopausal women over 50 years old and women at high risk of ovarian cancer.[53]

In September 2016, the FDA released a consumer safety alert noting that

despite extensive research and published studies, there are currently no screening tests for ovarian cancer that are sensitive enough to reliably screen for ovarian cancer without a high number of inaccurate results. However, over the years, numerous companies have marketed tests that claim to screen for and detect ovarian cancer.[54]

The agency further emphasized that the

FDA is concerned that women and their physicians may be misled by such claims and rely on inaccurate results to make treatment decisions. Based on the FDA's review of available clinical data from ovarian cancer screening trials and recommendations from healthcare professional societies and the U.S. Preventive Services Task Force, available data do not demonstrate that currently available ovarian cancer screening tests are accurate and reliable in screening asymptomatic women for early ovarian cancer. For example,

some women may receive test results that suggest ovarian cancer even though no cancer is present (a false-positive). These women may undergo additional medical tests and/or unnecessary surgery, and may experience complications related to both. Or, test results may not show ovarian cancer even though cancer is present (a false-negative), which may lead women to delay or not seek surgery or other treatments for ovarian cancer.[54]

The FDA's announcement was welcomed by the Ovarian Cancer Research Fund Alliance, which noted that

we all wish there were an effective screening test for ovarian cancer. Unfortunately, we haven't yet found a test proven to save women's lives. We share the FDA's concern that the ROCA Test, which is being marketed directly to women in 47 states, may do more harm than good. The money spent marketing tests of questionable benefit would be much better spent on research to find an effective test, better treatments and a cure[55]

and broadcast on its webpage.[56]

Although the effect of recent published medical guidelines, consumer safety alerts, and actions of advocacy groups on de-implementation of ineffective ovarian cancer screening tests is yet to be determined, the long-term goal is to reduce the utilization of ovarian cancer screening or diagnostic tests with unproven benefit.

CASES OF OVERUSE IN TREATMENT

Breast Cancer Management in the United States: Bilateral Mastectomy

Breast cancer is the most common non-skin cancer and the second leading cause of cancer deaths among women in the United States.[14] Breast-conserving surgery (lumpectomy) and surgical removal of the breast, also known as total mastectomy, are common for the treatment of breast cancer, with lumpectomy the most preferred recommendation when possible. Clinical applications of mastectomy are not limited to the breast harboring a malignancy; women with a genetic susceptibility to breast cancer or those diagnosed with cancer in only one breast may choose to remove their healthy breast(s). Greater than 97% of breast cancer cases arise in only one breast;[57] however, women may elect to have their opposite, healthy breast removed via contralateral prophylactic mastectomy despite the absence of evidence that doing so reduces the risk of death from breast cancer outside the situation of highly penetrant inherited genetic mutations such as *BRCA1* or *BRCA2*. Such decisions may be made for a variety of reasons, including physician recommendation, positive family history of breast cancer, fear of developing breast cancer in the healthy breast, and cosmetic symmetry if one breast has been removed.[58,59] In addition, women of younger age (<40 years), Caucasian race, and higher educational level are more likely to choose prophylactic mastectomy.[60-62]

Recent trends show a rise in the rates of bilateral mastectomies and increasing shift of this surgery from inpatient to ambulatory surgical centers. From 1998 to 2011, the rates of bilateral mastectomy in early stage breast (unilateral) cancer patients eligible for breast conservation surgery increased from 1.9% to 11.2%.[63] A 2016 federal analysis using the 2005–2013 Healthcare Cost and Utilization Project (HCUP) data from 13 states representing more than one-fourth of the US population reported a 21% increase in the overall rate of mastectomy and a 300% increase in the rate of bilateral mastectomy (from 10.0 in 2005 to 29.7 in 2013 per 100,000 adult women), whereas the incidence of breast cancer and rates of unilateral mastectomy remained relatively constant in adult women.[64] The rates of bilateral mastectomies in women with breast cancer tripled (10.5% in 2005 vs. 28.0% in 2013), and the proportion of bilateral mastectomies in the absence of breast cancer almost doubled (2.9% in 2005 vs. 4.9% in 2013). During the same time period, the rate of bilateral outpatient or "drive-by" mastectomies increased by more than 500% (from 1.9 to 10.0 per 100,000 adult women), while inpatient bilateral mastectomy rates increased by approximately 200% (from 8.1 to 19.7 per 100,000 adult women).[64] In addition, a comparison of 2003 to 2013 HCUP inpatient and outpatient hospital surgical data revealed that the proportion of mastectomies performed in a hospital outpatient setting increased from 22% to 45% during this period.[64,65]

The increase in the rate of bilateral mastectomy in women without highly penetrant germline mutations represents a case of overuse that increases harms and costs without commensurate benefit. During approximately the past 15 years,

the use of bilateral mastectomy has more than tripled despite evidence suggesting no survival benefit for women with unilateral breast cancer and no genetic abnormalities undergoing contralateral prophylactic mastectomy compared with breast-conserving surgery.[59,66,67] Bilateral mastectomy is associated with increased postoperative complications compared with unilateral surgeries.[68] These complications include wound infection, postoperative bleeding or hematoma, abdominal wall bulge, laxity, hernia requiring surgery, and implant removal.[68] Despite this evidence, women with no significant excess risk of contralateral breast cancer continue to choose contralateral prophylactic mastectomy in the misplaced belief that it extends life. A 2014 study comparing the health care costs of women treated for stage I–III breast cancer with or without contralateral prophylactic mastectomy reported that this procedure increased the mean total health care costs by 16% for women with unilateral breast cancer within the first 2 years of surgery.[69] The mean difference in health care expenditure between patients with and those without contralateral prophylactic mastectomy was $7,749 for total costs; $3,573 for clinician-related activities; and $4,176 for the technical component, including billing for facilities, supplies, and equipment.[69] These patient-level outcome and cost data should be used in future studies to evaluate their impact on patient decisions on whether or not to undergo bilateral mastectomy.

Localized Prostate Cancer Treatment in the United States: Proton Beam Therapy

Prostate cancer is a complex and heterogeneous disease with a broad spectrum of clinical behavior. Risk stratification predictors have been developed based on several factors, including biopsy Gleason score, PSA levels, and clinical stage, but all are relatively imprecise.[70,71] Low-risk prostate cancer, which comprises approximately 40% of newly diagnosed prostate cancers, is defined as Gleason score ≤6, PSA <10 ng/ml, and clinical stage T1c to T2a. The management of low-risk prostate cancer varies widely, driven as much by personal beliefs and tolerance of uncertainty as by empiric evidence.[72] This has created a controversy in the field.

Proton beam therapy (PBT), also known as proton beam radiation therapy or proton radiotherapy, is one of the controversial subclasses of external beam radiation therapy (EBRT) used in the initial treatment of localized prostate cancer. Not at all in question, however, is the high cost compared to standard radiotherapy. This emerging form of radiation therapy, which is used mainly in the United States, uses beams of protons to deliver virtually all of its ionizing energy to a specific tissue with minimal scatter compared to standard X-ray photon beams. A 2016 study, using the 2004–2012 National Cancer Data Base, reported that the rate of PBT use in patients diagnosed with nonmetastatic prostate cancer had increased from 2.3% to 4.8% during this period.[73] This intervention was much more likely to be offered to men who were White, younger, healthier, from metropolitan areas, from zip codes with higher median household incomes, visiting an academic medical center, and who were not diagnosed with an advanced stage prostate cancer.[73] It is heavily marketed to patients.

PBT has been investigated either as a radiation "boost," in combination with other forms of external beam radiotherapy, or as the sole radiation modality. Currently, the commonly used X-ray-based intensity-modulated radiotherapy (IMRT) is well tolerated in most older patients with localized prostate cancer, and it has been shown to produce high rates of local control.[74] The harms of IMRT include genitourinary and gastrointestinal toxicities and dysfunction that has been reported to be mostly manageable and occur at low rates. Although PBT has theoretical advantages over IMRT, no randomized controlled clinical trials have compared the benefit of PBT compared to IMRT in terms of survival, tumor control, or toxicity. Moreover, it is unclear whether proton beam affects healthy tissues in the case of smaller target volumes. Therefore, the current lack of direct comparative evidence on harms and benefits of PBT versus standard photon radiation, the rapid dissemination and marketing of this intervention to prostate cancer patients, varied physician beliefs on the effectiveness of this intervention, and the high cost of protons may lead to overuse, which may increase costs and harms without benefiting prostate cancer patients.

Early studies of PBT, as a combination radiation modality, reported contradictory findings on the role of this intervention in possibly improving the disease-free survival in patients with localized prostate cancer and its complication rates. In an observational study, Yonemoto and colleagues[75] prospectively examined the use of combined proton and photon radiation therapy for the treatment of locally advanced carcinoma of prostate cancer on treatment morbidity and tumor response. During a median follow-up of 20.2 months, the combined therapy yielded low incidence of late morbidity (12%), low rate of local recurrence (2.8%), and high actuarial rate of normalization (96% or 97%) with pretreatment PSA levels less than 20 ng/ml; morbidity outcomes were similar to those of traditional photon radiation therapy.[75] At approximately the same time, a randomized prospective trial evaluated the use of combined proton and photon radiation therapy versus conventional external beam irradiation in patients with stage T3 or T4 prostate cancer.[76,77] After a median follow-up of 61 months, proton boost (25.2 cobalt gray equivalent [CGE] by protons and 50.40 Gy by photons) improved local control of prostate cancer by 12% compared to the conventional dose of 67.2 Gy by photons, while the survival and recurrence-free survival were similar between the treatment arms.[77] Toxicities related to the gastrointestinal (GI) and genitourinary tracts were significantly higher among individuals who had proton boost therapy.[76,77]

In a 2009 systematic review of published peer-reviewed literature on the use of PBT to treat cancers, including localized prostate cancer, in comparison with conventional therapies, Brada and colleagues[78] concluded that the current literature lacked evidence of benefit in terms of survival, tumor control, or toxicity for PBT intervention. They further suggested that such lack of evidence should stimulate the scientific community to design appropriate trials to determine if there is incremental benefit using PBT for treating localized prostate cancer and to guide the future use of this therapy based on clear evidence rather than commercial influence. A 2010 analysis of an RCT of prostate cancer patients with T1b–T2b tumor stage and PSA ≤ 15 ng/ml who received either high dose (28.8 GyE protons followed by 50.4 GyE photons) or the conventional dose (19.8 GyE protons followed by 50.4 GyE photons) indicated that those in the high-dose arm were less likely to have local failures and had a lower rate of biochemical failure. However, no difference was detected in overall survival between the treatment arms after a median follow-up of 8.9 years.[78] A 2012 retrospective study compared morbidity and disease control of IMRT, proton therapy, and conformal radiation therapy for localized prostate cancer treatment using 2000–2007 Surveillance, Epidemiology, and End Results (SEER) Medicare-linked data.[79] Men who received IMRT versus proton therapy had very similar morbidity and disease control outcomes except for a lower rate of GI morbidity.[79]

In 2014, the Agency for Healthcare Research and Quality published an update of the 2008 systematic review for localized prostate cancer.[80] The report summarized the relative effectiveness and safety of treatment options, including PBT, EBRT, and radical prostatectomy, for clinically localized prostate cancer. Eight RCTs and 44 non-randomized comparative studies were included in the report. The authors concluded that "overall, the body of evidence for treating prostate cancer continues to evolve, but the evidence for most treatment comparisons is largely inadequate to determine comparative risks and benefits of therapies for clinically localized prostate cancer." This conclusion is similar to that of the 2008 review, which found that no single therapy can be considered the preferred treatment for localized prostate cancer because of limitations in the body of evidence as well as the likely trade-offs a patient must make between estimated treatment effectiveness, necessity, and adverse effects. Although limited evidence appears to favor surgery over watchful waiting or external beam radiotherapy, or favors three-dimensional conformal radiation therapy (3D-CRT) plus androgen-deprivation therapy over 3D-CRT alone, the patients most likely to benefit and the applicability of these study findings to contemporary patients and practice remain uncertain. More RCTs and better designed observational studies that can control for many of the known and unknown confounding factors that can affect long-term outcomes are needed to evaluate comparative risks and benefits of therapies for clinically localized prostate cancer.

Among all EBRT interventions, PBT is the most expensive. The cost of building a one-room proton therapy facility is approximately $20 million, and the cost of building a multiroom facility is approximately $200 million. These manufacturing and construction costs are much higher than those of similarly sized photon-based facilities.[81] According to a 2007 study using a Markov model, PBT was not found to be cost-effective in treating localized prostate cancer compared to standard IMRT therapy with respect to quality-adjusted life-year (QALY) differences.[82] The model included the assumption that patients treated with IMRT and PBT had the same utility and PBT could be used to escalate the dose while maintaining a similar toxicity profile to that of IMRT. At 15-year follow-up, the incremental cost-effectiveness ratios (ICER)

for a 60-year-old man and a 70-year-old man were $55,726/QALY and $63,578/QALY, respectively. The ICER values did not meet the requirements for cost-effectiveness (the accepted standard in 2007 was $50,000/QALY).[82] In addition, a recent economic evaluation of treatments for localized prostate cancer patients found that IMRT was more cost-effective that 3D-CRT and proton therapy.[83] Cost-effective estimates will change over the years as more prospective data shed light on the efficacy of PBT and as the cost of building PBT facilities declines over time. Therefore, estimates of the cost-effectiveness of PBT require frequent adjustments as information emerges. In addition, the patient-level outcome and cost-effectiveness data should be used in future studies to evaluate their impact on patient decisions regarding whether or not to undergo PBT.

FACTORS PROMOTING OVERUSE

Provider-Driven Factors

Several provider-driven factors may fuel overuse of medical care. The 2014 survey of 600 primary care physicians and specialists by the American Board of Internal Medicine Foundation identified multiple factors that contribute to unnecessary use of tests and procedures in the US health care system. Nearly 75% of the responders thought that use of unnecessary services was a serious problem. The reasons physicians stated they ordered unnecessary tests and procedures were "malpractice concerns" (52%), "just to be safe" (36%), "want more information to reassure myself" (30%), "patients insisting on test" (28%), "wanting to keep patients happy" (23%), "feel patients should make final decision" (13%), "not enough time with patients" (13%), "fee-for-service system" (5%), and "new technology in practice" (5%).[84] Although the findings of this survey highlighted important provider-driven factors contributing to medical overuse, they also suggested patients and systems-driven factors as crucial contributors to this issue. In their 2015 article "Setting a Research Agenda for Medical Overuse," Morgan and colleagues[2] reported several literature-identified provider-driven factors as causing medical overuse. These factors included " belief more care is better," "lack of knowledge of harm from overuse," "discomfort with uncertainty," "poor knowledge of patient preference," "regret for errors of omission greater than commission," "belief action better than inaction," "use of therapeutics off label," "over-reliance on pathophysiological and anatomical reasoning," and "desire for reassurance."[2] In a classic history of medical education in the 20th century, Kenneth Ludmerer[85] provides a detailed argument that a major driver of overuse of clinical testing and overtreatment has been the failure to train physicians in uncertainty and probabilistic thinking.

Patient-Driven Factors

Various patient-driven factors likely contribute to overuse of medical care. As noted previously, the 2014 survey of 600 primary care physicians and specialists by the American Board of Internal Medicine Foundation reported that approximately 50% of physicians stated that in their own practice, patients ask for unnecessary tests or procedures. Nearly 30% of physicians reported that this occurs at least several times per week.[84] In their previously mentioned report, Morgan and colleagues[2] also listed several literature-identified patient-driven factors as causes of medical overuse, including "belief more care is better," "lack of knowledge of harm from overuse," and "discomfort with uncertainty." It is not just physicians who have inadequate training in uncertainty and probabilistic thinking; each patient–physician encounter and discussion is imbued with this deficit.

Systems-Driven Factors

In addition to patient- and provider-driven pressures, systems-driven factors (at the community, organizational, and policy levels) also contribute to medical overuse. Morgan and colleagues[2] list several literature-identified extrinsic factors as causative agents. Prominent drivers include "financial—provider and hospital," "resource supply," "defensive medicine," "variation in medical and surgical practice," "process measures," "inadequate time," "positive publication bias," "guidelines promoting overuse," "medical culture," "lack of training in shared decision making," "advocacy groups," and "medicalization of non-disease (e.g., male-pattern baldness)." Systems-driven factors that contribute to patient-driven overuse include "financial—third party payment shielding from costs," "culture of avoiding mortality," "media misrepresentation of research," "advocacy groups," and "medicalization of non-disease."[2]

The supply-and-demand market forces that drive choices in most other sectors of the economy are disengaged in the medical sector. Financial incentives, at both the provider level and the hospital level, in prescribing an unnecessary test or medication have been identified as one of the key drivers of medical overuse. Fee-for-service payment models, in which physicians are reimbursed based on individual services provided to patients, have stirred up heated debates among health care policymakers in recent years. Under this model of "high-tech piecework" that emphasizes the quantity of care, there are strong incentives for physicians to invest in radiology clinics, clinical laboratories, pathology services, and radiation therapy centers and to engage in self-referrals that generate income. In their 2015 report "Physician Self-Referral: Regulation by Exceptions," Adashi and Kocher[86] summarize findings by the Government Accountability Office on the national state of physician self-referrals. Between 2004 and 2010, the number of magnetic resonance imaging (MRI), computed tomography (CT), pathology, and radiation therapy services prescribed by self-referring physician groups with financial interests in health care facilities offering advanced imaging, anatomic pathology, or radiation therapy services for the treatment of prostate cancer increased at a higher pace compared to those prescribed by non-self-referring groups. Physician self-referral as a driving force in MRI overuse has drawn particular attention in recent years. A 2013 study compared the likelihood of positive findings at knee MRI between physicians with financial interest in the imaging equipment and those with no financial interest. Doctors in the two study groups had similar training, and patients had similar age and gender demographics. Nevertheless, compared to patients of doctors with no financial interest in the MRI equipment, patients of self-referring physician groups that owned the MRI equipment were 33% more likely to get a negative test result, indicating that these physicians were more likely to send low-risk patients for unnecessary testing.[87] Similar findings have also been reported with regard to ordering MRIs of the lumbar spine, cervical spine, and shoulder.[88–90]

DOWNSTREAM CONSEQUENCES OF OVERUSE

Although the population-level and systems-level impacts of overuse in cancer screening, diagnostic tests, and treatment have received increased attention in recent years, a more limited body of literature has focused on identifying health outcomes and economic consequences. In this section, we provide a brief review of reported adverse effects of overuse in certain types of cancers. For more in-depth information on these cases as well as other types of cancer, refer to the case study section of this chapter. A prominent case with national consequences derives from the Republic of South Korea, where the incidence of thyroid cancer diagnosis increased by 15-fold from 1993 to 2011, while thyroid cancer mortality rates remained unchanged.[8] The increased incidence was primarily due to increased implementation of cancer screening programs that dramatically increased the rate of papillary thyroid carcinoma diagnosis, which is nonfatal. This phenomenon was a clear indication of overdiagnosis. More than half of screen-detected thyroid cancer patients received radical thyroidectomy, and nearly one-fourth of thyroid cancer surgeries were performed on patients harboring very small tumors despite guidelines that encouraged watchful waiting rather than immediate surgery. Thyroidectomy is a technically demanding surgery performed in an anatomic field containing the parathyroid glands and laryngeal nerves. It is therefore not surprising that hypoparathyroidism and vocal cord paralysis were among the important harms reported in the screening program.[7]

A second case involves PSA testing of asymptomatic men, triggering further testing and overtreatment of many clinically insignificant prostate cancer cases in the United States and throughout the world. A positive PSA test often leads to biopsies and treatment of incidental indolent or non-progressing tumors. The harms associated with biopsies include pain, bleeding, and infection. The harms associated with treatments such as radical prostatectomy and radiation therapy include permanent urinary, bowel, or erectile dysfunction.[23] In addition, the harms associated with false-positive PSA test results include complications of the biopsy and anxiety.

A third case involves the surgical removal of the healthy breast in women diagnosed with unilateral cancer, also known as contralateral prophylactic mastectomy, which has become increasingly common as MRIs are ordered to rule out small lesions in the opposite breast. Recent studies have indicated an increase in the number of women with breast cancer choosing this more aggressive surgery despite a very low risk of developing cancer in the healthy breast. Bilateral mastectomy (removal of both breasts) is associated with increased postoperative complications compared with unilateral surgeries, including wound infection, postoperative bleeding or hematoma, abdominal wall bulge, laxity, hernia requiring surgery, implant removal, loss of muscle strength, numbness, and sexual intimacy concerns.[68] In addition to reported harms, contralateral prophylactic mastectomy has been suggested to considerably increase financial burdens in women who choose to undergo this procedure. This procedure has been shown to increase the mean health care costs by more than 15% for women diagnosed with cancer in one of their breasts within the first 24 months of surgery.[69] Between patients who underwent contralateral prophylactic mastectomy and those who did not, the mean difference in billed costs was approximately $7,000, $3,500, and $4,000 for total costs, clinician-related activities, and technical components of the care, respectively.[69] These economic outcomes may incur serious financial hardships for cancer patients and certainly will contribute to the rise in health care costs.

STRATEGIES TO MITIGATE OVERUSE: CURRENT AND FUTURE RESEARCH

Strategies to mitigate use of low-value care can target clinicians or patients or both as part of a multilevel strategy (Figure 17.1). In addition, these strategies can be engineered at the individual, interpersonal (including clinical), community, organizational, or policy level to mediate change. Although most of the reported mitigation strategies have been studied or implemented in fields other than cancer, a few oncology-related examples have recently been reported. This section covers both oncology- and non-oncology-related strategies to provide readers with a broader view of the types of mitigation strategies used to reduce overuse of low-value care and their potential application in the cancer control continuum. A recent systematic review on the topic identified 10 subcategories of strategies described in 108 articles.[91] The highest proportion of effective strategies fell into the category of clinical decision support, followed by multicomponent strategies, clinical education, patient education, provider feedback, patient cost sharing, insurer restrictions, and pay-for-performance. The effectiveness of provider report cards and risk-sharing strategies was uncertain. Whereas greater than 60% of the identified

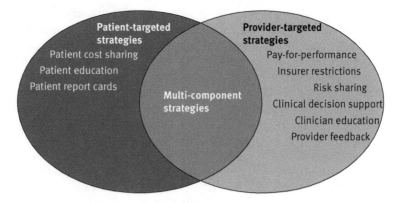

FIGURE 17.1   Tested strategies to mitigate overuse of low-value care.

articles addressed components of clinical decision support, multicomponent strategies, and patient cost sharing, very few articles focused on the remaining mentioned strategies. When mitigation strategies were stratified by targets, interventions related to medication use were the most common (56%), followed by radiology (12%), procedures (10%), and pathology and laboratory tests (10%). In the classification of medical care setting, most strategies were tested in hospitals (56%), followed by ambulatory care settings (20%) and health systems (16%).[91]

Provider-Targeted Strategies

CLINICIAN EDUCATION

This approach involves educating clinicians to distinguish low-value care with the goal of encouraging providers to emphasize high-value care in daily practice. A 2011 study investigated the effect of physician education on antibiotic prescription rates.[92] The education campaigns were led by local leaders and included focus group meetings, workshops, seminars, development of evidence-based guidelines, and practice-based education campaigns. The campaigns focused on establishing self-developed guidelines and improving parent and physician knowledge, diagnostic skills, and parent–physician communication skills to promote awareness of antibiotic overuse and resistance. The results of this cluster RCT indicated a 40% reduction in antibiotic prescription rates among patients treated by the study intervention physicians compared to the control group.[92]

PAY-FOR-PERFORMANCE

The pay-for-performance (P4P) strategy involves financially rewarding health care providers for services based on meeting a predefined quality, outcome, or efficiency metric. Because this strategy links quality of care directly to physician reimbursement, providers are incentivized to both lower costs and improve the quality of offered care. It has been implemented in several countries, including member countries of the Organization for Economic Co-operation and Development, with the goal of improving the quality of care provided by hospitals.[93] Although the impact of P4P is yet to be determined, it has been speculated that some of these programs may experience moderately positive effects.[93,94]

INSURER RESTRICTIONS

Insurance companies can act directly to reduce low-value care by coverage and reimbursement decisions. Prior authorizations and restricted network membership are the primary tools insurers use to discourage use of potentially low-value medical procedures or products.[95-97] Although prior authorization has been shown to reduce low-value care, it may also have unintended consequences. For example, one prior authorization strategy required pharmacists to deny antibiotic prescriptions if the request did not meet guidelines. As a result, the intervention decreased the use of a particular overused antibiotic, but prescriptions for other antibiotics soared.[98] Restricting physician network membership to high-value providers is another tool that insurers use to discourage low-value care. Such narrow networks have been shown to reduce costs and utilization by lowering readmission rates, surgical procedures, and expenditure.[99] Although these tools can supposedly be used to discourage the delivery of low-value services and reduce overuse in the cancer control continuum, the risk of service substitution for other low-value interventions should be considered and measured in assessment of their impacts.

RISK SHARING

This shared payer–provider risk payment model incentivizes providers to consider the value of delivered services using the tool of exposure to costs. To date, four approaches to shared risk have been identified and implemented by insurers: (1) bonus payment at risk, (2) market share risk, (3) risk of baseline revenue loss, and (4) financial risk for the whole or partial patient population. In the first approach, instituted by Blue Cross Blue Shield of Minnesota Preferred One, the shared risk is defined as putting the provider's bonus payment at risk, based on quality and/or efficiency performance. In the second approach, employed by Buyers Health Care Action Group, the shared risk is incentivized through lower copays and premiums to select certain providers and therefore exposing providers to a risk of market share loss. In the third approach, introduced by Blue Cross Blue Shield of Massachusetts, the Alternative Quality Contract (AQC), and Blue Cross Blue Shield of Illinois Advocate Health Care, shared risk is created through payment penalties if providers fail to meet certain cost or quality thresholds or if actual costs exceed a target cost. This approach was built on a fee-for-service model. Finally, in the fourth approach, used by the State Employees Health Commission of the state of Maine and Anthem/WellPoint companies, providers must manage patient treatment costs for all or a designated set of services within a predetermined payment stream, and providers are at risk for costs that exceed payments.[100] Although the effect of risk sharing on low-value care has not been investigated in detail, one study found that AQC was associated with an increase in the number of colonoscopies (considered to be a high-value care) and decreased total spending on imaging services.[101]

CLINICAL DECISION SUPPORT

This strategy, a form of "moral suasion," provides evidence-based information to clinicians to help inform decisions about a patient's care. To date, several clinical decision support tools have been developed, including the creation of disease-specific or sub-patient population-specific order sets, the provision of databases containing evidence summaries on certain conditions or patient populations, and the creation of reminder systems for preventive care appointments designed to reduce use of low-value care by preventing low-value or redundant testing and encouraging compliance with treatment guidelines. For example, a recent study found that adding a requirement for clinical justification to override support alerts for repeat CT orders decreased the number of repeat CT orders by 23% relative to the baseline assessment. This strategy prompted physicians to cancel redundant orders after receiving the support alert.[102]

Patient-Targeted Strategies
PATIENT COST SHARING

This implementation strategy involves shifting costs of low-value services to patients, engaging traditional market forces, thereby encouraging consumers to take into account service-related harms, benefits, and associated costs. In the past decade, several cost-sharing designs were introduced in the US health care system with the goal of communicating value information and incentivizing patients to avoid low-value care by offering differential copays, deductibles, and co-insurance.[103,104] Several studies have indicated that benefit designs that lower cost sharing for effective preventive services have increased the use of high-value care.[105–108] However, the impact of increased personal charges for low-value services on the use of low-value care is less understood.

PATIENT EDUCATION

The 2014 survey of physicians by the American Board of Internal Medicine Foundation found that approximately half of physicians reported patient requests as an important reasons for using unnecessary tests or procedures in their practices.[84] Therefore, patient education is a logical tool in mitigating low-value care. Patient education strategies can target patient subpopulations either directly through educational methods or via a collaborative arrangement between physicians and patients, referred to as shared decision-making. Several studies have examined the impact of direct patient education or shared decision-making on low-value care utilization. A 2002 study assessed whether sharing the uncertainty of the value of antibiotics for acute bronchitis in the form of written and verbal advice affects the likelihood of patients taking antibiotics and therefore reduces antibiotic overuse. Compared to the control group, the educated group was 24% less likely to take antibiotics.[109] However, an educational intervention that included use of videotaped messages or a waiting room poster targeting parents to reduce antibiotic prescription for their children did not change pediatric antibiotic prescription rates.[110-112] Similarly, providing patients with information about low-value prescription drugs in the Eliminating Medications Through Patient Ownership of End Results (EMPOWER) cluster randomized trial has been shown to reduce the use of these drugs.[113] With respect to shared decision-making, a recent randomized study indicated that patients who were assigned to health coaches (including registered nurses, licensed vocational nurses, dietitians, respiratory therapists, and pharmacists) received detailed information about their treatment options. They were engaged in discussions to further sort out their treatment preferences. This program resulted in 9.9% fewer preference-sensitive surgeries when the choice of treatment depended on preference of patients due to availability of several legitimate treatment options, including nonsurgical ones.[114]

Efforts to increase patient education through communication of harms and benefits associated with cancer screening have been shown to reduce overuse. In 2014, The Coalition of Doctors to Prevent Overdiagnosis of Thyroid Cancer in South Korea started a public educational campaign on the issue of overdiagnosis. Strategies included an open letter to the Korean public recommending against ultrasonography screening for thyroid cancer, hearings and broadcasted public debates on the subject of thyroid cancer overdiagnosis, and a large-scale mass media campaign along with the airing of short investigative reports.[11] Although the effect of these patient-centered educational efforts on thyroid cancer screening rates is not known, a recent follow-up study suggested a one-third reduction in the number of operations for thyroid cancer since the campaign began.[13]

PROVIDER REPORT CARDS

Provider report cards allow health care workers to compare their performance to that of other health professionals on specific measures of quality and cost information. They may also be used to aid consumers in choosing high-value providers, although this is often met with provider resistance. The effect of provider report cards on reducing low-value care is yet to be understood, but theoretically they can convey important information to end-users (i.e., content, design, and accessibility) in an effort to help them understand why some care is low value and to change their medical system consumption to improve their health.[115]

Multicomponent Strategies

In 2002 and 2003, a large-scale multicomponent strategies involving a patient–physician education campaign consisting of paid outdoor advertising and media and physician advocacy was implemented in two metropolitan communities in Colorado. Following the campaign, there was a 3.8% net reduction in retail pharmacy antibiotic dispenses.[116]

In their 2015 report, Morgan and colleagues[2] suggested several research objectives to inform how best to reduce overuse in health care systems. The first objective was to "understand the effect of low value lists on clinical practice and patient outcomes" and further investigate the impact of organizations and initiatives such as Right Care Alliance, Proven Best Choices, and Choosing Wisely on overuse in clinical practice and on patient outcomes. This involves first defining low-value care in the health care system. Although there have been attempts to define and measure low-value care, no consensus has been reached on what factors should be included in the definition.[1,117-123] Therefore, it is critical for the scientific community to concentrate its efforts on defining low-value care and subsequently identifying standardized indexes to measure overuse. This would greatly aid researchers in investigating the effect of low-value care and devising and evaluating implementation strategies. The second suggested objective was to "understand patient and clinician views on the acceptability and legitimacy of different methods to encourage appropriate care." Multicomponent strategies involving both patients and clinicians would likely have the greatest potential to reduce overuse. Several solutions have been suggested to mitigate the problem of overuse, including removing low-value care from reimbursement schedules, patient education, clinician education, and using clinical decision support.[91] However, the effectiveness and acceptability of such strategies to facilitate de-implementation are not clear from both patient's and provider's perspectives. Some may be politically infeasible. Perhaps surveys and other methods of obtaining feedback could provide crucial insights on such proposed strategies for de-implementation. The third suggested objective was to "investigate how patients understand overuse and the best methods for communicating its harms." The body of literature on why patients choose certain medical interventions despite lack of proven benefits or clear evidence of harms, their interpretation of overuse, and best communication strategies is sparse and often plagued by weak study design. Previously, we summarized "patient-driven factors" that encourage overuse. However, studies are needed to better understand how patients understand overuse and its consequences, as well as to determine the most effective methods to communicate these issues to them. The fourth suggested objective was to "examine the effect of shared decision

making and other patient focused interventions on overuse." It is not clear to what extent involving a patient in decision-making about receiving a certain intervention would change powerful misconceptions that drive overuse. We suggest a framework for prevention of medical overuse (Figure 17.2). This framework is adapted from the Social–Ecological Model (SEM), a systems model that is frequently used in understanding the multiple levels of a social system and the interactions between individuals and their environment within this system that determine behaviors. In addition, this framework aids in identifying leverage points at individual and organizational levels and their intermediaries for reducing medical overuse and consequently improving health. The framework has five hierarchical bands of influence: individual (patients and physicians), interpersonal, community, organizational, and policy. In this chapter, we described patient-, physician-, and systems-driven factors as causing overuse of medical care. We have summarized patient-, physician-, and multicomponent-targeted interventions that have been tested to reduce overuse. Whereas most of the tested interventions have targeted one level of SEM,

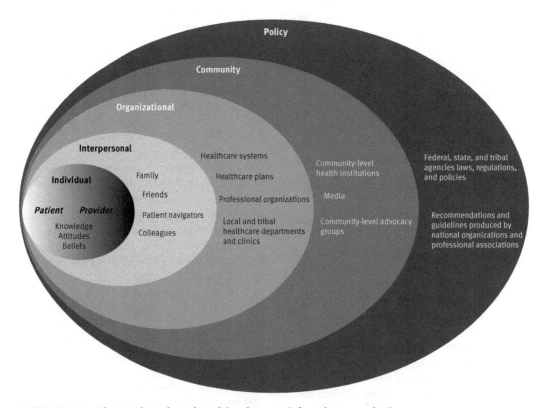

FIGURE 17.2   The Social–Ecological Model: A framework for reducing medical overuse.

other public health prevention studies (violence, nutrition, etc.) have involved both understanding the driving factors and implementing interventions at multiple levels of SEM to increase the likelihood of success.[124] Therefore, researching on how best to reduce overuse in health care systems should propose and test strategies at all bands of influence.

REFERENCES

1. Chassin MR, Galvin RW. The urgent need to improve health care quality: Institute of Medicine National Roundtable on Health Care Quality. *JAMA*. 1998;280(11):1000–1005.
2. Morgan DJ, Brownlee S, Leppin AL, et al. Setting a research agenda for medical overuse. *BMJ*. 2015;351:h4534.
3. Wennberg JE, Fisher ES, Skinner JS. Geography and the debate over Medicare reform. *Health Aff (Millwood)*. 2002;Suppl Web Exclusives:W96–W114.
4. Berwick DM, Hackbarth AD. Eliminating waste in US health care. *JAMA*. 2012;307(14):1513–1516.
5. Carter SM, Rogers W, Heath I, Degeling C, Doust J, Barratt A. The challenge of overdiagnosis begins with its definition. *BMJ*. 2015;350:h869.
6. Welch HG, Schwartz L, Woloshin S. *Overdiagnosed: Making People Sick in the Pursuit of Health*. Boston, MA: Beacon; 2011.
7. Ahn HS, Kim HJ, Welch HG. Korea's thyroid-cancer "epidemic"—Screening and overdiagnosis. *N Engl J Med*. 2014;371(19):1765–1767.
8. Torre LA, Bray F, Siegel RL, Ferlay J, Lortet-Tieulent J, Jemal A. Global cancer statistics, 2012. *CA Cancer J Clin*. 2015;65(2):87–108.
9. Waterhouse J, Muir C, Shanmugaratnam K, Powel J, eds. *Cancer Incidence in Five Continents*. Vol 4. Lyon, France: International Agency for Research on Cancer; 1982.
10. Harach HR, Franssila KO, Wasenius VM. Occult papillary carcinoma of the thyroid—a "normal" finding in Finland: A systematic autopsy study. *Cancer*. 1985;56(3):531–538.
11. What caused jump in thyroid cancer cases? *The Korea Times*. March 27, 2014. http://www.koreatimes.co.kr/www/news/culture/2014/03/319_154183.html.
12. Why is thyroid cancer so common here? *The Korea Times*. January 10, 2014. http://www.koreatimes.co.kr/www/news/culture/2014/01/319_149577.html.
13. Ahn HS, Welch HG. South Korea's thyroid-cancer "epidemic"—Turning the tide. *N Engl J Med*. 2015;373(24):2389–2390.

14. Siegel RL, Miller KD, Jemal A. Cancer statistics, 2016. *CA Cancer J Clin*. 2016;66(1):7–30.
15. Stanford JL, Stephenson RA, Coyle LM, et al. Prostate Cancer Trends 1973–1995, SEER Program. NIH Publication No. 99-4543. Bethesda, MD: National Cancer Institute; 1999.
16. US Preventive Services Task Force. Screening for prostate cancer: US Preventive Services Task Force recommendation statement. *Ann Intern Med*. 2008;149(3):185–191.
17. Moyer VA; US Preventive Services Task Force. Screening for prostate cancer: US Preventive Services Task Force recommendation statement. *Ann Intern Med*. 2012;157(2):120–134.
18. Andriole GL, Crawford ED, Grubb RL 3rd, et al. Mortality results from a randomized prostate-cancer screening trial. *N Engl J Med*. 2009;360(13):1310–1319.
19. Schroder FH, Hugosson J, Roobol MJ, et al. Screening and prostate-cancer mortality in a randomized European study. *N Engl J Med*. 2009;360(13):1320–1328.
20. Drazer MW, Huo D, Eggener SE. National prostate cancer screening rates after the 2012 US Preventive Services Task Force recommendation discouraging prostate-specific antigen-based screening. *J Clin Oncol*. 2015;33(22):2416–2423.
21. Jemal A, Fedewa SA, Ma J, et al. Prostate cancer incidence and PSA testing patterns in relation to USPSTF screening recommendations. *JAMA*. 2015;314(19):2054–2061.
22. Barocas DA, Mallin K, Graves AJ, et al. Effect of the USPSTF Grade D recommendation against screening for prostate cancer on incident prostate cancer diagnoses in the United States. *J Urol*. 2015;194(6):1587–1593.
23. Resnick MJ, Koyama T, Fan KH, et al. Long-term functional outcomes after treatment for localized prostate cancer. *N Engl J Med*. 2013;368(5):436–445.
24. American College of Obstetricians and Gynecologists. ACOG Practice Bulletin: Clinical management guidelines for obstetrician–gynecologists. Number 45, August 2003. Cervical cytology screening (replaces committee opinion 152, March 1995). *Obstet Gynecol*. 2003;102(2):417–427.
25. Saslow D, Runowicz CD, Solomon D, et al. American Cancer Society guideline for the early detection of cervical neoplasia and cancer. *CA Cancer J Clin*. 2002;52(6):342–362.
26. US Preventive Services Task Force. Screening for cervical cancer: Recommendations and rationale. *Am J Nurs*. 2003;103(11):101–102, 105–106, 108–109.

27. Vesco KK, Whitlock EP, Eder M, et al. *Screening for Cervical Cancer: A Systematic Evidence Review for the U.S. Preventive Services Task Force.* Rockville, MD: US Agency for Healthcare Research and Quality; 2011.

28. Sawaya GF, Kerlikowske K, Lee NC, Gildengorin G, Washington AE. Frequency of cervical smear abnormalities within 3 years of normal cytology. *Obstet Gynecol.* 2000;96(2):219–223.

29. Sawaya GF, McConnell KJ, Kulasingam SL, et al. Risk of cervical cancer associated with extending the interval between cervical-cancer screenings. *N Engl J Med.* 2003;349(16):1501–1509.

30. Auger M, Khalbuss W, Nayar R, et al. Accuracy and false-positive rate of the cytologic diagnosis of follicular cervicitis: Observations from the College of American Pathologists Pap Educational Program. *Arch Pathol Lab Med.* 2013;137(7):907–911.

31. Saslow D, Solomon D, Lawson HW, et al. American Cancer Society, American Society for Colposcopy and Cervical Pathology, and American Society for Clinical Pathology screening guidelines for the prevention and early detection of cervical cancer. *Am J Clin Pathol.* 2012;137(4):516–542.

32. Moyer VA; US Preventive Services Task Force. Screening for cervical cancer: US Preventive Services Task Force recommendation statement. *Ann Intern Med.* 2012;156(12):880–891, W312.

33. Cooper CP, Saraiya M, McLean TA, et al. Report from the CDC: Pap test intervals used by physicians serving low-income women through the National Breast and Cervical Cancer Early Detection Program. *J Womens Health (Larchmt).* 2005;14(8):670–678.

34. Saint M, Gildengorin G, Sawaya GF. Current cervical neoplasia screening practices of obstetrician/gynecologists in the US. *Am J Obstet Gynecol.* 2005;192(2):414–421.

35. Almeida CM, Rodriguez MA, Skootsky S, Pregler J, Steers N, Wenger NS. Cervical cancer screening overuse and underuse: Patient and physician factors. *Am J Manag Care.* 2013;19(6):482–489.

36. Choosing Wisely recommendation analysis: Prioritizing opportunities for reducing inappropriate care. Institute for Clinical and Economic Review website. http://icer-review.org/wp-content/uploads/2016/01/FINAL-Pap-testing-analysis-November-28.pdf. Accessed September 27, 2016.

37. Saraiya M, McCaig LF, Ekwueme DU. Ambulatory care visits for Pap tests, abnormal Pap test results, and cervical cancer procedures in the United States. *Am J Manag Care.* 2010;16(6):e137–e144.

38. Jacob BJ, Moineddin R, Sutradhar R, Baxter NN, Urbach DR. Effect of colonoscopy on colorectal cancer incidence and mortality: An instrumental variable analysis. *Gastrointest Endosc.* 2012;76(2):355–364.

39. Baxter NN, Goldwasser MA, Paszat LF, Saskin R, Urbach DR, Rabeneck L. Association of colonoscopy and death from colorectal cancer. *Ann Intern Med.* 2009;150(1):1–8.

40. US Preventive Services Task Force; Bibbins-Domingo K, Grossman DC, et al. Screening for colorectal cancer: US Preventive Services Task Force recommendation statement. *JAMA.* 2016;315(23):2564–2575.

41. Lieberman DA, Rex DK, Winawer SJ, et al. Guidelines for colonoscopy surveillance after screening and polypectomy: A consensus update by the US Multi-Society Task Force on Colorectal Cancer. *Gastroenterology.* 2012;143(3):844–857.

42. Johnson MR, Grubber J, Grambow SC, et al. Physician non-adherence to colonoscopy interval guidelines in the Veterans Affairs Healthcare System. *Gastroenterology.* 2015;149(4):938–951.

43. Murphy CC, Sandler RS, Grubber JM, Johnson MR, Fisher DA. Underuse and overuse of colonoscopy for repeat screening and surveillance in the Veterans Health Administration. *Clin Gastroenterol Hepatol.* 2016;14(3):436–444.

44. Saini SD, Powell AA, Dominitz JA, et al. Developing and testing an electronic measure of screening colonoscopy overuse in a large integrated healthcare system. *J Gen Intern Med.* 2016;31(Suppl 1):53–60.

45. Schoen RE, Pinsky PF, Weissfeld JL, et al. Utilization of surveillance colonoscopy in community practice. *Gastroenterology.* 2010;138(1):73–81.

46. Kruse GR, Khan SM, Zaslavsky AM, Ayanian JZ, Sequist TD. Overuse of colonoscopy for colorectal cancer screening and surveillance. *J Gen Intern Med.* 2015;30(3):277–283.

47. SEER stat fact sheets: Ovarian cancer. National Cancer Institute website. http://seer.cancer.gov/statfacts/html/ovary.html. Accessed September 22, 2016.

48. Halila H, Stenman UH, Seppala M. Ovarian cancer antigen CA-125 levels in pelvic inflammatory disease and pregnancy. *Cancer.* 1986;57(7):1327–1329.

49. Hung CL, Hung TC, Lai YH, Lu CS, Wu YJ, Yeh HI. Beyond malignancy: The role of

carbohydrate antigen 125 in heart failure. *Biomark Res.* 2013;1(1):25.

50. Seki K, Kikuchi Y, Uesato T, Kato K. Increased serum CA 125 levels during the first trimester of pregnancy. *Acta Obstet Gynecol Scand.* 1986;65(6):583–585.

51. Baldwin LM, Trivers KF, Matthews B, et al. Vignette-based study of ovarian cancer screening: Do U.S. physicians report adhering to evidence-based recommendations? *Ann Intern Med.* 2012;156(3):182–194.

52. Trends in potential overuse of three services among individuals with employer sponsored health insurance. 2016. American College of Physicians website. https://ahip.org/wp-content/uploads/2016/04/TrendsinOveruse_Report_3-21-16.pdf. Accessed September 29, 2016.

53. Ovarian cancer testing. Abcodia website. https://www.rocatest.com/roca-test/roca-test-for-ovarian-cancer-overview. Accessed September 22, 2016.

54. Ovarian cancer screening tests: Safety communication—FDA recommends against use. US Food and Drug Administration website. http://www.fda.gov/Safety/MedWatch/SafetyInformation/SafetyAlertsforHumanMedicalProducts/ucm519540.htm?source=govdelivery&utm_medium=email&utm_source=govdelivery. Accessed September 22, 2016.

55. OCRFA applauds Food and Drug Administration's statement on ovarian cancer screening test. Ovarian Cancer Research Fund Alliance website. http://www.ocrf.org/news/research/ocrfa-applauds-food-and-drug-administrations-statement-on-ovarian-cancer-screening-test. Accessed September 22, 2016.

56. OCRFA applauds FDA's statement on ovarian cancer screening test. Ovarian Cancer Research Fund Alliance website. http://www.ovariancancer.org/2016/09/07/ocrfa-applauds-fdas-statement-ovarian-cancer-screening-test. Accessed September 26, 2016.

57. Polednak AP. Bilateral synchronous breast cancer: A population-based study of characteristics, method of detection, and survival. *Surgery.* 2003;133(4):383–389.

58. Yi M, Meric-Bernstam F, Middleton LP, et al. Predictors of contralateral breast cancer in patients with unilateral breast cancer undergoing contralateral prophylactic mastectomy. *Cancer.* 2009;115(5):962–971.

59. Kurian AW, Lichtensztajn DY, Keegan TH, Nelson DO, Clarke CA, Gomez SL. Use of and mortality after bilateral mastectomy compared with other surgical treatments for breast cancer in California, 1998–2011. *JAMA.* 2014;312(9):902–914.

60. Arrington AK, Jarosek SL, Virnig BA, Habermann EB, Tuttle TM. Patient and surgeon characteristics associated with increased use of contralateral prophylactic mastectomy in patients with breast cancer. *Ann Surg Oncol.* 2009;16(10):2697–2704.

61. Tuttle TM, Habermann EB, Grund EH, Morris TJ, Virnig BA. Increasing use of contralateral prophylactic mastectomy for breast cancer patients: A trend toward more aggressive surgical treatment. *J Clin Oncol.* 2007;25(33):5203–5209.

62. Jones NB, Wilson J, Kotur L, Stephens J, Farrar WB, Agnese DM. Contralateral prophylactic mastectomy for unilateral breast cancer: An increasing trend at a single institution. *Ann Surg Oncol.* 2009;16(10):2691–2696.

63. Kummerow KL, Du L, Penson DF, Shyr Y, Hooks MA. Nationwide trends in mastectomy for early-stage breast cancer. *JAMA Surg.* 2015;150(1):9–16.

64. Steiner CA, Weiss AJ, Barrett ML, Fingar KR, Davis PH. Trends in bilateral and unilateral mastectomies in hospital inpatient and ambulatory settings, 2005–2013: Statistical Brief #201. Healthcare Cost and Utilization Project (HCUP) Statistical Briefs. Rockville, MD: US Department of Health and Human Services, Agency for Healthcare Research and Quality; 2006.

65. Russo CA, VanLandeghem K, Davis PH, Elixhauser A. Hospital and ambulatory surgery care for women's cancers. HCUP Highlight No. 2, AHRQ Publication No. 06-0038. September 2006. US Department of Health and Human Services, Agency for Healthcare Research and Quality website. http://archive.ahrq.gov/data/hcup/highlight2/high2.htm#Outpatient. Accessed September 30, 2016.

66. Wong SM, Freedman RA, Sagara Y, Aydogan F, Barry WT, Golshan M. Growing use of contralateral prophylactic mastectomy despite no improvement in long-term survival for invasive breast cancer. *Ann Surg.* 2017;265(3):581–589.

67. Pesce C, Liederbach E, Wang C, Lapin B, Winchester DJ, Yao K. Contralateral prophylactic mastectomy provides no survival benefit in young women with estrogen receptor-negative breast cancer. *Ann Surg Oncol.* 2014;21(10):3231–3239.

68. Momoh AO, Cohen WA, Kidwell KM, et al. Tradeoffs associated with contralateral

prophylactic mastectomy in women choosing breast reconstruction: Results of a prospective multicenter cohort. *Ann Surg.* 2017;266(1):158–164.

69. Deshmukh AA, Cantor SB, Crosby MA, et al. Cost of contralateral prophylactic mastectomy. *Ann Surg Oncol.* 2014;21(9):2823–2830.

70. Thompson I, Thrasher JB, Aus G, et al. Guideline for the management of clinically localized prostate cancer: 2007 update. *J Urol.* 2007;177(6):2106–2131.

71. D'Amico AV, Whittington R, Malkowicz SB, et al. Biochemical outcome after radical prostatectomy, external beam radiation therapy, or interstitial radiation therapy for clinically localized prostate cancer. *JAMA.* 1998;280(11):969–974.

72. Cooperberg MR, Broering JM, Carroll PR. Time trends and local variation in primary treatment of localized prostate cancer. *J Clin Oncol.* 2010;28(7):1117–1123.

73. Mahal BA, Chen YW, Efstathiou JA, et al. National trends and determinants of proton therapy use for prostate cancer: A National Cancer Data Base study. *Cancer.* 2016;122(10):1505–1512.

74. Jilani OK, Singh P, Wernicke AG, et al. Radiation therapy is well tolerated and produces excellent control rates in elderly patients with locally advanced head and neck cancers. *J Geriatr Oncol.* 2012;3(4).

75. Yonemoto LT, Slater JD, Rossi CJ Jr, et al. Combined proton and photon conformal radiation therapy for locally advanced carcinoma of the prostate: Preliminary results of a phase I/II study. *Int J Radiat Oncol Biol Phys.* 1997;37(1):21–29.

76. Benk VA, Adams JA, Shipley WU, et al. Late rectal bleeding following combined X-ray and proton high dose irradiation for patients with stages T3–T4 prostate carcinoma. *Int J Radiat Oncol Biol Phys.* 1993;26(3):551–557.

77. Shipley WU, Verhey LJ, Munzenrider JE, et al. Advanced prostate cancer: The results of a randomized comparative trial of high dose irradiation boosting with conformal protons compared with conventional dose irradiation using photons alone. *Int J Radiat Oncol Biol Phys.* 1995;32(1):3–12.

78. Brada M, Pijls-Johannesma M, De Ruysscher D. Current clinical evidence for proton therapy. *Cancer J.* 2009;15(4):319–324.

79. Tattam A. Patching up the NHS. *Nurs Times.* 1990;86(47):20–21.

80. Sun F, Oyesanmi O, Fontanarosa J, Reston J, Guzzo T, Schoelles K. *Therapies for Clinically Localized Prostate Cancer: Update of a 2008 Systematic Review.* Rockville, MD: Agency for Healthcare Research and Quality; 2014.

81. Verma V, Mishra MV, Mehta MP. A systematic review of the cost and cost-effectiveness studies of proton radiotherapy. *Cancer.* 2016;122(10):1483–1501.

82. Konski A, Speier W, Hanlon A, Beck JR, Pollack A. Is proton beam therapy cost effective in the treatment of adenocarcinoma of the prostate? *J Clin Oncol.* 2007;25(24):3603–3608.

83. Becerra V, Avila M, Jimenez J, et al. Economic evaluation of treatments for patients with localized prostate cancer in Europe: A systematic review. *BMC Health Serv Res.* 2016;16(1):541.

84. Unnecessary tests and procedures in the health care system: What physicians say about the problem, the causes, and the solutions. PerryUndem Research/Communication website. http://www.choosingwisely.org/wp-content/uploads/2015/04/Final-Choosing-Wisely-Survey-Report.pdf. Accessed September 28, 2016.

85. Ludmerer K.M., ed. *Time to Heal: American Medical Education from the Turn of the Century to the Era of Managed Care.* New York: Oxford University Press; 1999:516.

86. Adashi EY, Kocher RP. Physician self-referral: Regulation by exceptions. *JAMA.* 2015;313(5):457–458.

87. Lungren MP, Amrhein TJ, Paxton BE, et al. Physician self-referral: Frequency of negative findings at MR imaging of the knee as a marker of appropriate utilization. *Radiology.* 2013;269(3):810–815.

88. Paxton BE, Lungren MP, Srinivasan RC, et al. Physician self-referral of lumbar spine MRI with comparative analysis of negative study rates as a marker of utilization appropriateness. *AJR Am J Roentgenol.* 2012;198(6):1375–1379.

89. Amrhein TJ, Lungren MP, Paxton BE, et al. Journal Club: Shoulder MRI utilization: Relationship of physician MRI equipment ownership to negative study frequency. *AJR Am J Roentgenol.* 2013;201(3):605–610.

90. Amrhein TJ, Paxton BE, Lungren MP, et al. Physician self-referral and imaging use appropriateness: Negative cervical spine MRI frequency as an assessment metric. *AJNR Am J Neuroradiol.* 2014;35(12):2248–2253.

91. Colla CH, Mainor AJ, Hargreaves C, Sequist T, Morden N. Interventions aimed at reducing use of low-value health services: A systematic review. *Med Care Res Rev.* 2017;74(5):507–550.

92. Regev-Yochay G, Raz M, Dagan R, et al. Reduction in antibiotic use following a cluster randomized controlled multifaceted intervention: The Israeli judicious antibiotic prescription study. *Clin Infect Dis.* 2011;53(1):33–41.

93. Milstein R, Schreyoegg J. Pay for performance in the inpatient sector: A review of 34 P4P programs in 14 OECD countries. *Health Policy.* 2016;120(10):1125–1140.

94. Lin TY, Chen CY, Huang YT, Ting MK, Huang JC, Hsu KH. The effectiveness of a pay for performance program on diabetes care in Taiwan: A nationwide population-based longitudinal study. *Health Policy.* 2016;120(11):1313–1321.

95. Sinclair D, Saas M, Stevens JM. The effect of a symptom related "gating policy" on ANCA requests in routine clinical practice. *J Clin Pathol.* 2004;57(2):131–134.

96. Conant MM, Erdman SM, Osterholzer D. Mandatory infectious diseases approval of outpatient parenteral antimicrobial therapy (OPAT): Clinical and economic outcomes of averted cases. *J Antimicrob Chemother.* 2014;69(6):1695–1700.

97. Nyman JA, Feldman R, Shapiro J, Grogan C, Link D. Changing physician behavior: Does medical review of Part B Medicare claims make a difference? *Inquiry.* 1990;27(2):127–137.

98. MacCara ME, Sketris IS, Comeau DG, Weerasinghe SD. Impact of a limited fluoroquinolone reimbursement policy on antimicrobial prescription claims. *Ann Pharmacother.* 2001;35(7–8):852–858.

99. Burns J. Narrow networks found to yield substantial savings. *Manag Care.* 2012;21(2):26–30.

100. Promising payment reform: Risk-sharing with accountable care organizations. 2011. The Commonwealth Fund website. http://www.commonwealthfund. org/~/media/ files/publications/ fund-report/ 2011/jul/1530delbanco promisingpaymentreformrisksharing-2.pdf. Accessed November 11, 2016.

101. Song Z, Fendrick AM, Safran DG, Landon B, Chernew ME. Global budgets and technology-intensive medical services. *Healthc (Amst).* 2013;1(1–2):15–21.

102. O'Connor SD, Sodickson AD, Ip IK, et al. Journal Club: Requiring clinical justification to override repeat imaging decision support: Impact on CT use. *AJR Am J Roentgenol.* 2014;203(5):W482–W490.

103. Chernew ME., Rosen AB, Fendrick AM. Value-based insurance design. *Health Aff (Millwood).* 2007;26(2):w195–w203.

104. Colla CH. Swimming against the current—What might work to reduce low-value care? *N Engl J Med.* 2014;371(14):1280–1283.

105. Busch SH, Barry CL, Vegso SJ, Sindelar JL, Cullen MR. Effects of a cost-sharing exemption on use of preventive services at one large employer. *Health Aff (Millwood).* 2006;25(6):1529–1536.

106. Cassidy, A. Preventive services without cost sharing. 2010. Health Affairs website. http:// www.healthaffairs.org/healthpolicybriefs/brief. php?brief_id=37. Accessed November 1, 2016.

107. Chernew ME, Shah MR, Wegh A, et al. Impact of decreasing copayments on medication adherence within a disease management environment. *Health Aff (Millwood).* 2008;27(1):103–112.

108. Maciejewski ML, Farley JF, Parker J, Wansink D. Copayment reductions generate greater medication adherence in targeted patients. *Health Aff (Millwood).* 2010;29(11):2002–2008.

109. Macfarlane J, Holmes W, Gard P, Thornhill D, Macfarlane R, Hubbard R. Reducing antibiotic use for acute bronchitis in primary care: Blinded, randomised controlled trial of patient information leaflet. *Br Med J.* 2002;324(7329):91–94.

110. Taylor JA, Kwan-Gett TS, McMahon EM Jr. Effectiveness of a parental educational intervention in reducing antibiotic use in children: A randomized controlled trial. *Pediatr Infect Dis J.* 2005;24(6):489–493.

111. Wheeler JG, Fair M, Simpson PM, Rowlands LA, Aitken ME, Jacobs RF. Impact of a waiting room videotape message on parent attitudes toward pediatric antibiotic use. *Pediatrics.* 2001;108(3):591–596.

112. Ashe D, Patrick PA, Stempel MM, Shi Q, Brand DA. Educational posters to reduce antibiotic use. *J Pediatr Health Care.* 2006;20(3):192–197.

113. Tannenbaum C, Martin P, Tamblyn R, Benedetti A, Ahmed S. Reduction of inappropriate benzodiazepine prescriptions among older adults through direct patient education: The EMPOWER cluster randomized trial. *JAMA Intern Med.* 2014;174(6):890–898.

114. Veroff D, Marr A, Wennberg DE. Enhanced support for shared decision making reduced costs of care for patients with

preference-sensitive conditions. *Health Aff (Millwood)*. 2013;32(2):285–293.

115. Sinaiko AD, Eastman D, Rosenthal MB. How report cards on physicians, physician groups, and hospitals can have greater impact on consumer choices. *Health Aff (Millwood)*. 2012;31(3):602–611.

116. Gonzales R, Corbett KK, Wong S, et al. "Get smart Colorado": Impact of a mass media campaign to improve community antibiotic use. *Med Care*. 2008;46(6):597–605.

117. Feeley TW, Fly HS, Albright H, Walters R, Burke TW. A method for defining value in healthcare using cancer care as a model. *J Healthc Manag*. 2010;55(6):399–411.

118. Hoverman JR. Commentary: Hard times for oncologists? *J Oncol Pract*. 2011;7(6 Suppl), 82s–84s.

119. Porter ME. What is value in health care? *N Engl J Med*. 2010;363(26):2477–2481.

120. Torrance GW, Thomas WH, Sackett DL. A utility maximization model for evaluation of health care programs. *Health Serv Res*. 1972;7(2):118–133.

121. Chan KS, Chang E, Nassery N, Chang HY, Segal JB. The state of overuse measurement: A critical review. *Med Care Res Rev*. 2013;70(5):473–496.

122. Segal JB, Nassery N, Chang HY, Chang E, Chan K, Bridges JF. An index for measuring overuse of health care resources with Medicare claims. *Med Care*. 2015;53(3):230–236.

123. Segal JB, Bridges JF, Chang HY, et al. Identifying possible indicators of systematic overuse of health care procedures with claims data. *Med Care*. 2014;52(2):157–163.

124. Dahlberg LL, Krug EG. Violence—A global public health problem. In: Krug E, Dahlberg LL, Mercy JA, Zwi AB, Lozano R, eds. *World Report on Violence and Health*. Geneva, Switzerland: World Health Organization; 2002:1–56.

18

PARTNERSHIPS AND NETWORKS TO SUPPORT IMPLEMENTATION SCIENCE

Shoba Ramanadhan, Racquel E. Kohler, and K. Viswanath

PARTNERSHIPS BETWEEN researchers and stakeholders offer an important opportunity to leverage complementary expertise to improve the quality, value, and relevance of implementation science efforts and increase the application of findings.[1,2] For cancer prevention and control, research–stakeholder partnerships present an important opportunity to capitalize on a rich, but underutilized, evidence base and increase the impact of research evidence from the individual to the policy level and from primary prevention to survivorship.[3] In this chapter, we focus on research–stakeholder partnerships and networks in the context of implementation science, defined as the study of strategies that facilitate adoption and integration of research evidence into practice settings.[4] Partnerships between researchers and stakeholders are a natural fit for implementation science, given that (1) evidence-based programs, policies, practices, and interventions (EBIs) are expected to marry research evidence, end-user preferences, and expert opinion; (2) diverse expertise is required to solve complex, multilevel public health problems; and (3) the evidence base will only be utilized if it reflects the realities of practice.[5-7] Depending on the nature of the implementation science effort, a range of stakeholders may be suitable partners, including community members, patients/clients/publics, practitioners/providers, administrators, insurers, purchasers, policymakers, and government officials.[8,9] Relationships between researchers and stakeholders form the basis of partnership networks, facilitating the reciprocal flow of social influence and resources, which drive the spread, adoption, adaptation, and implementation of innovations in organizations and communities.[10,11]

This chapter highlights important considerations regarding partnerships and networks for implementation science to promote cancer prevention and control. First, we describe a continuum of engagement between researchers and stakeholders for implementation science efforts and discuss the benefits and challenges of participatory implementation science. Second, we consider partnerships for implementation science in a few key areas, including community, policy, public opinion, and public–private partnership domains. Third, we discuss methods by which implementation science partnerships can be evaluated, with an emphasis on social networks. We conclude with a series of questions for the field.

A CONTINUUM OF ENGAGEMENT FOR IMPLEMENTATION SCIENCE

There is a rich literature describing ways in which stakeholders can be engaged in research, including approaches such as community-engaged research, community-based participatory research (CBPR), and participatory action research.[12–14] These approaches have different philosophical and historical underpinnings and offer a range of intensities and depths for research–practice partnerships. There is no one-size-fits-all rule to stakeholder engagement, nor is the line among different types always clear. We thus present a continuum of engagement for researchers and stakeholders to consider for implementation science. Although a wide array of terms are used, the characterization offered by Biggs and expanded by Minkler and colleagues is a useful starting point.[1,15,16] The continuum of participation

can be characterized as follows: (1) contractual—stakeholders are involved, but not active, in the research study (e.g., providing a site or setting for an implementation study); (2) consultative—stakeholders are consulted initially or in an ongoing manner for specific goals (e.g., to facilitate recruitment); (3) collaborative—stakeholders and researchers work together, with researchers controlling decisions and resources; and (4) collegial/symmetric—diverse partners work together as colleagues, with power/resource sharing, capacity building, and benefits accruing to all partners.

Figure 18.1 highlights the ways in which researchers and stakeholders may engage in implementation science efforts, from the transactional to the transformational. Although a contractual model can facilitate the execution of cancer prevention and control research, interaction with a community or stakeholder site solely as a lab may suffer from many of the challenges inherent in the top-down approach that has been identified as a major driver of the research–practice chasm.[17,18] For this reason, we focus on the other models of engagement. As stakeholder engagement increases, so do opportunities for knowledge co-creation. In this way, the research–practice gap is framed not as a knowledge transfer issue but, rather, as a knowledge

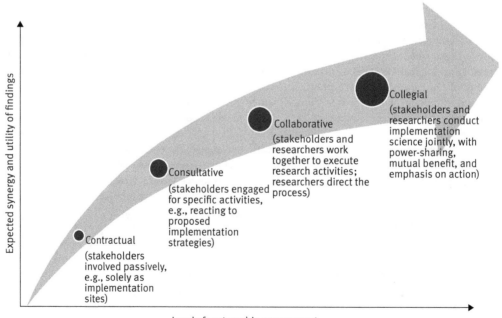

FIGURE 18.1   The continuum of engagement for implementation science.

production issue, which can be addressed through collaborative efforts to create knowledge grounded in the realities of practice.[14]

One example of a consultation-style model is to convene panels of stakeholders who can offer feedback on proposed research activities. For example, a panel of providers or patients could offer feedback on an implementation science proposal or study plan, ideally early enough in the process to allow researchers to react and recraft as needed. An example comes from the Meharry–Vanderbilt Community Engaged Research Core at the Vanderbilt Institute for Clinical and Translational Research, which offered *community engagement studios* as a service to affiliated researchers.[19] The Core created a pool of community experts to serve as representatives of a given community or population of interest and offer advice to researchers. Researchers presented their proposals and key questions (in lay terms) to a panel of community experts, who offered feedback in a session moderated by a facilitator. A toolkit to support replication of the program is available online.[20] For use with implementation science, community experts might include intended recipients of the EBI, as well as implementers, decision-makers, and others who can provide insight into the broader implementation context. As with any approach that relies on a subset of experts to represent a larger community, it is critical to utilize a systematic process to ensure that certain groups are not left out of the conversation. In addition, an opportunity exists to increase the bidirectionality of the effort—for example, providing a forum for stakeholders to identify important health issues for the community, which are then responded to by interested researchers.

Engagement in the collaboration style often includes efforts to solicit input from stakeholders over multiple phases of the research process but does not include a commitment to sharing power and resources to direct the research effort. For many projects, this may take the form of a community advisory board that provides researchers with information about community needs and preferences to support research. These advisory boards may offer recommendations or support for some or all parts of the research process, from study design to dissemination of findings.[21] For example, we recently conducted a study to assess the impacts of graphic health warnings on cigarette packages among vulnerable populations.[22] At the individual level, we assessed psychosocial and behavioral attributes; at the organization level, we explored requirements of community-based organizations to support national implementation of the warnings. We partnered with health-focused coalitions in each of the three study communities and provided a stipend, shared results, and created local dissemination materials. Our partners facilitated recruitment and retention, gave us advice on study design (e.g., the need to provide an audio-assist for our tablet-based survey), and supported data interpretation. As a contrast to our CBPR projects, for this effort, our partners did not participate in issue selection or jointly direct the study but instead partnered in a less intensive manner agreed upon at the outset of the project.

At the far end of the continuum, the collegial approach, which includes CBPR, is often considered the ideal but can be difficult to achieve. The CBPR approach emphasizes collaborative engagement among partners to utilize their strengths and resources to address a health issue of interest to the community and create knowledge and action, with explicit attention to health disparities.[23,24] By minimizing the distance between research and practice settings, CBPR studies are expected to produce research that is more relevant to communities and more likely to be utilized.[15] For implementation science, CBPR approaches are expected to yield a richer understanding of the implementation context and climate, be more sensitive to local culture and power structures, provide legitimacy to the EBI, and increase investment in the uptake of the EBI. These benefits are particularly critical in interventions that address health disparities when power structures of one kind or other are likely to be challenged.

An example comes from PLANET MassCONECT, a CBPR study focused on building capacity in community-based organizations for implementation of EBIs, with an emphasis on cancer control programs. In addition to providing training, tools, and mini-grants, the intervention supported network development among trainees trained to adapt and implement EBIs. Additional details about the intervention and the ways in which CBPR principles were operationalized are summarized elsewhere.[25] We formed a Community Project Advisory Committee that included leaders of health-focused coalitions in each of the partner communities. This group of partners was formed through an earlier grant and identified the capacity gap for EBI implementation that prompted the proposal to the National Cancer Institute (NCI). In addition to issue selection, the advisory committee provided critical insights for (1) intervention curriculum development (e.g., using an iterative design process, a focus on adult learning, provision of local examples, and emphasis on practice-focused tools), (2) recruitment (e.g., framing the training as professional development offered free to participants because it was subsidized by the NCI), (3) retention (e.g., contacting trainees to encourage them to continue to participate in networking activities and research surveys), (4) evaluation design (e.g., offering guidance on interview guides and surveys), (5) data interpretation (e.g., providing insight into trainee barriers to engagement or practice change), and (6) dissemination of findings (e.g., collaborating on a two-page brief for practitioners or scientific manuscripts).

As evidenced by these examples, an array of partnership and engagement levels can be utilized for researchers and stakeholders to bring their diverse expertise to address cancer prevention and control challenges. Using a *participatory implementation science* approach, researchers and stakeholders can identify a level of engagement that meets the needs of a given partnership or project, build on complementary expertise, and co-produce knowledge to support the integration of cancer prevention and control evidence into practice settings. Building off a growing literature linking engaged research and implementation science,[25-27] we argue that ongoing partnership between researchers and stakeholders (particularly at higher levels of engagement) can support achievement of both short-term goals (e.g., increasing integration of a specific cancer prevention EBI in community-based organizations) and long-term goals (e.g., systems change to support community-based organizations to integrate the broader/dynamic cancer prevention and control evidence base over time).

KEY BENEFITS OF PARTICIPATORY IMPLEMENTATION SCIENCE

There are several benefits to participatory implementation science, extending across research phases. Engaging stakeholders for knowledge creation, intervention/tool development, and evaluation increases the likelihood of generating practical, acceptable solutions to enhance adaptation and implementation[28-31] and heeds the call to generate practice-based evidence to support evidence-based practice.[32,33] Another benefit is that stakeholder engagement provides an automatic feedback loop that

can serve as the foundation for future implementation studies. For implementation science, collaboration with stakeholders can provide critical contextual information so that implementation packages can be customized to maximize appropriateness and utility. Researcher–stakeholder collaboration can increase the external validity of implementation science results and thereby increase the utility of those findings to professionals and policymakers interested in scaling cancer prevention and control EBIs up to different populations and settings than those initially studied.[34] As researchers move along the engagement continuum toward collegial forms, they can shift the focus from a decontextualized assessment of the "what" of implementation to the "how" of implementation for a specific setting and population and time.[35] At the same time, by including partner organizations serving or representing vulnerable subgroups, implementation scientists can develop implementation packages that actively address cancer disparities or, at a minimum, protect against creating or exacerbating disparities.

Participatory implementation science efforts can draw on CBPR approaches to emphasize building capacity among stakeholdres,[24] equipping partners to better handle current and future health challenges.[36] For implementation science, this can translate into increased capacity of stakeholders to engage with data, research evidence, and EBIs as they create change.[25] Building capacity allows stakeholders to engage more effectively with the cancer control evidence base has important implications for the sustainability of cancer prevention and control activities. For researchers, engagement can offer important insight into the "real-world" considerations that drive implementation efforts and can build capacity among research teams to appreciate and draw on evidence gained outside traditional scientific processes. In this way, participatory implementation science offers an opportunity to expand the definition of what evidence is brought to bear in supporting change in practice settings. Although the call by Green[7] to generate practice-based evidence in order to drive evidence-based practice is well received, it also prompts the question of what evidence "counts" in implementation science.[37] Partnerships afford implementation scientists the opportunity to identify and capitalize on evidence outside the realm of traditional scientific inquiry, which requires expanding the definition of "evidence" and what evidence is acceptable. The challenge is to apply rigorous methods to collect and analyze nontraditional data. Qualitative methods and process data may be of particular importance for such applications.

Participatory implementation science can offer partnerships and organizations, especially those working with vulnerable groups, important resources to support their work to address cancer disparities. For example, we have developed a model of engagement that utilizes human, social, and fiscal capital investments in our partner communities to support sustainable efforts to use research evidence to address cancer and other health disparities.[25] Another example comes from an assessment of the NCI's Community Networks Programs, an effort to use CBPR methods to build research infrastructure for cancer control in minority and disadvantaged communities. A survey of 22 of the 25 networks found that all networks facilitated access to resources for cancer services, 15 developed community leadership resources (through training and supporting community members), and all reported that community partners secured cancer programming grants, among other benefits.[38] An engaged approach is also likely to provide additional nontangible resources, such as legitimacy, endorsement, and advice, that can go a long way in enhancing the relevance and utility of implementation science findings to the vulnerable communities and the organizations that serve them.

KEY CHALLENGES OF PARTICIPATORY IMPLEMENTATION SCIENCE

Partnerships between researchers and stakeholders require an agreement to engage in a manner that is likely to be far from "business as usual" for any of the partners. Clear communication and planning for engagement and a structure that fosters engagement are critical, particularly as roles and responsibilities may change across stages of the partnership. One challenge when using a higher level of engagement in a research project relates to the investments required. For example, taking a CBPR approach is expected to be time- and resource-intensive because of the expected practice of joint decision-making, resource sharing, co-learning, and so forth. For implementation science, this can be a challenge if relationships need to be built and maintained among diverse partners. For this reason, it is useful to think of and find a place on the continuum of engagement that meets the needs, resources, and culture of the researchers

and partners involved. This can help bridge potential gaps, such as those between research teams with a project- or grant-based approach that have a tightly defined scope versus a team of stakeholders with competing priorities and needs that diffuse across sectors and health topics. Another solution may be technology-enhanced engagement, such as using new media technologies, particularly those that support user-generated content and interaction (e.g., blogs, wikis, and networking sites), to reinforce relationship development and maintenance as well as resource sharing.[39]

Another challenge relates to disconnects faced by stakeholders and researchers, compared to their usual way of working. For stakeholders, this may reflect an orientation to "doing" rather than "researching" and the perception that research diverts limited resources from practical goals. The tension between action and research may be particularly apparent in low-resource organizations with insufficient personnel, time, and money and far too many demands on existing resources. Fiscal challenges may make it difficult for them to meet their primary goals, much less expand to partner in research.[40] However, there is an opportunity to link implementation science (and the related capacity developed among partners) to larger organization goals, such as quality improvement. Cancer prevention and control researchers can learn from HIV prevention researchers, who have highlighted the important overlaps between capacity built for implementation science and capacity required for monitoring and evaluation efforts, management science, and continuous quality improvement. In this way, building capacity for implementation science can have important benefits for service delivery, particularly in low-resource settings.[41,42] Similarly, the idea of a "learning organization," or one in which the organization invests in staff and trains them to use problem-solving cycles, documentation, experimentation, and reflection to learn and improve in an ongoing manner,[43] may also have utility in linking capacity built through research activities with broader institutional goals.

On the researcher side, capacity for engaged research may be an issue because skills for engaged research are not routinely required for research training in public health.[44] A recent study of a clinical translational science center found that 58% of the researchers surveyed had CBPR experience, but half of this group reported needing additional skills in research methods, dissemination, and capacity-building activities and one-third of this group was interested in additional mentoring in this area. Across all investigators, approximately half reported needing training on funding, partnership development, evaluation, and dissemination.[45] In addition, funding mechanisms and researchers' requirements for career advancement often limit opportunities for community-engaged research.[46] Yet another challenge on the part of the researchers is a lack of or, at least, an insufficient orientation toward an understanding of the importance of community engagement in research. Research is often presented as specialized expertise leading to specification of problems and methods to study problems based on that expertise. The idea of collaborative definition and implementation with non-specialists requires a different mindset and a supportive environment.

Another challenge of engaged research relates to the ability to build and sustain partnerships. In addition to the time and other investments required, a lack of trust among potential partners is a common barrier to engaged research, and strategies to put structure around the partnership (e.g., through a memorandum of understanding or other commitments) can be important for relationship development.[37] However, implementation scientists may be in a strong position to build multiple connections with partner organizations as they engage with implementers, champions, leaders, and others. Again, by integrating with larger goals such as quality improvement, the research generates value for stakeholders, which is likely to increase the sustainability of the partnership.

STRATEGIC PARTNERSHIP COMPOSITION

A variety of partners may be appropriate for implementation science and may play critical roles at different points in the process. For example, a recent study highlighted the importance of policy partners in facilitating the adoption of a childhood obesity prevention EBI, whereas local implementers (including program coordinators, local government, and other key stakeholders) were critical for facilitating program delivery.[47] An important consideration for partnership composition is the question of which stakeholders are invited to participate and which stakeholders are excluded, whether intentionally or unintentionally. A strategic method for identifying partners is useful because creating

change in a practice setting requires supportive organizational, contextual, and policy environments. For example, one might draw on community reconnaissance techniques, methods to uncover underlying power dynamics in communities.[48,49] We used these techniques in a recent study to identify the range of key players needed to support EBI implementation for tobacco-related health disparities in a partner community. We started with a seed group of community leaders and asked them to nominate key leaders who are critical for creating local change, with a focus on recruiting across six sectors. Through this combination of positional and reputational approaches, we identified 33 diverse leaders and mapped their relationships using UCINET,[50] dedicated network analysis software. The resulting maps identified the relevant set of leaders in key sectors of the community and highlighted connections that could be utilized by our community partners to promote an agenda focused on addressing tobacco-related health disparities. This type of assessment was appropriate for a community-level change effort, particularly because public health practice efforts may include wide-ranging actors and systems, including community members; community-based/nongovernmental/private sector organizations; entities from a range of sectors, such as housing and transportation; and governmental structures at local and higher levels.[51] However, an institutional-level change effort could use a similar process at a much smaller (and more manageable) scale, with the important outcome of determining the key set of stakeholders necessary to ensure the success of the implementation effort.

PARTNERSHIPS IN A RANGE OF DOMAINS

Given that EBIs are implemented in a wide range of settings, it is useful to consider how partnerships and networks might function differently across domains. Much of the implementation science literature focuses on clinical settings, such as hospitals, clinics, and health systems.[52,53] We focus here on other realms for which partnerships and networks play an important role, such as community settings, public policy, public opinion, and public–private partnerships.

Community Settings

Community-based organizations are promising, but underutilized, channels for delivery of cancer control EBIs and are important partners to address cancer disparities given their reach and trust among vulnerable population subgroups.[54-56] Despite the potential health impact of improving EBI implementation in community settings and the opportunity offered by using engaged approaches, participatory implementation science in community settings is currently limited.[57,58] Implementation efforts in community settings are distinct from corollary work conducted in clinical settings in a few key ways. First, implementation efforts typically target a multisector network of organizations and stakeholders. Second, a broad range of types of knowledge are valued by stakeholders, including local knowledge and experiential knowledge. Third, advocacy can be a central part of collaborative activities.[58] Conducting implementation science in the context of coalitions and community-based organizations' partnerships brings a unique set of considerations. Each partner brings unique goals, constituents, and obligations. Thus, partnership development and maintenance is a continuous undertaking requiring careful attention.[59] Given the diversity of community organizations engaged in health promotion, working with coalitions (such as state and local cancer control coalitions) and obtaining member buy-in for a given set of objectives and programs may be quite different from implementation efforts in more homogeneous settings.

In community settings, a diverse range of partners may be engaged in cancer control. For example, best practice guidelines for tobacco control coalitions suggest that these coalitions should include representatives from each community sector, members of diverse racial/ethnic groups, community leaders, those most affected by tobacco use, national tobacco control partners, and organizations delivering health services. Leveraging the strength of diverse actors working in concert, tobacco control coalitions have effectively advocated for increasing tobacco taxes at state and local levels, reduce tobacco product advertising, and conducted counter-marketing campaigns, among other activities.[60]

In the context of cancer control, partnerships offer an important opportunity to promote community capacity building to use knowledge to develop, implement, and sustain EBIs that shift community behaviors and norms. The Participatory Knowledge Translation Framework offers a road map to use engaged approaches to build local "engines for change" through community capacity, ensuring that communities can leverage research evidence to address health issues of importance for the long term. The framework highlights the importance of a series of inputs (institutionalized participation, investments in human capital and social capital plus resource sharing, and knowledge production and transfer) that are applied in rapid learning cycles to build community infrastructure for knowledge translation (including implementation of EBIs).[25] Application of this and other frameworks for community-based implementation science[52,58,61] will be critical for furthering the knowledge base on partnered implementation science in community settings. There are, of course, challenges in engaged implementation science in community settings, including issues related to building trust,[62] sharing power,[63] funding sources,[64] equitable levels of community participation,[65] and collaboration readiness and capacity to implement EBIs.[66,67]

To move participatory implementation science forward in community settings, research emerging from community-identified priorities and in partnership with stakeholders will require changes to traditional approaches to research as well as supporting funding mechanisms. It will be critical to align funding reporting requirements, research milestones, and implementation timelines with necessary community processes.[68]

Policy

A critical element of implementation science is understanding how policies—codification of principles accompanied by a degree of regulatory authority—could facilitate practice espoused by EBIs or the evidence base more broadly writ. Policies can be a critical intermediate step between evidence and practice. They can take a variety of forms—from enactment of laws and regulations in the government to rules, procedures, and protocols in organizations—with the intention of applying the evidence base. Dissemination of the evidence base to promote policy change is by itself insufficient; instead, policy change requires mobilization across multiple sectors. Partnerships are critical in such mobilization because they bring resources, legitimacy, and an understanding of levers of power to enact changes. Freudenberg and Tsui[69] identify four principles for effective policy change, drawing on participatory approaches: (1) recognition that actions to make change work across "multiple levels and scales"; (2) appreciation of the role of political power in promoting policy change; (3) understanding that the definition, acceptability, and the role of evidence are subject to influence of power; and (4) acknowledgment that evidence and power play different roles leading to policy change.[69] In the realm of EBI-driven policy changes to address health equity, power plays a particularly critical role. This warrants a mapping of dynamics of power relationships in the community, current policies or problems that are a target of change, and potential agents of change.[70,71] The selection of stakeholders is vital to the process of generating support for and implementing the policy change.

An excellent example of gathering a strategic set of stakeholders to serve as advisors and partners derives from the CHOICES model, a project that assessed the cost-effectiveness of four childhood obesity prevention interventions with the goal of delivering information to key decision-makers in the United States.[72] Selection of the stakeholder group was one of seven key program components, and the 32-member group included policymakers, program delivery experts, and researchers focused on policy, nutrition, and physical activity. Stakeholders provided expert advice to support cost-effectiveness modeling (e.g., specifying interventions, identifying data sources, and supporting the analyses). They also reviewed the findings regarding issues of implementation and equity and considered "quality of evidence, equity, acceptability, feasibility, sustainability, side effects, and social and policy norms" (p. 104). The implementation and equity findings were combined with the results of the cost-effectiveness analysis to provide decision-makers with the information they needed. Researchers involved in this effort had previously identified policymakers' need to address cost-effectiveness, practical considerations related to implementation (feasibility and sustainability among them), and issues of equity (e.g., balancing reach and effectiveness).[73] The team built off similar models used in Australia[74] and adapted the methods for use in the United States. Use of a systems approach and corresponding methods allowed the team to meet the needs of the ultimate end-users, the policymakers.

Public Opinion

Complex, systems-driven issues such as cancer disparities require complementary work at multiple levels to create change at scale, challenge power structures, and address a climate or culture that may be less hospitable or even hostile to structural changes. Although implementation science is inherently system focused, the boundaries of research efforts are often limited to organizations or small systems. Despite the limited attention given to this area, partnerships and networks can also be activated to address the role of the media and the larger cultural understanding they engender, in the context of supporting and promoting the use of research evidence. One such example (Project IMPACT) is discussed in case study section in this volume. Here, we discuss the theory behind the case.

Studies in public opinion have long documented the role of media in developing public images or opinions about important issues[75-77] and, in fact, in shaping issues through framing.[78-81] Framing provides the prism through which different publics perceive an issue—for example, taxes to provide health insurance to the underserved or increasing taxes on sugar-sweetened beverages—and the policy preferences they support.[82] Media framing is also critical in mobilizing coalitions and starting and sustaining (or even negatively affecting) social movements,[83] which can promote structural changes such as tax reforms to deter risky behaviors (e.g., tax on tobacco or sugar-sweetened beverages) or changes in transportation policies to promote physical activity (e.g., encouraging biking or mass transit). Taking the example of taxes on tobacco, partnership mobilization through capacity building could potentially influence media agenda and framing. This, in turn, would influence public opinion to promote policy preferences that leverage the research evidence on tobacco taxation and result in improvement in tobacco control outcomes. Considerable evidence exists to suggest that media agendas are products of dynamic interaction between sources of news, "frame sponsors,"[84,85] as well reporters.[86] In health media coverage, it has been shown that scientists, professional journals, and news releases are critical sources of ideas for reporters.[87-89] A sophisticated understanding of how this dynamic may be tapped to promote change in the climate for implementation of research evidence related to policy and structural changes, as well as the key role of partnerships in promoting agenda setting, is ripe for more research.

Public–Private Partnerships

Increasingly, public health partnerships are engaging the private and non-profit sectors to employ diverse resources and improve intervention planning, implementation, and impact. These cross-sector partnerships are a popular tool being used to promote healthy workplaces, deliver health services, and develop and finance health system infrastructure. Functioning program infrastructure is particularly important to capacity, implementation, and sustainability. Public–private partnerships (PPPs) combine private sector strengths (e.g., innovation, entrepreneurship, and scale) with the goals of the public sector (e.g., public accountability and health equity) and the non-profit sector (e.g., fundraising and advocacy).[90] Various PPP models exist to implement programs, increase capacity, and improve infrastructure, although most are business models. These partnerships can maximize potential health outcomes and cost savings, but the collaborative nature of the partnerships may be limited.[91] For example, many PPPs operate as contractual partnerships, so the social, political, and legal environments may greatly influence governance, trust, capacity to share resources, and sustainability. Still, there is much variation in engagement, risk sharing, decision-making, and benefits between members.

The business nature of these partnerships can create complex power dynamics. Although programs may be implemented through local- and state-level private, public, and informal members, they may be centrally coordinated at a national level. In many low- and middle-income countries, international donor organizations and for-profit partners join with national governments to organize and support programs. Program funding may be donor driven, but local context, partner relationships, and capacity ultimately affect implementation and PPP success.[92] For example, Pink Ribbon Red Ribbon is a PPP focused on improving breast and cervical cancer control in multiple low- and middle-income countries. The non-profit organization builds upon the US President's Emergency Plan for AIDS Relief (PEPFAR) platform and leverages multilateral and local private and public investments in global health.[93] Within each country, Pink Ribbon Red Ribbon partners with the private sector, national governments, and in-country leadership to adapt cancer control solutions to local resources, needs, and capacities. Local challenges related to member capacity, stakeholder priorities, and communication and coordination across sectors require different partnership arrangements and implementation approaches. Therefore, each country-led PPP model is unique, with Pink Ribbon Red Ribbon providing resources and technical assistance to help country partnerships create relevant policies; adapt guidelines; train health workers; and increase access to services for breast and cervical cancer prevention, screening, and treatment. Innovative partnership models across and within private and public sectors, governments, and communities are being deployed to meet population health goals. Because of the multisector interactions that affect cancer prevention and control, we must understand how different programs and sectors can work together to improve EBI implementation within PPPs. Because PPPs are increasingly becoming a way of doing business and engaging the community to prevent cancer, it is critical to use implementation science to evaluate various strategies as well as their replicability and scalability. Research on the context of various PPP models will help us understand how and why certain collaborations are successful and sustainable, as well as which designs and arrangements are needed to create a positive environment for partner co-learning and scaling-up EBIs.

ASSESSING PARTNERSHIPS AND NETWORKS

Social Network Approaches

When considering the role of partnerships and networks in implementation science, it is natural to turn to social network analysis—the theories and methods that support the study of social relationships among actors in a given system.[94] Examining networks held by implementers, change agents, researchers, and other actors can have important impacts on implementation efforts. Social network analysis can support implementation science through network description and visualization, assessing prominence of particular actors, and modeling implementation outcomes.[95] These methods can be applied at different stages of implementation studies to support network ethnography, network interventions, network diagnostics, and network surveillance, as detailed by Valente and colleagues.[96] We present a series of examples of network analysis applications across the life course of implementation science efforts.

Network mapping efforts can be a useful component of formative research for an implementation science effort. By mapping existing relationships, researchers can assess available social capital, identify implementation barriers and facilitators at multiple levels, and gather contextual data about the community and organizations involved in/affected by the implementation effort.[96] As described under Strategic Partnership Composition, researchers can be strategic and proactive in partnership development to ensure that all the necessary partners are engaged and early network mapping can facilitate these activities. Figure 18.2 offers examples of network visualizations. Data are from the community reconnaissance sampling effort described previously, with the goal of identifying leaders from a range of sectors who could play pivotal roles in addressing health disparities in the partner community. The visual on the left shows the overall map of connections and highlights the position of a government leader as central to the network. It also shows the ways in which leaders tended to cluster by sector. Another way in which data from that study were visualized is depicted on the right side of Figure 18.2, using the example of intra- and intersectoral connections held by leaders of the grassroots sector.[70]

As part of early network mapping, it can be useful to determine the set of network functions of interest. For example, a recent study of community–clinical linkages to support implementation of EBIs for tobacco cessation and other prevention issues in Massachusetts highlighted key functions of interagency network members: sharing information/best practices, sending/receiving referrals, sharing resources, provision of services, and conducting outreach.[97] A collaboration between the National Cancer Institute's Center for Global Health and the non-profit organization Global Oncology offers another example. The Global Cancer Project Map is an interactive map to visualize international cancer control efforts and catalyze collaborations.[98,99]

Social network analysis can also support examination of infrastructure development, both during and after an implementation science study. Network infrastructure can be an important (but easily missed) outcome of partnered approaches to implementation science. For example, we created the Massachusetts Community Network for Cancer Education, Research, and Training (MassCONECT) through the Community Networks Program funded by the NCI. The goal of the project was to use CBPR approaches to support diverse local stakeholders (including researchers, policymakers, leaders of health-focused coalitions, media, and local and state government officials) to collaborate and apply the best available research evidence to address cancer disparities in three partner communities.[101,102] At the suggestion of community partners, we conducted a social network analysis to document infrastructure development to support action against cancer disparities. We studied the network of MassCONECT participants and focused on intersectoral connections—the relationships between network members from different sectors, such as community-based organizations and researchers. We found an increase in

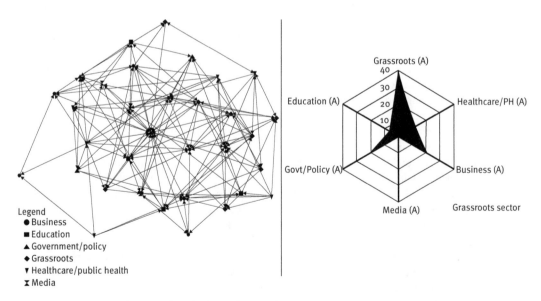

FIGURE 18.2   Exemplar uses of network visualization for partnership assessment, including overall network map (left) and chart describing intra- and intersectoral connections (right).

connections within the network over 4 years, as well as increases in the number of intersectoral connections and the extent to which intersectoral connections were reciprocated. Intersectoral connections were positively associated with outcomes of interest to diverse partners, such as community cancer prevention activities, grants and publications, and policy activities.[102] Findings such as these underscore the importance of multilevel and multisectoral connections, but they also highlight the tremendous investment required to build and sustain such relationships. Given the challenges faced by so many public health initiatives in terms of having insufficient time to demonstrate impact on health outcomes, infrastructure development in the form of social networks may be an important intermediate marker by which to assess progress and requirements for sustainability. For projects using a CBPR approach, this type of infrastructure development supports the goals of creating systems change and supporting iterative efforts to create change through partnerships.[24,103]

Researchers can also utilize social network analysis to examine the impact of networks on implementation outcomes. For example, a recent mixed-methods study analyzed connections among agency directors considering adopting EBIs. The assessment included details of drivers of network connections (e.g., roles and friendship ties), the resources that flow across the network (e.g., information about EBIs and influence to promote EBI adoption), and the relationship between network metrics and implementation of EBIs at 2-year follow-up.[104]

In the context of implementation science, social network analysis supports researchers to examine (1) partnerships supporting implementation, (2) the network characteristics of implementers and other important stakeholders, and (3) the program delivery context.[96] As the literature in this area grows, it will become increasingly possible to conduct network interventions[96,105] to support implementation science goals, such as identifying important individuals (e.g., opinion leaders) to promote implementation or identifying network structures that are more likely to support implementation outcomes.

Evaluating Partnerships

As part of the effort to improve cancer prevention and control through research–practice partnerships, it is useful to assess how partnerships function, what

can be improved, and what will aid sustainability. Although the diversity of partners is a strength and justification for collaboration, differences in perspectives, interpretations, priorities, and definitions of success create challenges and conflict in selecting indicators to assess partnership impact.[106] Outcome measures must be responsive to shared and individual goals of partners and allow for evaluation across multiple levels. A range of quantitative, qualitative, and mixed-methods approaches can be used to evaluate partnership functioning. Qualitative data collection may play an important role in eliciting critical local and experiential knowledge from stakeholders,[107] including insights into partnership processes over time.[108] A mixed-methods approach, which integrates qualitative and quantitative data to leverage the complementary strengths of each,[109] can be useful for the study of partnership as one of the implementation processes that impacts implementation outcomes.[110] Using mixed methods also helps provide a comprehensive picture of how well a partnership is functioning and implementing EBIs while recognizing multiple and multilevel organizational perspectives, local context, and cultural influences.[111]

To analyze partnerships for implementation science, it is useful to draw on the broader partnerships literature. This perspective prompts attention to studying infrastructure components (e.g., characteristics of members, lead agency/organization, staffing, and funding) in light of the context (e.g., organizational, social, and political climates; collaboration history; and leadership). A review of 26 partnerships, including cancer control-focused initiatives, identified 55 measures including six coalition-building factors that were positively correlated with effectiveness in more than five studies (i.e., formalization/rules, leadership style, active member participation, diverse membership, member agency collaboration, and group cohesion).[112] Norms and attitudes, organizational structures, resources, policies, and networks and linkages[113] are important contextual factors often considered in determining "fit" but are rarely reported upon. Explicit reporting of contextual factors is needed, especially in light of the multidimensional and interactive nature of partnerships. In a review of coalition functioning measurements and tools, Granner and Sharpe[114] found a wide range of tools and measures to assess individual and group characteristics, but they noted that few studies report the psychometric properties of the measures used.

As noted previously, it is a challenge to build and sustain research–practice partnerships for implementation science. However, a long-term, systems view suggests that the investment is worthwhile. As highlighted by the Dynamic Sustainability Framework, one can consider implementation as an ongoing evolution of an EBI to ensure continued/increasing fit between interventions and the broader implementation context.[115] With that perspective, research–practice partnerships provide an excellent base from which to study and guide ongoing iterations of EBIs and can contribute to the pool of data describing context-driven adaptations and EBI evolution that will be critical to supporting scale-up of EBIs.[116,117] The literature includes various conceptualizations and operational definitions of sustainability of partnerships, most of which focus on member relationships and collaborative engagement.[118] Measuring trust, interest, and involvement is critical throughout partnership activities. They may be difficult to capture, but they provide insight into the life and interactions of a partnership. These measures are especially helpful in understanding why members leave or the partnership dissolves. Other common measures include the structure and frequency of partner meetings as well as communications channels and frequency, problem-solving or conflict resolution, and staff and leadership capacity. Modeling techniques can be applied to study the impacts of longitudinal data linking the overall network, interactions between partners, and characteristics of partners with sustainability markers.[118] As described previously, sustainable research–practice networks offer critical infrastructure to support integration of the cancer control evidence base over the long term.

SUMMARY AND NEXT STEPS

Partnerships between researchers and stakeholders must be strategically developed and sustained to improve the integration of cancer prevention and control evidence into practice settings. However, the use of participatory implementation science approaches is still rare, prompting several important areas for inquiry. First, we recognize the challenge in conducting research among and within dynamic networks/partnerships and utilizing ever-evolving EBIs. Research designs and methods will need to allow for these challenges to traditional methods and approaches. Viewing an EBI as a dynamic event in a system supports inquiry that allows for the evolution of both the context and the innovation under study.[116,119] The use of methods such as dynamic social network analysis and agent-based modeling will allow researchers to understand the influence of changing connection patterns among important actors on implementation processes and outcomes.[120] Second, although participatory approaches to implementation science can increase the relevance and utility of research results, it remains a challenge to make findings accessible and usable to diverse stakeholders. Partnerships can and should be utilized to paint a full picture of implementation context, which should increase the ability to support adaptation and implementation efforts. Third, research–practice partnerships can offer important insight into the way researchers define the evidence base that needs to be accessed and utilized. This includes the study of the implementation of EBIs, evidence-based approaches (e.g., those offered by the Centers for Disease Control and Prevention's Community Guide[121]), and high-quality practice-based evidence. Research–practice partnerships offer an important way to build the scientific literature regarding how evidence is defined and applied in diverse practice settings, prompting researchers to design vehicles for sharing evidence that can be applied more easily in practice settings. Last, research–practice partnerships offer the important opportunity to tackle implementation science challenges across levels and sectors (e.g., in clinical, community, and public health settings but also related to policy, public opinion, and the private sector), which is critical for addressing the complex, systems-level challenges of cancer prevention and control.

Implementation science lends itself to partnered research. It is necessary to study content, context, and process in partnership with those who have expertise in these areas in order to create sustainable change. Through participatory implementation science, it may be possible to improve the knowledge production process and generate rigorous, relevant research as well as tools to support their integration into practice settings at scale.

REFERENCES

1. Sibbald SL, Tetroe J, Graham ID. Research funder required research partnerships: A qualitative inquiry. *Implement Sci.* 2014;9(1):1.
2. Wallerstein N, Yen IH, Syme SL. Integration of social epidemiology and community-engaged

interventions to improve health equity. *Am J Public Health*. 2011;101(5):822–830.

3. Emmons KM, Colditz GA. Realizing the potential of cancer prevention—The role of implementation science. *N Engl J Med*. 2017;376(10):986–990.

4. National Institutes of Health. *Dissemination and Implementation Research in Health (R01)*. Bethesda, MD: National Institutes of Health; 2016.

5. Sackett DL, Rosenberg WM, Gray JM, Haynes RB, Richardson WS. Evidence based medicine: What it is and what it isn't. *BMJ*. 1996;312(7023):71–72.

6. Chambers DA, Azrin ST. Research and services partnerships: Partnership: A fundamental component of dissemination and implementation research. *Psychiatr Serv*. 2013;64(6):509–511.

7. Green LW. Making research relevant: If it is an evidence-based practice, where's the practice-based evidence? *Fam Pract*. 2008;25(Suppl 1):i20–i24.

8. Mendel P. Interventions in organizational and community context: A framework for building evidence on dissemination and implementation in health services research. *Adm Policy Ment Health*. 2008;35(1–2):21–37.

9. Damschroder LJ, Aron DC, Keith RE, Kirsh SR, Alexander JA, Lowery JC. Fostering implementation of health services research findings into practice: A consolidated framework for advancing implementation science. *Implement Sci*. 2009;4(1):50.

10. Rogers E. *Diffusion of Innovations*. 5th ed. New York: Free Press; 2003.

11. Valente TW, Chou CP, Pentz MA. Community coalitions as a system: Effects of network change on adoption of evidence-based substance abuse prevention. *Am J Public Health*. 2007;97(5):880–886.

12. Israel BA, Eng E, Schulz AJ, Parker EA, eds. *Methods for Community-Based Participatory Research for Health*. 2nd ed. San Francisco, CA: Wiley; 2013.

13. Whyte WF, Greenwood DJ, Lazes P. Participatory action research: Through practice to science in social research. *Am Behav Scientist*. 1989;32(5):513.

14. Van de Ven AH, Johnson PE. Knowledge for theory and practice. *Acad Manage Rev*. 2006;31(4):802–821.

15. Minkler M, Salvatore AL. Participatory approaches for study design and analysis in dissemination and implementation research. In: Brownson RC, Colditz GA, Proctor EK, eds. *Dissemination and Implementation Research in Health*. New York: Oxford University Press; 2012:192–212.

16. Biggs S. Resource-poor farmer participation in research: A synthesis of experiences from national agricultural research systems. OFCOR-Comparative study (Netherlands) No 3; 1989.

17. Orleans CT. Increasing the demand for and use of effective smoking-cessation treatments reaping the full health benefits of tobacco-control science and policy gains—In our lifetime. *Am J Prev Med*. 2007;33(6 Suppl):S340–S348.

18. Viswanath K. Public communication and its role in reducing and eliminating health disparities. In: Thomson GE, Mitchell F, WIlliams MB, eds. *Examining the Health Disparities Research Plan of the National Institutes of Health: Unfinished Business*. Washington, DC: Institute of Medicine; 2006:215–253.

19. Joosten YA, Israel TL, Williams NA, et al. Community engagement studios: A structured approach to obtaining meaningful input from stakeholders to inform research. *Acad Med*. 2015;90(12):1646-1650.

20. Community engagement studio toolkit. 2015. Meharry–Vanderbilt Community Engaged Research Core website. https://medschool. vanderbilt.edu/meharry-vanderbilt/files/ meharry-vanderbilt/public_files/CES-Toolkit-web.pdf. Accessed November 16, 2016.

21. Newman SD, Andrews JO, Magwood GS, Jenkins C, Cox MJ, Williamson DC. Community advisory boards in community-based participatory research: A synthesis of best processes. *Prev Chronic Dis*. 2011;8(3):A70.

22. Ramanadhan S, Nagler R, McCloud R, Kohler RE, Viswanath K. Graphic health warnings as activators of social networks: A field experiment among individuals of low socioeconomic position. *Social Sci Med*. 2017;175:219–227.

23. Kellogg Health Scholars: About us—Community health track. 2001. WK Kellogg Foundation website. http://www. kellogghealthscholars.org/about/community. php. Accessed April 12, 2010.

24. Israel BA, Schulz AJ, Parker EA, Becker AB. Review of community-based research: Assessing partnership approaches to improve public health. *Annu Rev Public Health*. 1998;19:173–201.

25. Ramanadhan S, Viswanath K. Engaging communities to improve health: Models, evidence, and the Participatory Knowledge Translation (PaKT) framework. In: Fisher EB, ed. *Principles and Concepts of*

Behavioral Medicine: A Global Handbook. New York: Springer; in press.

26. Gagliardi AR, Berta W, Kothari A, Boyko J, Urquhart R. Integrated knowledge translation (IKT) in health care: A scoping review. *Implement Sci.* 2016;11(1):38.

27. Minkler M, Salvatore AL, Chang C. Participatory approaches for study design and analysis in dissemination and implementation research. In: Brownson RC, Colditz GA, Proctor EK, eds. *Dissemination and Implementation Research in Health.* 2nd ed. New York: Oxford University Press; 2018:175–190.

28. Viswanathan M, Ammerman A, Eng E, et al. Community-based participatory research: Assessing the evidence. *Evid Rep Technol Assess.* 2004;(99):1–8.

29. Minkler M, Wallerstein N, eds. *Community Based Participatory Research in Health.* 2nd ed. San Francisco, CA: Jossey-Bass; 2008.

30. Israel BA, Schulz AJ, Parker EA, Becker AB, Allen AJ III, Guzman R. Critical issues in developing and following CBPR principles. In: Minkler M, Wallerstein N, eds. *Community-Based Participatory Research for Health: From Process to Outcomes.* 2nd ed. San Francisco, CA: Jossey-Bass; 2008:47–66.

31. Israel BA, Schulz AJ, Parker EA, Becker AB. Review of community-based research: Assessing partnership approaches to improve public health. *Annu Rev Public Health.* 1998;19:173–202.

32. Stamatakis KA, Vinson CA, Kerner JF. Dissemination and implementation research in community and public health settings. In: Brownson RC, Colditz GA, Proctor EK, eds. *Dissemination and Implementation Research in Health.* New York: Oxford University Press; 2012:359–383.

33. Green LW. Making research relevant: If it is an evidence-based practice, where's the practice-based evidence? *Fam Pract.* 2008;25(Suppl 1):i20–i24.

34. Green LW, Nasser M. Furthering dissemination and implementation research: The need for more attention to external validity. In: Brownson RC, Colditz GA, Proctor EK, eds. *Dissemination and Implementation Research in Health.* New York: Oxford University Press; 2012:305–326.

35. Glasgow RE, Green LW, Taylor MV, Stange KC. An evidence integration triangle for aligning science with policy and practice. *Am J Prev Med.* 2012;42(6):646–654.

36. Hawe P, Noort M, King L, Jordens C. Multiplying health gains: The critical role of capacity-building within health promotion programs. *Health Policy.* 1997;39(1):29–42.

37. Wallerstein N, Duran B. Community-based participatory research contributions to intervention research: The intersection of science and practice to improve health equity. *Am J Public Health.* 2010;100(Suppl 1):S40–S46.

38. Braun KL, Nguyen TT, Tanjasiri SP, et al. Operationalization of community-based participatory research principles: Assessment of the National Cancer Institute's community network programs. *Am J Public Health.* 2012;102(6):1195–1203.

39. Robinson TE, Rankin N, Janssen A, Mcgregor D, Grieve S, Shaw T. Collaborative research networks in health: A pragmatic scoping study for the development of an imaging network. *Health Res Policy Systems.* 2015;13(1):1.

40. Mason M, Rucker B, Reed M, et al. "I know what CBPR is, now what do I do?" Community perspectives on CBPR capacity building. *Prog Community Health Partnersh.* 2013;7(3):235–241.

41. Schackman BR. Implementation science for the prevention and treatment of HIV/AIDS. *J Acquir Immun Defic Syndr.* 2010;55(Suppl 1):S27.

42. Norton WE, Amico KR, Cornman DH, Fisher WA, Fisher JD. An agenda for advancing the science of implementation of evidence-based HIV prevention interventions. *AIDS Behav.* 2009;13(3):424–429.

43. Garvin D. Building a learning organization. *Harv Bus Rev.* 1993:78–91.

44. Gehlert S, Colditz GA. Cancer disparities: Unmet challenges in the elimination of disparities. *Cancer Epidemiol Biomarkers Prev.* 2011;20(9):1809–1814.

45. DiGirolamo A, Geller AC, Tendulkar SA, Patil P, Hacker K. Community-based participatory research skills and training needs in a sample of academic researchers from a clinical and translational science center in the Northeast. *Clin Transl Sci.* 2012;5(3):301–305.

46. Lobb R, Colditz GA. Implementation science and its application to population health. *Annu Rev Public Health.* 2013;34:235.

47. Laws R, Hesketh K, Ball K, Cooper C, Vrljic K, Campbell K. Translating an early childhood obesity prevention program for local community implementation: A case study of the Melbourne InFANT Program. *BMC Public Health.* 2016;16(1):748.

48. Nix HL. *The Community and Its Involvement in the Study Planning Action Process.* Atlanta, GA: US Department of Health Education and Welfare,

Public Health Service, Centers for Disease Control and Prevention; 1977.

49. Nix HL, Seerley NR. Community reconnaissance method: A synthesis of functions. *Commun Dev Soc.* 1971;2(2):62–69.

50. UCINET for windows: Software for social network analysis [computer program]. Lexington, KY: Analytic Technologies; 2005.

51. Trochim WM, Cabrera DA, Milstein B, Gallagher RS, Leischow SJ. Practical challenges of systems thinking and modeling in public health. *Am J Public Health.* 2006;96(3):538–546.

52. Jenkins EK, Kothari A, Bungay V, Johnson JL, Oliffe JL. Strengthening population health interventions: Developing the CollaboraKTion Framework for Community-Based Knowledge Translation. *Health Res Policy Syst.* 2016;14(1):65.

53. Harrison MB, Graham ID. Roadmap for a participatory research–practice partnership to implement evidence. *Worldviews Evid Based Nurs.* 2012;9(4):210.

54. Saidel JR. Dimensions of interdependence: The state and voluntary-sector relationship. *Nonprofit Voluntary Sector Q.* 1989;18(4):335–347.

55. Maibach EW, Van Duyn MA, Bloodgood B. A marketing perspective on disseminating evidence-based approaches to disease prevention and health promotion. *Prev Chronic Dis.* 2006;3(3):A97.

56. Rabin BA, Glasgow RE, Kerner JF, Klump MP, Brownson RC. Dissemination and implementation research on community-based cancer prevention: A systematic review. *Am J Prev Med.* 2010;38(4):443–456.

57. Teal R, Bergmire DM, Johnston M, Weiner BJ. Implementing community-based provider participation in research: An empirical study. *Implement Sci.* 2012;7:41.

58. Kothari A, Armstrong R. Community-based knowledge translation: Unexplored opportunities. *Implement Sci.* 2011;6:59.

59. Provan KG, Veazie MA, Staten LK, Teufel-Shone NI. The use of network analysis to strengthen community partnerships. *Public Adm Rev.* 2005;65(5):603–613.

60. Center for Tobacco Policy Research–George Warren Brown School of Social Work at Washington University. *Best Practices for Comprehensive Tobacco Control Programs: User Guide—Coalitions.* Atlanta, GA: US Department of Health and Human Services, Centers for Disease Control and Prevention; 2007.

61. Wilson M, Lavis J, Travers R, Rourke S. Community-based knowledge transfer and exchange: Helping community-based organizations link research to action. *Implement Sci.* 2010;5:33.

62. Wallerstein N, Duran B. Community-based participatory research contributions to intervention research: The intersection of science and practice to improve health equity. *Am J Pub Health.* 2010;100:S40–S46.

63. Schulz AJ, Israel BA, Lantz P. Instrument for evaluating dimensions of group dynamics within community-based participatory research partnerships. *Eval Program Plann.* 2003;26(3):249–262.

64. Paige C, Peters R, Parkhurst M, et al. Enhancing community-based participatory research partnerships through appreciative inquiry. *Prog Community Health Partnersh.* 2015;9(3):457–463.

65. Becker AB, Israel BA, Allen A. Strategies and techniques for effective group process in CBPR partnerships. In: Israel BA, Eng E, Schulz AJ, Parker EA, eds. *Methods in Community-Based Participatory Research for Health.* San Francisco, CA: Jossey-Bass; 2005:52–72.

66. Andrews JO, Newman SD, Meadows O, Cox MJ, Bunting S. Partnership readiness for community-based participatory research. *Health Educ Res.* 2012;27(4):555–571.

67. Kegler MC, Rigler J, Honeycutt S. How does community context influence coalitions in the formation stage? A multiple case study based on the Community Coalition Action Theory. *BMC Public Health.* 2010;10(1):1.

68. Chambers D, Simpson L, Hill-Briggs F, et al. Proceedings of the 8th Annual Conference on the Science of Dissemination and Implementation. *Implement Sci.* 2016;11(2):100.

69. Freudenberg N, Tsui E. Evidence, power, and policy change in community-based participatory research. *Am J Public Health.* 2014;104(1):11–14.

70. McCauley MP, Ramanadhan S, Viswanath K. Assessing opinions in community leadership networks to address health inequalities: A case study from Project IMPACT. *Health Educ Res.* 2015;30(6):866–881.

71. Thompson B, Molina Y, Viswanath K, Warnecke R, Prelip ML. Strategies to empower communities to reduce health disparities. *Health Aff (Millwood).* 2016;35(8):1424–1428.

72. Gortmaker SL, Long MW, Resch SC, et al. Cost effectiveness of childhood obesity interventions: Evidence and methods for CHOICES. *Am J Prev Med.* 2015;49(1):102–111.

73. Gortmaker SL, Swinburn BA, Levy D, et al. Changing the future of obesity: Science, policy, and action. *Lancet.* 2011;378(9793):838–847.

74. Haby M, Vos T, Carter R, et al. A new approach to assessing the health benefit from obesity interventions in children and adolescents: The Assessing Cost-Effectiveness in Obesity Project. *Int J Obes.* 2006;30(10):1463–1475.

75. Katz E, Lazarsfeld, P. *Personal Influence. The Part Played by People in the Flow of Mass Communications.* New York: Free Press; 1955.

76. McCombs ME, Shaw DL. The evolution of agenda-setting research: Twenty-five years in the marketplace of ideas. *J Commun.* 1993;43(2):58–67.

77. Watts DJ, Dodds PS. Influentials, networks, and public opinion formation. *J Consumer Res.* 2007;34(4):441–458.

78. Goffman E. *Frame Analysis: An Essay on the Organization of Experience.* Cambridge, MA: Harvard University Press; 1974.

79. Entman RM. Framing: Toward clarification of a fractured paradigm. *J Commun.* 1993;43(4):51–58.

80. Tewksbury D, Scheufele DA. News framing theory and research. In: Bryant J, Oliver M, eds. *Media Effects: Advances in Theory and Research.* 3rd ed. Hillsdale, NJ: Erlbaum; 2009:17–33.

81. Scheufele DA. Agenda-setting, priming, and framing revisited: Another look at cognitive effects of political communication. *Mass Commun Soc.* 2000;3(2–3):297–316.

82. Bleich S. Is it all in a word? The effect of issue framing on public support for US spending on HIV/AIDS in developing countries. *Harvard Int J Press/Politics.* 2007;12(2):120–132.

83. Gitlin T. *The Whole World Is Watching: Mass Media in the Making & Unmaking of the New Left.* Berkeley: University of California Press; 1980.

84. Kosicki GM. Problems and opportunities in agenda-setting research. *J Commun.* 1993;43(2):100–127.

85. Cappella JN, Jamieson KH. *Spiral of Cynicism: The Press and the Public Good.* New York: Oxford University Press; 1997.

86. Weaver DH, Beam RA, Brownlee BJ, Voakes PS, Wilhoit GC. *The American Journalist in the 21st Century: US News People at the Dawn of a New Millennium.* Mahwah, NJ: Erlbaum; 2009.

87. Viswanath K, Blake KD, Meissner HI, et al. Occupational practices and the making of health news: A national survey of US health and medical science journalists. *J Health Commun.* 2008;13(8):759–777.

88. Wallington SF, Blake KD, Taylor-Clark K, Viswanath K. Challenges in covering health disparities in local news media: An exploratory analysis assessing views of journalists. *J Community Health.* 2010;35(5):487–494.

89. McCauley MP, Blake KD, Meissner H, Viswanath K. The social group influences of US health journalists and their impact on the newsmaking process. *Health Educ Res.* 2013;28(2):339–351.

90. Roehrich JK, Lewis MA, George G. Are public–private partnerships a healthy option? A systematic literature review. *Soc Sci Med.* 2014;113:110–119.

91. Fawcett S, Schultz J, Watson-Thompson J, Fox M, Bremby R. Building multisectoral partnerships for population health and health equity. *Prev Chronic Dis.* 2010;7(6):A118.

92. Whyle EB, Olivier J. Models of public–private engagement for health services delivery and financing in southern Africa: A systematic review. *Health Policy Plann.* 2016;31(10):1515–1529.

93. Oluwole Z, Kraemer J. Innovative public–private partnership: A diagonal approach to combating women's cancers in Africa. *Bull World Health Organ.* 2013;91(9):691–696.

94. Valente TW, Gallaher P, Mouttapa M. Using social networks to understand and prevent substance use: A transdisciplinary perspective. *Subst Use Misuse.* 2004;39(10–12):1685–1712.

95. Luke DA, Stamatakis KA. Systems science methods in public health: Dynamics, networks, and agents. *Annu Rev Public Health.* 2012;33:357–376.

96. Valente TW, Palinkas LA, Czaja S, Chu K-H, Brown CH. Social network analysis for program implementation. *PLoS One.* 2015;10(6):e0131712.

97. Program HCPHR. Independent evaluation of Prevention Wellness Trust Fund Initiative. Report submitted to the Massachusetts State Legislature. Boston, MA; in press.

98. Chisti A, Sharara N, Gupta M, et al. A global cancer project map integrating global cancer staCtistics to guide international efforts. *J Global Oncol.* 2016;2(3 Suppl):9s–10s.

99. Trimble EL, Chisti AA, Craycroft JA, et al. Launching an interactive cancer projects map: A collaborative approach to global cancer research and program development. *J Global Oncol.* 2015;1(1):7–10.

100. Koh HK, Oppenheimer SC, Massin-Short SB, Emmons KM, Geller AC, Viswanath K. Translating research evidence into practice to reduce health disparities: A social

determinants approach. *Am J Public Health.* 2010;100(S1):S72–S80.

101. Emmons KM, Viswanath K, Colditz GA. The role of transdisciplinary collaboration in translating and disseminating health research: Lessons learned and exemplars of success. *Am J Prev Med.* 2008;35(2S):S204–S210.

102. Ramanadhan S, Salhi C, Achille E, et al. Addressing cancer disparities via community network mobilization and intersectoral partnerships: A social network analysis. *PLoS One.* 2012;7(2):e32130.

103. Wallerstein N, Oetzel J, Duran B, Tafoya G, Belone L, Rae R. What predicts outcomes in CBPR? In: Minkler M, Wallerstein N, eds. *Community-Based Participatory Research for Health: From Process to Outcomes.* 2nd ed. San Francisco, CA: Jossey-Bass; 2008:371–392.

104. Palinkas LA, Holloway IA, Rice E, Fuentes D, Wu Q, Chamberlain P. Social networks and implementation of evidence-based practices in public youth-serving systems: A mixed-methods study. *Implement Sci.* 2011;6:113.

105. Valente TW. Network interventions. *Science.* 2012;337(6090):49–53.

106. Caplan K, Jones D. Partnership indicators: Measuring effectiveness of multi-sector approaches to service provision. BPD Water and Sanitation Cluster Practitioner note series: Partnership indicators; 2002.

107. Kitson A, Powell K, Hoon E, Newbury J, Wilson A, Beilby J. Knowledge translation within a population health study: How do you do it? *Implement Sci.* 2013;8(1):1.

108. Palinkas LA, Aarons GA, Horwitz S, Chamberlain P, Hurlburt M, Landsverk J. Mixed method designs in implementation research. *Adm Policy Ment Health.* 2011;38(1):44–53.

109. Creswell JW, Plano Clark VL. *Designing and Conducting Mixed Methods Research.* Thousand Oaks, CA: Sage; 2007.

110. Green CA, Duan N, Gibbons RD, Hoagwood KE, Palinkas LA, Wisdom JP. Approaches to mixed methods dissemination and implementation research: Methods, strengths, caveats, and opportunities. *Adm Policy Ment Health.* 2015;42(5):508–523.

111. Creswell JW, Klassen AC, Plano Clark VL, Smith KC. *Best Practices for Mixed Methods Research in the Health Sciences.* Bethesda, MD: National Institutes of Health; 2011.

112. Zakocs RC, Edwards EM. What explains community coalition effectiveness? A review of the literature. *Am J Prev Med.* 2006;30(4):351–361.

113. Mendel P, Meredith LS, Schoenbaum M, Sherbourne CD, Wells KB. Interventions in organizational and community context: A framework for building evidence on dissemination and implementation in health services research. *Adm Policy Ment Health.* 2008;35(1):21–37.

114. Granner M, Sharpe P. Evaluating community coalition characteristics and functioning: A summary of measurement tools. *Health Educ Behav.* 2004;19:514–532.

115. Chambers DA, Glasgow RE, Stange KC. The dynamic sustainability framework: Addressing the paradox of sustainment amid ongoing change. *Implement Sci.* 2013;8:117.

116. Chambers DA, Norton WE. The adaptome: Advancing the science of intervention adaptation. *Am J Prev Med.* 2016;51(4 Suppl):S124–S131.

117. Holmes BJ, Finegood DT, Riley BL, Best A. Systems thinking in dissemination and implementation research. In: Brownson RC, Colditz GA, Proctor EK, eds. *Dissemination and Implementation Research in Health.* New York: Oxford University Press; 2012:175–191.

118. Manning MA, Bollig-Fischer A, Bobovski LB, Lichtenberg P, Chapman R, Albrecht TL. Modeling the sustainability of community health networks: Novel approaches for analyzing collaborative organization partnerships across time. *Transl Behav Med.* 2014;4(1):46–59.

119. Hawe P, Shiell A, Riley T. Theorising interventions as events in systems. *Am J Community Psychol.* 2009;43(3–4):267–276.

120. Brown CH, Kellam SG, Kaupert S, et al. Partnerships for the design, conduct, and analysis of effectiveness, and implementation research: Experiences of the Prevention Science and Methodology Group. *Adm Policy Ment Health.* 2012;39(4):301–316.

121. The Community Guide: Cancer prevention and control. 2011. Centers for Disease Control and Prevention website. http://www.thecommunityguide.org/cancer/index.html. Accessed March 27, 2012.

19

COST-EFFECTIVENESS ANALYSIS IN IMPLEMENTATION SCIENCE

Heather Taffet Gold

IMPLEMENTATION SCIENCE has as its goal to rigorously establish and evaluate the integration of evidence-based health care practices and interventions into everyday use to improve population health. However, to improve the value and relevance of implementation science itself,

information on costs and resources required to deliver an intervention are essential, and often the first question asked by potential decision-makers. All too often, there are no data to answer this question, despite existing methods, and, when present, cost-of-intervention information, for example, is often non-standardized and often does not take the perspective of a potential adopting organization.[1p50]

Cost-effectiveness analysis is a tool used to systematically and quantitatively compare trade-offs between health outcomes and costs of alternative health care interventions with standards set for the United States,[2,3] yet many recommendations may

not coalesce with implementation science methods and do not focus on the implementation process itself. There is a lack of consensus for economic evaluation in implementation science that has resulted in conflicting norms and conventions, which in turn make analyses difficult to compare, raise quality concerns, and may put the relevance of research into question.[4-7] Some implementation studies have emphasized costs and cost analysis and can inform and encourage future investigators to include costs in their implementation analysis.[8-11] This chapter outlines areas for future research and standardization for cost-effectiveness analysis in implementation science.

The Second Panel on Cost-Effectiveness in Health and Medicine provides significant recommendations for the base-case, standardized analyses, referred to as reference cases, and analytic perspectives to improve comparability across studies.[2] The panel now endorses two cost-effectiveness analyses of the same intervention—one from the societal perspective and one from the health care sector perspective. The perspective determines in large part what costs

Table 19.1. Costs to Include by Analytic Perspective

COSTS	SOCIETAL[2,13]	HEALTH CARE SECTOR[2,13]	PATIENT	OTHER PAYER OR PROVIDER[a]
Implementation strategy costs (e.g., staff training, administration, planning, intervention adaptation)	X	X		X
Intervention-specific costs				
Third-party payer costs (e.g., health insurance, county health department) for health care intervention	X	X		P
Patient out-of-pocket costs	X		X	
Patient time costs	X		X	
Productivity costs	X		X	
Informal caregiver costs	X			
Transportation costs	X		X	P
Other costs				
Third-party payer costs (e.g., health insurance, county health department) for future health care consumption	X	X		P
Future productivity costs	X		X	
Other sector costs (e.g., judiciary system, social services, education)	X			P

[a]Examples include a county health department, physician group, community health center, and hospital.
X, include costs; P, potentially include costs, depending on specific payer.

and effects are included in the analysis (Table 19.1). Beyond the analytic perspectives, further guidance for conducting cost-effectiveness analysis in implementation science should be provided for implementation and program costs, health outcomes, incremental cost-effectiveness ratios, time horizon, sensitivity analyses, and possible temporal changes in the intervention.

ANALYTIC PERSPECTIVES

The societal perspective requires that all costs and effects of the alternative interventions be included, regardless of who or what pays or accrues them. The comprehensive, societal perspective requires the following cost categories be included: health care sector costs, intervention-specific costs including the implementation strategy (or strategies), patient and informal caregiver costs (e.g., transportation time and cost), productivity costs (e.g., time lost from work), non-health care costs (e.g., other sectors affected, such as judiciary or police), and future related and unrelated costs (i.e., every downstream cost because someone lives longer). The importance of the societal perspective is that it includes all the "ripple" effects when comparing interventions. For example, one intervention might require more time away from work or more frequent office visits (i.e., patient time), whereas another might burden the judiciary system or informal caregivers more. These impacts can only be evaluated in a societal perspective analysis, in which one considers all the potential upfront and downstream impacts associated with the alternative interventions.

Unlike the societal perspective, the health care sector perspective is much narrower and includes only health care costs paid by third-party payers (e.g., insurance companies) and patient out-of-pocket costs, including downstream health care costs that are consequences of consumption of the initial interventions. This perspective is relevant for decision-makers considering only the health care sector impact when comparing interventions on costs and effectiveness.

In implementation science, it is often the health care system, county health department, hospital, health center, or physician organization that decides whether to adopt a new intervention. Therefore, the costs from these perspectives may be more relevant for consideration by such decision-makers to optimize their choices, and the societal or health care sector perspectives are less informative and useful. Whatever entity implements the new program is responsible for the implementation costs. The health care system or organization perspective is relevant for system-level administrators deciding whether to use an implementation strategy in concert with a health care intervention for their panel of patients and would include all costs (and savings) accrued to the organization and exclude patient out-of-pocket costs. A county health department perspective would include costs incurred only by the health department and not the entire health care sector. The patient or participant perspective is important if patient time, transportation, and out-of-pocket costs would affect uptake or sustainability of the intervention and therefore the success of the intervention. It is critical for the analytic perspective to be stated clearly and follow rules for costs to include so that analyses can be compared fairly.

PROGRAM COSTS TO INCLUDE

Implementation science focuses on studying the implementation of evidence-based interventions or programs to improve population health. Previous work provides guidance for which programmatic costs to include.[11] Program or intervention costs that are required to implement the program elsewhere (e.g., administration, training, and, sometimes, recruitment) should be included and are sometimes called implementation or organizational process costs.[8,10,12] The analysis should answer the question, What would it cost to carry out this intervention in a site somewhere else in the country? This implies that one should exclude research and development costs for the intervention. However, one must include costs associated with adapting the intervention or implementing relevant organizational processes for a new site or population. Pre-implementation costs, such as planning or staffing for the intervention or holding a staff training meeting, should be included in organizational costs,[10] as should the cost of bringing in technical expertise if unavailable on site.[8] Sustaining the implementation might incur follow-up training or intervention adaptation, and those costs associated with sustainability or enhancing fidelity should be included as intervention costs in the analysis.[10] Note that if the relative order of magnitude of costs is large (e.g., phone call vs. hospitalization), the analyst must consider the burden and expense of estimating the much smaller costs if they will not have much impact on the analysis.[13]

Furthermore, although decision-makers may be interested in overall value, their budgets often take a short view, and the upfront implementation costs[12] and possibly 1-year costs for a previously proven implementation strategy or intervention are what matter most in decision-making. In addition, subdividing costs by the relevant analytic perspectives, such as assessing overall societal costs, health care sector costs, and patient or participant costs, can aid in framing the decision and assessing the likelihood of success from those many perspectives. By creating standards for cost-effectiveness analysis, results become generalizable across settings, and decision-makers can assess intervention feasibility in their own environments and for their respective audiences.[10,13]

HEALTH OUTCOMES AND INCREMENTAL COST-EFFECTIVENESS RATIOS

The ultimate outcome in a cost-effectiveness analysis is the incremental cost effectiveness ratio (ICER). This is represented as $[(cost_1 - cost_2)/(outcome_1 - outcome_2)]$, where two interventions are being compared. The Second Panel recommends using the quality-adjusted life-year (QALY) as the primary health outcome in the denominator for the reference case cost-effectiveness analysis.[2] The QALY is calculated by multiplying patient quality of life, in the form of utility values ranging from 0 (death) to 1 (perfect health), by life expectancy. However, in implementation science, researchers may be more concerned with implementing an evidence-based intervention and therefore may not follow patients over the long term—that is, through mortality. It is possible to estimate a QALY through 1 year of follow-up, but that also requires eliciting or estimating patient quality of life, which could burden staff or participants depending on the intervention. Note that some implementation strategies focus on providers or health systems and not on patients or program participants, making quality-of-life and mortality assessment especially challenging.

Because quality of life may be too burdensome to estimate or potentially irrelevant (i.e., the intervention target is not the patient) and follow-up may be short, the comparative analysis must be rethought for implementation science. As a first step, one can conduct a comparative cost analysis by calculating the costs associated with each implementation strategy arm through the end of follow-up, using the perspective of the decision-maker(s) as outlined previously, and keeping an inventory of categories of costs (e.g., cost type, such as training, supplies, brochure printing, physician visits; perspective-related costs, such as health care sector costs, informal health care sector costs, patient/participant costs including lost productivity, and non-health care sector costs; and possibly by phases such as planning, initial rollout, and full implementation). Second, one should calculate the total cost per participant in the study by implementation strategy arm, including implementation costs, and note that the "participant" is defined by whatever target(s) the implementation strategy intends. This might be patients, clinicians, hospitals, physician practices, or others. To get the comparative cost per participant, subtract the average cost per participant of one implementation strategy from that of the other implementation strategy to obtain the incremental cost per participant of using one implementation strategy instead of the other.[6]

Ideally, patient health outcomes can be integrated with the cost analysis to conduct a cost-effectiveness analysis, leading to the analytic outcome of cost per [health unit] gained, or the incremental cost per incremental improvement in health outcome unit. Determining the health outcome to use depends on (1) the intervention implemented and (2) whether the analysis will include long-term follow-up and/or simulation modeling such as decision analysis. The disease-specific health outcome should relate to the intervention. For example, if one were studying tobacco cessation, then cost per tobacco quit would be relevant. If one were studying weight loss, then the outcome might be cost per person achieving goal weight, cost per person achieving healthy body mass index, or cost per person achieving 5% weight loss. One issue to note with the last example is that the analysis would not account for participants who gain weight. For a program improving physicians' adherence to clinical guidelines for cancer screening, the outcome could be cost per physician adhering to guidelines, with some potential patient-level analysis of cost per patient receiving guideline-concordant screening. These shorter term outcomes are useful for comparing implementation strategies for evidence-based interventions only within the same disease or health behavior category.

Ultimately, however, the goal is to link short-term health outcomes (e.g., cost per tobacco quit and cost per tumor identified) to the proven long-term health benefit of the evidence-based intervention in order to compare strategies across a multitude of health conditions and be able to prioritize interventions given a limited budget. Importantly, the analyst should estimate how much money must be spent to obtain an increase in population health outcomes, such as improved life expectancy or quality-adjusted life expectancy. For this, one must either follow patients (either directly or through the recipient of the intervention, such as the provider or health system) to a mortality outcome or consider simulation modeling (discussed in the next section).

TIME HORIZON

With implementation science, the limited duration of follow-up of a given intervention makes downstream costs and effects difficult to measure. One suggestion is to estimate at least 1 year of follow-up—that is, plan for a minimum 1-year time horizon, even if intervention follow-up is less than 1 year. One can estimate the downstream costs and effects through complementary data sources, if necessary.

It is difficult to know the true value of an intervention if only short-term outcomes are assessed, however. There may be a spillover of the intervention's effects to other health conditions besides the immediate ones or a substitution of services more probable with the new intervention. For example, getting people to quit smoking prior to surgery will not only decrease short-term risks, such as long hospital stays or surgical complications, but also reduce lung cancer and heart disease risks later in life. An intervention to increase human papillomavirus vaccination would increase upfront office or health department visits but reduce downstream utilization of surgery and hospitalization for cervical cancer.

As a solution, simulation modeling to the ultimate outcome of cost per QALY gained may be preferable when many expected intervention impacts are beyond follow-up. Building one's own model for the condition under study, collaborating with investigators who have already built a relevant simulation model, or adapting a published model are all solutions to modeling to this long-term outcome.

EXTENSIVE SENSITIVITY ANALYSIS

As outlined by the Second Panel,[13] sensitivity analysis and transparency are key to credibility in cost-effectiveness analysis. Any analysis or model is based on a multitude of decisions—which costs to include, which effects to include, and how to obtain the estimates of each—and therefore must be detailed fully so that the analysis can be replicated. Several issues are particularly relevant for cost-effectiveness analyses in implementation science: program or intervention capacity, cost categories to include, time horizon, potential target population, and setting and location where the intervention is implemented.

Because interventions can take time and experience to build to full capacity, the analyst may want to consider aspects of program capacity in primary and sensitivity analyses. First, it is important to examine the rollout of the intervention in stages and identify if it is working at full capacity following initial implementation and throughout the intervention. For example, are all intervention staff working at full capacity, or could they serve more patients (or other intervention target)? Is there an initial rollout period running at reduced volume while staff learns the intervention? If so, the initial startup period and subsequent program periods should be analyzed as separate components until the program is at full capacity; analysis by month can be very useful for assessing volume changes. If the intervention never appears to run at full capacity, in addition to a standard analysis, the analyst should approximate optimal capacity and estimate a cost per outcome as if the program were at full capacity—that is, vary the size of the target population to answer the question, What is the maximum size target population for the same total cost?

Using national average cost estimates provides important information for decision-makers considering implementing a new program in a different geographic location from the original study. This conforms to the societal perspective because it is more generalizable and represents average wages throughout the country rather than a localized wage rate. In addition, applying a range of cost values from lowest possible program cost to highest possible cost—for example, by using ranges of wage rates—represents a best case versus worst case scenario that can be helpful for decision-makers. Furthermore, for wage estimates, national average wage rates plus fringe (i.e., the cost of benefits)[13] by worker type for each staffperson yield a relevant, generalizable cost estimate, and sensitivity analysis should consider substitution of workers or setting that might change the cost of an intervention (e.g., social worker/psychologist/mental health counselor; and physician office/hospital/public health clinic). Separating cost categories and providing category estimates allow decision-makers to modify estimates to the local setting or exclude explicitly some cost categories that might be irrelevant to their setting.

DECISION ABOUT WHETHER TO CONDUCT COST-EFFECTIVENESS ANALYSIS

There are two points at which cost-effectiveness analysis can be used to drive implementation: initial or local implementation and broader scale-up. Prior to implementation, there should be data suggesting that an intervention is efficacious. A cost-effectiveness analysis could then be conducted to determine whether the intervention implemented under optimal conditions is valuable and therefore should be scaled widely. Sensitivity analyses would highlight whether under all scenarios the intervention remains cost-effective and which variables change the optimal decision and therefore need either more study on effectiveness or to be explored in wider implementation. For example, there might be economies of scale (i.e., larger target population) or learning curves (e.g., efficiency gains with more staff experience) that decrease costs or increase effectiveness; these factors could be explored more fully in an implementation study. The cost-effectiveness analysis with a long-term time horizon, and potentially a value-of-information analysis building on the analytic model, may inform sample size or adaptation of the implementation strategy and the intervention for broader implementation.

The other point at which to consider cost-effectiveness analysis is when the initial implementation project is completed. If in that scenario the implemented intervention is not cost-effective, or is never cost-effective through all reasonable assumptions, then the intervention should not be further scaled-up because its value is not proven.

As the field of implementation science matures, one can think about fully integrating cost-effectiveness analysis into it. Researchers seeking to include cost-effectiveness analysis in their studies might consider attending to some of the following recommendations:

1. Include experts in cost-effectiveness analysis on teams for implementation studies to assess the value of research findings for subsequent implementation and scale-up.

2. Expand the focus of cost-effectiveness analysis to include implementation strategies for evidence-based interventions.

3. Consider inclusion of both societal and sectoral perspectives by carefully considering decision-makers' perspectives and types of costs that are likely to affect adoption, implementation, fidelity, and sustainability.

4. Be explicit about each included category and type of cost data, its source, and how it is calculated in order to enhance transparency and improve adoption decisions by others. Develop and use an expanded Impact Inventory as outlined by the Second Panel to clarify scope and boundaries of analyses.[2]

5. Make all assumptions in cost-effectiveness analyses clear and unambiguous, from durability of the implemented intervention's effect to time

horizon, analytic perspective(s), and reasons for including or excluding specific costs. Test the robustness of results and the impact of these assumptions through extensive sensitivity analyses.

6. Conduct future research that considers relevant and appropriate cost-effectiveness thresholds and the effects of using multiple analytic perspectives on decision-making.

7. Consider conducting a budget impact analysis, combining the total population eligible and the cost per unit, to assess the affordability and sustainability of the implemented intervention for the payer.[14]

8. Consider cost-effectiveness analyses alongside other emerging themes in implementation science (e.g., de-implementation, local adaptation, sustainability, and genomic medicine).

SUMMARY

In order to assess the value of implementing evidence-based interventions to improve population health, we need standards and guidelines for analysis to improve the quality, rigor, transparency, and, ultimately, comparability of cost-effectiveness analyses in implementation science. Much work needs to focus on adapting and building on current guidelines, taking as a starting point the Second Panel on Cost-Effectiveness in Health and Medicine[13] and then going beyond by explicitly including costs of implementation strategies themselves in the analysis.

REFERENCES

1. Neta G, Glasgow RE, Carpenter CR, et al. A framework for enhancing the value of research for dissemination and implementation. *Am J Public Health*. 2015;105(1):49–57. doi:10.2105/AJPH.2014.302206

2. Sanders GD, Neumann PJ, Basu A, et al. Recommendations for conduct, methodological practices, and reporting of cost-effectiveness analyses. *JAMA*. 2016;316(10):1093. doi:10.1001/jama.2016.12195

3. Gold MR, Siegel JE, Russell LB, Weinstein MC. *Cost-Effectiveness in Health and Medicine*. New York: Oxford University Press; 1996.

4. Grimshaw J, Thomas R, MacLennan G, et al. Effectiveness and efficiency of guideline dissemination and implementation strategies. *Health Technol Assess*. 2004;8(6):1–72. doi:10.3310/hta8060

5. Hoomans T, Severens JL. Economic evaluation of implementation strategies in health care. *Implement Sci.* 2014;9(1):168. doi:10.1186/s13012-014-0168-y

6. Lau R, Stevenson F, Ong BN, et al. Achieving change in primary care—Effectiveness of strategies for improving implementation of complex interventions: Systematic review of reviews. *BMJ Open.* 2015;5(12):e009993. doi:10.1136/bmjopen-2015-009993

7. Peek CJ, Glasgow RE, Stange KC, Klesges LM, Purcell EP, Kessler RS. The 5 R's: An emerging bold standard for conducting relevant research in a changing world. *Ann Fam Med.* 2014;12(5):447–455. doi:10.1370/afm.1688

8. Liu C-F, Rubenstein L V, Kirchner JE, et al. Organizational cost of quality improvement for depression care. *Health Serv Res.* 2009;44(1):225–244. doi:10.1111/j.1475-6773.2008.00911.x

9. Proctor E, Silmere H, Raghavan R, et al. Outcomes for implementation research: Conceptual distinctions, measurement challenges, and research agenda. *Adm Policy Ment Health.* 2011;38(2):65–76. doi:10.1007/s10488-010-0319-7

10. Saldana L, Chamberlain P, Bradford WD, Campbell M, Landsverk J. The Cost of Implementing New Strategies (COINS): A method for mapping implementation resources using the stages of implementation completion. *Child Youth Serv Rev.* 2014;39:177–182. doi:10.1016/j.childyouth.2013.10.006

11. Ritzwoller DP, Sukhanova A, Gaglio B, Glasgow RE. Costing behavioral interventions: A practical guide to enhance translation. *Ann Behav Med.* 2009;37(2):218–227. doi:10.1007/s12160-009-9088-5

12. Lang JM, Connell CM. Measuring costs to community-based agencies for implementation of an evidence-based practice. *J Behav Health Serv Res.* 2017;44(1):122–134. doi:10.1007/s11414-016-9541-8

13. Neumann PJ, Sanders GD, Russell LB, Siegel JE, Ganiats TG. *Cost-Effectiveness in Health and Medicine.* 2nd ed. New York: Oxford University Press; 2017.

14. Brown PM, Cameron LD, Ramondt S. Sustainability of behavioral interventions: Beyond cost-effectiveness analysis. *Int J Behav Med.* 2015;22(3):425–433. doi:10.1007/s12529-014-9437-z

20

FUTURE DIRECTIONS IN IMPLEMENTATION SCIENCE ACROSS THE CANCER CONTINUUM

Wynne E. Norton, Cynthia A. Vinson, and David A. Chambers

THE FIELD of implementation science in health has made considerable progress in the past decade, including in cancer control and prevention. Researchers, practitioners, policymakers, patients, and funding agencies have all played a critical role in acknowledging the need for more evidence-based practices and moving toward identifying ways in which such practices can more quickly and efficiently be integrated into routine health care and public health settings. As the field reflects on accomplishments and advancements, one must also consider emerging challenges and outstanding issues in need of additional research.

In this chapter, we provide an overview of three issues in implementation science in health that warrant additional consideration and attention: minimum criteria for implementation, implementation strategies 2.0, and generalizability of implementation science (Table 20.1). These topics have been mentioned in the literature briefly, and some have already become mainstream in other scientific disciplines (e.g., reproducibility in psychology,

economics, and cancer biology).[1-3] Our goal is to increase focus on these areas of inquiry and highlight some specific challenges and concerns that implementation science may encounter. We take a critical yet constructive approach to these issues and, in doing so, hope to challenge the field to begin to address these topics.

MINIMUM CRITERIA TO WARRANT IMPLEMENTATION OF EVIDENCE-BASED INTERVENTIONS

The evidence base for health-focused interventions, practices, programs, guidelines, and treatments is traditionally conceptualized as a hierarchy,[4,5] ranging from least rigorous evidence in support of (or against) an intervention to most rigorous evidence in support of (or against) an intervention. The level of evidence is broadly based on the ability of the research design to minimize bias and increase the probability that results from the study accurately reflect the phenomena under examination (i.e.,

Table 20.1. Overview of Select Implementation Science Topics Areas for Future Research

TOPIC AREA	KEY ISSUES
Minimum criteria for implementation of evidence-based interventions	• Is there a minimum level of evidence needed to justify implementation of evidence-based interventions? • What is the process for determining the minimum level of evidence? What criteria should be used (e.g., sample size, effect size, confidence interval, and study design)? • Should the standard of evidence be consistent across types of interventions?
Implementation strategies 2.0	• What is the optimal level of fidelity for implementation strategies? What are some validated measures for assessing fidelity of implementation strategies? • What types of strategies are most appropriate and effective for broad (*vs.* limited) scale-up? • What strategies are needed during the sustainability phase?
Generalizability of implementation science	• How can we maximize the generalizability of implementation science? What are some aspects of implementation science that limit external validity (e.g., selection bias) and how can they be overcome? • How can issues related to reproducibility and replication be addressed in implementation science? • How can we better address questions that are of importance to practitioners and systems in addition to patients?

Does this intervention change a health outcome or health behavior among participants?). Evidence hierarchies are often interpreted as prioritizing internal validity to the detriment of external validity. Recently developed study approaches—such as pragmatic trials—make an effort to simultaneously maximize internal validity by using rigorous study designs (e.g., experimental and quasi-experimental designs such as randomized controlled trials, cluster-randomized controlled trials, interrupted time series, and regression discontinuity[6]) and maximize external validity by attending to various elements in the design of the trial (e.g., recruitment strategies, participants, and planned analyses[7]). Examples at the lower end of the evidence hierarchy include evidence derived from anecdotes, consensus panels, and expert opinion.[4,5] Evidence derived from observational study designs (e.g., case controlled studies and cohort studies) is in the middle range of the hierarchy.[4,5] Evidence derived from experimental and quasi-experimental study designs is considered at the upper end of the evidence hierarchy, with meta-analyses and systematic reviews at the top of the hierarchy.[4,5]

The quality and amount of evidence needed to justify implementation of a practice, program, or intervention, however, have yet to be a mainstream topic in implementation science. Of course, researchers, practitioners, and funding agencies alike prefer to see some type of evidence to support the use of a practice, program, or intervention that is the focus of an implementation study. Standards for the minimum quality and amount of evidence needed to warrant proceeding to an implementation study, however, are non-existent. There are certainly strong arguments for and against setting a minimum standard of evidence for an intervention prior to broader implementation, as summarized in Table 20.2.

There are many arguments against establishing minimum standards of evidence for interventions before broader use. One argument is that evidence standards may need to be applied consistently across all interventions or at least a subset of interventions; if it is the latter, the set of interventions that are

Table 20.2. Key Questions and Select Considerations for Establishing Minimum Evidence Criteria for Implementation

QUESTION	SELECT CONSIDERATIONS
What should be the minimum quality of evidence needed to justify implementation of an intervention in a study?	• Is evidence from a randomized study design necessary, sufficient, and/or feasible? • Should there be a minimum effect size, sample size, confidence interval, or other metric of impact to warrant broader implementation?
What should be the minimum quantity of evidence needed to justify implementation of an intervention in a study?	• How many randomized trials are needed to justify implementation? • Is evidence from several observational studies sufficient to warrant implementation?
Should the quality and/or amount of evidence needed to justify implementation vary by type of intervention (e.g., diagnostic test, surgical procedure, drug/medication, behavioral therapy, media campaign, and physical activity program)?	• Should biomedical interventions (e.g., drugs, surgical procedures, and diagnostic tests) have a higher standard of evidence given increased potential for harmful side effects compared to public health interventions? • Should the standard of evidence be higher for interventions that are used more frequently than those used less often?
Should the quality and/or amount of evidence needed to justify implementation vary by type of target population or delivery setting?	• What are the ethical considerations for requiring the same quality and/or amount of evidence for understudied or traditionally marginalized populations? • Should the evidence standard be higher to reduce the likelihood for de-implementation? Should it be lower to make interventions more readily available?

encompassed within a minimum evidence standard may be challenging and at some point obviate the objective of setting standards. For example, should cancer prevention interventions (e.g., physical activity, diet, and sun safety) be subject to one minimum evidence standard (e.g., at least one pre–post study with a minimum of 200 participants, 9-month follow-up, and medium effect size) and cancer treatment interventions subject to another standard (e.g., at least three randomized controlled clinical trials with a minimum combined sample size of 8,500 patients, 3-year follow-up, and medium effect size)? Should the same minimum level of evidence be set for interventions across target populations, which may disproportionately disadvantage populations for whom health conditions or diseases are rare (e.g., aggressive natural killer cell leukemia), emergent, and/or racial and ethnic minority populations for whom fewer interventions exist?

There are certainly many arguments in favor of establishing a minimum level of evidence for interventions to justify broader implementation. These arguments center on preventing the need for future de-implementation of the intervention, to the extent that it is found to be harmful, ineffective, and/or of low value in future studies. Thus, establishing a minimum level of evidence before widespread use may prevent—or at least reduce—the need for future de-implementation of that intervention. Of course, newer, cheaper, more efficient, and more effective interventions will continue to be developed and tested, but setting strong, minimum standards of evidence may reduce the probability of needing to de-implement at least some interventions in the future. Relatedly, implementing interventions before establishing a minimum standard of evidence may be a poor use of resources, to the extent that an intervention requires resources to be de-implemented in the future or if the intervention has a small effect size and thus limited resources may be better allocated to an intervention with a greater impact on outcomes. Implementing interventions prematurely—without a strong level of evidence—increases the likelihood of a medical reversal,[8,9] which, over time, may erode public trust in the biomedical research enterprise.

Currently, there exist many compendiums of interventions that must meet certain eligibility criteria—often including, but not limited to, a minimum level of evidence. For example, the National Cancer Institute's (NCI) Research-Tested Intervention Programs (RTIPs) compendium only includes interventions that have a positive effect on one or more behavioral or psychological outcomes and have been tested using an experimental or quasi-experimental study design, among other criteria.[10] The Centers for Disease Control and Prevention's (CDC) compendium of HIV-focused interventions is assessed and rated for "best-evidence" or "good-evidence" based on a priori criteria (e.g., strength of evidence and study design) established by the Prevention Research Synthesis team.[11,12] The Substance Abuse and Mental Health Services Administration's National Registry of Evidence-based Programs and Practices (NREPP) has minimum requirements that must be met to be considered for the compendium, including (1) assessment of substance use- or mental health-related outcome, (2) experimental or quasi-experimental study design, (3) no-treatment control group, and (4) publication in peer-reviewed journal or comparable scientific outlet.[13] The US Preventive Services Task Force (USPSTF) uses a grading system to rate the quality of research on health services and practices (i.e., Grades A, B, C, D, and I) and make corresponding suggestions for actual use in practice (i.e., Grades A and B: Offer or provide service; Grade C: Offer or provide service for selected patients; Grade D: Discourage use of service; Grade I [Insufficient]: Consult clinical considerations section of USPSTF Recommendation Section to inform use).[14] Importantly, grades influence whether practices and services are covered and paid for by commercial payers,[14] thereby influencing the extent to which a practice or service will be adopted and integrated into routine settings.

Although criteria are not standardized, these compendiums have similar requirements for minimum level of evidence to support use in practice. However, the extent to which these or similar criteria may be used across all types of health practices, programs, interventions, guidelines, and policies is questionable and has yet to be addressed. If established, the minimum standard of evidence may change over time, depending on advances in interventions, needs among target populations, and evolution in thinking in what constitutes an evidence base. Future efforts may begin to grapple with whether and, if so, how to set minimum standards of evidence to warrant implementation.

IMPLEMENTATION STRATEGIES 2.0

Research has identified, operationalized, and evaluated approaches for facilitating the adoption, implementation, and sustainability of evidence-based practices, programs, interventions, and guidelines—otherwise known as implementation strategies.[15] Indeed, as detailed by Powell and colleagues, more than 70 discrete implementation strategies have been identified through a combination of expert input and systematic review;[16,17] many of these have been tested in experimental or quasi-experimental trials, and the field is beginning to identify combinations of strategies that significantly increase the use of practices in routine settings. Moreover, researchers have provided guidance on how best to define, describe, and operationalize implementation strategies[15,18] and have reported guidelines for publication in peer-reviewed journals.[19] As Gold explores in Chapter 19 of this volume, cost-effectiveness of implementation strategies—separate from cost-effectiveness of evidence-based interventions—is in the early stages of development. Certainly, cost-effectiveness of implementation strategies has important practical implications as one seeks to scale up not only evidence-based practices but also the corresponding implementation strategies through which they are scaled. In addition to cost-effectiveness, several other aspects of implementation strategies may be ripe for future research, including fidelity, scale-up, and sustainability.

Fidelity of Implementation Strategies

Although traditionally conceptualized in the literature as the extent to which evidence-based interventions are delivered as originally intended,[20,21] and differentiating between core intervention components and peripheral intervention components that may or may not be moderately versus significantly adapted while retaining impact,[22,23] the concept of fidelity can also be applied to implementation strategies. Strategies such as coaching, external facilitation, organizational change, and audit and feedback[17] are undoubtedly delivered with varying degrees of fidelity within and outside of the context of a study. For example, research assistants may serve as external facilitators and coaches in a trial comparing a compilation of implementation strategies to an implementation-as-usual condition. Per protocol, research assistants would be trained in external facilitation and coaching, and they would deploy such strategies (in the experimental arm of the trial) to increase the adoption, implementation, and sustainability of motivational interviewing[24] delivered by oncologists to increase physical activity among ovarian cancer patients, for example. Fidelity assessments would determine the extent to which oncologists are able to effectively deliver motivational interviewing to patients per prespecified minimal fidelity criteria[25,26] and ideally assess any change in patients' physical activity as a measure of both intervention effectiveness and implementation fidelity.

The extent to which research assistants (in a relatively explanatory implementation trial[7,27]) or everyday personnel from professional societies, practice organizations, or consultants (in a relatively pragmatic implementation trial[7]) deliver implementation strategies with fidelity has received relatively little attention in the literature to date. As with interventions targeting individual-level behavior change across the cancer control continuum (e.g., adherence to chemoprevention, increase in physical activity, reduction in sugar intake, completion of home-based colorectal cancer screening tests, and completion of treatment),[10] so, too, are implementation strategies likely to have some minimum level of fidelity with which they should be delivered. Emerging work has focused on ways to select and tailor implementation strategies[18] and ways to document what changes occur to interventions during the adaptation process;[21] a natural extension would be to focus on adaptation and fidelity of implementation strategies and the degree to which these aspects affect implementation outcomes. Identifying an optimal balance between adaptation

of implementation strategies to improve contextual fit and the fidelity with which strategies should be delivered to maximize impact may be a topic for future research.

Scaling-Up Implementation Strategies

Scaling-up evidence-based practices and requisite implementation strategies is another important area in implementation science. The robust literature on scale-up[28–31] includes frameworks, barriers, facilitators, and strategies for bringing an evidence-based practice to the regional, national, or international level. Future research may focus on the extent to which implementation strategies are needed, appropriate, and feasible for local delivery among relatively few clinics, organizations, or public health settings (e.g., 50 or fewer sites) compared to strategies that are needed, appropriate, and feasible for scale-up at the state, regional, national, or international level (e.g., greater than 50 sites, often hundreds or thousands). Moreover, research is needed on how best to package and deploy implementation strategies coupled with evidence-based practices. For example, "implementation toolkits" are commonly developed strategies used to support adoption, implementation, and sustainability of evidence-based practices.[17] To some extent, such implementation toolkits are reminiscent of intervention manuals or "interventions-in-a-box" that, although helpful, are likely insufficient to lead to widespread use. Should we expect implementation toolkits to be different? If not, can we apply the same principles used to optimally package and disseminate evidence-based practices to implementation strategies? What alternative dissemination outlets can be leveraged to distribute effective implementation strategies? Certainly, as with interventions, peer-reviewed publications and conference presentations are a good start, but they often do not reach the intended end-user. Stakeholder organizations involved in the development and testing of the implementation toolkit are certainly primed to use it beyond the research study, but what efforts can or should be made to extend the reach to other potential adopters of the toolkit and corresponding intervention? These are just a few of the many questions about the scalability of implementation strategies ripe for future research.

Sustainability of Implementation Strategies

Research is also needed on the sustainability of implementation strategies. Typical studies on sustainability examine the extent to which an evidence-based intervention is delivered over time following the use of implementation strategies to facilitate adoption and implementation.[32,33] Although time frames vary (e.g., sustainability of an evidence-based program has been studied between 6 months and 6 years), recommendations suggest that sustainability should be studied no sooner than 1 year post-completion of study funding.[31] To what extent do implementation strategies need to be delivered over time to ensure the sustainability of evidence-based interventions? Outside the context of a study, by whom would such strategies be delivered, and how would those organizations be trained to deliver them? What would trigger the need for implementation strategies to be deployed during the sustainability phase—hiring new staff, availability of a new and more cost-effective evidence-based intervention, poor fidelity with which an intervention is being delivered, organizational restructuring, or change in providers' scope of work? What type of strategies are most needed over time, how might those strategies change over time, and when should they be delivered?

As with the sustainability of evidence-based practices, there are several challenges in studying the sustainability of implementation strategies. First, it is difficult to study the long-term sustainability of strategies within the limited time frame of typical grant opportunities. Second, studying sustainability of implementation strategies necessitates that (1) the evidence-based intervention is implemented and (2) an infrastructure exists for strategies to be delivered over time. Finally, trials to test approaches to facilitate the sustainability of implementation strategies may be neither generalizable nor feasible outside the context of a well-funded study.

The next wave of research may seek to address fidelity, scale-up, and sustainability of implementation strategies. Issues that have been raised with respect to evidence-based interventions—fidelity, scale-up, sustainability, cost-effectiveness, adaptation, and others—are certainly applicable to implementation strategies. For example, efforts to expand the use of evidence-based interventions in practice may similarly guide the use of evidence-based strategies. Compendiums of implementation strategies—complete with interactive tools for identifying the most appropriate and effective compilation of strategies by intervention type, delivery setting, resource availability, and context—may serve to accelerate the spread of strategies into community and delivery settings. As with evidence-based practices, such an approach would create the opportunity for researchers to study the process of selecting, adapting, deploying, and sustaining strategies *in vivo*. Designing implementation strategies with end-users in mind is also applicable, to the extent that well-resourced, effective, yet highly impractical strategies are tested in trials. Research designs that incorporate the specific elements for pragmatic designs[7] into implementation trials will develop more actionable and purposeful results compared to those with explanatory elements. The divide between research and practice lies not only between evidence-based interventions and everyday settings but also between evidence-based implementation strategies and everyday delivery. As we move toward implementation strategies 2.0, the field can benefit from advances it has already made in the development, testing, and dissemination of health-focused practices, programs, and interventions.

GENERALIZABILITY OF IMPLEMENTATION SCIENCE

A major theme throughout implementation science is external validity—essentially, the extent to which the results of a study are generalizable to similar or comparable populations and settings.[6] Indeed, implementation science is built on the need for more practice-based research—research that is actionable, applicable, and relevant to patients, providers, organizations, systems, and populations.[34,35] Generally speaking, implementation science acknowledges the importance of internal validity, but it places equal or greater weight on external validity, to the extent that findings from implementation science are intended to generate information that can improve population health outcomes and address practical yet vexing issues. Classifications of types of research to understand and address important applied questions (compared to pure basic research) have been suggested by Stokes[36] and Chalmers and colleagues.[37] Moreover, efforts to increase external validity while maintaining internal validity have led to calls for more pragmatic study designs, partnership research, multidisciplinary teams, and stakeholder engagement to increase the relevance and application of research to everyday settings.

Certainly, efforts in implementation science to move beyond the traditional highly resourced, artificially situated, expertly conducted efficacy trials have generated invaluable knowledge. But are there other ways in which we might increase the external validity and generalizability of implementation studies? As we enter a more mature state of the science, how can implementation science maximize external validity while maintaining internal validity? Here, we offer a few considerations.

Diversity of Participants and Partnerships

Implementation science studies are conducted with a variety of provider, team, and organizational participants. Examples include Federally Qualified Health Centers (FQHCs), NCI-designated cancer centers, community oncology practices (e.g., the NCI Community Oncology Research Program [NCORP]), public health departments,[38] and academic–community partnerships (e.g., the CDC- and NCI-funded Cancer Prevention and Control Research Network [CPCRN]). These settings and providers are invaluable networks and sites in which implementation science studies take place, especially with respect to cancer control and prevention.

Enrolling diverse participants (i.e., individuals or patients) in trials is important to ensure the applicability of study findings to broader populations who would benefit from the research. But how reflective are providers, organizations, and settings that participate in implementation studies of the overall population from which they are sampled? To what extent is there a selection bias in the types of providers, organizations, and settings that are willing and able to participate in implementation studies, and what can be done to expand participation among traditionally understudied settings? Is there a selection bias that favors providers and organizations that are likely to score high on readiness to implement an evidence-based practice, and how might that constrain the generalizability to other settings that might score lower on readiness? As with understudied target populations, are there particular approaches that can be adapted (e.g., community-based participatory research) to increase participation among understudied providers, organizations, and settings? Attention to these issues and deliberate efforts to increase the diversity of participation of providers, organizations, and settings will help expand the application and generalizability of implementation science.

Reproducibility of Results

Related to both the minimum level of evidence needed to warrant implementation and the generalizability of research findings, the reproducibility of research is an important issue that has received relatively little attention among the implementation science community to date. Reproducibility can be defined as

> the ability of a researcher to duplicate the results of a prior study using the same materials as were used by the original investigator. That is, a second researcher might use the same raw data to build the same analysis files and implement the same statistical analysis in an attempt to yield the same results.[39]

Relatedly, replication is defined as "the ability of a researcher to duplicate the results of a prior study if the same procedures are followed but new data are collected."[39] The National Institutes of Health has increasingly focused on enhancing the reproducibility of research results including policies to support reproducibility in the form of enforced registration of clinical trials, transparency, results reporting, and grant application criteria.[40] Prominent biomedical journals, per policy from the International Committee of Medical Journal Editors, will soon require data sharing statements and data sharing plans as criteria for publication.[41] Reproducibility and replication are critical processes in science; although they have received attention in other fields,[2,42] they have yet to become mainstream in the field of implementation science.

To the extent that implementation science may be subject to the same biases and external pressures as have been found in other scientific disciplines,[43,44] future work is needed to increase transparency and reproducibility in implementation studies. Researchers and funding agencies alike can support data sharing policies, registration of trial protocols, and a supportive scientific culture that embraces best practices in the conduct of research to increase accuracy and potential health impact.[43] Replicating implementation studies—and trials in particular—may be quite time-intensive, costly, and logistically challenging; instead, enhancing transparency and reproducibility of results may be a more appropriate goal.

Prominent questions regarding transparency and reproducibility in implementation science overlap significantly with those in other research areas. For example, what type of data should researchers share? Who should have access to these data? Should researchers be required to share trial protocols and receive feedback from the research community prior to recruitment and enrollment? How can we engender a supportive environment that encourages and rewards transparency and reproducibility without attacking the credibility of research teams or the field?

There are also questions that are more unique to implementation science. For example, what are some ethical issues to consider when sharing data from implementation studies, particularly with respect to multilevel data from individuals/patients, providers, organizations, systems, and communities? How can confidentiality and privacy be respected when conducting partnership research in which data are derived from participating health care or public health organizations and the communities that they serve? As these issues become more prominent in other scientific disciplines, implementation science will need to consider how transparency, reproducibility, and data sharing can be adopted as best practices in the research enterprise.

Practitioner-Centered Research

Patient-centered research, broadly interpreted as conducting research with patients on topics and issues important to the patients,[45–48] has become an increasingly common theme throughout health care and public health research. Implementation science can extend this type of thinking to practitioners, teams, organizations, delivery settings, and systems, such that research questions are those identified and prioritized not only by patients but also by those entities entrusted to deliver evidence-based practices and services. Infrastructure (e.g., a web-based system for submitting and collating ideas) or surveys (e.g., annual surveys of major health care and public health practitioners in cancer control and prevention) could be developed to systematically capture practitioners' questions or concerns; subsequently, these questions could be reviewed by research teams and also be a research–practice matchmaking service. The concept of practice-based research should expand beyond

patients' input and research in everyday settings; it should include practitioner-, team-, and organizational-based research to answer questions about pressing issues with regard to the experiences of those in these everyday settings, some but not all of which may directly concern patient–provider interaction. Increasing the involvement of cancer prevention and control practitioners, agencies, and organizations in the conduct of research *and* the generation of research questions may help advance the field while simultaneously reducing the research-to-practice gap.

SUMMARY

In this chapter, we identified several emerging issues for the field to consider as it continues to evolve and mature. To accelerate the research-to-practice transition, we focused our suggestions on considerations for establishing a minimum level of evidence to warrant implementation of interventions, advancing implementation strategies (i.e., fidelity, scale-up, and sustainability), and maximizing the generalizability of implementation science. We hope these are but some of the many issues that the research and practice communities will consider exploring in more depth in the future.

REFERENCES

1. Managing and Adapting Practice (MAP). 2017. PracticeWise website. https://www.practicewise.com/Community/MAP.
2. Errington TM, Iorns E, Gunn W, Tan FE, Lomax J, Nosek BA. An open investigation of the reproducibility of cancer biology research. *Elife* 2014;3:e04333.
3. Hamermesh DS. Replication in economics. *Can J Econ.* 2007;40:715–733.
4. Ball C, Sackett D, Phillips B, Haynes B, Straus S, Dawes M. Levels of evidence and grades of recommendations. 2001. Centre for Evidence-based Medicine website. http://cebm jr2.ox.ac.uk/docs/levels html.
5. Evidence-Based Medicine Working Group. Evidence-based medicine: A new approach to teaching the practice of medicine. *JAMA* 1992;268:2420.
6. Cook TD, Campbell DT, Day A. *Quasi-experimentation: Design & Analysis Issues for Field Settings.* Boston, MA: Houghton Mifflin; 1979.
7. Loudon K, Treweek S, Sullivan F, Donnan P, Thorpe KE, Zwarenstein M. The PRECIS-2

tool: Designing trials that are fit for purpose. *BMJ.* 2015;350:h2147.

8. Prasad V, Vandross A, Toomey C, Cheung M, Rho J, Quinn S, Chacko SJ, Borkar D, Gall V, Selvaraj S. A decade of reversal: An analysis of 146 contradicted medical practices. *Mayo Clin Proc.* 2013;88(8):790–798.

9. Prasad V, Gall V, Cifu A. The frequency of medical reversal. *Arch Intern Med.* 2011;171:1675–1676.

10. Research-Tested Intervention Programs. 2017. National Cancer Institute website. https://rtips.cancer.gov/rtips/index.do.

11. Collins CB Jr, Sapiano TN. Lessons learned from dissemination of evidence-based interventions for HIV prevention. *Am J Prev Med.* 2016;51:S140–S147.

12. Collins CB Jr, Wilson KM. CDC's dissemination of evidence-based behavioral HIV prevention interventions. *Transl Behav Med* 2011;1:203–204.

13. National Registry of Evidence-based Programs and Practices (NREPP). 2017. Substance Abuse and Mental Health Services Administration website. https://www.samhsa.gov/nrepp.

14. US Preventive Services Task Force website. 2017. https://www.uspreventiveservicestaskforce.org.

15. Proctor EK, Powell BJ, McMillen JC. Implementation strategies: Recommendations for specifying and reporting. *Implement Sci.* 2013;8:139.

16. Powell BJ, Proctor EK, Glass JE. A systematic review of strategies for implementing empirically supported mental health interventions. *Res Soc Work Pract.* 2014;24:192–212.

17. Powell BJ, Waltz TJ, Chinman MJ, Damschroder LJ, Smith JL, Matthieu MM, Proctor EK, Kirchner JE. A refined compilation of implementation strategies: Results from the Expert Recommendations for Implementing Change (ERIC) project. *Implement Sci.* 2015;10:21.

18. Powell BJ, Beidas RS, Lewis CC, Aarons GA, McMillen JC, Proctor EK, Mandell DS. Methods to improve the selection and tailoring of implementation strategies. *J Behav Health Serv Res* 2017;44:177–194.

19. Pinnock H, Barwick M, Carpenter CR, et al. Standards for Reporting Implementation Studies (StaRI) statement. *BMJ.* 2017;356:i6795.

20. Schoenwald SK, Garland AF, Chapman JE, Frazier SL, Sheidow AJ, Southam-Gerow MA. Toward the effective and efficient measurement of implementation fidelity. *Adm Policy Ment Health* 2011;38:32–43.

21. Stirman SW, Miller CJ, Toder K, Calloway A. Development of a framework and coding system for modifications and adaptations of evidence-based interventions. *Implement Sci.* 2013;8:65.

22. Chambers DA, Glasgow RE, Stange KC. The dynamic sustainability framework: Addressing the paradox of sustainment amid ongoing change. *Implement Sci.* 2013;8:117.

23. Castro FG, Barrera M Jr, Martinez CR Jr. The cultural adaptation of prevention interventions: Resolving tensions between fidelity and fit. *Prev Sci.* 2004;5:41–45.

24. Miller WR, Rollnick S. *Motivational Interviewing: Helping People Change.* New York: Guilford; 2012.

25. Miller WR, Mount KA. A small study of training in motivational interviewing: Does one workshop change clinician and client behavior? *Behav Cogn Psychother.* 2001;29:457–471.

26. Moyers TB, Martin T, Manuel JK, Hendrickson SM, Miller WR. Assessing competence in the use of motivational interviewing. *J Subst Abuse Treat* 2005;28:19–26.

27. Norton, WE, Loudon, K, & Zwarenstein, M. Extension of the PRECIS-2 Tool to Assist in Planning Trials of Multi-Level Interventions. Oral conference presentation, Society for Clinical Trials Annual Meeting, May 23rd. Portland, Oregon; 2018.

28. Barker PM, Reid A, Schall MW. A framework for scaling up health interventions: Lessons from large-scale improvement initiatives in Africa. *Implement Sci.* 2016;11:12.

29. Hanson K, Ranson MK, Oliveira-Cruz V, Mills A. Expanding access to priority health interventions: A framework for understanding the constraints to scaling-up. *J Int Dev.* 2003;15:1–14.

30. Mangham LJ, Hanson K. Scaling up in international health: What are the key issues? *Health Policy Plann.* 2010;25:85–96.

31. McCannon CJ, Berwick DM, Massoud MR. The science of large-scale change in global health. *JAMA.* 2007;298:1937–1939.

32. Scheirer MA, Dearing JW. An agenda for research on the sustainability of public health programs. *Am J Public Health.* 2011;101:2059–2067.

33. Wiltsey Stirman S, Kimberly J, Cook N, Calloway A, Castro F, Charns M. The sustainability of new programs and innovations: A review of the empirical literature and recommendations for future research. *Implement Sci.* 2012;7:17.

34. Green LW. Making research relevant: If it is an evidence-based practice, where's

the practice-based evidence? *Fam Pract.* 2008;25:i20–i24.

35. Green LW, Glasgow RE. Evaluating the relevance, generalization, and applicability of research: Issues in external validation and translation methodology. *Eval Health Professions.* 2006;29:126–153.

36. Stokes DE. *Pasteur's Quadrant: Basic Science and Technological Innovation.* Washington, DC: Brookings Institution; 2011.

37. Chalmers I, Bracken MB, Djulbegovic B, Garattini S, Grant J, Gulmezoglu AM, Howells DW, Ioannidis JP, Oliver S. How to increase value and reduce waste when research priorities are set. *Lancet.* 2014;383:156–165.

38. Allen P, Sequeira S, Jacob R, et al. Promoting state health department evidence-based cancer and chronic disease prevention: A multi-phase dissemination study with a cluster randomized trial component. *Implement Sci.* 2013;8:141.

39. Cacioppo JT, Kaplan RM, Krosnick JA, Olds JL, Dean H. Social, behavioral, and economic sciences perspectives on robust and reliable science. 2015. National Science Foundation website. https://www.nsf.gov/sbe/AC_Materials/SBE_Robust_and_Reliable_Research_Report.pdf.

40. Collins FS, Tabak LA. NIH plans to enhance reproducibility. *Nature.* 2014;505:612.

41. Taichman DB, Sahni P, Pinborg A, et al. Data sharing statements for clinical trials. *BMJ.* 2017;357:j2372.

42. Ioannidis JPA. The reproducibility wars: Successful, unsuccessful, uninterpretable, exact, conceptual, triangulated, contested replication. *Clin Chem.* 2017;63:943–945.

43. Fanelli D, Costas R, Ioannidis JP. Meta-assessment of bias in science. *Proc Natl Acad Sci USA.* 2017;114:3714–3719.

44. Bruns SB, Ioannidis JP. p-Curve and p-hacking in observational research. *PLoS One.* 2016;11:e0149144.

45. Berwick DM. What "patient-centered" should mean: Confessions of an extremist. *Health Aff.* 2009;28(4):w555-6.

46. Stewart M. *Patient-Centered Medicine: Transforming the Clinical Method.* Abingdon, UK: Radcliffe; 2003.

47. Gerteis M, Edgman-Levita S, Daley J, Delbanco TL, eds. *Through the Patient's Eyes: Understanding and Promoting Patient-Centered Care.* San Francisco, CA: Jossey-Bass; 1993.

48. Selby JV, Beal AC, Frank L. The Patient-Centered Outcomes Research Institute (PCORI) national priorities for research and initial research agenda. *JAMA.* 2012;307:1583–1584.

RESOURCES

Annual Conference on the Science of Dissemination and Implementation in Health
- Website: http://www.academyhealth.org/events/site/10th-annual-conference-science-dissemination-and-implementation-health
- Brief description: This conference intends to support collective understanding of the research agenda to incorporate these challenges into dissemination and implementation (D&I) research through a combination of plenaries, concurrent, and poster sessions that will present research findings and identify the next set of research priorities, setting the field up for the next decade.

Cancer Control P.L.A.N.E.T. (Plan, Link, Act, Network with Evidence-based Tools)
- Website: https://cancercontrolplanet.cancer.gov
- Brief description: The Cancer Control P.L.A.N.E.T. portal provides access to data and resources that can help planners, program staff, and researchers design, implement, and evaluate evidence-based cancer control programs.

Cancer Prevention and Control Research Network (CPCRN)
- Website: http://cpcrn.org
- Brief description: The CPCRN is a national network of academic, public health, and community partners who work together to reduce the burden of cancer, especially among those disproportionately affected. Its members conduct community-based participatory cancer research across its eight network centers, crossing academic affiliations and geographic boundaries.

Coalition for Evidence Based Policy
- Website: http://toptierevidence.org
- Brief description: This is a validated resource for distinguishing research-proven social programs from everything else. The non-profit, nonpartisan Coalition for Evidence-Based Policy launched the Top Tier Evidence initiative in 2008, in consultation with senior federal officials, to identify social programs meeting the top tier evidence standard.

Cochrane Effective Practice and Organisation of Care (EPOC) Group
- Website: http://epoc.cochrane.org
- Brief description: The EPOC Group is a Cochrane Review Group. The scope of the EPOC Group is to undertake systematic reviews of educational, behavioral, financial, regulatory, and organizational interventions designed to improve health professional practice and the organization of health care services.

Community Guide
- Website: https://www.thecommunityguide.org
- Brief description: The Guide to Community Preventive Services (The Community Guide) is a collection of evidence-based findings of the Community Preventive Services Task Force. It is a resource to help one select interventions to improve health and prevent disease in one's state, community, community organization, business, health care organization, or school.

Comprehensive Cancer Control National Partnership (CCCNP)
- Website: http://www.cccnationalpartners.org
- Brief description: Through coordination and collaboration, the CCCNP assists comprehensive cancer control (CCC) coalitions to develop and sustain implementation of CCC plans at the state, tribe, territory, US Pacific Island Jurisdiction, and local levels.

Consolidated Framework for Implementation Research (CFIR) Technical Assistance Website
- Website: http://cfirguide.org
- Brief description: This site was created for individuals considering using the CFIR to evaluate an implementation or design an implementation study.

Consortium for Implementation Science (CIS)
- Website: http://consortiumforis.org
- Brief description: CIS is a joint endeavor of RTI International and the University of North Carolina Gillings School of Global Public Health that facilitates collaborations to advance implementation science. The consortium provides resources to build knowledge and skills in implementation research, foster new collaborations with methodological and content experts, and inform the design and evaluation of new study interventions.

- CIS also publishes a monthly e-newsletter with the latest research, news and opportunities from the field.

Dissemination and Implementation Core, Adult and Child Consortium for Health Outcomes Research and Delivery Science (ACCORDS), University of Colorado School of Medicine
- Website: https://goo.gl/VMKuLb
- Brief description: The ACCORDS D&I Program provides local consultation and collaborative learning to enable increased funding success and to drive evidence-based programs into practice more quickly and successfully. Includes online and published resources for funding, study planning, and evaluation in D&I.

Dissemination & Implementation Models in Health Research & Practice
- Website: http://dissemination-implementation.org
- Brief description: This interactive website was designed to help researchers and practitioners to select the D&I model that best fits their research question or practice problem, adapt the model to the study or practice context, fully integrate the model into the research or practice process, and find existing measurement instruments for the model constructs.

Global Implementation Conference (GIC)
- Website: https://gic.globalimplementation.org
- Brief description: The biennial GIC was launched in 2011 with a focus on implementation.

Implementation Science
- Website: https://implementationscience.biomedcentral.com
- Brief description: *Implementation Science* aims to publish research relevant to the scientific study of methods to promote the uptake of research findings into routine health care in clinical, organizational, or policy contexts.

Implementation Science Exchange (IMPSCIX).
- Website: https://impsci.tracs.unc.edu
- Brief description: A one-stop resource for implementation researchers.

Leadership and Organizational Change for Implementation (LOCI)
- Website: http://implementationleadership.com

- Brief description: LOCI is a multilevel leadership and organizational change strategy to improve implementation of a new innovation. LOCI can be tailored for specific settings and clinical interventions and generally spans between 9–12 months.

National Cancer Institute (NCI) Implementation Science
- Website: https://cancercontrol.cancer.gov/IS/index.html
- Brief description: Housed within the Office of the Director in the Division of Cancer Control and Population Sciences at the NCI, the Implementation Science (IS) team is engaged in a variety of activities to advance research and practice in implementation science. The mission of the IS team is to develop and apply the implementation science knowledge base to improve the impact of cancer control and population science on the health and health care of the population and also to foster rapid integration of research, practice, and policy.

National Collaborating Center for Methods and Tools (NCCMT)
- Website: http://www.nccmt.ca
- Brief description: NCCMT is one of six National Collaborating Centers for Public Health in Canada. NCCMT facilitates and supports the development of knowledge and capacity to use the best available evidence in practice among public health professionals.

RE-AIM (Reach, Effectiveness, Adoption, Implementation, and Maintenance)
- Website: http://re-aim.org
- Brief description: The goal of RE-AIM is to encourage program planners, evaluators, readers of journal articles, funders, and policymakers to pay more attention to essential program elements, including external validity, that can improve the sustainable adoption and implementation of effective, generalizable, evidence-based interventions.

Research-Tested Intervention Programs (RTIPs)
- Website: https://rtips.cancer.gov/rtips/index.do
- Brief description: RTIPs is a searchable database of evidence-based cancer control interventions and program materials and is designed to provide program planners and public health practitioners with easy and immediate access to research-tested materials.

Society for Implementation Research Collaboration (SIRC)
- Website: https://societyforimplementationresearchcollaboration.org
- Brief description: SIRC is dedicated to facilitating communication and collaboration between implementation research teams, researchers, and community providers. SIRC aims to bring together researchers and stakeholders committed to the rigorous evaluation of implementation of evidence-based psychosocial interventions.

US Department of Veterans Affairs Quality Enhancement Research Initiative (QUERI)
- Website: https://www.queri.research.va.gov
- Brief description: QUERI is a quality improvement program that has become a central component of the US Department of Veterans Affairs' commitment to improving the quality of veterans' health care.

World Health Organization Special Program for Research and Training in Tropical Diseases (TDR) Implementation Research Toolkit

- Website: http://www.who.int/tdr/publications/topics/ir-toolkit/en
- Brief description: This toolkit was designed to help people learn a standard process that leads to results that can be compared across regions and countries. It is designed to help identify system bottlenecks and the stakeholders to be involved, formulate appropriate research questions, conduct the research, and develop a plan for implementing the study results.

GLOSSARY

adaptation (of evidence-based interventions) The degree to which an evidence-based intervention is changed or modified by a user during adoption and implementation to suit the needs of the setting or to improve the fit to local conditions.[1,2]

adoption (of evidence-based interventions) A decision to make full use of an innovation, intervention, or program as the best course of action available.[1] Also defined as the decision of an organization or community to commit to and initiate an evidence-based intervention.[1-3]

big data Data generated during health care delivery that are too large, too diverse, and too rapidly changing to be analyzed by traditional, human-driven research methods and that need the assistance of computer-driven analytics.[4]

cancer care delivery research Multidisciplinary field of scientific investigation that studies how social factors, financing systems, organizational structures and processes, health technologies, and health care provider and patient behaviors affect access to cancer care, the quality and cost of cancer care, and ultimately the health and well-being of cancer patients and survivors.[5]

clinical decision support systems Computer systems designed to impact clinician decision-making about individual patients at the point in time when these decisions are made.[6]

clinical practice guidelines Systematically developed statements used to inform care delivery and assess the appropriateness of specific health care decisions, services, and outcomes.[7,8]

community engagement Process of inclusive participation that supports mutual respect of values, strategies, and actions for authentic partnership of people affiliated with or self-identified by geographic proximity, special interest, or similar situations to address issues affecting the well-being of the community of focus.[9,10]

community-based participatory research (CBPR) A collaborative approach to research that equitably involves all partners in the research process and recognizes the unique strengths that each brings. CBPR begins with a research topic of importance to the community and has the aim of combining knowledge with action and achieving social change to improve health outcomes and eliminate health disparities.[11] See additional definitions.[12–14]

cost-effectiveness analysis Systematic and quantitative comparisons of trade-offs between health outcomes and costs of alternative health care interventions with standards set for the United States.[15,16]

de-implementation Reducing or stopping the use of a health service or practice provided to patients by health care practitioners and systems.[17] See associated definitions.[18–20]

diffusion of innovations A process in which an innovation is communicated through certain channels over time among the members of a social system.[1]

dissemination science, dissemination research Scientific study of targeted distribution of information and intervention materials to a specific public health or clinical practice audience. The intent is to understand how best to spread and sustain knowledge and the associated evidence-based interventions.[21]

evidence-based interventions Health-focused intervention, practice, program, or guideline with evidence demonstrating the ability of the intervention to change a health-related behavior or medicine. See variations of this definition from other sources.[2,20,22,23]

evidence-based medicine The conscientious, explicit, and judicious use of current best evidence in making decisions about the care of the individual patient.[22–24]

evidence-based public health Defined by several key characteristics that include making decisions based on evidence-based interventions, using data and information systems systematically, applying program planning frameworks, engaging the community in assessment and decision-making, conducting sound evaluation, and disseminating what is learned to key stakeholders and decision-makers.[25]

evidence-informed decision-making Process of distilling and disseminating the best available evidence from research, context, and experience (political and organizational) and using that evidence to inform and improve public health practice and policy.[25]

experimental design A study in which an intervention is deliberately introduced to observe its effects.[26,27]

external validity The generalizability of the results of a research study to the actual phenomenon as it occurs outside the context of a research study.[26,28]

fidelity (of evidence-based interventions) Degree to which an intervention or program is implemented as intended by the developers and as prescribed in the original protocol.[2,29]

formative evaluation Evaluative activities undertaken during the design and pretesting of programs to guide the design process.[30] See additional references.[31,32]

implementation outcomes Effects of deliberate and purposive actions to implement new treatments, practices, and services. First, implementation outcomes serve as indicators of the implementation success. Second, they are proximal indicators of implementation processes. Third, they are key intermediate outcomes in relation to service system or clinical outcomes in treatment effectiveness and quality of care research. Implementation outcomes include acceptability, adoption, appropriateness, costs, feasibility, fidelity, penetration, and sustainability.[33]

implementation science, implementation research Scientific study of the use of strategies to adopt and integrate evidence-based health interventions into clinical and community settings to improve patient outcomes and benefit population health.[21]

implementation strategies Methods or techniques used to enhance the adoption, implementation, and sustainability of a clinical program or practice.[34,35]

internal validity The ability to draw sound conclusions about what causes any observed differences in a dependent (outcome) measure or variable.[25,28,36]

intervention mapping Framework for effective decision-making at each step in the intervention development process and provides a system for the integration of theory, empirical findings from the literature, and information collected from the target population. The intervention mapping process includes five fundamental steps: (1) creating matrices of proximal program objectives from performance objectives and determinants of behavior and environmental conditions, (2) selecting theory-based intervention methods and practical strategies, (3) designing and organizing programs, (4) specifying adoption and implementation plans, and (5) generating an evaluation plan.[37]

knowledge translation Dynamic and iterative process that includes synthesis, dissemination, exchange, and ethically sound application of knowledge to improve health, provide more effective health services and products, and strengthen the health care system.[38,39]

low-value care Services that provide little or no clinical benefit on average[40] or a service for which the potential for harm exceeds the possible benefit.[41]

mixed methods research Research in which the investigator collects and analyzes data, integrates the findings, and draws inferences using both qualitative and quantitative approaches or methods in a single study or program of inquiry.[42]

overuse Provision of a health service under circumstances in which its potential for harm exceeds the possible benefit.[41]

palliative care Care given to improve the quality of life of patients who have a serious or life-threatening disease. The goal of palliative care is to prevent or treat as early as possible the symptoms of a disease; side effects caused by treatment of a disease; and psychological, social, and spiritual problems related to a disease or its treatment. Also called comfort care, supportive care, and symptom management.[43]

patient navigation (in cancer) Support and guidance ("intervention") offered to persons with abnormal cancer screening results or cancer, with the goal of improving access and coordination of timely care.[44] Patient navigation typically includes five characteristics: (1) provided to individual patients for a defined episode of cancer-related care; (2) an endpoint when the services provided are complete; (3) targets a defined set of health services that are required to complete an episode of cancer-related care; (4) focuses on the identification of individual patient-level barriers to accessing cancer care; and (5) aims to reduce delays in accessing the continuum of cancer care services.[45] Patient navigators may be nurses, laypersons or peers, social workers, health educators, and cancer survivors, among others.[46] See other definitions and conceptualizations.[47,48]

patient-centered care Care that is respectful of and responsive to individual patient preferences, needs, and values and that ensures that patient values guide all clinical decisions.[49,50]

patient-reported outcomes (PROs) Any report on the status of a patient's health condition that comes directly from the patient, without interpretation of the patient's response by a clinician or anyone else.[51] PROs include any treatment or outcome evaluation obtained directly from patients through interviews, self-completed questionnaires, diaries, or other data collection tools such as hand-held devices and web-based forms.[52,53]

pragmatic trials Trials primarily designed to determine the effects of an intervention under the usual conditions in which it will be applied. Contrasts with explanatory trials, which are primarily designed to determine the effects of an intervention under ideal circumstances.[53–56]

precision medicine Tailoring of medical treatment to the individual characteristics of each patient[57] or prevention and treatment strategies that take individual variability into account.[58]

precision public health Provision of the right intervention to the right population at the right time.[59]

quality improvement Efforts by health care professionals, patients and their families, researchers, payers, planners, and educators to make the changes that will lead to better patient outcomes (health), better system performance (care), and better professional development (learning).[60] Also defined as systematic and continuous actions that lead to measurable improvement in health care services and health status of patients.[61,62]

quasi-experimental design An experimental study design in which units are not assigned to conditions randomly.[27] Examples of quasi-experimental designs include interrupted time series, regression discontinuity, and non-equivalent control group design.[25,27]

randomized experimental design An experimental study in which units are assigned to receive the treatment or an alternative condition by a random process.[25,27] Examples of randomized experimental designs include the randomized controlled trial (RCT), cluster randomized controlled trial (cRCT), and pragmatic randomized controlled trial (pRCT).

replication The ability of the researcher to duplicate the results of a prior study if the same procedures are followed but new data are collected.[63] See related definitions and explanations.[64,65]

reproducibility The ability of a researcher to duplicate the results of a prior study using the same materials as were used by the original investigator. That is, a second researcher might use the same raw data to build the same analysis files and implement the same statistical analysis in an attempt to yield the same results.[63] See related definitions and explanations.[64,65]

scale-up or scaling-up Efforts to increase the impact of innovations successfully tested in pilot or experimental projects so as to benefit more people and to foster policy and program development on a lasting bases.[66] See variations of this definition from other sources.[67,68]

shared decision-making (SDM) Collaborative process through which health care professionals share information about the benefits and harms of proposed interventions, and patients (and possibly family and friends) share information about their relevant preferences and values.[69] SDM traditionally includes four key characteristics: (1) involves at least two participants—the provider and the patient; (2) both participants (provider and patient) take steps to participate in the process of treatment decision-making; (3) information sharing is a prerequisite to SDM; and (4) treatment decision is made, and both parties agree to the decision.[70]

social determinants of health Conditions in which people are born, grow, live, work, and age. These circumstances are shaped by the distribution of money, power, and resources at global, national, and local levels. The social determinants of health are mostly responsible for health inequities—the unfair and avoidable differences in health status seen within and between countries.[71,72]

stepped wedge design Study design in which an intervention is rolled out sequentially to trial participants (e.g., individuals, groups, organizations, clinics, and communities) or clusters of trial participants over different time periods. Participants or clusters of participants receive the intervention at a randomly assigned time point such that all participants receive the intervention by the end of the trial.[73-76]

sustainability of evidence-based interventions The continued use of program components and activities for the continued achievement of desirable program and population outcomes.[77] See additional definitions.[78,79]

REFERENCES

1. Rogers EM. *Diffusion of Innovations.* New York: Simon & Schuster; 2010.
2. Rabin BA, Brownson RC, Haire-Joshu D, Kreuter MW, Weaver NL. A glossary for dissemination and implementation research in health. *J Public Health Manag Pract.* 2008;14(2):117–123.
3. Sussman S, Valente TW, Rohrbach LA, Skara S, Ann Pentz M. Translation in the health professions: Converting science into action. *Eval Health Prof.* 2006;29(1):7–32.
4. Adapted from Raghupathi W, Raghupathi V. Big data analytics in healthcare: Promise and potential. *Health Inf Sci Syst.* 2014; 2:3. http://doi.org/10.1186/2047-2501-2-3.
5. Kent EE, Mitchell SA, Castro KM, et al. Cancer care delivery research: Building the evidence base to support practice change in community oncology. *J Clin Oncol.* 2015;33(24):2705–2711.
6. Berner ES. *Clinical Decision Support Systems.* Vol 233. New York: Springer; 2007.
7. Lohr KN, Field MJ. *Clinical Practice Guidelines: Directions for a New Program.* Vol 90. Washington, DC: National Academies Press; 1990.
8. Lohr KN, Field MJ. *Guidelines for Clinical Practice: From Development to Use.* Washington, DC: National Academies Press; 1992.
9. Ahmed SM, Palermo AG. Community engagement in research: Frameworks for education and peer review. *Am J Public Health.* 2010;100(8):1380–1387.
10. Moini M, Fackler-Lowrie N, Jones L. *Community Engagement: Moving from Community Involvement to Community Engagement—A Paradigm Shift.* Santa Monica, CA: PHP Consulting; 2005.
11. Program goals and competencies. Community Health Scholars website. 2007.
12. Faridi Z, Grunbaum JA, Gray BS, Franks A, Simoes E. Community-based participatory research: Necessary next steps. *Prev Chronic Dis.* 2007;4(3):A70.
13. Viswanathan M, Ammerman A, Eng E, et al. Community-based participatory research: Assessing the evidence. *Evid Rep Technol Assess.* 2004; (99):1–8.
14. Minkler M, Wallerstein N. *Community-Based Participatory Research for Health: From Process to Outcomes.* New York: Wiley; 2011.
15. Weinstein MC, Siegel JE, Gold MR, Kamlet MS, Russell LB. Recommendations of the Panel on Cost-effectiveness in Health and Medicine. *JAMA.* 1996;276(15):1253–1258.
16. Sanders GD, Neumann PJ, Basu A, et al. Recommendations for conduct, methodological practices, and reporting of cost-effectiveness analyses: Second Panel on Cost-Effectiveness in Health and Medicine. *JAMA.* 2016;316(10):1093–1103.
17. Norton WE, Kennedy AE, Chambers DA. Studying de-implementation in health: An analysis of funded research grants. *Implement Sci.* 2017;12(1):144.
18. Niven DJ, Mrklas KJ, Holodinsky JK, et al. Towards understanding the de-adoption of low-value clinical practices: A scoping review. *BMC Med.* 2015;13:255.
19. Prasad V, Ioannidis JP. Evidence-based de-implementation for contradicted, unproven, and aspiring healthcare practices. *Implement Sci.* 2014;9:1.
20. Brownson RC, Colditz GA, Proctor EK. *Dissemination and Implementation Research in Health: Translating Science to Practice.* New York: Oxford University Press; 2017.

21. Dissemination and implementation research in health. 2017. National Institutes of Health website. https://grants.nih.gov/grants/guide/pa-files/PAR-18-007.html.

22. Sackett DL, Rosenberg WM, Gray JM, Haynes RB, Richardson WS. Evidence based medicine: What it is and what it isn't. *BMJ*. 1996;312(7023):71–72.

23. Guyatt G, Cairns J, Churchill D, et al. Evidence-based medicine: A new approach to teaching the practice of medicine. *JAMA*. 1992;268(17):2420–2425.

24. Ball C, Sackett D, Phillips B, Haynes B, Straus S, Dawes M. Levels of evidence and grades of recommendations. 2001. Centre for Evidence-based Medicine website. https://www.cebmjr2oxacuk/docs/levels html.

25. Brownson RC, Fielding JE, Green LW. Building capacity for evidence-based public health: Reconciling the pulls of practice and the push of research. *Annu Rev Public Health*. 2018;39:27–53.

26. Cook TD, Campbell DT. The design and conduct of true experiments and quasi-experiments in field settings. In: Mowday RT, Steers RM, eds. *Research in Organizations: Issues and Controversies*. Culver City, CA: Goodyear; 1979.

27. Cook TD, Campbell DT, Shadish W. *Experimental and Quasi-experimental Designs for Generalized Causal Inference*. Boston, MA: Houghton Mifflin; 2002.

28. Campbell DT. Factors relevant to the validity of experiments in social settings. *Psychol Bull*. 1957;54(4):297.

29. Dusenbury L, Brannigan R, Falco M, Hansen WB. A review of research on fidelity of implementation: Implications for drug abuse prevention in school settings. *Health Educ Res*. 2003;18(2):237–256.

30. Rossi PH, Lipsey MW, Freeman HE. *Evaluation: A Systematic Approach*. Thousand Oaks, CA: Sage; 2003.

31. Stetler CB, Legro MW, Wallace CM, et al. The role of formative evaluation in implementation research and the QUERI experience. *J Gen Intern Med*. 2006;21(Suppl 2):S1–S8.

32. Patton MQ. Evaluation of program implementation. *Eval Stud Rev Annu*. 1979;4(3):318–345.

33. Proctor E, Silmere H, Raghavan R, et al. Outcomes for implementation research: Conceptual distinctions, measurement challenges, and research agenda. *Adm Policy Ment Health*. 2011;38(2):65–76.

34. Powell BJ, McMillen JC, Proctor EK, et al. A compilation of strategies for implementing clinical innovations in health and mental health. *Med Care Res Rev*. 2012;69(2):123–157.

35. Proctor EK, Powell BJ, McMillen JC. Implementation strategies: Recommendations for specifying and reporting. *Implement Sci*. 2013;8:139.

36. Reis HT, Judd CM. *Handbook of Research Methods in Social and Personality Psychology*. New York: Cambridge University Press; 2000.

37. Bartholomew LK, Parcel GS, Kok G. Intervention mapping: A process for developing theory and evidence-based health education programs. *Health Educ Behav*. 1998;25(5):545–563.

38. Graham ID, Logan J, Harrison MB, et al. Lost in knowledge translation: Time for a map? *J Contin Educ Health Prof*. 2006;26(1):13–24.

39. Straus SE, Tetroe J, Graham I. Defining knowledge translation. *Can Med Assoc J*. 2009;181(3–4):165–168.

40. Schwartz AL, Landon BE, Elshaug AG, Chernew ME, McWilliams JM. Measuring low-value care in Medicare. *JAMA Intern Med*. 2014;174(7):1067–1076.

41. Chassin MR, Galvin RW. The urgent need to improve health care quality: Institute of Medicine National Roundtable on Health Care Quality. *JAMA*. 1998;280(11):1000–1005.

42. Tashakkori A, Creswell JW. *The New Era of Mixed Methods*. Thousand Oaks, CA: Sage; 2007.

43. NCI dictionary of cancer terms. 2017. National Cancer Institute website. https://www.cancer.gov/publications/dictionaries/cancer-terms/def/palliative-care.

44. Jean-Pierre P, Hendren S, Fiscella K, et al. Understanding the processes of patient navigation to reduce disparities in cancer care: Perspectives of trained navigators from the field. *J Cancer Educ*. 2011;26(1):111–120.

45. Wells KJ, Battaglia TA, Dudley DJ, et al. Patient navigation: State of the art or is it science? *Cancer*. 2008;113(8):1999–2010.

46. Paskett ED, Harrop J, Wells KJ. Patient navigation: An update on the state of the science. *CA Cancer J Clin*. 2011;61(4):237–249.

47. Freeman HP, Rodriguez RL. History and principles of patient navigation. *Cancer*. 2011;117(Suppl 15):3537–3540.

48. Freund KM, Battaglia TA, Calhoun E, et al. Impact of patient navigation on timely cancer care: The Patient Navigation Research Program. *J Natl Cancer Inst*. 2014;106(6):dju115.

49. Baker A. Crossing the quality chasm: A new health system for the 21st century. *BMJ.* 2001;323(7322):1192.

50. Institute of Medicine. *Crossing the Quality Chasm: A New Health System for the 21st Century.* Washington, DC: National Academies Press; 2001.

51. US Department of Health and Human Services, Food and Drug Administration, Center for Drug Evaluation and Research, Center for Biologics Evaluation and Research, Center for Devices and Radiological Health. Guidance for industry: Patient-reported outcome measures: Use in medical product development to support labeling claims: draft guidance. *Health Qual Life Outcomes.* 2006;4:1–20.

52. Patrick DL, Guyatt GH, Acquadro C. Patient-reported outcomes. *Cochrane HandbSyst Rev Interv.* 2008:531-545.

53. Haynes RB, Sackett DL, Guyatt GH, Tugwell P. *Clinical Epidemiology: how to do clinical practice research.* 3rd ed. Philadelphia, PA: Lippincott Williams & Wilkins; 2006.

54. Schwartz D, Lellouch J. Explanatory and pragmatic attitudes in therapeutical trials. *J Clin Epidemiol.* 1967;20(8):637–648.

55. Thorpe KE, Zwarenstein M, Oxman AD, et al. A Pragmatic–Explanatory Continuum Indicator Summary (PRECIS): A tool to help trial designers. *J Clin Epidemiol.* 2009;62(5):464–475.

56. Roland M, Torgerson DJ. Understanding controlled trials: What are pragmatic trials? *BMJ.* 1998;316(7127):285.

57. Council NR. *Toward Precision Medicine: Building a Knowledge Network for Biomedical Research and a New Taxonomy of Disease.* Washington, DC: National Academies Press; 2011.

58. Collins FS, Varmus H. A new initiative on precision medicine. *N Engl J Med.* 2015;372(9):793–795.

59. Khoury MJ, Iademarco MF, Riley WT. Precision public health for the era of precision medicine. *Am J Prev Med.* 2016;50(3):398–401.

60. Batalden PB, Davidoff F. What is "quality improvement" and how can it transform healthcare? *Qual Saf Health Care.* 2007;16(1):2–3.

61. Marshall M, Pronovost P, Dixon-Woods M. Promotion of improvement as a science. *Lancet.* 2013;381(9864):419–421.

62. Davidoff F, Batalden P, Stevens D, Ogrinc G, Mooney S. Publication guidelines for quality improvement in health care: Evolution of the SQUIRE project. *BMJ Qual Saf.* 2008;17(Suppl 1):i3–i9.

63. Cacioppo JT, Kaplan RM, Krosnick JA, Olds JL, Dean H. Social, Behavioral, and Economic Sciences Perspectives on Robust and Reliable Science. Alexandria, VA: National Science Foundation; 2015.

64. Goodman SN, Fanelli D, Ioannidis JP. What does research reproducibility mean? *Sci Transl Med.* 2016;8(341):341ps312.

65. Ioannidis JP, Fanelli D, Dunne DD, Goodman SN. Meta-research: Evaluation and improvement of research methods and practices. *PLoS Biol.* 2015;13(10):e1002264.

66. Simmons R, Fajans P, Ghiron L. *Scaling Up Health Service Delivery: From Pilot Innovations to Policies and Programmes.* Geneva, Switzerland: World Health Organization; 2007.

67. Mangham LJ, Hanson K. Scaling up in international health: What are the key issues? *Health Policy Plann.* 2010;25(2):85–96.

68. Barker PM, Reid A, Schall MW. A framework for scaling up health interventions: Lessons from large-scale improvement initiatives in Africa. *Implement Sci.* 2016;11:12.

69. Elwyn G, Lloyd A, May C, et al. Collaborative deliberation: A model for patient care. *Patient Educ Couns.* 2014;97(2):158–164.

70. Charles C, Gafni A, Whelan T. Shared decision-making in the medical encounter: What does it mean?(or it takes at least two to tango). *Social Sci Med.* 1997;44(5):681–692.

71. Marmot M, Friel S, Bell R, Houweling TA, Taylor S; Commission on Social Determinants of Health. Closing the gap in a generation: Health equity through action on the social determinants of health. *Lancet.* 2008;372(9650):1661–1669.

72. Marmot M, Wilkinson R. *Social Determinants of Health.* New York: Oxford University Press; 2005.

73. Brown CA, Lilford RJ. The stepped wedge trial design: A systematic review. *BMC Med Res Methodol.* 2006;6(1):54.

74. Gambia Hepatitis Study Group. The Gambia Hepatitis Intervention Study. *Cancer Res.* 1987;47(21):5782–5787.

75. Hussey MA, Hughes JP. Design and analysis of stepped wedge cluster randomized trials. *Contemp Clin Trials.* 2007;28(2):182–191.

76. Hemming K, Haines T, Chilton P, Girling A, Lilford R. The stepped wedge cluster randomised trial: Rationale, design, analysis, and reporting. *BMJ.* 2015;350:h391.

77. Scheirer MA, Dearing JW. An agenda for research on the sustainability of public

health programs. *Am J Public health.* 2011;101(11):2059–2067.

78. Pluye P, Potvin L, Denis J-L. Making public health programs last: Conceptualizing sustainability. *Eval Prog Plann.* 2004;27(2):121–133.

79. Shediac-Rizkallah MC, Bone LR. Planning for the sustainability of community-based health programs: Conceptual frameworks and future directions for research, practice and policy. *Health Educ Res.* 1998;13(1):87–108.

INDEX

Page numbers followed by *f* and *t* indicate figures and tables, respectively. Numbers followed by *b* indicate boxes.